HEALTH SCIENCES

D1145003

Critical Care THE REQUISITES IN ANESTHESIOLOGY

SERIES EDITOR

Roberta L. Hines, M.D.
Chair and Professor
Department of Anesthesiology
Yale University School of Medicine
New Haven, Connecticut

OTHER VOLUMES IN THE REQUISITES™ SERIES

Adult Perioperative Anesthesia

Pediatric Anesthesia

Cardiac and Vascular Anesthesia

Regional Anesthesia

Obstetric and Gynecologic Anesthesia

Pain Medicine

Ambulatory Anesthesia

Critical Care

THE REQUISITES IN ANESTHESIOLOGY

Peter J. Papadakos, MD, FCCM, FCCP

Director of Critical Care Medicine
Professor of Anesthesiology, Surgery and Neurosurgery
University of Rochester
Rochester, New York
Professor and Medical Director
Respiratory Care
State University of New York
Genesee College
Batavia, New York

James E. Szalados, MD, JD, MBA, MHA, FCCP, FCCM

Partner, Westside Anesthesiology Associates of Rochester, LLP
Attending in Anesthesiology, Critical Care and Medicine
Medical Director of Respiratory Care
Unity Health System at Park Ridge Hospital
Adjunct Clinical Professor, Rochester Institute of Technology
Rochester, New York

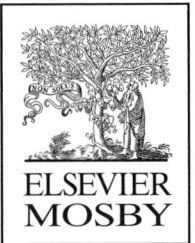

ELSEVIER
MOSBY

WO 200
PAPADAKOS
H0506681

ELSEVIER
MOSBY

1600 John F. Kennedy Blvd.
Ste 1800
Philadelphia, PA 19103-2899

THE REQUISITES ™
THE REQUISITES
THE REQUISITES
THE REQUISITES
THE REQUISITES

THE REQUISITES is a proprietary trademark
of Mosby, Inc.

CRITICAL CARE: THE REQUISITES IN ANESTHESIOLOGY   ISBN 0-323-02262-6
Copyright © 2005, Mosby, Inc.

All rights reserved. No part of this publication may be reproduced or transmitted in any form or by any means, electronic or mechanical, including photocopying, recording, or any information storage and retrieval system, without permission in writing from the publisher. Permissions may be sought directly from Elsevier's Health Sciences Rights Department in Philadelphia, PA, USA: phone: (+1) 215 239 3804, fax: (+1) 215 239 3805, e-mail: healthpermissions@elsevier.com. You may also complete your request on-line via the Elsevier homepage (http://www.elsevier.com), by selecting 'Customer Support' and then 'Obtaining Permissions'.

NOTICE

Knowledge and best practice in this field are constantly changing. As new research and experience broaden our knowledge, changes in practice, treatment and drug therapy may become necessary or appropriate. Readers are advised to check the most current information provided (i) on procedures featured or (ii) by the manufacturer of each product to be administered, to verify the recommended dose or formula, the method and duration of administration, and contraindications. It is the responsibility of the practitioner, relying on their own experience and knowledge of the patient, to make diagnoses, to determine dosages and the best treatment for each individual patient, and to take all appropriate safety precautions. To the fullest extent of the law, neither the Publisher nor the Editors assumes any liability for any injury and/or damage to persons or property arising out or related to any use of the material contained in this book.

Library of Congress Cataloging-in-Publication Data

Critical care : the requisites in anesthesiology / [edited by] Peter J. Papadakos, James E. Szalados.—1st ed.
    p. ; cm. — (Requisites in anesthesiology series)
  ISBN 0-323-02262-6
    1. Anesthesiology. 2. Critical care medicine. 3. Intensive care units.
  I. Papadakos, Peter. II. Szalados, James E. III. Series.
    [DNLM: 1. Critical Care—methods. 2. Anesthesia, General. 3. Anesthesiology — methods.
  4. Critical Illness. 5. Intensive Care Units. 6. Perioperative Care. WX 218 C93647 2005]
  RD81.C828 2005
  617.9′6–dc22

                                                                2004059742

Acquisitions Editor: Natasha Andjelkovic
Developmental Editor: Anne Snyder
Project Manager: David Saltzberg
Design Manager: Steven Stave
Marketing Manager: Emily McGrath-Christie

Printed in the United States of America

Last digit is the print number: 9 8 7 6 5 4 3 2 1

Working together to grow
libraries in developing countries

www.elsevier.com | www.bookaid.org | www.sabre.org

ELSEVIER   BOOK AID International   Sabre Foundation

I would like to thank all those who have believed in my dreams, supported my aspirations, and tolerated my pursuit of them. To my parents, whose spirit of discovery, determination, and resilience in the face of challenge instilled in me a desire to always do my best and make the world a better place; and to my sister Elisabeth, her husband Michael, and their children Justin, Benjamin, and Nathan who are the future; and most of all to my wife Doris for always being there for me.

J. E. Szalados, M.D.

I wish this work to honor the many teachers, students, residents, and fellows who over the years have made me think and grow in the subject of critical care. I especially wish to honor the contributions of two great teachers: the late Dr. Thomas Iberti M.D. who taught me to ask the key question of clinical medicine, "why?"; and Prof. Dr. Lachmann who made me into a scientist. To truly balance one's life we need love and support, and without the great love of my wife Susan and son Yanni I would not be able to find my inner strength. And to my father who taught and guided me that with hard work you always win, a special thanks. Also to my friends Allan Ross and Anne Snyder at Elsevier who supported me in this and many other projects, we did it again.

P. J. Papadakos, M.D.

Contributors

Michael J. Apostolakos, MD
Associate Professor of Medicine
Director, Adult Critical Care
University of Rochester Medical Center
Rochester, New York

Timothy J. Barreiro, DO
Assistant Clinical Professor
Department of Medicine
Northeast Ohio College of Medicine
Youngstown, Ohio

Rinaldo Bellomo, MD, FRACP, FCCP
Professorial Fellow
University of Melbourne Medical School
Melbourne
Victoria, Australia
Director of Intensive Care Research
Austin Hospital
Melbourne
Victoria, Australia

Ali Borhan, MD
Urology Resident
University of Rochester Medical Center
Rochester, New York

Lynn K. Boshkov, MD
Associate Professor of Pathology and Medicine
Department of Pathology
Oregon Health & Science University
Portland, Oregon

Ewan M. Cameron, MD
Clinical Assistant Professor of Anesthesiology
Tufts Medical School
Boston, Massachusetts
Senior Physician
Lahey Clinic
Burlington, Massachusetts

Sanjeev V. Chhangani, MD, MBA
Associate Professor of Anesthesiology
University of Rochester School of Medicine
    and Dentistry
Rochester, New York
Medical Director
Surgical Intensive Care Unit,
Rochester General Hospital
Rochester, New York

Ashwani Chhibber, MD
Associate Professor
Anesthesiology and Pediatrics
Vice Chair Anesthesiology
University of Rochester
Rochester, New York

Guglielmo Consales, MD
Senior Specialist
Department of Anesthesia and
    Intensive Care
University of Florence
Azienda Ospedaliero-Universitaria Careggi
Florence
Italy

Susan E. Dantoni, MD, FACOG
Clinical Assistant Professor of Obstetrics
    and Gynecology
University of Rochester
Rochester, New York
Clinical Adjunct Professor Health Professions
Rochester Institute of Technology
Rochester, New York
Attending Physician
Highland Hospital, Strong Memorial Hospital,
    Park Ridge Hospital
Rochester, New York

A. Raffaele De Gaudio, MD
Professor of Anesthesiology and Intensive Care
Director, Section of Anesthesiology and
  Intensive Care
Azienda Ospedaliero-Universitaria Careggi
University of Florence
Florence
Italy

Joseph Dooley, MD
Associate Professor of Anesthesiology
  and Neurosurgery
University of Rochester
Rochester, New York
Attending Physician, Anesthesiology
  and Critical Care Medicine
University of Rochester Medical Center
Rochester, New York

D. Jay Duong, MD
Resident in Anesthesiology
University of Rochester
Rochester, New York

Jason Dziak, MD
Assistant Professor
Department of Anesthesiology
University of Rochester
Rochester, New York

Dina M. Elaraj, MD
Senior Resident
Department of Surgery
University of Rochester
Rochester, New York

Erdal Erturk, MD
Professor of Urology
Director of Kidney Stone
  Treatment Center
University of Rochester Medical Center
Rochester, New York

Curtis E. Haas, PharmD
Assistant Professor
Department of Pharmacy Practice
University of Pharmacy and
  Pharmaceutical Sciences
University of Buffalo
Buffalo, New York
Clinical Assistant Professor
Department of Surgery
School of Medicine and Dentistry
University of Rochester
Rochester, New York

Jack J. Haitsma, MD, PhD
Visiting Research Fellow
Division Critical Care Medicine
University of Rochester
Rochester, New York
Member Department of Anesthesiology
Erasmus MC-Faculty
Rotterdam
The Netherlands

David Kaufman, MD, FCCM
Associate Professor of Surgery, Anesthesia,
  Medicine and Medical Humanities
University of Rochester
Medical Director, Surgical Intensive
  Care Unit
Strong Memorial Hospital
Rochester, New York

John A. Kellum, MD, FACP, FCCP
Associate Professor of Critical Care Medicine,
  Anesthesiology and Medicine
University of Pittsburgh
Department of Critical Care Medicine
CRISMA (Clinical Research Investigation
  and Systems Modeling of Acute Illness)
Pittsburgh, Pennsylvania
Intensitist, Cardiothoracic and Liver Transplant
  Intensive Care Units
University of Pittsburgh Medical Center
Pittsburgh, Pennsylvania

Heidi B. Kummer, MD, MPH
Assistant Clinical Professor of
  Anesthesiology
Tufts Medical School
Boston, Massachusetts
Senior Physician
Lahey Clinic
Burlington, Massachusetts

Burkhard Lachmann, MD, PhD
Director of Anesthesia Research
Professor of Anesthesiology
Erasmus MC-Faculty
Rotterdam
The Netherlands

Jaclyn M. LeBlanc, PharmD
Critical Care Pharmacy
  Research Fellow
College of Pharmacy
The Ohio State University
Columbus Ohio

Christopher W. Lentz, MD, FACS
Director, Strong Regional Burn Center
Associate Professor, Department of Surgery
    and Pediatrics
University of Rochester
Rochester, New York

Xavier M. Leverve, MD, PhD
Laboratoire de Bioénergétique Fondamentale
    et Appliqué
Université Joseph Fourier
Also: Service de Réanimation Médicale
Hospital A. Michallon
Centre Hospitalier Universitaire
Grenoble
France

Carlos J. Lopez III, MD
Associate Professor of Anesthesiology and
    Critical Care
Section Chief, Anesthesia Critical Care
Upstate Medical University
Syracuse, New York
Attending Intensitist, Attending Anesthesiologist
Co-Director, Surgical Intensive Care Unit
University Hospital at
    Upstate Medical University
Syracuse, New York

Stephen M. Luczycki, MD, MBA
Assistant Professor
Department of Anesthesiology
Yale University School of Medicine
New Haven, Connecticut

Stewart J. Lustik, MD
Associate Professor of Anesthesiology
University of Rochester School of Medicine
    and Dentistry
Rochester, New York
Strong Memorial Hospital
Rochester, New York

Ralph Madeb, MD
Urology Resident
University of Rochester Medical Center
Rochester, New York

Edward M. Messing, MD, FACS
W.W. Scott Professor
Professor of Oncology and Pathology
Chairman, Department of Urology
Deputy Director, James P. Wilmot Cancer Center
University of Rochester Medical Center
Rochester, New York

†**Iqbal Mustafa,** MD, PhD
Professor of Anesthesiology
Intensive Care Unit
Harapan Kita Cardiaovascular Center
Jakarta
Indonesia

Roger R. Ng, MD
Resident
Department of Anesthesiology
University of Rochester
Rochester, New York

Craig Nicholson, MD
Urology Resident
University of Rochester Medical Center
Rochester, New York

Peter J. Papadakos, MD, FCCP, FCCM
Director, Division of Critical
    Care Medicine
Professor of Anesthesiology, Surgery,
    and Neurosurgery
University of Rochester School of Medicine
    and Dentistry
Rochester, New York

Charles R. Phillips, MD
Assistant Professor of Medicine
Department of Pulmonary and Critical
    Care Medicine
Oregon Health and Science University
Portland, Oregon

Simone Rinaldi, MD
Research Fellow in Anesthesiology and
    Intensive Care
University of Florence
Florence
Italy

Claudio Ronco, MD, PhD
Lecturer
University of Padua Medical School
Padua
Italy
Director of Nephrology
San Bortolo Hospital,
Vicenza
Italy

†Deceased

Marc J. Shapiro, MD, FACS, FCCM
Professor of Surgery and Anesthesiology
State University of New York
Stony Brook, New York
Chief, General Surgery Trauma, Critical Care and Burns
University Hospital
Stony Brook, New York

Jeffrey Spike, PhD
Associate Professor of Medical Humanities
Florida State University College of Medicine
Tallahassee, Florida

David Story, MD, FANZCA
Department of Anaesthesia
Austin & Repatriation Medical Centre
Melbourne
Victoria, Australia

James E. Szalados, MD, JD, MBA, MHA, FCCP, FCCM
Partner, Westside Anesthesiology Associates of
  Rochester, LLP
Attending in Anesthesiology, Critical Care and Medicine
Medical Director of Respiratory Care
Unity Health System at Park Ridge Hospital
Adjunct Clinical Professor, Rochester Institute
  of Technology
Rochester, New York

Judit Szolnoki, MD
Assistant Professor of Anesthesiology and Critical Care
Department of Anesthesiology
Upstate Medical University
Syracuse, New York
Attending Anesthesiologist
VA Hospital of Syracuse and University Hospital
  in Syracuse
Syracuse, New York

Per A. J. Thorborg, MD, PhD
Associate Professor
Department of Anesthesiology and
  Perioperative Medicine
Oregon Health and Science University
Portland, Oregon

Jean-Louis Vincent, MD, PhD
Professor of Intensive Care
Free University of Brussels
Brussels
Belgium
Head, Department of Intensive Care
Erasme University Hospital
Brussels
Belgium

Jacek A. Wojtczak, MD, PhD
Associate Professor of Anesthesiology
University of Rochester School of Medicine
  and Dentistry
Rochester, New York

Preface

It is an incontrovertible fact that anesthesiology is the practice of medicine. Therefore, anesthesiologists must be fluent in the theories and techniques of preoperative medical assessment, intraoperative cardiopulmonary life support, and postoperative critical care intervention. Anesthesiology is the synthesis of the basic medical sciences, including anatomy, physiology, biochemistry, pharmacology, and epidemiology; and is a bridge that spans the disciplines of medicine and all its subspecialties, surgery, and obstetrics. The making of an anesthesiologist is therefore the culmination of premedical and medical schooling, a four-year intense postgraduate clinical residency program, and possibly thereafter a subspecialized fellowship. Most importantly, there then follows a lifetime commitment to learning and further honing of technical skills.

It is likely that no person will ever trust anyone else to the extent that they trust their anesthesiologist. The patient undergoing surgery will depend on the anesthesiologist for safety and comfort during a time when their body is subjected to extreme stress. It is a remarkable fact that most patients accept the risks of anesthesia without questions, are incognizant of the fact that they will fully be on "life support" for the duration of their operation, and most do not remember the experience or even the name of their anesthesiologist. That the public at large can have such trust and high expectations from medical professionals who will only be transiently involved in their care is a testament to the training, professionalism, and skill of anesthesiologists as well as a reflection of the many technological advances in medical science which have made modern anesthesiology a safer experience.

In order for the anesthesiologist to provide the level of medical care that will result in the best outcome for the patient, the anesthesiologist must be comfortable in the role of a "perioperative physician." That physician who cares for patients as they undergo the stress of surgery is best positioned to understand the preoperative and postoperative issues. Every preoperative patient requires that the anesthesiologist perform a careful and detailed assessment of their medical condition including coexisting illnesses, physical limitations, and their general fitness for anesthesia and surgery. It is a seldom-voiced tacit understanding among anesthesiologists that each and every patient who undergoes elective surgery becomes critically ill, albeit perhaps only for a limited time period. Of course, those patients who come to the operating room in the setting of severe trauma, overwhelming organ dysfunction due to illness, or patients who present with severe comorbidities for emergency surgery are de facto critically ill and are likely to remain so for some time postoperatively. There was once a time when patients could be deemed "too sick for surgery." However, this adage is seldom employed today and anesthesiologists, surgeons, as well as patients and their families in weighing the risks against the potential benefits often determine that the short and intense stress of surgery compares favorably to the alternative. Patients come to the operating room in septic shock for the control of their septic source, following an acute myocardial infarction for emergency coronary revascularization, in multiple organ failure and end-stage liver disease for liver transplantation, and after massive trauma; each patient's condition can be further complicated by systemic diseases such as chronic lung disease, severe atherosclerotic coronary and vascular disease, renal failure, diabetes mellitus, malnutrition, and others. Therefore, anesthesiology is unique in that there is no other specialty of medicine where every single patient encounter requires both knowledge and application of advanced life-support skills. All these patient groups will require elements of mechanical ventilation, sedation and analgesia, neuromuscular blockade, intravascular volume replacement, management of electrolytes, hemodynamic support and monitoring, monitoring of and replacement of blood and coagulation factors, as well as related monitoring and interventions directed at minimizing secondary injuries.

It is because anesthesiology is *also* the practice of *critical care medicine* that this textbook summarizes for anesthesiologists the state-of-the-art and the standard of care for the management of critically ill patients. It is incumbent on anesthesiologists to understand and apply the principles of critical care medicine that are relevant to the management of intraoperative patients as well as their continued postoperative care. We recognize that not all anesthesiologists will participate in the care of patients in the intensive care unit. However, all anesthesiologists will use critical care principles in the operating room. Therefore, new advances in modes of mechanical ventilation, new understanding regarding optimization of oxygen delivery to tissues, new perspectives on the evaluation and management of severe comorbidities, as well as preparedness for emerging threats such as biological and chemical terrorism are matters of interest to all anesthesiologists. Finally, for those physicians who also practice in the intensive care unit, this book is intended to highlight established principles, evolving standards of care, and new opportunities to provide excellence in patient care.

Peter J. Papadakos, M.D.
James E. Szalados, M.D.

Contents

GENERAL PRINCIPLES OF THE INTENSIVE CARE UNIT

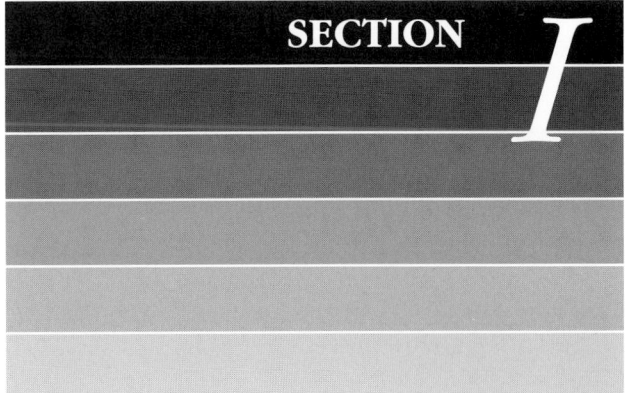

SECTION

I

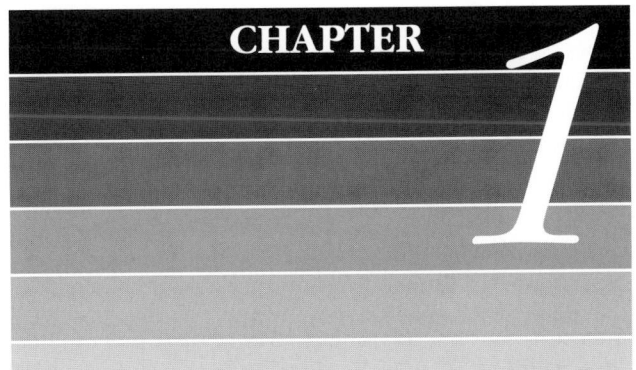

CHAPTER 1

Sepsis: The Systemic Inflammatory Response

JEAN-LOUIS VINCENT, M.D., Ph.D

Sepsis, the inflammatory response to infection, is perhaps the most common disease encountered by the critical care physician, complicating some 30 to 40% of intensive care unit (ICU) admissions and accounting for considerable morbidity and mortality. The exact incidence of sepsis is difficult to determine because of differences in definitions and populations. An international study across eight countries involving 14,364 ICU patients reported that there were 3034 infectious episodes giving a crude incidence of infections of 21.1%. Interestingly, one-fifth of these infections did not fit into any of the definition categories proposed by the ACCP/SCCM classification, which has been widely used in studies of sepsis. The mortality rate in patients with repeated infectious episodes was 53.6% compared to 16.9% in non-infected patients. A recent study, the Sepsis Occurrence in Acutely Ill Patients (SOAP), involving 3147 patients in 24 European countries, reported that 37.4% of patients were infected at some point during their ICU stay. Interestingly, the occurrence of sepsis ranged from 17.5 to 72.5% between countries. Importantly, the incidence of sepsis seems to be increasing with one study reporting an annual increase of 8.7% in the USA, from 82.7 cases per 100,000 population in 1979 to 240.4 per 100,000 population in 2000. Thus, although the risk of death per individual case may be falling, overall mortality rates are increasing as the size of the problem increases. This chapter briefly considers some of the basic features and the latest developments in this critically important field of sepsis in terms of diagnosis, pathophysiology, and management.

DEFINITION AND DIAGNOSIS

For many years definitions of sepsis have relied on those proposed by the ACCP/SCCM consensus conference published back in 1992. This conference introduced the systemic inflammatory response syndrome (SIRS) concept, whereby a patient was said to have SIRS if they met two or more of the following conditions: temperature greater than 38°C or less than 36°C, tachycardia, tachypnea, white blood cell count greater than 12,000 cells/mm^3 or less than 4000 cells/mm^3. Sepsis was then defined as infection plus SIRS, severe sepsis as sepsis plus organ dysfunction, and septic shock as severe sepsis with hypotension despite adequate fluid resuscitation and evidence of perfusion abnormalities. However, the SIRS criteria are very sensitive, and are met by most ICU patients and many general ward patients, making them of little practical value in identifying the patient with sepsis.

Recently, a sepsis definitions conference involving 29 physicians from Europe and North America was held in Washington, DC, to improve and standardize definitions in the field of sepsis. The conference participants agreed with the 1992 definitions in that sepsis should be defined as infection plus signs of systemic inflammation, but felt that the SIRS criteria were too non-specific and proposed rather a much longer list of possible signs of sepsis (Table 1-1). Unfortunately, as yet, no individual sign is specific for sepsis and clinical diagnosis relies on the combined presence of several signs and symptoms that together confirm the likelihood of sepsis as the diagnosis.

Table 1-1   Diagnostic Criteria for Sepsis

Infection, documented or suspected, and some of the following:
General variables
　　Fever or hypothermia
　　Tachycardia
　　Tachypnea
　　Significant edema or unexplained positive fluid balance
Inflammatory variables
　　Leukocytosis or leukopenia
　　Increased plasma C-reactive protein (CPR), procalcitonin (PCT)
　　　or interleukin-6 (IL-6) levels
Hemodynamic alterations
　　Arterial hypotension
　　Hyperkinetic state (high cardiac index – high SvO₂)
　　Decreased capillary refill or mottling
　　Hyperlactatemia
Organ dysfunction variables
　　Arterial hypoxemia
　　Creatinine increase or acute oliguria
　　Altered mental status
　　Thrombocytopenia – coagulation abnormalities
　　Hyperbilirubinemia
　　Ileus
　　Hyperglycemia in the absence of diabetes

Definitions of severe sepsis and septic shock remained unchanged from the 1992 publication.

In addition to discussing problems of definition, the participants at the Washington conference also developed a new system to characterize and stage patients with sepsis, to enable patients to be stratified according to their baseline risk of an adverse outcome and their potential to respond to therapy. Such systems are used widely in other areas of medicine, the prototypical system perhaps being the tumor/nodes/metastases (TNM) staging system for malignant tumors developed by Pierre Denoix in the 1940s. The PIRO system stratifies patients according to their Predisposing conditions, the nature and extent of the Insult, the nature and magnitude of the host Response, and the degree of concomitant Organ dysfunction (Table 1-2).

Predisposing conditions – As with any disease process, there are certain conditions that predispose a patient to developing sepsis. These include individual characteristics, such as age, presence of chronic disease processes (e.g., cancer), chronic administration of certain medications (e.g., immunodepressant drugs), history of alcohol abuse, etc., which may influence a patient's response to infection and/or suggest which therapies may be most appropriate in that patient. Recent attention has focused on genetic polymorphisms that may influence a patient's susceptibility to develop sepsis or affect their outcome if they do develop it. Various potential genetic factors have already been elucidated. A polymorphism of the tumor necrosis factor alpha (TNF-α) gene, the TNF-2 allele, is associated with increased serum levels of TNF and a greater risk of mortality from septic shock. A polymorphism within the intron 2 of the interleukin-1 receptor antagonist (IL-1ra) gene (IL-1RN*2) has been associated with reduced IL-1ra production and increased mortality rates. Similarly polymorphisms of the Toll-like receptor 4 (TLR4) and mannose-binding lectin (MBL) genes that seem to increase susceptibility to sepsis have also been identified. Gender may also influence susceptibility to and outcome from sepsis. Clearly, this is an area of ongoing research and the complex interaction of these predisposing factors requires more research to determine which carry most weight and how knowledge of increased risks can be translated into improved clinical outcomes.

Insult – The insult in sepsis is infection and specific characteristics of the infection that will influence the patient's immune response to that infection and likely outcome and response to treatment include the site of infection (e.g., urinary tract versus respiratory versus intra-abdominal), the specific organism (e.g., Gram-positive versus Gram-negative), the size of the inoculum, the susceptibility of the organism to antimicrobial agents, and the severity of the infection.

Response – The host response to sepsis can be assessed according to the presence or absence of various

Table 1-2 The PIRO System		
	Clinical	Laboratory
P: predisposition	Age, alcoholism, chronic diseases, steroid or immunosuppressive therapy, gender, etc.	Genetic factors
I: insult	Site (urinary tract, lungs, abdomen, etc.)	Bacteriology, assay of microbial products (lipopolysaccharide, mannan, bacterial DNA, etc.)
R: response	Temperature, heart rate, respiratory rate, arterial pressure, etc.	White blood cell count, blood lactate, C-reactive protein, procalcitonin, etc.
O: organ dysfunction	Arterial pressure, urine output, Glasgow coma scale, etc.	PaO₂/FIO₂, creatinine, bilirubin, platelet count, etc.

signs and symptoms and to the degree of elevation of, for example, white cell count, C-reactive protein, procalcitonin, etc. Importantly, initial suggestions that sepsis was simply an uncontrolled inflammatory response and could be treated by blocking or removing any or several of the inflammatory cytokines have been supplanted by the realization that the inflammatory response is a normal and necessary response to infection, and interrupting that response at any point may do more harm than good. Indeed, the early hyperinflammatory phase of sepsis is soon replaced by a hypoinflammatory state. Each individual will mount a different response pattern depending on various factors including those outlined in the predisposing factors and insult sections above, and patients who die from sepsis often have a prolonged hypoimmune stage (Figure 1-1). This differentiation is important in therapeutic terms, as anti-inflammatory therapies may be harmful if given to a patient who is already in the hypoinflammatory phase; such a patient may benefit rather from a pro-inflammatory therapy to boost their immune system.

Organ dysfunction – Organ dysfunction can be measured using scores such as the sequential organ failure assessment (SOFA; Table 1-3). This system uses parameters that are routinely available in all ICUs to assess the degree of dysfunction for six organ systems, respiratory, cardiovascular, renal, coagulation, neurologic, and hepatic, with a scale of 0 (no dysfunction) to 4 for each organ. Importantly, organ dysfunction can be recorded for each organ separately or a composite score can be calculated. Thus with repeated scores, a dynamic picture of the effects of sepsis on individual or global organ dysfunction can be developed and followed. Sequential assessment of SOFA during the first few days of ICU admission has been shown to be a good indicator of prognosis, with an increase in SOFA score during the first 48 hours in the ICU predicting a mortality rate of at least 50%.

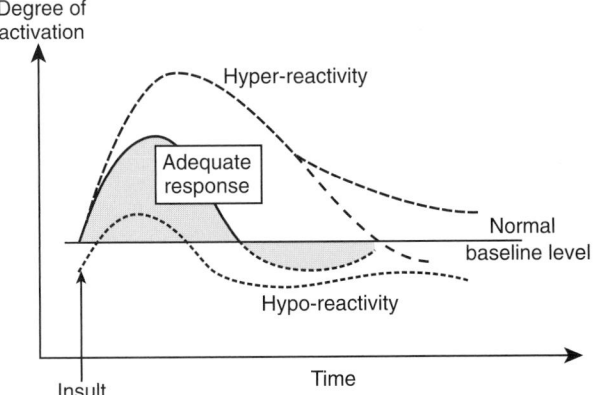

Figure 1-1 Graph shows prolonged hypoimmune stage response.

The PIRO system is newly developed and each item requires weighting and validation in septic patients. However, one could envisage patients receiving a PIRO stage, e.g., $P^2I^2R^1O^3$, which would help determine prognosis and direct treatment. This is an important advance in this field and, in addition to characterizing individual patients, will facilitate comparison of patient populations for clinical trial purposes, and help focus clinical research. Importantly, as new developments are made in gene mapping, or new markers of disease presence and severity are identified, the relevant component of the PIRO system would need to be modified accordingly.

PATHOPHYSIOLOGY

Inflammatory Mediators

The pathophysiology of sepsis is complex and although huge advances have been made, many facets remain unclear; indeed, while each new discovery provides new understanding, it also reveals new intricacies requiring further clarification. Essentially, the sepsis response is initiated directly by an invading organism, or by particular products or features of the organism, such as endotoxin (Gram-negative), peptidoglycan, and lipotiechoic acid (Gram-positive). These microbial products stimulate endothelial damage, the release of cytokines, the generation of complement, the activation of coagulation, and a range of other effects, both directly and via so-called mediators of sepsis. The activities and identities of many of the mediators of sepsis have been widely studied, but many features of the response remain unclear. Initiation occurs as microbial components are recognized by soluble or cell-bound pattern recognition molecules or receptors, such as CD14 and TLRs. For Gram-negative organisms, endotoxin (lipopolysaccharide, LPS) binds to a specific LPS-binding protein (LPB) in the plasma, which carries the LPS to a macrophage membrane receptor, CD14. The LPS/CD14 complex then interacts with a signal-transducing receptor in the membrane, TLR4, and MD-2. Activation of TLR4 induces the transcription of inflammatory and immune response genes via a nuclear factor-κB (NF-κB)-mediated mechanism, resulting in the release of cytokines. Pro-inflammatory cytokine release then attracts further macrophages and monocytes and the cycle repeats. The LPS/LBP complex can also bind to a soluble CD14 receptor present in the serum that promotes LPS binding to endothelial cells, again via TLRs. For Gram-positive and fungal organisms, the sequence is probably similar with cell-wall components such as lipoteichoic acid or peptidoglycan binding to CD14, which then binds to TLR2, again stimulating cytokine release. Bacterial components can also act directly to stimulate the coagulation (see below) and complement

Table 1-3 The Sequential Organ Failure Assessment (SOFA) Score

SOFA score	0	1	2	3	4
Respiration					
PaO_2/FIO_2, mmHg	>400	≤400	≤300	≤200 (with respiratory support)	≤100 (with respiratory support)
Coagulation					
Platelets × $10^3/mm^3$	>150	≤150	≤100	≤50	≤20
Liver					
Bilirubin, mg/dL (μmol/L)	<1.2 (<20)	1.2–1.9 (20–32)	2.0–5.9 (33–101)	6.0–11.9 (102–204)	>12.0 (>204)
Cardiovascular					
Hypotension	No hypotension	MAP <70 mmHg	Dopamine ≤5 or dobutamine (any dose)*	Dopamine >5 or epinephrine ≤0.1 or norepinephrine ≤0.1*	Dopamine >15 or epinephrine >0.1 or norepinephrine >0.1*
Central nervous system					
Glasgow coma score	15	13–14	10–12	6–9	<6
Renal					
Creatinine, mg/dL (μmol/L) or urine output	<1.2 (<110)	1.2–1.9 (110–170)	2.0–3.4 (171–299)	3.5–4.9 (300–440) or <500 ml/d	>5.0 (>440) or <200 ml/d

* Adrenergic agents administered for at least one hour (doses given are in μg/kg/min).

systems; the overall host response is thus a complex interaction between multiple factors.

Pro-inflammatory Cytokines

Cytokines are produced by a variety of cell types under normal and pathological conditions, and have systemic and local effects. They are commonly divided into pro- or anti-inflammatory cytokines although some may have both effects at different times or on different cells or tissues. Some of the key pro-inflammatory cytokines are TNF and IL-1, -6, and -8.

The TNF family is primarily involved in the regulation of cell proliferation and apoptosis, but TNF-α also recruits and activates neutrophils, macrophages, and lymphocytes, and stimulates the release of other pro-inflammatory cytokines and acute-phase proteins. TNF-α exerts its actions by binding to two distinct TNF receptors (TNFR1 and TNFR2). TNFR1 stimulation leads to classic TNF effects, while TNFR2 stimulation facilitates binding of TNF-α to the TNFR1 receptor.

IL-1 includes two related proteins, IL-1α and IL-1β, which activate the same receptors and thus have similar biological actions. The spectrum of activity of IL-1 is similar to that of TNF-α, although it generally produces less severe effects; these two cytokines work synergistically to give a greater effect than stimulation of either alone.

IL-6 is released largely under the influence of TNF-α and IL-1, and is involved in stimulating the release of acute-phase proteins, such as C-reactive protein (CRP), by the liver. It also induces B-cell growth and T-cell differentiation, and has been implicated in the myocardial depression seen in septic shock. IL-6 levels correlate more closely than other cytokines with the severity and outcome of septic shock.

IL-8 is released predominantly on stimulation by TNF-α and IL-1. Its major role is as a chemokine, i.e., it recruits inflammatory cells to the site of injury. It promotes recruitment and activation of leukocytes, upregulates expression of adhesion molecules, and enhances degranulation.

Anti-inflammatory Cytokines

Anti-inflammatory cytokines are released alongside the pro-inflammatory cytokines to modulate the inflammatory response. IL-10 is synthesized by monocytes, macrophages, T cells and B cells. IL-10 inhibits the release of TNF, IL-1, and IL-6, and suppresses monocyte procoagulant activity. Soluble TNF receptors are present in septic patients and bind to TNF, thus acting to limit TNF activity. IL-1 receptor antagonist (IL-1ra) is a competitive inhibitor of the IL-1 receptor and is produced by sepsis-activated monocytes and polymorphonuclear cells.

Other Mediators

Many other sepsis mediators are involved in the propagation or control of the septic response; some of the key agents are platelet activating factor (PAF), interferon (IFN)-γ, IL-4, macrophage inhibitory factor, high mobility group (HMG) proteins, transforming growth factor (TGF)-β, arachidonic acid metabolites, reactive oxygen species, nitric oxide, and cell adhesion molecules.

Coagulation and Inflammation

One of the key concepts that has changed our view, and indeed management, of sepsis is new understanding of the interaction of inflammation, coagulation, and fibrinolysis. The imbalance in hemostatic mechanisms may manifest as disseminated intravascular coagulopathy (DIC) and microvascular thrombosis and could be a key factor in the development of organ dysfunction, ultimately leading to multiple organ failure and death.

Essentially, the cycle starts with early endothelial damage initiated both directly by endotoxins and other infectious products, and indirectly by the initial components of the inflammatory response to the invading microorganism, including TNF-α and IL-1. Subendothelial structures are exposed and collagenases are released. Exposed tissue factor triggers the extrinsic coagulation cascade and accelerates the production of thrombin. At the same time, the endothelial damage further exacerbates inflammation, with neutrophil activation, neutrophil-endothelial cell adhesion, and continued elaboration of inflammatory cytokines, which in turn produce more endothelial damage, compromising microvascular function. Endogenous modulators of homeostasis, such as protein C and antithrombin, are consumed as the body attempts to return to a normal functional state. Under normal conditions, the endothelial surface proteins, thrombomodulin and endothelial protein C receptor (EPCR), activate protein C and its modulating effects; however, in sepsis the endothelial damage impairs this function of thrombomodulin and EPCR, thereby contributing to the loss of control. In addition to activated coagulation, fibrinolysis is suppressed, with increased levels of two of the key inhibitors of fibrinolysis: plasminogen activator inhibitor 1 (PAI-1) and thrombin activatable fibrinolysis inhibitor (TAFI). There is thus a cascade of inflammation and coagulopathy that drives the sepsis response, leading to multiple organ failure and death for many patients.

MANAGEMENT OF SEPSIS

Hemodynamic Stabilization

The basic management of sepsis involves appropriate and rapid antimicrobial therapy, surgical removal of any infectious nidus, and hemodynamic stabilization following the VIP (ventilate, infuse, pump) principles. The optimal hemodynamic management of septic shock has been the subject of some debate, in particular regarding the choice of fluid and vasoactive agents. Patients with septic shock can be successfully resuscitated with crystalloid or colloid, and when crystalloids and colloids are titrated to the same level of filling pressure they restore tissue perfusion to the same degree. However, because of their propensity for leakage into the extravascular space, to achieve the same effect approximately three times greater volume of crystalloid is required than colloid, and slightly longer infusion periods may be necessary to achieve comparable hemodynamic endpoints. The choice of fluid is probably less important than the quantity given, with cardiac output and systemic oxygen delivery increasing in proportion to the degree of intravascular volume expansion achieved. Repeated fluid challenges, in which a predefined amount of fluid is infused over a set time and the chosen clinical endpoints and pressure safety limits monitored, can be conducted to assess the adequacy of fluid resuscitation (Table 1-4).

Colloid solutions are much more expensive than crystalloid solutions, even when taking into account the reduced volumes required. Crystalloids are often regarded as first-line fluids for the hemodynamically stable patient and colloids are administered in addition to rather than in lieu of crystalloids. However, when the patient is hemodynamically compromised many clinicians prefer colloids. With several recent studies suggesting that new generation hydroxyethyl starches may reduce the inflammatory response and directly improve tissue oxygenation, the precise choice of fluid may become more important; however, further study is needed to confirm these observations.

The choice of vasoactive agent similarly has been the subject of some debate, with a keen search to determine which agent, if any, has direct beneficial effects on the microcirculation. However, there remains no evidence in favor of one agent or another, with dopamine and norepinephrine both valid choices as first-line agents.

One of the key features of hemodynamic stabilization in septic patients is that it should be done early. Early goal-directed therapy in patients with severe sepsis and septic shock improves mortality rates compared to standard therapy.

Immunomodulating Therapy

The recognition of the important interaction between the coagulation system and the inflammatory response outlined above led to the development of the first immunomodulating therapy to be shown to reduce mortality in patients with severe sepsis. A recombinant form of activated protein C, known as drotrecogin-alfa (activated), given at a dose of 24 µg/kg/hour for 96 hours improves organ dysfunction and decreases mortality in patients with severe sepsis and septic shock. The mechanisms of action of this drug are still uncertain, but combine anticoagulant properties and direct effects on the inflammatory response. Activated protein C can reduce LPS-induced TNF release, inhibit leukocyte adhesion, decrease leukocyte activation, inhibit NF-κB formation, and inhibit induction of inducible nitric oxide synthase (iNOS), all key factors in the systemic inflammatory response to sepsis. Activated protein C also has anti-apoptotic effects. As expected, drotrecogin alfa (activated) administration is associated with an increase in the risk of bleeding, although this is mostly associated with use of invasive procedures. It is therefore contraindicated in patients with active internal bleeding, recent hemorrhagic stroke, intracranial or intraspinal surgery, severe head trauma, presence of an epidural catheter, intracranial neoplasm, or evidence of cerebral herniation (Table 1-5). Care should be taken in other

Table 1-4 Clinical Example of Fluid Challenge

Strategy	Patient with Arterial Hypotension (MAP 65 mmHg, CVP 12 mmHg)
Select type of fluid	Ringer's lactate
Select rate of infusion	1000 ml/30 min
Select clinical end-points	MAP 75 mmHg
Select pressure safety limits	CVP 15 mmHg

Results	Baseline	Fluid Challenge	Fluid Challenge		Fluid Challenge
MAP	65	70	75		65
CVP	12	14	15	OR	15
Urine output	0	20	20		0
Skin	Mottled	OK	OK		Mottled
Action		**Continue**	**Stop**		**Stop**

Table 1-5	Contraindications and Cautions for the Use of Drotrecogin Alfa (Activated) in Patients with Severe Sepsis and Septic Shock

CONTRAINDICATIONS

Active internal bleeding
Trauma with risk of life-threatening bleeding (spleen, liver, retroperitoneal, etc.)
Central nervous system (CNS)
    Recent hemorrhagic stroke (3 months)
    Recent CNS surgery or head trauma (2 months)
    Intracranial mass
    Epidural catheter

CAUTIONS

Abnormal coagulation
    Bleeding diathesis
    Platelet count < 30,000/mm^3
    Very prolonged INR
    Full heparin therapy
    Recent thrombolytic therapy
Significant risk of bleeding
    Polytrauma
    Active ulcer
    Esophageal varices
Recent ischemic stroke (3 months)

groups of patients at high risk of bleeding, and infusion should be interrupted for surgery or invasive interventions. Although costly, its cost-effectiveness ratio compares well with other widely used healthcare strategies.

Another strategy that has been shown to be beneficial in patients with septic shock is the administration of moderate doses of corticosteroids. In patients with septic shock the adrenal response may be insufficient, and in such patients moderate doses of corticosteroids (50 mg IV hydrocortisone every 6 hours) have been shown to improve survival rates. Similarly, septic shock is associated with a relative deficiency of vasopressin and administration of low doses of vasopressin may be beneficial although this has yet to undergo randomized clinical trials, and thus cannot be recommended for routine use.

CONCLUSION

Severe sepsis and septic shock are common causes of morbidity and mortality, and their incidence is increasing. Improved understanding of the pathophysiology of the sepsis response, in particular regarding the interaction between inflammation and coagulation, has seen a major advance in the treatment options with the development of drotrecogin alfa (activated). Importantly, as other effective immunomodulatory strategies become available,

strategies to characterize the patient with sepsis, such as the PIRO system, will become increasingly important to help determine which therapy or therapies should be given to which patient and when.

SELECTED READING

Alberti C, Brun-Buisson C, Burchardi H et al: Epidemiology of sepsis and infection in ICU patients from an international multicentre cohort study. Intensive Care Med 28:108-121, 2002.

Angus DC, Linde-Zwirble WT, Clermont G et al: Cost-effectiveness of drotrecogin alfa (activated) in the treatment of severe sepsis. Crit Care Med 31:1-11, 2003.

Annane D, Sebille V, Charpentier C et al: Effect of treatment with low doses of hydrocortisone and fludrocortisone on mortality in patients with septic shock. JAMA 288:862-871, 2002.

Appoloni O, Dupont E, Andrien M et al: Association of TNF2, a TNFα promoter polymorphism, with plasma TNFα levels and mortality in septic shock. Am J Med 110:486-488, 2001.

Bernard GR, Vincent JL, Laterre PF et al: Recombinant human protein C Worldwide Evaluation in Severe Sepsis (PROWESS) study group. Efficacy and safety of recombinant human activated protein C for severe sepsis. N Engl J Med 344:699-709, 2001.

Bossink AW, Groeneveld J, Hack CE et al: Prediction of mortality in febrile medical patients: How useful are systemic inflammatory response syndrome and sepsis criteria? Chest 113:1533-1541, 1998.

Eachempati SR, Hydo L, Barie PS: Gender-based differences in outcome in patients with sepsis. Arch Surg 134:1342-1347, 1999.

Ferreira FL, Bota DP, Bross A, Melot C, Vincent JL: Serial evaluation of the SOFA score to predict outcome in critically ill patients. JAMA 286:1754-1758, 2001.

Hotchkiss RS, Karl IE: Pathophysiology and treatment of sepsis. N Engl J Med 348:138-150, 2003.

Joyce DE, Grinnell BW: Recombinant human activated protein C attenuates the inflammatory response in endothelium and monocytes by modulating nuclear factor-κB. Crit Care Med 30:S288-S293, 2002.

Levy MM, Fink MP, Marshall JC et al: 2001 SCCM/ESICM/ACCP/ATS/SIS International Sepsis Definitions Conference. Crit Care Med 31:1250-1256, 2003.

Martin GS, Mannino DM, Eaton S et al: The epidemiology of sepsis in the United States from 1979 through 2000. N Engl J Med 348:1546-1554, 2003.

Members of the American College of Chest Physicians/Society of Critical Care Medicine Consensus Conference Meeting: Definitions for sepsis and organ failure and guidelines for the use of innovative therapies in sepsis. Crit Care Med 20:864-874, 1992.

Rivers E, Nguyen B, Havstad S et al: Early Goal-Directed Therapy Collaborative Group. Early goal-directed therapy in the treatment of severe sepsis and septic shock. N Engl J Med 345:1368–1377, 2001.

Vincent JL, Moreno R, Takala J et al: The SOFA (Sepsis-related Organ Failure Assessment) score to describe organ dysfunction/failure. On behalf of the Working Group on Sepsis-Related Problems of the European Society of Intensive Care Medicine. Intensive Care Med 22:707–710, 1996.

Wichmann MW, Inthorn D, Andress HJ et al: Incidence and mortality of severe sepsis in surgical intensive care patients: the influence of patient gender on disease process and outcome. Intensive Care Med 26:167–172, 2000.

CHAPTER 2

Acute Respiratory Failure

MICHAEL J. APOSTOLAKOS, M.D.

Hypoxemia
Hypoxemia: Management
Hypercapnia
Hypercapnia: Management
Summary

Respiratory failure is a condition in which the respiratory system fails in one or both of its gas-exchanging functions (oxygenation of or carbon dioxide removal from mixed venous blood). Thus, respiratory failure is a syndrome rather than a specific disease.

Respiratory failure may be acute or chronic. Acute respiratory failure is associated with life-threatening alterations in arterial blood gases and acid–base status whereas chronic respiratory failure is a more indolent process. This chapter focuses on acute respiratory failure.

Respiratory failure may be divided into two broad categories: hypoxemic (type 1) and hypercapnic (type 2). Hypoxemic respiratory failure is defined as an arterial PO_2 less than 55 mmHg when the fraction of inspired air (FIO_2) is 0.60 or greater. Hypercapnic respiratory failure is defined as an arterial PCO_2 greater than 45 mmHg. Disorders that initially cause hypoxemia may be complicated by respiratory pump failure and hypercapnia (Table 2-1). Conversely, diseases that produce respiratory pump failure are frequently complicated by hypoxemia due to secondary pulmonary parenchymal processes (e.g., pneumonia) or vascular disorders (e.g., pulmonary embolism).

HYPOXEMIA

Hypoxemia may be broadly divided into four major categories:

1. Ventilation/perfusion ($\dot{V}/\dot{Q}$) mismatch
2. Shunt
3. Diffusion limitation
4. Hypoventilation and low FIO_2

These will now be addressed individually in reverse order.

Hypoventilation and low FIO_2 are rare causes of hypoxemia in the intensive care unit (ICU). One should suspect hypoventilation as the cause of hypoxemia in patients with elevated $PaCO_2$. Oversedation or hypercarbic respiratory failure are common causes of this condition. Low FIO_2 should not be a cause of this condition in the ICU unless there is an inadvertent oxygen disconnection. Hypoventilation and low FIO_2 may be separated from the other causes of hypoxemia in that they are the only ones associated with a normal alveolar-arterial (A-a) PO_2 gradient (Table 2-2).

The A-a PO_2 gradient represents the difference between alveolar and arterial PO_2. The A-a PO_2 gradient may be calculated from the following equation: A-a PO_2 gradient = $FIO_2(P_B P_{H_2O}) - (PaCO_2/R) - PaO_2$, where FIO_2 is the fraction of inspired O_2, P_B is the barometric pressure, P_{H_2O} is the partial pressure of water, and R is the respiratory quotient. The A-a PO_2 gradient is normally less than 10 mmHg on room air. In adults over the age of 65, normal values may extend up to 25 mmHg.

Table 2-1 Common Causes of Hypoxemia and Hypercapnia	
Hypoxemia	**Hypercapnia**
Pneumonia	Muscle weakness
Acute respiratory distress syndrome	Increased CO_2 production
Congestive heart failure	Airway obstruction
Pulmonary embolism	Narcotic overdose

Table 2-2 Type 1 Respiratory Failure Mechanisms, Responsiveness to Supplemental O₂, and Presence of A-a Gradient

Mechanism	Responds to Added O₂	Increased A-a PO₂ Gradient
Decreased FIO_2	Yes	No
Hypoventilation	Yes	No
Shunt	No	Yes
V/Q Mismatch	Yes	Yes
Diffusion Limitation	Yes	Yes

An example of the usefulness of calculating an A-a PO_2 gradient is demonstrated by this case. A 21-year-old patient is admitted from the emergency department (ED) with a drug (narcotic) overdose. On presentation to the ED the patient's respiratory rate is 4 breaths per minute. Initial ABG is pH 7.1, $PaCO_2$ = 80 mmHg, PaO_2 = 40 mmHg, O_2 sat = 70%. The patient is intubated and transferred to the ICU. The A-a PO_2 gradient calculated from the equation above is:

$$\text{A-a } PO_2 \text{ gradient} = 0.21(747 - 47) - (80/0.8) - 40 = 147 - 100 - 40$$
$$= 7 \text{ (i.e., } \leq 10 \text{ on room air)}$$

The normal A-a PO_2 gradient supports the fact that this patient's hypoxemia is due solely to hypoventilation and that no other cause of hypoxemia, such as pneumonia, needs to be implicated. The normal A-a PO_2 gradient separates this category of hypoxemia from the other three categories.

Diffusion limitation is a very rare cause of hypoxemia in the ICU. The alveolar capillary unit has about 1 second in which to exchange carbon dioxide for oxygen. This normally occurs within the first 0.3 seconds. This leaves approximately 0.7 seconds as a buffer. This protects against hypoxemia during exercise (which increases cardiac output and hence decreases available time for gas exchange) and/or to overcome diseases which cause diffusion limitation. Except for severe end-stage lung disease (e.g., fibrosis, emphysema), this is a very rare occurrence and, hence, a very rare cause of acute hypoxemia. Diffusion limitation, in general, is something that is handled by the pulmonary specialist over a long period of time.

$\dot{V}/\dot{Q}$ mismatch is the most common cause of hypoxemia. With reference to hypoxemia, only perfusion with reduced or absent ventilation leads to hypoxemia. Ventilation without perfusion is simply deadspace ventilation and by itself does not lead to hypoxemia. If severe, it may lead to CO_2 retention.

To understand this completely, one needs to call to mind the following equations:

$$\dot{V}_E = \dot{V}_D + \dot{V}_A$$

$$PaCO_2 = k \times \dot{V}CO_2/\dot{V}_A$$

where $\dot{V}_E$ equals total minute ventilation, $\dot{V}_D$ equals deadspace minute ventilation, $\dot{V}_A$ equals alveolar minute ventilation, and $\dot{V}CO_2$ equals CO_2 production. Normally $\dot{V}_D$ and $\dot{V}_A$ represent 30% and 70% respectively of total ventilation. Also, as k is a constant and $\dot{V}CO_2$ can generally be considered constant, $PaCO_2$ is inversely proportional to $\dot{V}_A$ (i.e., $PaCO_2 \sim 1/\dot{V}_A$). This will become important to understand when adjusting ventilator settings.

When assessing hypoxemia it is important to understand the normal physiology of the lung (Figure 2-1A). The pulmonary artery is the only artery in the body that delivers unoxygenated blood. A normal blood gas obtained from the pulmonary artery is pH 7.35/PCO_2 = 45 mmHg/PO_2 = 40 mmHg/O_2 sat = 75%. The alveolar PO_2 is approximately 110 mmHg (obtained from the alveolar-arterial gas equation), and alveolar PCO_2 is 40 mmHg. A perfectly matched alveolar capillary unit will produce pulmonary venous blood with a pH of 7.4/PCO_2 = 40 mmHg/PO_2 = 110 mmHg, and O_2 sat = 100%. However, a "normal" arterial blood gas obtained peripherally will yield something like: pH = 7.4/$PaCO_2$ = 40 mmHg/PaO_2 = 95 mmHg/O_2 sat = 98%. The difference between the pulmonary venous blood and the arterial blood gas is due to anatomic shunt. Approximately 2% of venous return from the systemic circulation is returned to the left side of the circulation without going through the pulmonary circulation. Two major contributors to this shunt are the bronchial circulation and the thebesian veins of the heart. A combination of 98% of pulmonary venous blood and 2% anatomic shunt (systemic venous) blood yields the "normal" peripheral ABG.

$\dot{V}/\dot{Q}$ mismatch leads to hypoxemia when perfused alveolar units have reduced oxygen levels in the alveolar space due to reduced ventilation. This reduced ventilation is generally due to some obstruction (bronchiolar edema or mucus related to infection, bronchospasm secondary to asthma, etc.). $\dot{V}/\dot{Q}$ mismatch, however, may be overcome with additional FIO_2 (Figure 2-1B). Shunt is simply the extreme of $\dot{V}/\dot{Q}$ mismatch where there is no ventilation but perfusion persists. (Remember ventilation without perfusion is deadspace ventilation.) Shunt will not be overcome by additional FIO_2 (Figure 2-1C).

HYPOXEMIA: MANAGEMENT

Quite simply there are two major ways to improve oxygenation: (i) increase FIO_2 and (ii) increase mean airway pressure.

Increasing FIO_2 is simple and can only be done one way. Increasing mean airway pressure can be done by a multitude of ways. Increasing mean airway pressure improves oxygenation by recruiting partially or fully collapsed alveoli, thus better matching ventilation to perfusion and reducing shunt. Mean airway pressure may be

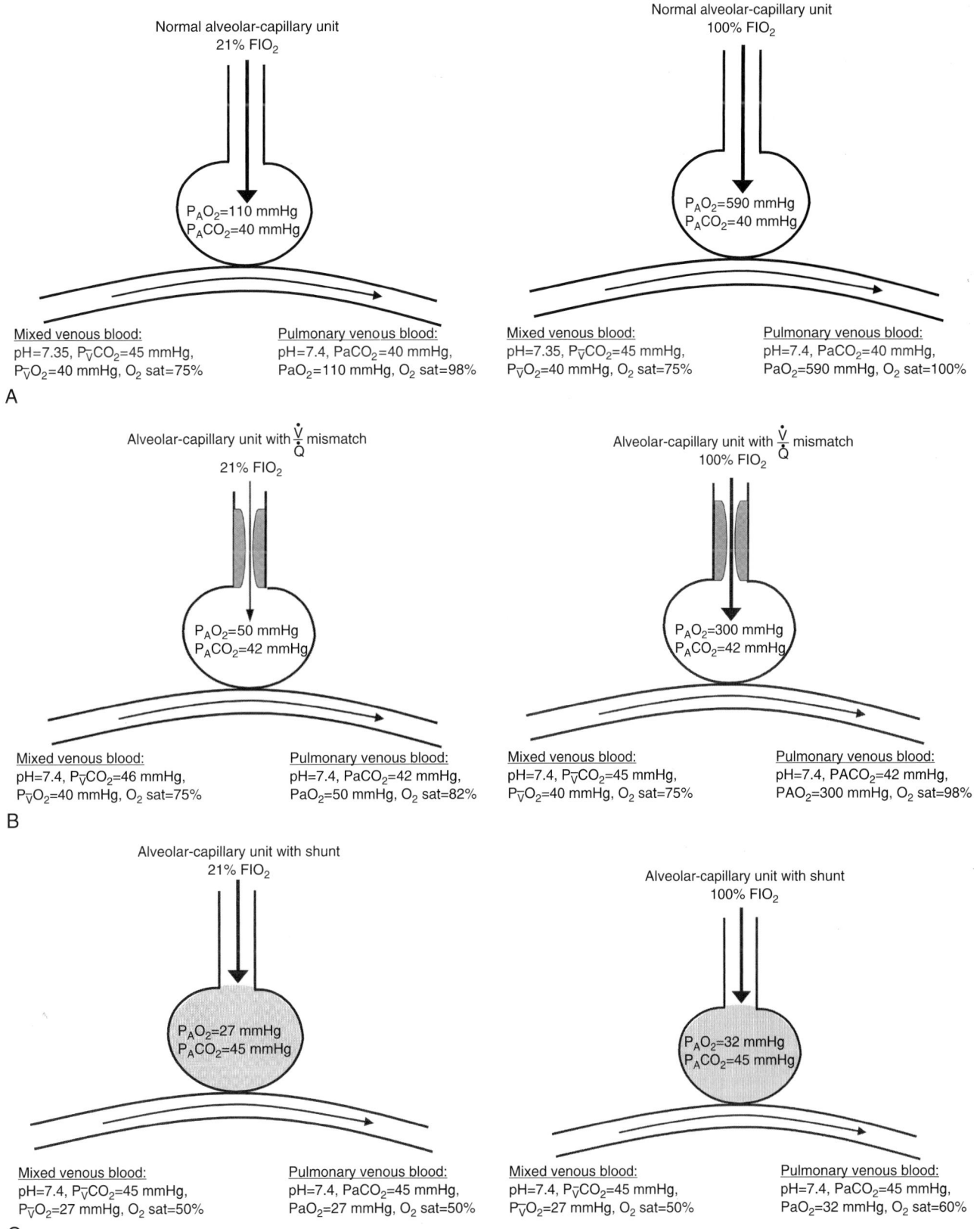

Figure 2-1   Physiology of oxygenation in the lung under normal circumstances (**A**), during V/Q mismatch (**B**), and shunt (**C**). See text for details. (Adapted from Apostolakos MJ: The critically ill patient: overview of respiratory failure and oxygen delivery. In Apostolakos MJ, Papadakos PJ, editors: *The Intensive Care Manual*, New York: McGraw-Hill, 2001, pp 1–13.)

increased either invasively or non-invasively. Non-invasive means include the use of continuous positive airway pressure ventilation (CPAP). CPAP utilizes a tightfitted nasal or naso-oral mask (to reduce leaks). The CPAP machine provides a continuous pressure to the airway to assist in recruiting alveoli and improving oxygenation. Usual starting pressures are 3–8 cmH₂O and may be titrated to 10–15 cmH₂O to improve oxygenation. Issues of comfort limit the pressure that can be used. Contraindications to the use of CPAP include poor mental status or patients with increased risk of aspiration (such as those patients with ileus or bowel obstruction).

Another way to increase mean airway pressure is through invasive mechanical ventilation which utilizes an endotracheal tube. The easiest way to increase mean airway pressure for a patient on invasive mechanical ventilation is to increase positive end expiratory pressure (PEEP). This is the back pressure that the ventilator provides during the exhalation phase to prevent alveolar collapse. Inverse ratio ventilation (IRV) is another maneuver that increases mean airway pressure by increasing the normal inspiratory/expiratory ratio from 1:2 to 1:1 or 2:1. This change keeps the positive pressure in the chest for longer periods of time. Some believe that this technique simply adds to the PEEP by not allowing enough time for exhalation. This has led to the term "sneaky PEEP" being used in reference to IRV. High-frequency JET ventilation and oscillating ventilation are "high tech" ways of increasing mean airway pressure and oxygenation. Two less commonly used ways to improve oxygenation, prone positioning and inhaled nitric oxide, work by improving $\dot{V}/\dot{Q}$ matching.

HYPERCAPNIA

Besides oxygenation, the other major function of the respiratory system is ventilation (CO₂ removal). At a constant rate of CO₂ production ($\dot{V}CO_2$), PaCO₂ is determined by the level of alveolar ventilation. The relationship between alveolar ventilation, rate of CO₂ production, and PaCO₂ is:

$$\dot{V}_A = K \times \dot{V}CO_2/PaCO_2$$

where $\dot{V}_A$ = alveolar minute ventilation, K = a constant, and $\dot{V}CO_2$ = rate of CO₂ production. When $\dot{V}CO_2$ is constant a patient's PaCO₂ will be inversely proportional to $\dot{V}_A$ in a linear fashion.

One also needs to remember that $\dot{V}_E = \dot{V}_D + \dot{V}_A$, where $\dot{V}_E$ = total minute ventilation, $\dot{V}_D$ = deadspace minute ventilation, and $\dot{V}_A$ = alveolar minute ventilation. Normally deadspace ventilation represents approximately 30% of total ventilation. This, however, can increase in certain conditions such as chronic obstructive pulmonary disease (COPD) or acute respiratory distress syndrome

(ARDS). At times, deadspace ventilation may approach 70% or more of total ventilation. If this occurs, the relative amount of alveolar ventilation is reduced and total ventilation must be increased if PCO₂ is to be maintained constant. When this demand cannot be met, hypercapnia ensues. Abnormalities of the airways or alveoli as described above increase the demand as well as increased metabolic rate or elevated respiratory quotient ($\dot{V}CO_2/\dot{V}O_2$) (Table 2-1).

The other side of the supply/demand equation that can lead to hypercapnia is when the supply side is adversely affected. The supply side is made up of the neuromuscular system. Normally the respiratory system can sustain approximately half of the maximum voluntary ventilation (MVV). This is called the maximal sustainable ventilation (MSV). A 70-kg adult under basal conditions has a minute ventilation of approximately 6 l/min, MSV of 80 l/min, and MVV of 160 l/min. When certain conditions intervene (Table 2-1) the body's ability to supply increases in ventilation are compromised and therefore hypercapnia can ensue. This may lead to respiratory failure.

Abnormalities of the central nervous system, peripheral nervous system, chest wall, airways, or alveoli can all lead to hypercapnic respiratory failure. Narcotic overdose, meningoencephalitis, vascular abnormalities, or strokes affecting medullary control centers can lead to hypoventilation and subsequently to hypercapnic respiratory failure.

A wide variety of disorders that affect peripheral nerves, neuromuscular junction, and chest wall are associated with weakness and ineffective ventilation and thus with hypercapnic respiratory failure. Guillain-Barré syndrome, myasthenia gravis, polymyositis, muscular dystrophies, and metabolic disorders are the most common neuromuscular causes of hypercapnic respiratory failure.

Primary disorders of the chest wall constitute another important category of neuromuscular respiratory failure. These conditions include severe kyphoscoliosis, flail chest, extensive thoracoplasty, morbid obesity, and massive abdominal distention secondary to distended loops of bowel or ascites. These conditions place respiratory muscles at mechanical disadvantage and tidal volume drops. Despite increases in respiratory rate, alveolar ventilation drops and hypercapnia ensues.

Obstructed airways are another common cause of hypercapnia. Causes of obstruction include aspirated foreign objects, tracheal tumor, COPD, and asthma. The airway narrowing leads to greater transthoracic pressure gradient required for inspiratory flow. The resistive component of the work of breathing is increased, and the increase is associated with increased oxygen consumption. In addition tidal volume falls and deadspace ventilation increases. Respiratory muscle fatigue and hypercapnia develops.

HYPERCAPNIA: MANAGEMENT

When hypercapnia occurs ventilatory demand outstrips supply. Therefore choices of treatment are in two categories: augment ventilatory capacity (supply) or decrease workload (demand).

If airway obstruction is an issue such as it is in COPD or asthma, bronchodilators (e.g., beta agonists), anti-inflammatories (e.g., steroids), and secretion elimination are effective in decreasing airway resistance and hence the workload. Thus, demand on ventilation is reduced.

Correcting electrolyte disturbances (e.g., hypokalemia, hypocalcemia, hypomagnesemia, and hypophosphatemia) may improve respiratory pump function and thus augment ventilatory supply. Improving nutritional parameters can have similar effects.

CLINICAL CAVEAT

Non-invasive Ventilation in Acute Respiratory Failure
- Reduces need for invasive ventilation.
- Stabilizes gas exchange and vital signs.
- Decreases hospital mortality.

If the above fails, augmentation of the patient's spontaneous ventilation can be achieved by either invasive or non-invasive techniques. Non-invasive ventilation includes bi-level positive airway pressure (BiPAP). Nasal or naso-oral masks may be used. Settings include inspiratory pressures (generally 8–15 cmH$_2$O) and expiratory pressures (generally 3–8 cmH$_2$O). Inspiratory pressures augment alveolar ventilation and thus this pressure is adjusted upward to increase tidal volumes and reduce PCO$_2$ levels. Expiratory pressures are adjusted to optimize oxygenation. Contraindications to BiPAP are the same as CPAP above. The use of this form of ventilation has resulted in a reduced need for invasive ventilation, more rapid stabilization of gas exchange and vital signs, and a decrease in hospital mortality.

Invasive mechanical ventilation is reserved for patients who cannot tolerate or who do not improve with non-invasive ventilation. Increasing respiratory rate and/or tidal volumes on the mechanical ventilator will increase alveolar minute ventilation and thus reduce PCO$_2$.

CURRENT CONTROVERSY

Non-invasive Ventilation
- Characterization of which patients may benefit from non-invasive forms of ventilation remains unclear.
- The question as to which patients are not candidates for non-invasive ventilation is controversial.

SUMMARY

Acute respiratory failure is divided into type 1 hypoxemic respiratory failure and type 2 hypercapnic respiratory failure. Type 1 hypoxemic respiratory failure is subdivided into four major categories that have unique characteristics with respect to the presence of A-a PO$_2$ gradient and response to supplemental oxygen. Type 2 hypercapnic respiratory failure occurs when ventilatory supply is outstripped by demand.

Treatment of respiratory failure focuses on reversing the underlying cause of respiratory failure. Barring that, supportive measures incude increasing FIO$_2$ and mean airway pressure to improve oxygenation and the use of BiPAP or invasive ventilation to reduce PCO$_2$.

CASE STUDY

A 72-year-old white female with history of COPD and coronary artery disease is one day status post an uneventful open cholecystectomy. Pain control is an issue despite escalating doses of narcotics. During the evening shift the patient is found "gurgling" in bed, O$_2$ saturation is 50% on room air, and the patient is only responsive to painful stimuli with groaning. An arterial blood gas is checked with the following results on room air: pH = 7.18, PCO$_2$ = 65, PO$_2$ = 32, O$_2$ saturation = 52%.

QUESTIONS

1. What is the A-a PO$_2$ gradient?
2. Is the cause of the respiratory failure simply narcotic overdose or is there a superimposed cause of hypoxemia such as pneumonia?
3. How can this respiratory failure be managed?

SELECTED READING

Apostolakos MJ: The critically ill patient: overview of respiratory failure and oxygen delivery. In Apostolakos MJ, Papadakos PJ, editors: *The Intensive Care Manual*, New York: McGraw-Hill, 2001, pp 1–13.

Brochard L, Mancebo J, Wysocki M et al: Non-invasive ventilation for acute exacerbations of chronic obstructive pulmonary disease. N Engl J Med 333:817–822, 1995.

Criner GJ: Respiratory failure. In Criner GJ and D'Alonzo GE, editors: *Pulmonary Pathophysiology*, Madison: Fence Creek Publishing, 1999, pp 171–190.

Grippi MA: Respiratory failure: an overview. In Fishman AP, Elias JA, Fishman JA, Grippi MA, Kaiser LR, Senior RM, editors: *Fishman's Pulmonary Diseases and Disorders*, New York: McGraw-Hill, 1998, pp 2525–2535.

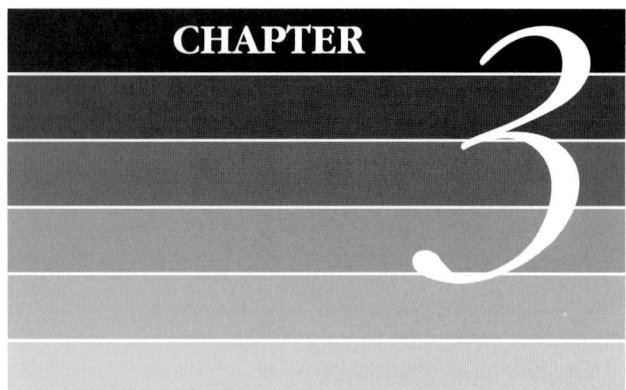

CHAPTER 3

Vascular Access and Hemodynamic Monitoring

JAMES E. SZALADOS, M.D., J.D., M.B.A.

MONITORING STANDARDS OF CARE

The intensive care unit (ICU) is defined by the intensity of monitoring (technology and personnel) and the aggressiveness of diagnostic and therapeutic interventions aimed at optimizing patient care and outcome. Teamwork facilitates the complex care processes, increases the level of vigilance, and provides multiple tiers of backup for safety. Since all ICU patients are inherently unstable with respect to dysfunctional organ system status, the typical feedback loop of monitoring and evaluation, through therapeutic intervention, and then back to re-evaluation is extremely tight.

The most important potential complication of patient monitoring is that of erroneous decisions based on inadequate or flawed data. Monitors are only as useful as the people who operate them and interpret the data. Whenever the data do not reconcile with the clinical picture, they must be questioned. For this reason, physicians must closely and personally participate in all aspects of data collection and be completely familiar with all monitoring protocols, tools, and data presentation. It is a fallacy to believe that the role of the physician can be separated from moment-to-moment bedside patient care in the ICU.

Therefore, reliable information is vital to effective clinical decision-making. In the critically ill patient immediately actionable information frequently determines their survival. The greater the complexity of any individual ICU patient, the greater is the need for data.

In order for a monitor to have both utility and effectiveness, it must be (1) capable of detecting a physiologically useful signal, (2) capable of responding rapidly to physiologic changes, (3) able to process the data and display it in such a way that the user can rapidly interpret it, and, preferably, (4) able to track trends. Therefore, monitors must provide *valid* information: information that accurately represents the state of the patient; and monitors must provide *reliable* information: data that are precise and reproducible. Monitors must also be equipped with alarm systems which should never be disabled; and, whenever possible, alarm systems should be redundant and also should be graduated so that problems trigger more than one alarm and increase rapidly in intensity of warning. The level of monitoring must be commensurate with the patient's severity of illness and underlying organ dysfunction. More importantly, skilled, alert, and prepared staff must be ready to respond immediately to the alarms.

It is generally accepted that critically ill patients must receive continuous monitoring. However, monitoring standards for ICU patients have not yet been universally codified, as they have by the American Society of Anesthesiologists for intraoperative patient monitoring. The typical physiologic monitors in the ICU include continuous electrocardiography (ECG), pulse oximetry, apnea/respiratory rate, urine output, and blood pressure. Respiratory rate can be easily obtained from modern ECG monitoring which should be configured to detect apnea, especially in patients receiving sedation, or in patients who are mechanically ventilated. Hourly urine output is a standard of care for all patients at risk of shock. A minimally acceptable urine output of 0.5 cm³/kg/hour suggests, but does not guarantee, that renal perfusion is adequate. Blood pressure monitoring should occur at an interval that accounts for a patient's potential for decompensation, recent trends, and therapeutic regimen. Invasive and noninvasive monitoring of cardiovascular status is thus a backbone to the delivery of critical care.

More complicated patients who receive additional levels of critical care may require general or organ-specific monitors; these may include, for example, capnography (monitoring of end tidal CO_2 concentrations), peripheral nerve stimulation (monitoring of the level of neuromuscular blockade), intracranial pressure monitoring, or abdominal compartment pressure monitoring. Additionally, ICU patients who are mechanically ventilated require ventilator monitoring such as spirometry, and most ICU patients receive aggressive biochemical monitoring by frequent blood sampling as indicated by their condition.

ELECTROCARDIOGRAPHY

Basic telemetry requires continuous ECG monitoring of heart rate and rhythm. The choice of the lead that is monitored during ECG determines diagnostic sensitivity. Since the electrical axis of lead II runs parallel to the atria, lead II accentuates P wave morphology changes and also enhances the diagnosis of dysrhythmias and inferior wall, or right ventricular, ischemia. V5 at the level of the fifth intercostal space in the left axillary line is especially useful for the detection of lateral wall, or left ventricular, ischemia. Whenever only one lead is displayed, the choice of lead depends upon clinical history and an index of suspicion.

ST–T wave changes cannot be reliably detected on telemetry; both false positive and false negative errors are possible. A 12-lead ECG should be performed to verify any suspected changes.

PULSE OXIMETRY

The importance of pulse oximetry is that it is inexpensive, easy to use, reliable, and it has been definitively shown to increase greatly patient safety; therefore, pulse oximetry must be used for every critically ill patient. Pulse oximetry estimates the saturation of arterial blood by using changes in light absorption and reflectance from vascular beds. Oximetry is based on the principle of reflectance spectrophotometry whereby light passed through a solution is differentially absorbed based on solute concentration, solute characteristics, the path length of transmitted light, and solution-specific extinction coefficients. For a solution containing hemoglobin (Hb), the relative concentrations of oxyhemoglobin and

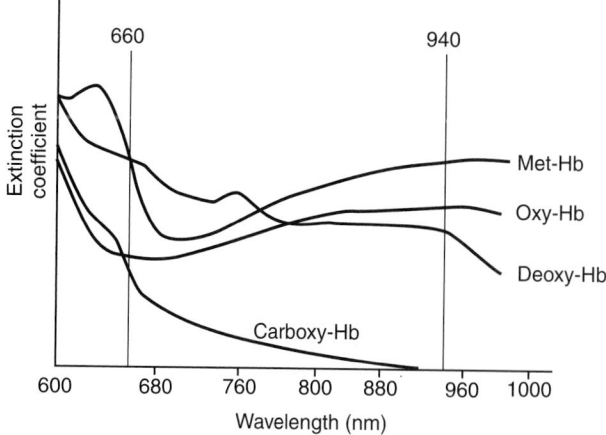

Figure 3-1 Hemoglobin extinction curves. Extinction coefficient plotted as a function of the absorption spectral wavelength of transmitted light is shown for four hemoglobin species. Points at which two species of hemoglobin have the same extinction coefficient are known as isobestic points. For example, at 805 nm the extinction coefficients for oxyhemoglobin and reduced hemoglobin are the same. Met-Hb, methemoglobin; Oxy-Hb, oxyhemoglobin; Deoxy-Hb, deoxyhemoglobin; Carboxy-Hb, carboxyhemoglobin. See text for details.

deoxyhemoglobin can be determined because the hemoglobin moieties differ in their absorption coefficients to red and infrared light; this technology is based on the Beer–Lambert law. Specifically, oxyhemoglobin absorbs more infrared light (990 nm) than does deoxyhemoglobin, which instead absorbs more red light (660 nm) and thus visually appears blue or cyanotic (Figure 3-1). When changes in light absorption during arterial pulsation are compared as a ratio using microprocessor technology, both plethysmographic and oxygen saturation (SpO_2) data are derived. The value for oxygen saturation is displayed by the pulse oximeter is correctly referred to as the SpO_2 in order to differentiate it from the SaO_2 which is obtained from blood gas analysis.

Mathematically, the determination of *functional* SpO_2 is represented by the following equation:

$$SpO_2 = \frac{HbO_2}{HbO_2 + Hb} \times 100$$

where SpO_2 is the saturation of hemoglobin with oxygen as measured by pulse oximetry, HbO_2 is the oxyhemoglobin concentration of blood, and $HBO_2 + Hb$ is the total hemoglobin concentration of blood. Mathematically, the determination of *fractional* saturation is represented by the following equation:

$$SpO_2 = \frac{HbO_2}{HbO_2 + DeoxyHb + CarboxyHb + MetHb} \times 100$$

Based on the oxyhemoglobin dissociation curve, an SpO_2 of 90% reliably corresponds to an arterial or partial pressure of oxygen (PaO_2) of 60 torr (or mmHg); and an SpO_2 of 75% corresponds to a PaO_2 of 40 torr. The SpO_2 as displayed by most pulse oximeters in clinical use can be expected to be within 2% of the value for oxyhemoglobin concentration of blood determined using a co-oximeter. Therefore, there is an approximately 2% error associated with pulse oximetry measurements. Anemia, as long as the hematocrit is above 15%, does not interfere with the accuracy of pulse oximetry. Clinically detectable cyanosis generally occurs at an SpO_2 of 80%, which correlates with a deoxyhemoglobin concentration of 5 g-%. However, the reliability of most pulse oximeters in clinical use deteriorates very rapidly when the saturation value is < 75%. Therefore, there is very little physiologic meaning attached to clinical documentation of saturations significantly below 75%.

SpO_2 values that are obtained in the absence of a plethysmographic waveform are unreliable – the heart rate by the oximeter must correlate with the heart rate as displayed by the ECG. Therefore, the use of pulse oximetry is limited in patients with severe peripheral vasoconstriction, since there is frequently inadequate peripheral perfusion to obtain a reliable plethysmographic waveform. In the setting of profound peripheral vasoconstriction, alternative sites for measurement of pulse oximetry are available such as the earlobe, tongue, or cheek. Additionally, warming the extremity is frequently effective. Pulse oximeters are also prone to failure under some ambient light conditions as well as in the presence of certain colors of fingernail polish (e.g., dark blue). Finally, pulse oximeters may be unreliable during periods of tachycardia and other arrhythmias. New technology, by Masimo[R] for example, allows computer-assisted extraction of pulse oximeter signals from ambient noise and increases reliability and accuracy.

Since carboxyhemoglobin and oxyhemoglobin both absorb light at identical frequencies, 660 nm, pulse oximeters that compare only two wavelengths of light will provide falsely high readings of SpO_2 in patients with carbon monoxide poisoning. In these cases, a co-oximeter is necessary to determine SpO_2 accurately (Figure 3-1). On the other hand, met-hemoglobin absorbs light and red and infrared wavelengths with the same absorption coefficient; this results in a 1:1 absorption ratio which then corresponds to an SpO_2 reading of 85%. Met-hemoglobinemia causes falsely low saturations when the actual arterial saturation is >85% and causes falsely elevated SpO_2 readings when the actual arterial saturation is <85%. Met-hemoglobinemia occurs in patients with severe septic shock due to increased nitric oxide production and it is also common following excessive topical administration of benzocaine spray.

The use of pulse oximetry to determine the saturation of mixed venous blood return from the brain, known as jugular venous bulb oximetry, is used as an indicator of global oxygen kinetics in the brain. A fiber-optic catheter containing fiber-optic sensors is passed retrograde via the jugular vein to the point of the jugular venous bulb where it continuously measures the saturation of ambient blood. When the saturation of blood falls, there is increased oxygen utilization in the brain and the data can be used to estimate the cerebral oxygen extraction ratio. This technology is commonly employed in neurosurgical and trauma ICUs to guide therapy.

CAPNOGRAPHY

Capnography and capnometry refer to the monitoring of CO_2 concentration in exhaled gases. Capnometry refers to the determination of a simple numerical value for CO_2 concentration in expired gas. Capnography provides exhaled CO_2 concentrations as a continuous waveform display in addition to a numerical value for end-tidal CO_2 ($ETCO_2$) concentration. Reliable CO_2 determination in exhaled gas generally requires a closed ventilator circuit. However, the use of capnography as a general monitor of respiration, e.g., during sedation when a patient is receiving oxygen by nasal cannulae, is widely accepted and encouraged as long as the associated limitations are understood. The concentration of CO_2 in exhaled gas is measured using either an infrared analyzer or by mass spectrometry. The infrared analyzer determines CO_2 concentration using infrared light absorption and is more readily available, less costly, and allows for real-time sampling. The mass spectrometer is more complex and costly, is not portable, but is more accurate. Since capnography provides significantly more information, it has displaced capnometry as a standard for CO_2 monitoring. Capnography thus allows for (1) real-time assessment of the adequacy of alveolar ventilation, (2) an indirect assessment of pulmonary perfusion, (3) early detection of ventilator malfunction or systems disconnections, and (4) waveform analysis that correlates with conditions such as bronchospasm. CO_2 detection in expired gases is essential to document correct endotracheal tube placement following endotracheal intubation. Ordinarily, single-breath detection devices are used for this purpose; however, under some circumstances (such as ambient air insufflation into the stomach, or recent consumption of carbonated beverages) single-breath detection is misleading. Note that while continuous capnography can reliably detect esophageal intubation or verify airway intubation, it cannot detect endobronchial intubation.

The early return of CO_2 in expired gases during resuscitation from cardiac arrest correlates with outcome. Additionally, patients who are receiving sedation without a secure airway may become apneic for prolonged periods of time during which pulse oximetry values do not show hypoxemia; therefore, exhaled CO_2 monitoring should be considered in all patients prone to apnea. When $ETCO_2$ values are used in conjunction with arterial $PaCO_2$ estimation of the deadspace ventilation fraction is also possible. The deadspace to tidal volume ratio can be calculated from the Bohr equation:

$$\frac{V_D}{V_T} + \frac{PaCO_2 - P_ECO_2}{PaCO_2}$$

where $PaCO_2$ is the partial pressure of CO_2 in arterial blood and P_ECO_2 is the partial pressure of CO_2 in expired gas.

Note that $ETCO_2$ is not in itself an accurate indicator of $PaCO_2$. However, once an individual patient's $ETCO_2$ to $PaCO_2$ has been determined, under relatively stable physiologic conditions, the relationship should be relatively constant and therefore $ETCO_2$ can be used as a substitute for arterial blood gas monitoring to assess the adequacy of ventilation. In most patients the normal arterial-$ETCO_2$ gradient is 2–5 torr.

NONINVASIVE BLOOD PRESSURE MONITORING

Arterial blood pressure can be measured using auscultation (the Riva-Rocci method) whereby a compressed artery is auscultated using a stethoscope and the turbulent flow within the blood vessel walls causes characteristic Korotkoff sounds. Korotkoff sounds cannot be heard during the range of cuff deflation between systolic and diastolic pressures; this is known as the "auscultatory gap." Typically, a sphygmomanometer is used to inflate a cuff to a set pressure and then slowly deflate the cuff while ausculating for Korotkoff sounds. Visual–auscultatory correlation of the sounds with the pressure in the cuff (manometry) allows bedside determination of systolic and diastolic pressures. Although auscultated blood pressure measure is now relatively seldom used, it plays a very important role in the rapid verification of blood pressures when automated methods fail.

Noninvasive blood pressure (NIBP) measurements are more typically obtained using automated cuffs which rely on the oscillometric technique. The DINAMAP (*d*evice for *i*ndirect *n*oninvasive *a*utomatic *me*an *a*rterial blood *p*ressure) is the most commonly used NIBP system. The oscillometric technique for determining blood pressure either uses two cuffs placed in series, one includes the artery proximally, while the other detects the onset of pulsations; or, as in the DINAMAP system, a single cuff is alternately rapidly inflated and deflated. Oscillometry actually measures mean arterial pressure, MAP, which corresponds to the point of maximal cuff deflation. Despite its common usage, noninvasive oscillometric blood pressure measurements are relatively inaccurate measures of diastolic blood pressure. Also, oscillometric blood pressure measurement is very difficult to use in patients with arrhythmias or severe bradycardia. Furthermore, blood pressure measurements which rely on cuff bladders are subject to error based on relative cuff-arm sizing, the conical anatomy of obese extremities, and alterations in the blood volume of the ipsilateral extremity induced by repeated cuff inflation. Generally, a cuff that is 20% wider than the diameter of the limb must be used to obtain reliable noninvasive cuff blood pressures, and this is not always feasible. Blood pressures measured by automated cuffs are most reliable with respect to systolic blood pressure and MAP, whereas invasively obtained blood pressures are more reliable with respect to MAP as well as the diastolic blood pressure.

Doppler measurements of blood pressure are usually obtained as an adjunct to sphygmomanometry during profound hypotension or to auscultate specifically flow properties within an artery. The Doppler principle creates a sound wave by applying electrical potential to a crystal. When the sound wave passes through tissue and encounters a moving object, such as blood, the frequency of the reflected sound is altered in a manner proportionate to the velocity of the reflecting material. Therefore, "hissing" arterial pressures can be easily differentiated from venous "hums." Additionally, amplification of the Doppler signal allows the determination of flow which cannot be otherwise auscultated during periods of hypotension.

GENERAL PROCEDURAL PRINCIPLES

Each year in the USA more than 150 million intravascular devices such as peripheral venous catheters, arterial catheters, dialysis catheters, and central venous catheters (CVCs) are inserted. Of these, more than 5 million are CVCs. Therefore, these statistics underscore the dependence of modern inpatient medical care on intravenous access.

Credentialing

Procedural credentialing is generally accepted to be specialty- as well as institution-specific. Providers who are not credentialed to perform a procedure independently must be supervised. The level of supervision of non-credentialed providers that is typically required is "immediately available," a legal term which is commonly interpreted to mean that the supervisor is gowned, gloved, and ready to assume redirection or the full completion of the procedure at an instant's notice. The supervising or teaching physician assumes full responsibility for all and any complications. There is a presumption that providers credentialed to perform independently a procedure be able to recognize and treat or obtain immediate back-up in treating the more common complications associated with the procedure.

Justification

No critically ill patient should be without secure and functional intravenous access. Intravenous access is required for the therapeutic administration of medications, fluids, blood or blood products, and for diagnostic monitoring. On the other hand, arterial blood pressure monitoring is indicated for specific reasons in unstable patients. Every invasive procedure has an associated risk–benefit analysis associated with its use. Therefore, justification requires that the potential benefit to the patient be weighed against the short- and long-term risks to the patient. Risk–benefit analysis is not the same as cost–benefit analysis which has no role in emergency procedural justification. The justification or indication for a given intervention or procedure should be documented in the patient chart together with the procedural consent.

Preparation

Prior to considering any elective invasive procedure, the provider must be intimately acquainted with the patient's anatomy and physiology. Anatomic considerations include any lesions at or near the proposed operative site, prior surgery, or positioning contraindications. For example, CVCs should not be placed near sites of active infection, adjacent to arterial reconstructions, or near prior hardware placement. Physiologic considerations might include pre-existing coagulopathy, or cardiac conduction abnormalities such as a left bundle branch block (LBBB). Where there is a pre-existing coagulopathy, such as in the setting of active anticoagulant therapy, liver disease, uremia, or thrombocytopenia, vessels that can easily be compressed with external pressure (internal jugular, femoral) should be chosen for access over those that cannot be externally controlled if a hemorrhage occurs (subclavian). Additionally, since irritation of the right heart by catheter, or by the guide wire during placement, can precipitate right-sided conduction abnormalities and complete heart block or asystole, temporary pacing may be required in patients with LBBB.

Informed Consent

Patients and/or their surrogate decision-makers have the right to consent to or refuse treatment. Treatment without consent may represent assault and/or battery. Informed consent has two components: first, an explanation of the risks, benefits, and alternatives to the proposed procedures; and second, clear acceptance or denial of permission by a decision-maker after careful consideration. Patients who have received psychoactive medications, have an organic brain syndrome, or are confused due to their underlying disease cannot give their valid informed consent and they are considered to lack capacity. In such situations the healthcare proxy or surrogate decision-maker must give their consent on behalf of the patient, expressing the patient's wishes as they understand them to be. Even so, medical providers must be careful to avoid the use of jargon and technical language that may not be clearly understood during the consent process; a clear concise presentation decreases the possibility of misunderstanding and confusion. Consent must always be documented in writing. The documentation of consent may be limited to a brief note in the patient chart relating the informed consent discussions, the issues considered, and the outcome or decision and plan. However, a simple signed standard consent form placed within the body of the chart is traditionally acceptable, but less adequate. Frequently, during the care of unstable patients in the ICU, time pressures in the setting of life-threatening illness, non-communicative patients, or unavailability of proxy decision-makers, limit practitioners' ability to obtain informed consent and 'implied consent' may temporarily suffice. In such instances, the inability to obtain consent should be documented. In some instances, consent may be obtained by telephone, these versions of verbal consents should always be verified and witnessed, and similarly documented in the record.

Analgesia and Sedation

Patient comfort during procedures is important for both humanistic as well as practical purposes. A history of allergies or reactions should be determined prior to administering any medication. Local anesthesia or systemic analgesia and/or anxiolysis may be appropriate. When local anesthesia is used it may be used copiously as long as it does not distort the surrounding anatomy. Note that 10 cm^3 of 2% plain lidocaine that is inadvertently administered intravenously will have minimal cardiovascular effects under normal circumstances. Infiltration with local anesthesia must involve both superficial and deep structures; however, the majority of pain receptors will be in the subcutaneous tissues. Lidocaine 1–2% is typically used for infiltration. In some instances epinephrine in a concentration of 1:100,000 or 1:200,000 may be used to decrease cutaneous bleeding. However, local anesthetics containing epinephrine must never be injected in the proximity of arteries, especially end-arteries, because of the risk of vasospasm and distal ischemia. Therefore, providers must personally verify that the local anesthetic used for radial arterial line placement does not contain epinephrine.

In critically ill patients sedation needs to be considered carefully; in particular, bolus dosing of sedatives can precipitate hemodynamic compromise because all sedatives decrease autonomic tone. Bolus doses are more likely than infusions to result in high plasma concentrations and resulting side effects. In those patients who are maintaining cardiovascular homeostasis through an endogenous catecholamine release, even small doses of systemic sedation may acutely cause significant cardiovascular depression. Procedural sedation with fentanyl alone or small doses of intravenous etomidate are likely to provide the most sedation with the least hemodynamic compromise. Dexmetomidine provides hypnosis and analgesia but does not suppress respirations and only minimally alters cardiovascular status and is an excellent alternative. Patient immobility during delicate procedures is important for technical efficiency as well as for patient safety.

Sterile Technique

Sterile technique is fundamental to procedural medicine. The components of sterile technique are handwashing, sterile attire (gowns, gloves, mask, hat), sterile field containment, and recognition of breaches in sterile technique. The importance of handwashing in the ICU cannot be over-emphasized. The cost of using sterile technique is minimal compared to the cost of iatrogenic infection. In the ICU all invasive procedures should be performed using sterile technique, as opposed to simpler aseptic techniques, because of the propensity of ICUs to harbor ubiquitous pathogenic organisms. In most instances a breach in sterile technique is easier to correct by re-gloving, for example, than to have to address an infectious complication later.

Procedural Positioning

Central veins must be cannulated with the patient in at least 15 degree Trendelenburg (head-down) position because when veins are open to air above the level of the phlebostatic axis (the level of the right atrium) there is an increased risk for venous air entrainment and venous air embolism (VAE). The Trendelenburg position during CVC placement both decreases the incidence of VAE and also facilitates line placement because of venous engorgement.

The risk of VAE is especially great in those patients who are hypovolemic, breathing spontaneously, and generating significant intrathoracic pressure, or when large-bore catheters are used. When the intrathoracic pressure is negative relative to atmospheric pressure and the catheter is open, air can be entrained at the rate of 100 cm^3 per second and is capable of producing a fatal air embolus within one second in an adult. The air that enters the central venous system will pass through the right heart and cause an acute right ventricular outflow tract obstruction. Smaller amounts of air may pass through a patent foramen ovale, and precipitate a stroke in patients with this abnormality. The Trendelenburg position is also indicated for every removal of indwelling vascular catheters for the same reasons; central catheters must never be removed while the patient is in the upright or sitting position.

Infectious Complications

Implanted foreign bodies are especially predisposed to bacterial infection. More than 200,000 nosocomial bloodstream infections occur each year in the USA, with most of these being related to intravascular access devices. The case-fatality rate of catheter-related sepsis ranges from 14 to 19%. The mortality rate for *Streptococcus aureus*-related sepsis alone is 8.2%. Infected foreign bodies cannot be sterilized and must be removed. Indwelling vascular cannulae have been shown to develop a thin biofilm coating shortly after intravascular insertion. The biofilm is composed of thrombin and fibrin which serves as a nidus for microthrombus formation and clot propagation, as well as for bacterial colonization. Therefore, increasingly, catheters are impregnated with heparin, antibiotics, or both to decrease the microfilm coating and minimize the possibility of catheter colonization or infection.

Catheters may be infected hematogenously during septicemia or episodes of bacteremia. Typically, following hematogenous colonization or infection, bacterial cultures reveal enteric organisms such as enterococcus or Enterobacter; pulmonary organisms such as Pseudomonas, *S. pneumoniae*, or Haemophilus; or genitourinary organisms such as *E. coli* or Proteus. Fungal catheter colonization is increasingly common in ICU patients but very difficult to detect on routine blood and catheter cultures.

Most catheters are infected by cutaneous organisms which translocate through the catheter insertion tract. These organisms, such as *S. epidermidis* and *S. aureus* are the most common organisms isolated from catheter tip cultures. Catheters intended for long-term use are usually tunneled subcutaneously prior to intravenous insertion, a technique that decreases the incidence of infection from cutaneous sources.

The *gut motor hypothesis* proposes that bacterial translocation occurs across the intestinal mucosal barrier during periods of splanchnic hypoperfusion, as occurs during shock. Bacteria have been identified in the submucosal lymphatics and venous plexus of patients with splanchic ischemia. In addition to being a potential secondary source for systemic inflammation, re-initiation, or propagation (the *second hit hypothesis*), the gut is a potential source of enteric organisms and sepsis.

The rate of catheter infection increases at 1–2% per day after the first 72 hours. The number of manipulations of the closed infusion-catheter system may be a more important determinant of infection than the duration of catheterization. Erythema or exudate at the insertion site requires immediate line removal. Signs of vasculitis are even more ominous. Patients who are immune-compromised such as those with hematologic malignancies, malnutrition, or diabetes are especially vulnerable to iatrogenic line infections. Indwelling catheters must be monitored daily for evidence of infection.

Additionally, the placement of indwelling catheters should be minimized in patients with prostheses such as cardiac valves or orthopedic hardware. Routine catheter changes are not recommended since the incremental risk of infection from breaches of sterile technique during insertion may equal or surpass the risk of infection from an already indwelling catheter. Femoral venous central lines should be avoided in trauma patients because of the high risk of distal venous thrombosis. Additionally, whenever possible, total parenteral nutrition should not be infused through femoral venous catheters because of the significantly increased incidence of line infection.

Differentiation between catheter tip infection and catheter tip colonization is important for optimal antibiotic management. Catheter-related sepsis is diagnosed when the same organism is simultaneously isolated from the tip of the catheter and from blood cultures. Catheter colonization occurs when organisms are isolated from the catheter only. Both the diagnosis and optimal treatment of catheter sepsis are controversial and antibiotic therapy is based on local antibiograms and local epidemiologic data.

Semiquantitative cultures of catheter tips provide a guide to differentiating between catheter sepsis and catheter colonization, the latter requiring therapy less intensely and less often. Catheter infection is confirmed when there are greater than 15 colony-forming units (cfu) in semiquantitative culture analysis or more then 100 cfu/ml in quantitative culture analysis from catheter tips (Table 3-1).

Where the catheter is either infected or colonized, in the absence of catheter-related sepsis, a simple catheter change over a guide wire is appropriate unless there is otherwise evidence of infection at the insertion site. However, whenever possible, catheter change over guide wires in the setting of suspected catheter-related infection should be avoided. Other related infectious syndromes related to intravenous catheters include phlebitis and pocket infections (infected fluid in a subcutaneous pocket surrounding an implanted vascular device).

Table 3-1 Differentiating Between Catheter Sepsis and Catheter Infection

Blood Culture	Catheter Tip Colony Count	Interpretation
Positive	>15 cfu	Catheter sepsis
	<15 cfu	Catheter hematogenously seeded
Negative	>15 cfu	Catheter infection
	<15 cfu	Catheter position

Septic thrombosis refers to the development of an infected clot which may present as phlebitis, abscess, periodic drainage, or a pseudoaneurysm.

Each episode of catheter sepsis will typically increase the cost of a hospitalization by at least US$15,000–US$20,000 based on the additional hospital days, antibiotic therapy, and additional monitoring blood work. Where the catheter infection is due to especially dangerous organisms such as a resistant *S. aureus* or enterococcus, not only is the cost of hospitalization higher but the associated morbidity and mortality are also concomitantly significantly increased.

Wound and Dressing Care

Evidence demonstrates that wound and dressing care subsequent to procedures is a key element in the prevention of infectious complications. Pooled or dried blood on or around the catheter insertion site is an obvious nidus for bacterial colonization; dressings should not be applied over blood if it is at all possible. Intravenous catheters are at significantly higher risk of infection than are arterial catheters, possibly because the higher PaO_2 of arterial blood deters bacterial growth. The type of dressing used and the frequency with which it is changed is also related to the infection rate. The use of bacteriocidal creams and ointments over the insertion site is no longer favored because these preparations can macerate the skin and increase the risk of local infection.

Latex Allergy

The ubiquitous use of latex gloves over the past 20–30 years has resulted in increased prevalence of sensitization to latex in both patients and healthcare providers. In the general population the incidence of latex allergy is estimated to be approximately 1%, and in healthcare providers it is thought to be at least 10%; however, in patients who are chronically institutionalized the incidence can range from 28 to 67%. Inhalation of latex particles within the cornstarch dust that coats many latex gloves is the most common and significant route of exposure.

Percutaneous exposure to latex is unlikely to trigger a systemic anaphylactic reaction, but such an adverse reaction should be recognized and treated immediately. Therefore, a high index of suspicion is important. In patients with a history of latex allergy or where there is a high probability of prior subsidization, alternatives to latex barriers and tourniquets should be used. The treatment of any allergic reaction includes rapid initiation of intravascular volume resuscitation, airway support, epinephrine, inhaled bronchodilators, systemic steroids, an intravenous antihistamine such as diphenhydramine, and an H-2 antagonist such as ranitidine.

Needlestick Injuries

Barriers such as gloves, masks, eye shields, and gowns that are used during "sterile technique" also protect the operator from percutaneous exposure to body fluids. However, obviously sharp objects will penetrate most of these barriers, and, since vascular access cannot presently be performed without sharp cannulae, providers must use special precautions in the use and disposal of sharp objects. At least 20 different pathogens have been conclusively shown to be transmitted by needlestick injuries. These include HIV, human T cell lymphotropic virus (HTLV), hepatitis, Creutzfeldt–Jakob, and cytomegalovirus (CMV). The risk of transmission of HIV infection is estimated to be approximately 0.4% per single percutaneous exposure to body fluids from an HIV-infected patient. However, it is unethical for healthcare providers to decline to perform necessary procedures on patients infected with HIV or hepatitis.

The provider who is performing the procedure is responsible for the proper disposal of all contaminated objects. The premise behind the use of "universal precautions" is that any patient may be an unrecognized carrier of latent infection. Although the risk of transmission of blood-borne pathogens through percutaneous exposure or by needlestick injury is relatively low, the implications for healthcare workers are potentially devastating. Inadvertent needlestick injuries are thought to occur in as many as 80% of cases of inexperienced practitioners performing invasive procedures. However, it is estimated that less than 25% of injuries are documented. Documentation of inadvertent exposure to infectious agents is important for the management of occupational health risks, early initiation of appropriate treatment, and support for future disability. The CDC has guidelines regarding testing and prophylaxis following inadvertent needlestick injury. Hospital policies should also be consulted and followed.

Radiologic Verification

Vascular catheters are typically constructed of polymers such as polyurethane, polytetrafluoroethylene (Teflon), polyethylene, or siliconized polypropylene. Most catheters in common use are made radio-opaque by impregnation with barium or tungsten salts to facilitate their intravascular localization by radiography. Typically, radiographic confirmation is used to verify the positioning of centrally placed venous catheters, endotracheal tubes, and feeding and nasogastric tubes.

Although the radiation exposure from portable x-ray machines is greater than that of fixed x-ray machines, the beam is less concentrated, there is significantly greater scatter of radiation, and therefore the total or focused exposure may be less significant. The scatter of radiation from portable x-ray machines increases exponentially at distances of greater than 6 ft from the source. However, radiographs are routinely performed in ICUs and therefore providers receive potentially higher levels of cumulative exposure than staff outside the ICU. When indicated, maintaining a safe distance, lead shielding, or dosimeter monitoring may be considered. When there is a possibility of pregnancy in either the patient or the provider, appropriate lead shielding is encouraged.

Malposition of CVCs occurs in as many as 15% of cases, even when inserted by experienced clinicians. Therefore, a chest radiograph is indicated to check for catheter positioning as well as to rule out complications. Catheters placed via the internal jugular (IJ) approach are statistically less likely to be malpositioned than those placed by the subclavian route. Examples of malpositioned CVCs are those that are placed arterially or subcutaneously, within the cardiac chambers, or subclavian lines that inadvertently pass retrograde into the internal jugular vein.

ICU radiographs for central line placement are usually AP films. Since upright expiratory films decrease relative lung volume, they are most useful to exclude a small pneumothorax. Pneumothorax is air within the pleural space. A pneumothorax is not always located at the lung apex and this is especially true when supine chest x-rays are used. A pneumothorax may not be immediately evident following pleural injury and may take 24–48 hours to become sufficiently large as to be clearly visualized. The size of a pneumothorax will develop much more rapidly when pleural injury occurs in patients receiving positive pressure ventilation. When there are clinical signs of a significant pneumothorax, or tension pneumothorax, occurring in the setting of clinical index of suspicion, the diagnosis should never await chest x-ray confirmation prior to treatment. The emergency treatment for tension pneumothorax is the insertion of a large-bore catheter, such as a 16- or 14-gauge IV, into the second intercostal space, above the rib, in the anterior midclavicular line. Thereafter, following evacuation of the tension, a tube thoracostomy can be placed semi-electively.

The CVC tip should lie within the superior vena cava. When the catheter tip is in a subclavian vein, the risk of thrombus formation or vessel occlusion is increased.

Furthermore, when the catheter tip is within the right atrium, or within the cardiac silhouette on the chest radiograph, there is increased risk of right atrial perforation and cardiac tamponade and arrhythmias. In some instances, usually following left subclavian catheterization, a catheter tip will be seen to abut the wall of the superior vena cava. A catheter tip left in this position can erode and perforate the vena cava causing death by acute hemothorax.

Catheters and Thrombosis

Stasis predisposes to coagulation. By definition, the blood flow in cannulated vessels is diminished because of the decreased effective luminal size. Therefore, intravascular catheters must be flushed regularly with sterile fluids or anticoagulant solution to maintain catheter and luminal patency. Typically, pressure transducers infuse a flushing solution at the rate of 3 cm^3/hour. Although dilute heparin (100 units/ml) has been used ubiquitously to prevent the clotting of catheters, frequent or repeated exposure to heparin may precipitate heparin-induced thrombocytopenia (HIT), or heparin-associated thrombocytopenia (HAT), through platelet sensitization. HIT is a devastating complication and practitioners should have a high index of suspicion for HIT when the platelet count acutely drops following heparin exposure. Furthermore, the incidence of HIT in the general population is increasing rapidly as more patients are sensitized to heparin and are returning for repeat episodes of medical care.

An acceptable alternative to heparin is the use of sodium citrate in catheter flushes. Since citrate binds calcium, it prevents completion of the coagulation cascade. Sodium citrate is the anticoagulant used to prevent clotting of banked blood. The key advantage of sodium citrate is that it does not produce HIT. Furthermore, the negligible amount of citrate does not usually contribute to the development of metabolic alkalosis.

Patients with underlying malignancies tend to be hypercoagulable at baseline and therefore are at increased risk for catheter-related thrombosis. Thrombosis of the subclavian vein should be considered whenever there is unilateral upper extremity edema which may be related to an indwelling vascular catheter.

Polytetrafluoroethylene (Teflon) catheters are significantly less thrombogenic than are catheters made of polypropylene, polyvinyl chloride, or polyethylene. Therefore, the choice of catheter material may also influence complication rates.

ARTERIAL CANNULATION

Percutaneous arterial cannulation is most often performed for the purpose of continuous monitoring of blood pressure. Continuous beat-to-beat blood pressure monitoring is essential in patients with rapidly changing hemodynamic status and patients receiving rapidly acting cardiovascular agents. Under some circumstances, such as extreme obesity, arterial blood pressure monitoring may necessarily and appropriately take the place of non-invasive pressure monitoring. Arterial cannulation is also indicated when there is a need for frequent blood biochemical analyses, especially arterial blood gas analysis. It is generally accepted that if a patient will require more than six arterial punctures over their admission, convenience and safety favor an indwelling cannula.

The primary sites for arterial cannulation for blood pressure monitoring are the radial artery, the femoral artery, and the dorsalis pedis artery. However, the radial artery is the most common site for percutaneous arterial cannulation because it is superficial, technically easy to access, and is well collateralized. The ulnar artery is a dominant artery to the hand in up to 90% of patients. Under some circumstances the axillary artery may also be used as an alternative. However, the risk of thrombotic or air embolic stroke during flushing of the catheter is significantly greater with axillary artery lines because the tip of the cannula is very close to the carotid artery. End-arteries are never cannulated, since in the absence of collateral flow tissue distal to the end-artery will become ischemic. Surgical arterial cutdown should be used only in extreme circumstances because of the need for distal ligation and the high incidence of thrombosis and infection.

The Allen test is used to evaluate collateral flow to the hand when the radial artery is occluded; it is therefore a test for the patency of the ulnar artery. Under normal circumstances blanching following release of the ulnar artery during the Allen test should resolve in approximately 7–10 seconds. Although universally recommended, the Allen test does not have any proven validity.

Insertion technique is an important determination of complications. Typically, a 20-gauge catheter is inserted using the Seldinger technique under aseptic, and preferably sterile, conditions. Repeated attempts to cannulate the artery may cause vasospasm, laceration, or thrombosis and even permanent occlusion. Arterial occlusion has been documented in up to 25% of arterial cannulations and the occlusion may be permanent in up to 3% of these cases. Ischemic necrosis of the digits is extremely rare, but since the thumb is at risk, closed monitoring of distal perfusion is important. Therefore, arterial cannulation is not a benign procedure. Pre-existing arterial disease may be a risk factor for distal ischemia. Due to the right-handed dominance of the majority of patients, the left hand may be the preferred site for radial cannulation if the patient's "handedness" is unknown. It is estimated that the critical wrist circumference to safely accommodate a 20-gauge radial arterial catheter is 15 cm; smaller wrists require smaller catheters. Raynaud's disease is a special contraindication to instrumentation of distal arteries.

The dorsalis pedis artery is especially useful for monitoring when the upper extremities are inaccessible due to patient position, infection or burns, or trauma. The dorsalis pedis artery has a relatively higher incidence of thrombotic occlusion than does the radial artery. Additionally, the cannulation of arteries, the dorsalis pedis artery especially, should be carefully considered in patients with diabetes or severe peripheral vascular disease. Since the arterial branch points distal to a dorsalis pedis arterial cannula are inevitably close to the point of cannulation, systolic amplification of the arterial waveform is of more significant concern.

Inexperienced operators commonly find arterial cannulation challenging (Figure 3-2). The following technical considerations may be helpful: (1) the artery is generally very superficial and usually lies 0.5 cm or less from the skin; (2) the artery can be more easily pinned when the angle of approach is more acute, such as 45-60°; (3) at the point of entry into the lumen of the artery and the subsequent "flashback" of blood, usually only the steel tip of the cannula is within the artery, and premature withdrawal of the steel needle will result in a failed attempt because the plastic catheter cannot be forced through the relatively thick arterial wall; and (4) immediately following the "flashback" the angle of approach must be dropped to 30° or less so that the plastic catheter can enter the lumen without the steel needle passing through the posterior wall. Initial attempts at cannulation should be made distally, since iatrogenic vasospasm may preclude subsequent attempts more distally.

The reliability of the arterial blood pressure readings obtained via indwelling catheters depends on a large number of variables. Catheter "whip" will overestimate the systolic pressure. When blood flow velocity is relatively high, as in patients with low arterial compliance, reflected pressure waves return in diffuse with the systolic component of the next pressure waves. This produces an increase in the systolic pressure, catheter "whip," and a decrease in a diastolic pressure. Such systolic amplification is common in ICU patients. Over-damping and under-damping will alter the arterial waveform as well as provide erroneous blood pressure values. The transducer, which should be placed at the level of the phlebostatic axis, the right atrium, will erroneously provide higher blood pressure values if the transducer is placed too low, and it will provide erroneously low blood pressures if it is vertically higher than the patient. Since the numerical values obtained by transduction reflect pressure data that have been converted into electrical signals for monitoring, calibration prior to use is essential. The accuracy of pressures obtained via transducer systems also depends upon calibration

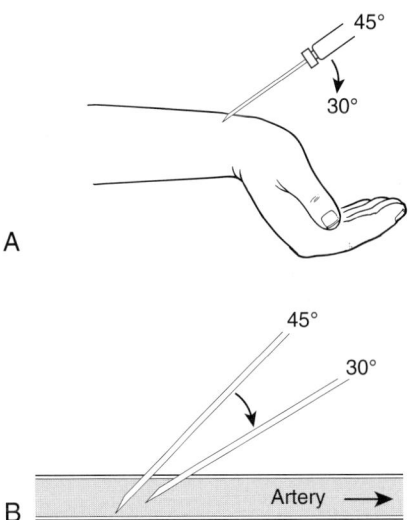

Figure 3-2 The technique of radial artery cannulation. (**A**) The wrist is dorsiflexed but not overly hyper-extended (which may compromise radial artery flow and increase the difficulty of cannulation). The initial angle of approach is 45°. Following "flashback" the angle is immediately dropped to 30° prior to advancing the catheter or the guide wire. (**B**) The steel cannula enters the thick wall of the artery before the plastic catheter does. Further advancement of the catheter at 45° will pierce the posterior wall of the artery. Advancement of the guide wire at 45° may be difficult and cause "kinking." When the catheter is dropped to 30° with gentle advancement so as to place the guide wire and the plastic catheter comfortably within the arterial lumen the technique is almost always successful.

and zeroing, and positioning with respect to the phlebostatic axis.

The shape of the arterial waveform can also provide clues regarding hemodynamic states. For example, the rate of upstroke may correlate with cardiac contractility; the rate of downstroke may correlate with peripheral vascular resistance; and exaggerated variations in waveform amplitude size with respirations may indicate hypovolemia.

As the arterial pressure waveform moves distally away from the aorta, the systolic pressure increases and the diastolic pressure decreases; the mean pressure remains relatively constant. Furthermore, amplification of the systolic pressure reading is common in patients with "stiff" arteries. Moreover, distortion of waveforms via under-damping of a resonant system can produce falsely elevated systolic blood pressure readings. Damping refers to the tendency of a waveform to die down.

MAP is directly related to the cardiac output (CO) and the total peripheral resistance: MAP = CO × TPR, where TPR or systemic resistance represents left ventricular afterload, mainly as reflected in arteriolar tone. Therefore, reliance on blood pressure alone is extremely dangerous when patients are clinically in shock (Figure 3-3). Notice that the MAP remains constant while the CO decreases and the TPR increases, or the MAP remains constant

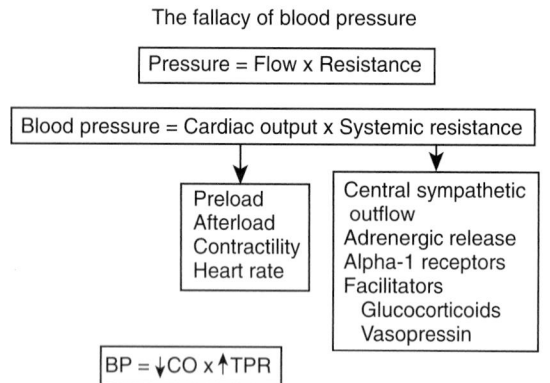

Figure 3-3 The fallacy of blood pressure. See text for details.

while the TPR drops and CO increases. In both the scenarios global tissue perfusion can be severely compromised in the face of a normal MAP.

The mean arterial blood pressure can be determined electronically by integrating the area under the arterial pressure waveform and dividing by the duration of the cardiac cycle; MAP can also be estimated as diastolic pressure is one-third of the pulse pressure. Mean arterial blood pressure is the driving pressure for peripheral blood flow and a key determinant of tissue perfusion (Box 3-1). The MAP represents the standing pressure in the arterial circuit, "averaging" the phasic nature of systolic and diastolic variations. Mathematically it is given by:

$$MAP = \frac{SBP + (2 \times DBP)}{3}$$

Pulse pressure is the difference between the systolic and diastolic pressures and reflects both cardiac stroke volume and vascular compliance. Pulse pressure narrowing, less than 30 torr, is associated with tachycardia, constrictive pericarditis, pleural effusions, and aortic stenosis. Widening of the pulse pressure is associated with aortic regurgitation, patent ductus arteriosus, arteriovenous shunting, coarctation of the aorta, and thyrotoxicosis.

Box 3-1 Examples Where MAP Reflects Driving Pressure for Perfusion

1. Cerebral Perfusion Pressure:
   CPP = MAP − ICP
   (ICP is the intracranial pressure)
2. Coronary Perfusion Pressure:
   CPP = MAP − LVEDP
   (LVEDP is the left ventricular end-diastolic pressure)
   MAP = mean arterial blood pressure.

Normally, there is little or no variation in the amplitude of arterial waves. However, respiratory variation, usually a decrease in the amplitude of arterial waves with inspiration (pulsus alternans), correlates well with hypovolemia.

When arterial catheters are flushed manually after sampling, heparinized fluid is infused into the artery under high pressure (250–300 torr). During flushing, the area supplied by the artery is frequently observed to blanch visibly. However, there is also retrograde flow of flush solution and with continued flushing, saline, air bubbles, and debris can be flushed into the central arterial circulation. This is an important consideration with axillary arterial catheters but can be significant even with radial or femoral arterial lines. Flushing of arterial catheters is an extremely important consideration in pediatric patients both with respect to flush volume as well as the possibility of cerebral embolization.

The presence of an indwelling arterial catheter is independently correlated with the frequency of blood work drawn from any one particular patient. Therefore, arterial catheters correlate with the cost of ICU care. Biochemical laboratory analyses are frequently most easily drawn from arterial catheters. Routine monitoring of blood chemistries may phlebotomize an adult ICU patient at the rate of one unit of packed red blood cells per week. Whenever possible adult ICU patients should have all their blood work drawn in pediatric tubes. Arterial cannulation should be avoided for blood sampling purposes alone and the use of venous blood gases coupled with pulse oximetry should be used to monitor oxygenation and ventilation status. Finally, arterial catheters must be clearly labeled to minimize the possibility that vasoconstrictive substances be inadvertently injected or infused.

CENTRAL VENOUS CANNULATION

Overview

CVCs are essential for the management of critically ill patients. A large variety of catheters are available for venous access and the choice of catheter must be based on its intended purpose. CVCs are used for the infusion of vasoactive substances, intravascular volume replacement, total parenteral nutrition (TPN), hemodialysis, and hemodynamic monitoring. CVCs are routinely placed in many clinical settings; however, they are probably more frequent in operating rooms and ICUs. Large-bore single-lumen catheters are best suited for rapid infusion of fluid, whereas multi-lumen catheters are important when multiple infusions of a potentially incompatible nature must be administered simultaneously. It is estimated that at least 8–12% of hospitalized patients receive percutaneous central venous cannulation.

Vasoactive drugs should always be infused via secure CVCs since inadvertent infiltration of vasoactive substances subcutaneously or into deep tissue spaces will cause vasospasm, severe tissue necrosis, and even loss of limb or limb function. The insertion of catheters into central veins, because of their larger size and more rapid vascular flow, is also indicated for the administration of hyperosmotic substances such as for chemotherapy or TPN. Hyperosmotic substances irritate small vessels and predispose to thrombophlebitis (venous inflammation) and phlebothrombosis (intravascular clotting).

Peripherally inserted central catheters (PICC lines) are increasingly used for intravenous access in hospitals. PICC lines are long catheters that are used for the basilic or cephalic vein at the antecubital fossa. Generally, the basilic vein (medial) is preferred because it follows a straighter course into the thorax and is less likely to have venous valvular obstruction (Figure 3-4). PICC lines have lower nosocomial infection rates than do other short-term CVCs. Therefore, PICC lines have important advantages in those instances where the need for central access is based on medication infusions, TPN, or even intravenous therapy in the home care setting. PICC lines do retain their favorable comparison to other CVCs with respect to the incidence of venous thrombosis. PICC lines are completely inadequate for monitoring or for acute intravascular volume expansion.

However, the maximum fluid infusion rate is determined by the size of the catheter and not by the size of the vein that is cannulated. For example, the maximum flow rate through a 9-French introducer sheath is approximately 247 cm³/minute, through 14-gauge peripheral IV the maximum flow rate is 195 cm³/minute, and through the 16-gauge port of a typical triple-lumen catheter the maximum flow rate is only 54 cm³/minute. In reality, the most important limitation of flow rate through a 9-French introducer is the diameter and length of the IV tubing and not the catheter itself. The Advanced Cardiac Life Support protocol of the American Heart Association advocates venous cannulation of the antecubital veins for cardiac resuscitation as the preferred IV access site.

The rate of flow through a cylinder such as a catheter or tube is described mathematically by the Poiseuille–Hagen formula which states that flow is directly proportional to the fourth power of the radius and inversely proportional to the length of the catheter and the viscosity of the fluid. This formula is expressed as:

$$Q = \frac{\pi r^4}{8\eta L}$$

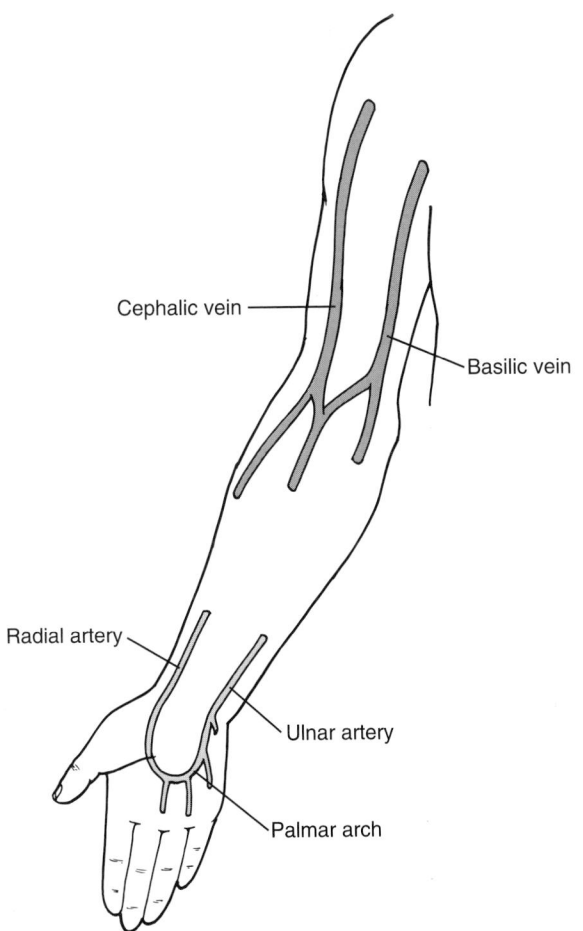

Figure 3-4 The vascular anatomy of the arm and forearm. The cephalic vein runs medial to the basilica vein in the arm. The radial and ulnar arteries together provide the blood supply to the hand via the palmar arches.

where Q is the rate of flow, r is the internal radius of the catheter, η is the viscosity of the fluid or gas flowing through the catheter or tube, and L is the catheter length. Therefore, for the purpose of rapid infusion of volume, because of length considerations, a short peripheral catheter is a better choice than an identical gauge longer centrally inserted catheter such as a PICC line. Alternatively, a large-bore CVC such as an 8.5 or 9 Fr percutaneous introducer sheath, which is both of short length and of large gauge, is the access of choice for rapid intravascular volume expansion. Furthermore, the relationship also makes it clear that viscous fluids such as packed red blood cells will infuse more rapidly if diluted with a crystalloid to decrease viscosity. Of note, packed red blood cells transfused through catheters of 20-gauge or smaller, especially when transfused under pressure, are extremely likely to hemolyze on infusion.

Additional considerations regarding catheter size are related to other specific indications for catheter placement. An introducer sheath is necessary for a pulmonary artery catheter placement, and a different type of introducer is required for passage of a temporary transvenous pacemaker wire. Hemodialysis catheters are typically large-bore catheters that have two ports to facilitate high-volume flow during hemodialysis.

Central venous lines directly administer fluid and medications to the right heart. Catheterization of the femoral vein is not technically *central* venous cannulation because it infuses fluid and medications into the inferior vena cava, which is far removed from the right heart. Additionally, femoral venous access during cardiac arrest and external thoracic compressions is notoriously ineffective for the delivery of vasoactive substances to the heart. Moreover, in trauma patients infusion of substances through a femoral venous catheter may be ineffective in the setting of inferior vena cava disruption or hepatic trauma. Finally, central venous pressure (CVP) cannot be reliably measured via a femoral venous catheter.

Cannulation of the external jugular (EJ) vein is not considered an appropriate approach for CVC placement in ICU patients because the vein is technically difficult to catheterize and therefore does not represent secure access, venous valves prevent successful catheter passage in most instances, and the catheter often does not pass into the thorax past the level of the clavicle. Venous valves are also prone to injury during EJ cannulation.

Catheters sizes are expressed in either gauge or French units which are measures of external diameter. The largest catheter diameters are those with the smallest gauge designation but with the largest French size. Mathematically, French size is defined as the outside catheter diameter in millimeters multiplied by three.

Central Venous Catheter Placement Procedure

CVCs are typically placed using the Seldinger technique, which refers to a "catheter-over-guide wire" method that is typical to vascular access and other invasive procedures. Typically, the guide wire has both a straight tip, and a flexible "J-wire" tip which is inserted intravascularly to prevent vascular injury.

Cannulation of the central circulation, which typically refers to the great veins within the thorax, is usually accomplished via the internal jugular (IJ) or subclavian vein (SV) approaches (Figure 3-5).

The IJ vein can be cannulated via at least three different approaches: (1) the anterior approach, anterior to the lateral belly of the sternocleidomastoid muscle (SCM); (2) the posterior approach, posterior to the lateral belly of the SCM; and (3) a supraclavicular approach at the midpoint of the anterior triangle immediately above the clavicle. The two heads of the SCM and the clavicle form the three sides of triangle which contains IJ vein, the carotid artery, and the vagus nerve. In almost any patient, except the extremely obese or edematous, the IJ vein can be located using a 25-gauge "finder" needle. The IJ runs deep to the lateral or posterior head of the SCM in a direction parallel to a line drawn between the mastoid process and the ipsilateral nipple when the neck is turned slightly (30°) to the opposite side. The large introducer needle should never be used for initial localization. If a paresthesia is obtained in an awake patient, the needle is injuring the cervical segment of the brachial plexus and needle location is too far posterior. The carotid artery runs close and medial to the IJ. Moreover, "cutting-tip" needles should never be repositioned subcutaneously because of the risk of lacerating vital structures; successive attempts requiring redirection of the needle tip must always be initiated *at the* level of the skin. Recently, the use of bedside ultrasound technology such as the Site-Rite^R can help better locate the IJ vein, decrease the incidence of pneumothorax and arterial puncture, and also improve patient comfort.

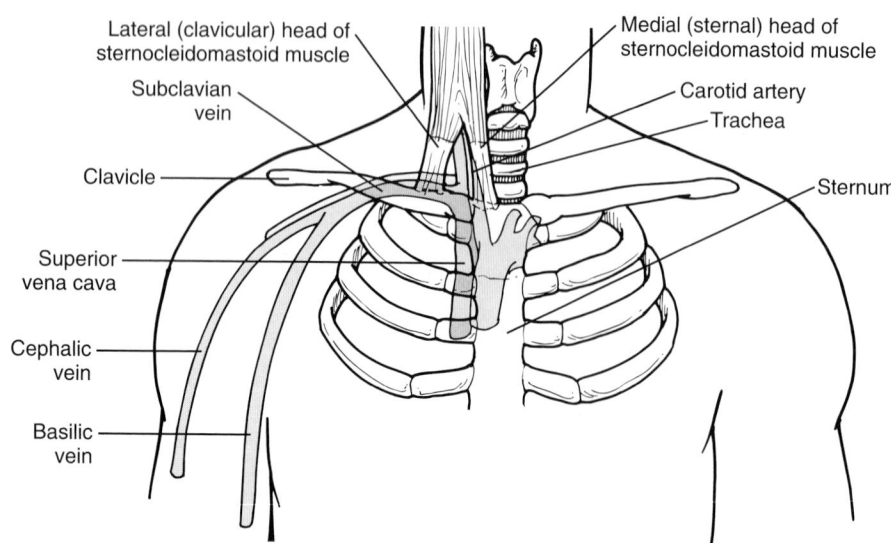

Lateral (clavicular) head of sternocleidomastoid muscle

Medial (sternal) head of sternocleidomastoid muscle

Subclavian vein

Carotid artery

Trachea

Clavicle

Sternum

Superior vena cava

Cephalic vein

Basilic vein

Figure 3-5 Approaches to central venous access: (1) the anterior approach to the IJ vein in the high to mid-anterior triangle of the neck; (2) the supraclavicular approach; (3) the common entry point into the subclavian vein; (4) the posterior approach to the IJ vein. See text for details. Note that the carotid artery runs medial to the IJ vein. Also note that the cupula of the lung extends approximately 2.5 cm above the clavicle into the neck.

However, such bedside ultrasound technology is rarely available in emergencies and therefore practitioners should be able to place reliably CVCs without the aid of such a device. When the possibility of a carotid arterial puncture is suspected, the needle or catheter should either be transduced, or blood should be drawn for a comparison in color to an arterial sample. Acute embolic cerebrovascular accidents (CVAs) have been reported with a single carotid puncture with a 25-gauge finder needle. Acute CVAs are rare, however, and every attempt must be made to ascertain venous location prior to passing subsequently the larger-bore catheters via the Seldinger technique. CVC kits usually contain both a soft plastic catheter and a larger steel needle, either of which can be used to pass the J-wire. The catheter may be more appropriate for the IJ approach, since it can be inserted with minimal trauma and is more easily secured prior to guide wire placement. On the other hand, the catheter will bend and kink under the clavicle and therefore only the steel needle should be used for the subclavian approach. Following insertion of the guide wire, with the J-tip leading, the introducer needle or catheter is withdrawn and a dilator is inserted. A scalpel is used to cut the skin at the insertion site and facilitate passage of the dilator and, ultimately, the catheter. The smaller the cut, the smaller the chance of lacerating the EJ vein, or cutting into the IJ vein. The scalpel tip should always be aimed laterally so that the chance of carotid puncture with the scalpel tip is minimized. If the dilator does not pass easily, it must not be forced since the possibility of lacerating a thin-walled vein exists. Thereafter, the CVC should be passed to an appropriate depth.

The SV is most often cannulated via an infraclavicular approach. Supraclavicular approaches are only more likely to cause a pneumothorax when attempted by inexperienced operators. The SV begins at the outer aspect of the first rib as a continuation of the axillary vein, passes anterior to the scalenus anterior muscle and its insertion point on the first rib, then passes caudally and anteriorly to join the IJ to form the brachial cephalic trunk. As the SV passes over the first rib, it is anterior to the subclavian artery and brachial plexus and only separated from them by the thin scalenus anterior muscle. In general, in order to access the SV, the insertion site should be at least 2 cm in and inferior to the clavicle in order to optimize the angle approach and minimize the possibility of passing inferior to the vein. A frequent choice for initial needle placement is at the level of the clavicular notch, the point at which the clavicle turns posteriorly. The clavicular notch lies at the junction of the outer one-third and the medial two-thirds of the clavicle. This point also generally coincides with the insertion point of the SCM on the clavicle. The direction in which the needle is pointed is directly toward the sternal notch. The left SV is anatomically preferable to the right SV for pulmonary artery catheter insertion because the acute angulation from the right subclavian vein makes PAC passage into the right atrium technically more difficult.

Typically, the CVC should be passed to a depth of 15-16 cm via the right IJ approach, 13-15 cm via the right subclavian approach, 15-16 cm via the left subclavian approach, and 16-17 cm via the left IJ approach. Radiographic verification is used to confirm proper catheter tip location and to exclude pneumothorax or hemothorax. Data suggest that the incidence of pneumothorax is not different between the IJ and subclavian approaches. The tip of the pleura, the cupula of the lung, extends approximately 2.5-3 cm above the clavicle into the anterior triangle. Therefore, lower approaches, especially when the needle is misdirected posteriorly, may puncture the pleura. However, inadvertent arterial cannulation is slightly more likely with the anterior IJ approach, because the carotid artery runs immediately medial to the IJ vein higher in the neck. The left-sided IJ approach carries an increased risk for thoracic duct injury, since the duct is anatomically located underneath the left IJ vein.

The femoral vein runs medial to the femoral artery within the femoral sheath. The femoral vein is a direct continuation of the popliteal vein and becomes the external iliac vein at the level of the inguinal ligament. The femoral vein is cannulated inferior to the inguinal ligament, and is usually located 1-2 cm medial to the palpated femoral artery pulsation.

Central Venous Pressure Monitoring

Vascular accesses are also used for monitoring purposes, and CVCs allow for the measurement of venous pressure within the thorax. Preload is defined by the volume of blood in the cardiac ventricle just prior to contraction and represents the sum of venous filling and residual volume following the previous contraction. CVP correlates with jugular venous distention and jugular venous pulsation on bedside clinical examination. The CVP, like the arterial waveform, must be measured at the level of the right atrium, or the phlebostatic axis. The phlebostatic axis is defined as the only point within the cardiovascular system where intravascular pressure reaches zero.

A typical CVP waveform consists of three positive deflections (*a*, *c*, *v* waves) and two descents (*x* and *y*) (Figure 3-6). The *a* wave represents the increasing venous pressure generated by each atrial contraction. The *c* wave is generated when the tricuspid valve is displaced into the right atrium during initial ventricular contraction. The *v* wave is produced by the increasing atrial pressure which occurs when venous return continues despite closure of the tricuspid valve. The *x* descent is the rapid decrease in CVP which corresponds to the period of

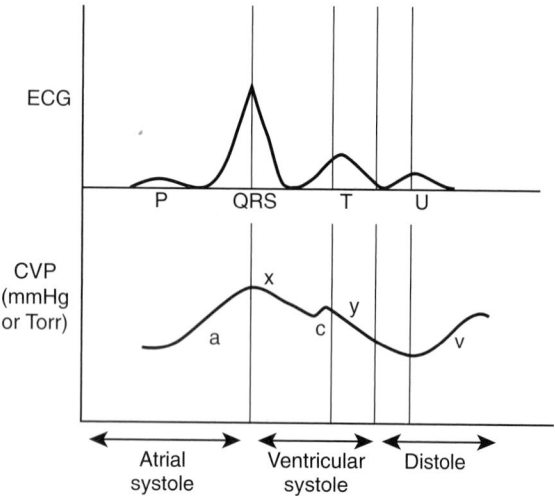

Figure 3-6 Correlation of CVP waveform monitoring with the electrocardiogram. See text for details.

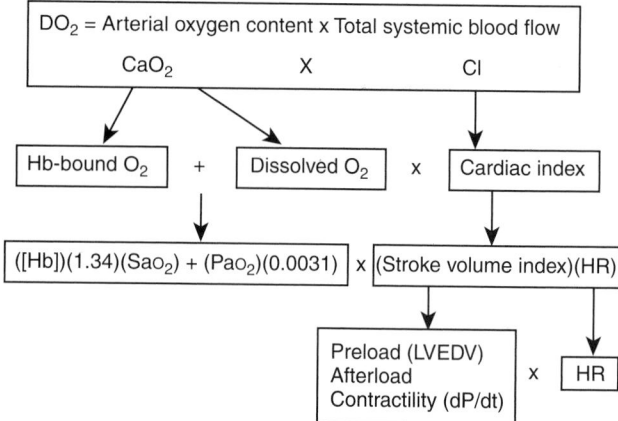

Figure 3-7 The determinants of oxygen delivery, DO_2.

ventricular ejection. The y descent occurs when the tricuspid valve opens at the end of ventricular contraction and blood again enters the ventricle. The importance of these waveforms is in their correlation with pathophysiologic processes. An absence of the a wave is characteristic of atrial fibrillation, where the x descent is also often absent. Amplified, or "cannon," a waves occur in the presence of mitral stenosis. Finally, both the x and y descents are frequently exaggerated in the presence of constrictive pericarditis whereas cardiac tamponade magnifies the x descent and abolishes the y descent.

PULMONARY ARTERY CATHETERIZATION

Shock is defined as a state of diminished tissue perfusion, where tissue blood flow is inadequate to meet the substrate (oxygen) needs of metabolizing tissues. *The longer a patient is in shock, the more likely it is that the patient will die.*

The importance of cardiac output determination in critically ill patients is reflected in the formula for oxygen delivery:

$$DO_2 = ([Hb] \times SpO_2 \times 1.34) \times (PaO_2 \times 0.0031) \times CI$$

In a simplified form, $DO_2 = CaO_2 \times CI$, the product of arterial oxygen content and cardiac output. From this formula it is clear that cardiac index and the hemoglobin concentration and saturation are the key determinants of global systemic oxygen delivery (Figure 3-7).

The determinants of cardiac output are preload, afterload, contractility, and heart rate. The ventricular function curve shows that cardiac performance increases almost linearly with increasing preload to a point, after which it levels off and may actually be impaired – a point of "fluid overload" (Figure 3-8).

Therefore, hypovolemic shock reflects a low cardiac output state which can be treated with intravascular volume expansion. Since oxygen delivery is most effectively improved by increasing cardiac output, clinical strategies to monitor and improve cardiac output must be implemented.

Therefore, hemodynamic monitoring is necessary to determine the pathophysiologic basis of the shock state. Hypovolemic shock is treated by improving venous return, CVP, pulmonary capillary wedge pressure (PCWP), and cardiac preload. Cardiogenic shock is treated by optimizing, often decreasing, cardiac preload to prevent ventricular overdistention and through the use of inotropic

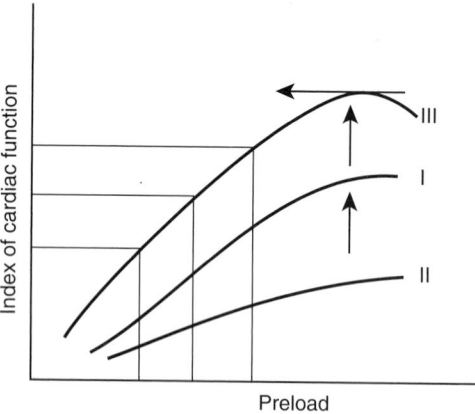

Figure 3-8 A "family" of left ventricular function curves. Cardiac function is dependent upon preload. Indices of cardiac function including cardiac output, ejection fraction, stroke volume, or left ventricular stroke work index. Indices of preload include CVP, PCWP, LVEDP, and LVEDV. Curve I represents a "normal" cardiac function curve whereby serial increases in preload generate progressive improvement in cardiac function to a point. Curve II represents cardiac failure. Curve III represents a hyperdynamic ventricle. In order to move from curve II to I to III, an inotrope can be administered. In order to move from left to right, from a point of relative excessive preload to a more "normal" ventricular filling pressure, a diuretic or vasodilator can be administered.

therapy to improve contractility. Where pharmacologic intervention does not improve cardiac output in cardiogenic shock, intra-aortic counter pulsation may be necessary. Obstructive shock, such as in cardiac tamponade, is treated by relieving the obstruction via pericardiocentesis, or surgical intervention, whereas pulmonary embolism requires thrombolytic therapy or urgent surgery (Trendelenburg procedure). Preload must be maintained at an elevated level during cardiac tamponade, whereas the load elevation is dangerous where there is embolic right ventricular outflow tract obstruction and in these cases inotropes are important adjunctive therapy to prevent acute right heart failure. Finally, distributive shock states, such as sepsis or anaphylaxis, respond well to fluid therapy, inotropic support, and etiology-specific adjunctive pharmacotherapy. Since the various shock states differ in terms of their effect on hemodynamic variables, cardiovascular monitoring is frequently necessary. The clinician's ability to utilize, understand, and act upon hemodynamic data is an important determinant of patient survival. Alternatively, ventricular function is correlated inversely with afterload and therefore afterload reduction in either the pulmonary or systemic circuits improves cardiac output (Figure 3-9).

Right heart catheterization using a pulmonary artery catheter (PAC or Swan-Ganz catheter) is used to guide volume resuscitation and vasoactive therapy in critically ill patients. The PAC is a long thin catheter, inserted via a larger bore central line, an "introducer," and is advanced through the central veins and the right cardiac chambers into the pulmonary outflow tract (Figure 3-10). Since the placement of the catheter is flow-directed, advancement of the catheter with each beat facilitates passage. Only rarely is fluoroscopic assistance necessary, but it should be considered if a recent transvenous pacer has been placed, if selective right or left pulmonary artery

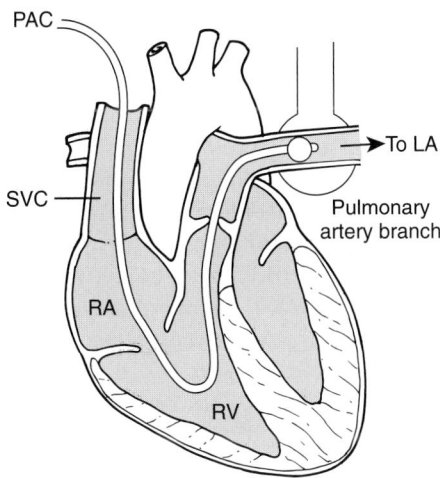

Figure 3-10 A schematic view of the anatomy of pulmonary catheterization.

catheterization is necessary, or unusual cardiac anatomy exists. If the catheter is advanced without a common evidence of waveform progression (Figure 3-11), then it should be suspected that the catheter is either coiling within the cardiac chambers or has passed into the inferior vena cava. When the catheter tip is in the distal pulmonary outflow tract, inflation of the balloon at the tip of the PAC occludes blood flow past the catheter tip. At this point the catheter tip is considered to be in the "wedged" position. "Pseudo-wedging" may occur if the catheter becomes entrapped underneath the pulmonary valve, trabeculae, or between pampering muscles. A pulmonary artery tip that is in a pseudo-wedged position reveals a flattened waveform, which appears almost identical to a catheter tip that is in a true "wedge" position. However, whereas a normal wedge tracing occurs after the tip of the catheter has passed through the pulmonary artery, a pseudo-wedge tracing is typically encountered out of sequence, often before the catheter tip has passed through the right ventricle and the pulmonary artery.

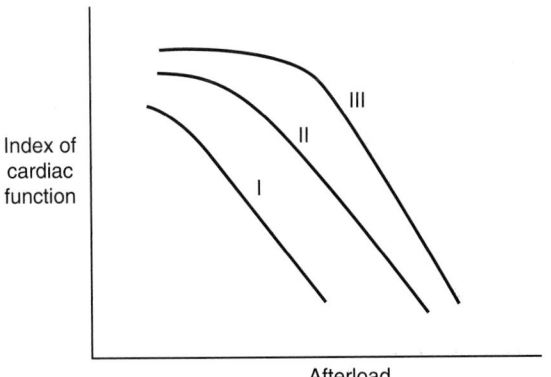

Figure 3-9 The relationship between cardiac function and afterload. Curve III represents a normal ventricular response to increasing afterload. Following an initial period of compensation, there is progressive decrease in left ventricular performance. Curve II represents a failing ventricle or it can also represent a normal right ventricular curve. Curve I represents a failed ventricle. Decreasing afterload improves cardiac performance.

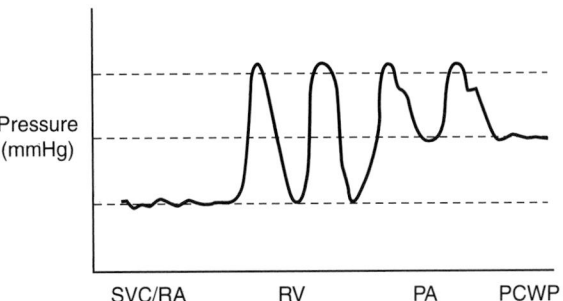

Figure 3-11 Sequential waveform changes during advancement of the pulmonary artery catheter from the superior vena cava (SVC) through the right atrium (RA), to the right ventricle (RV), into the pulmonary artery (PA), and finally into the "wedge position" (PCWP). Note that catheter migration from the RV into the PA is heralded by a change in diastolic pressure.

A pseudo-wedge tracing also resembles an "over-wedged" catheter tip with an elevated pressure reading. Since there is no blood flow past the tip of the PAC, the pressure transducer at the tip of the catheter distal to the balloon will transduce pressure from a theoretically static column of blood extending from that particular pulmonary arteriole through to the left atrium. During diastole, when the mitral valve is open, the pressure transduced by the PAC tip may approximate the left ventricular end-diastolic pressure (LVEDP). Therefore, the measured pressure is known as the pulmonary artery occlusion pressure (PAOP), or, more commonly, the PCWP.

The information obtained through the use of a PAC is complex and includes differential cardiac chamber pressure information, transduced waveforms, measures of cardiac output, and the oximetry-derived saturation of venous blood.

The PAC directly measures right heart pressures, thermodilution, right heart cardiac output, and mixed venous oxygen saturation. The utility of the PAC is that it allows for bedside construction of serial ventricular function ("Starling") curves. The ventricular function curve relates indices of cardiac function as dependent variables to indices of estimated preload.

Derived indices of cardiac function include CO, cardiac index (CI), stroke volume (SV), ejection fraction (EF), or ventricular stroke work index. Measured indices of estimated preload include CVP or PAOP or PCWP. The cardiac index is the cardiac output divided by the body surface area: $CI = CO/BSA$; the units are $l/minute/m^2$.

It is important to realize that in physiologic terms, preload is actually a volume, which causes stretching of cardiac sarcomeres to various points of contractility. More accurately, preload is a wall tension that results from the LVEDV, which causes myofibril stretch. Optimal pre-contraction sarcomere length is 2.2 times the resting sarcomere length. When the sarcomeres are stretched beyond 3.0 times their resting length, they are overstretched and cardiac contractility is impaired; this may account for the negative slope of the ventricular function curve during volume overload. However, it is very difficult to obtain clinically accurate bedside measurements of ventricular volumes. Therefore, pressures are measured and these pressures are used to estimate preload. Pressure and volume are related mathematically through compliance ($C = \Delta V/\Delta P$). Where preload acutely exceeds the ability of cardiac contractility to move the blood forward, the excessive preload precipitates signs and symptoms of heart failure. However, the causes of pulmonary edema are many. The CVP measures right-sided cardiac pressures, and the PCWP extrapolates LVEDP by measuring the back pressure at the point of right heart pulmonary capillaries via a catheter lodged in the right heart. Therefore, volume is estimated from pressure measurements without accounting for compliance. Furthermore, the assumption that the PCWP is directly related to LVEDP is flawed since pressures are measured across the pulmonary circuit, the left atrium, and the left ventricle.

$$CVP \propto RVEDP \propto PCWP \propto LAP \propto LVEDP \propto LVEDV$$

Contractility can be improved using inotropic agents. Examples of inotropic agents include β-1 agonists such as epinephrine, dopamine, or dobutamine; phosphodiesterase-III inhibitors such as milrinone; or more general inotropes such as digoxin or calcium. When contractility is improved, the cardiac function at any given level of preload is increased.

Tachycardia is often seen in hypovolemic states in physiologic effort to maintain cardiac output, a response mediated by endogenous catecholamine release. Also, β-1 agonists have chronotropic action in addition to their inotropic effects. Tachycardia may not be desirable because it increases myocardial oxygen demand and consumption and also may compromise cardiac output due to a rate-related impairment of diastolic ventricular filling. Patients with either fixed coronary obstruction or those with dynamic left ventricular outflow tract obstruction do not tolerate tachycardia well. Additionally, patients who are receiving beta-blocker therapy may not manifest a compensatory tachycardia in hypovolemic states; these patients will instead retain a controlled slower heart rate and the only sign of hypovolemia may be progressive hypotension.

Cardiac output was at one time determined using indicator dye methods (Fick principle) or manual thermodilution measurements using iced saline. Most catheters currently in use have instead a heater-coil which allows continuous automated cardiac output determination without the variability introduced by manual injections. The principle of thermodilution remains founded on a temperature gradient between the heater-coil and a more distally placed temperature sensor. The greater the cardiac output, the faster the blood flow around the catheter, and the less and more transient the change in blood temperature (Figure 3-12).

It is important to realize that the SVR is not measured but is calculated. Additionally, it is calculated using the cardiac output, to which the SVR is inversely related by the formula $SVR = [(MAP - CVP)/CO] \times 80$. The term "SVR" is frequently and erroneously used to refer to the total peripheral resistance (TPR) in the vascular circuit, which is related to a quantity different from the *calculated* SVR. Moreover, SVR does not in itself describe "afterload" which is a more specific term referring to the impedance to forward cardiac output.

Complications that are relatively unique to PAC use include catheter knotting and pulmonary artery rupture. The inadvertent knotting of a PAC occurs when the catheter does not pass easily through the cardiac

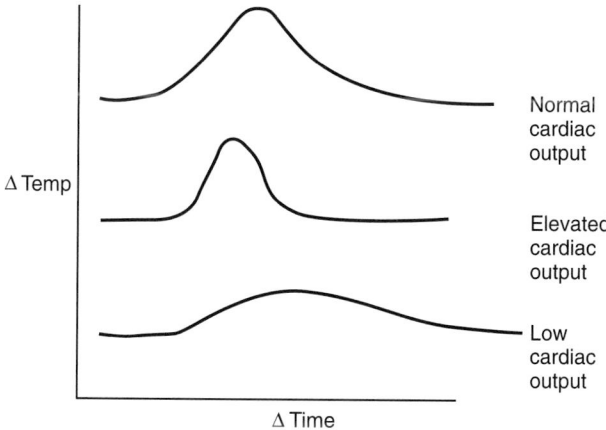

Figure 3-12 Thermodilution cardiac output. The rate of change in temperature as a function of time correlates mathematically with ambient blood flow and therefore cardiac output.

chambers and instead redundant catheter is entangled upon itself. Knotted catheters must be removed by invasive radiology techniques. Pulmonary artery rupture is probably the most feared complication of pulmonary artery catheterization and may result from either patient-specific pathology or operator error, or both. Pulmonary artery rupture has an overall incidence of less than 1% but is relatively more common in patients with pulmonary hypertension. Other factors associated with increased incidence of pulmonary artery rupture include age greater than 60 years, female gender, hypothermia, anticoagulation, catheter tip location >5 cm lateral to the mediastinum, frequent wedge pressure determinations, and mitral valve disease. Patients with pre-existing left bundle branch block may develop complete heart block as the catheter tip passes through the right ventricular wall and stimulates the right bundle branch system. In these cases, the immediate availability of transcutaneous pacing should be considered. However, most catheter-related arrhythmias are transient.

A PAC may, under normal circumstances, migrate distally into smaller pulmonary artery segments with continued normal pulmonary blood flow. When the balloon tips of these catheters are subsequently inflated, there is initially a typical "over-wedging" waveform indicative of excessive balloon pressures. If balloon inflation is inadvertently continued under these circumstances, iatrogenic rupture of the pulmonary artery is likely. Acute hemoptysis is the usual presenting sign of a pulmonary artery rupture. Generally accepted recommendations include leaving the catheter in place to tamponade bleeding, placing the patient with the affected side down, and emergent cardiothoracic consultation. Under usual circumstances, a pulmonary artery catheter will preferentially float into the right lung. Placement of a double-lumen endotracheal tube to allow for independent ventilation may also be necessary. Pulmonary infarction is also a frequently unrecognized

complication of PAC use whereby either an uninflated catheter tip migrates into a distal pulmonary artery and occludes blood flow or when the PAC is intermittently left inflated after determination of PCWP. Pulmonary infarction does not typically occur in the absence of lapses in appropriate patient monitoring. A PAC waveform that is persistently in wedge position should be a signal which triggers repositioning of the PAC, or simply deflation of the balloon, before a segment of lung becomes ischemic. Subsequent infarction of a watershed segment around the tip of a PAC may appear on subsequent chest radiography. Infarcted lung areas can later become hemorrhagic.

Ventilation–perfusion zones within the lung may be described in terms of West zones, which describe the relationship between alveolar pressure (P_A), pulmonary capillary pressure (P_C), and mean pulmonary artery pressure (Pa) (Figure 3-13). P_C resembles pulmonary venous pressure (Pv), which numerically approximates left atrial pressure P_{LA}. Due to gravitational effects, dependent lung zones receive better perfusion, whereas non-dependent lung zones receive less perfusion and relatively more ventilation. Thus, alveolar pressure (P_A) exceeds both capillary (P_C) and arteriolar (Pa) pressures in zone I, and pulmonary arteriolar pressure (Pa) exceeds alveolar pressure (P_A) and capillary pressure (P_C) in zone III. The influence of vascular pressure in dependent lung zones helps explain the development of pulmonary edema during failing contractility or acute hypervolemia. Since the pulmonary artery catheter is placed blindly, blood flow normally places the PAC tip in either zone II or, more likely, zone III of the lung. It is when the catheter tip is

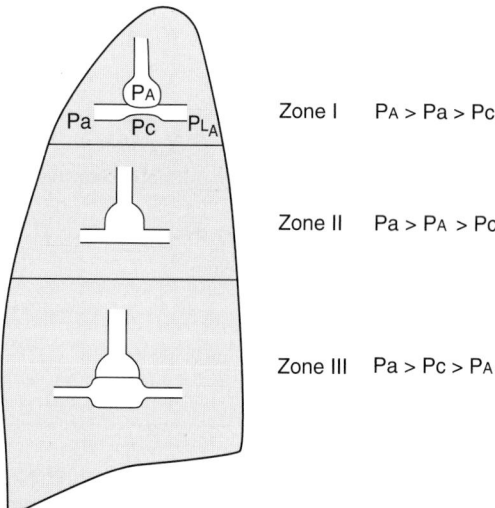

Figure 3-13 West zones of the lung. West zones depict relationships between ventilation and perfusion in different areas of the lung. Dependent lung zones receive more perfusion and non-dependent lung zones receive more ventilation. P_A, alveolar pressure; Pa, pulmonary arterial pressure; P_C, pulmonary capillary (or pulmonary venous) pressure.

within zone III that the reliability of the PCWP is greatest. Only in zone III is there a constant, uninterrupted column of blood between the catheter tip, through the pulmonary capillary circuit, through to the left heart. However, zone distributions change with patient positioning changes. Zone III is gravitationally defined so that it is in the dependent lung, for whatever position in which the patient is placed. Note that lung zones cannot be actually determined by chest radiography and catheter tip positioning is instead determined physiologically.

Zone I is especially vulnerable to high airway pressures. When positive end-expiratory pressure (PEEP) is applied then there is a greater likelihood that the PCWP will be falsely elevated by the airway pressures when the catheter tip is in zone I. Since many patients who have required PAC placement in the past have also required mechanical ventilation with higher airway pressure and PEEP, the PCWP may have inadvertently been misinterpreted. The relationship between PEEP and PCEP is not linear but can be estimated by:

$$PCWP = PCWP_M - 0.5(PEEP - 10)$$

where $PCWP_M$ is the PCWP measured at any level of PEEP.

In order for the PAC to provide meaningful measurements of PCWP, the PCWP must always be measured at end-expiration in the respiratory cycle. Intrathoracic pressure variations differ between spontaneously breathing and mechanically ventilated patients (Figure 3-14).

The saturation of the blood within the pulmonary capillaries, immediately prior to reoxygenation in the alveolar capillaries, is known as the mixed venous oxygen saturation S_VO_2. Since the diffusion of oxygen from oxyhemoglobin into the tissues follows a concentration gradient, tissues with greater metabolic rates utilize more oxygen and blood flowing from these tissues is more "desaturated." Additionally, blood that is flowing at lower rates, as in low cardiac output states, is more likely to be "desaturated." Therefore, the oxyhemoglobin saturation of "desaturated" blood accurately reflects the combined effects of peripheral tissue extraction and cardiac output (flow).

Normally, peripheral oxygen consumption, or uptake, is independent of oxygen delivery. Peripheral oxygen extraction is linearly related to oxygen delivery.

The oxygen extraction ratio, O_2 ER, is a calculation that determines global oxygen utilization based on the difference between the oxygen that is delivered to tissues in the oxygen concentration in mixed venous blood:

$$O_2 \ ER = VO_2/DO_2$$

The pulmonary artery catheter has recently fallen into disfavor. Outcome studies are ambivalent regarding the benefit of the PAC in critically ill patients. Perhaps an important response to the skepticism is that repeated studies demonstrate that many clinical practitioners have a flawed or incomplete understanding of the physiology and the assumptions involved in PAC placement and data interpretation. Furthermore, practitioners frequently treat absolute numbers such as the wedge pressure or the CVP in isolation from the cardiac output, and in isolation of the rest of the clinical picture. The key assumptions, that right heart function and compliance, that the catheter tip is reliably placed within lung zone II or III, that transpulmonary pressures are linearly related to the PCWP, and that left-sided volumes can be reliably estimated by using right-sided pressures, *must* be accounted for within the global clinical context.

Situations where the PCWP is likely to be significantly greater than LVEDP include mitral stenosis, pulmonary venous instruction or hypertension, left atrial myxoma, or elevated pulmonary alveolar pressure. Situations where the PCWP is likely to be significantly less than LVEDP include instances of diminished left ventricular compliance (infarction, ischemia, chronic left ventricular failure) or aortic insufficiency. A classic finding with the PAC occurs with cardiac tamponade where there is "equalization of pressures" and the CVP, mean PA pressure, and PCWP all become equal.

Where oxygen delivery (DO_2) is decreased past the point at which metabolically active tissues can compensate, oxygen uptake (VO_2) decreases linearly in proportion to DO_2. When tissues become hypoxic, and VO_2 falls, oxygen metabolism changes from oxidative phosphorylation to anaerobic glycolysis. Anaerobic glycolysis is a significantly less effective metabolic pathway and produces substantially less ATP per molecule of oxygen; lactate

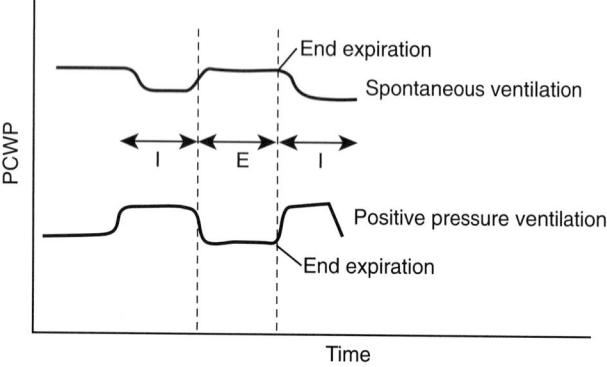

Figure 3-14 Determination of wedge pressure (PCWP). PCWP is determined at the end expiration. However, in spontaneously ventilating patients end expiration corresponds with positive intrathoracic pressure and therefore PCWP is measured at the end of a plateau. In patients receiving positive pressure ventilation end expiration corresponds with negative intrathoracic pressure, prior to the next breath, and is measured at the end of a "valley."

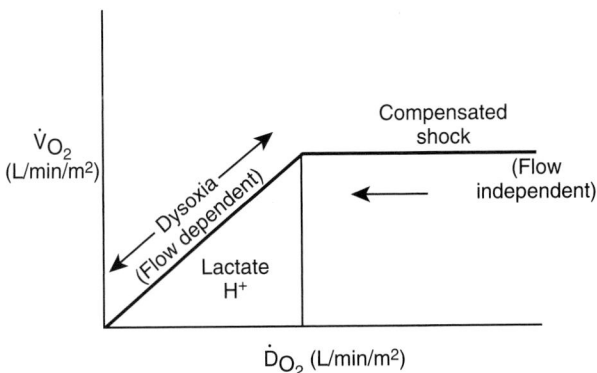

Figure 3-15 The classic DO_2-VO_2 relationship. Progressive decrease in oxygen delivery is compensated for by local tissue regulation and cellular oxygen kinetics. However, when DO_2 reaches a critical point, the curve's inflection point, cellular dysoxia occurs and there is progressive accumulation of cellular lactate and hydrogen as metabolic by-products.

and acid production are by-products of tissue hypoxia (Figure 3-15).

Serum lactate and serum base excess are therefore important indicators of global tissue hypoxia in the setting of shock (Figure 3-16). Since the peripheral oxygen extraction is elevated in the setting of diminished delivery, the saturation of blood returning to the lungs is profoundly diminished.

NONINVASIVE HEMODYNAMIC MONITORING

Despite its alleged drawbacks, invasive thermodilution is still the reference method for clinical determination of CO in critically ill patients. A large number of noninvasive hemodynamic monitors are available and marketed for

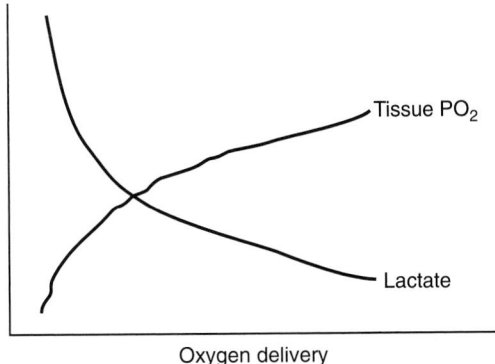

Figure 3-16 The relationship between tissue PO_2 and serum lactate. Serum lactate is a biochemical marker for anaerobic glycolysis and tissue dysoxia. It is a global marker rather than a tissue-specific or organ-specific indicator.

intraoperative or ICU use. The three primary technological approaches are (1) pulsed esophageal Doppler ultrasound, (2) partial CO_2 re-breathing using the Fick principle, and (3) thoracic bioimpedance. All methods that derive stroke volume from the blood flow velocity, Fick data, or relative amplitude of the bioimpedance signal rely on empirical data to calibrate the algorithms. These algorithms are not perfect and provide misleading information in critical pathophysiologic states. Additionally, where there is an inability to actually view the waveforms provided by the noninvasive device, there is no way of ensuring that adequate or appropriate waveforms are being analyzed. The simplicity of the PAC cannot be approximated by these newer noninvasive techniques.

Esophageal ultrasound technology is based on aortic blood flow velocity which helps determine both cardiac output and afterload. The advantage of the ultrasound-based technology is that it does not depend on an estimation of CVP. Disadvantages include difficulty and variability in probe positioning, difficulty in placement in awake patients, and difficulty in obtaining reliable data regarding cardiac preload. Thoracic bioimpedance is based on the principal that changes in thoracic blood volume alter the thoracic resistance to an electrical current. When bioimpedance changes are correlated with ventricular depolarization, stroke volume can be continuously and relatively reliably determined. Generally, four pairs of electrocardiographic electrodes pulse microcurrents across the thorax and sense the changes in resistance or conduction. A primary limitation of bioimpedance technology is that it also cannot independently determine cardiac filling pressures. In fact, cardiac function parameters determined using bioimpedance devices require an independent estimation of CVP. Therefore, invasive monitoring is either required, or the clinician must make a numerical approximation based on judgment.

ECHOCARDIOGRAPHY

Increasingly, echocardiography is available as a bedside monitoring device. Anesthesiologists are trained in the use of transesophageal echocardiography (TEE) in the operating room and this is a skill that can easily be transferred to the ICU. Experience in the use of TEE is especially important when other invasive hemodynamic monitoring, such as the PAC, is impossible, impractical, or likely to be unreliable.

Ultrasound waves are generated during electrical stimulation of piezoelectric crystals. The sound waves differentially penetrate tissues of varying density and allow the localization and visualization of these densities. Additionally, echocardiographic monitoring is now almost universally equipped with Doppler ultrasound which is extremely useful to image blood flow. In perioperative liver transplantation patients TEE can also easily image hepatic blood flow and serve as a useful adjunct to clinical and laboratory data regarding graft patency.

TEE is extremely useful in the direct visualization of cardiac chamber size and dynamic contractility. In patients with hypovolemia the end-systolic volume (ESV) and the end-diastolic volume (EDV) can be easily visualized with TEE to guide diagnosis and therapy. In hypovolemia the left ventricle contracts down upon itself almost completely. Computer-assisted TEE imaging allows for reliable determination of cardiac ejection fraction by comparison of EDV and ESV. However, the determination of cardiac ejection fraction based on chamber size comparisons alone is unreliable if there are associated valvular abnormalities or intracardiac shunts.

In patients with impaired contractility dynamic imaging will clearly reveal areas of wall motion abnormality, segmental wall motion defects (SWMAs). The SWMA will correlate with the anatomic distribution of ischemia and frequently will demonstrate reversibility with therapy. Since SWMAs are much earlier and more sensitive indicators of cardiac ischemia than are either the PAC or the ECG, TEE is an important clinical monitor.

TEE can also help visualize anatomic abnormalities such as valvular abnormalities and function, tumor or clot within the cardiac chambers, or aortic pathology. Pulsed Doppler ultrasound is especially useful when examining cardiac valves to look for valvular gradient abnormalities, prosthetic valve dysfunction or perivalvular leak, regurgitant ejection fraction, and pulmonary blood flow; this is known as color-flow mapping. When Doppler technology is combined with rapid ejection of agitated saline or agitated albumin the microbubbles can help delineate intracardiac shunting; which may be more sensitive than Doppler technology alone. TEE can also help visualize valvular endocarditis lesions. Pulsed Doppler evaluation of aortic blood flow velocity is an important adjunctive evaluation of cardiac function.

Important limitations regarding the use of TEE in ICU patients include a secure airway, coagulopathy, hiatal hernia, esophageal variceal disease, or recent esophagogastric surgery.

SELECTED READING

Bellomo R, Uchino S: Cardiovascular monitoring tools: use and misuse. Curr Opin Crit Care 9(3):225–229, 2003.

Branson PK, McCoy RA, Phillips BA, Clifton GD: Efficacy of 1.4 percent sodium citrate in maintaining arterial catheter patency in patients in a medical ICU. Chest 103(3):882–885, 1993.

Calvert N, Hind D, McWilliams RG et al. The effectiveness and cost-effectiveness of ultrasound locating devices for central venous access: a systematic review and economic evaluation. Health Technol Assess 7(12):1–84, 2003.

Connors AF, Speroff T, Dawson NV et al: The effectiveness of right heart catheterization in the initial care of critically ill patients. JAMA 276:889, 1996; Crit Care Med 28(8):2812–2818, 2000.

Davis N, Pohlman A, Gehlbach B et al: Improving the process of informed consent in the critically ill. JAMA 289(15):1963–1968, 2003.

Denault AY, Couture P, McKenty S et al: Perioperative use of transesophageal echocardiography by anesthesiologists: impact in noncardiac surgery and in the intensive care unit. Can J Anaesth 49(3):287, 2002.

Domino KB, Bowdle TA, Posner KL et al: Injuries and liability related to central vascular catheters: a closed claims analysis. Anesthesiology 100(6):1411–1418, 2004.

Hind D, Calvert N, McWilliams R et al: Ultrasonic locating devices for central venous cannulation: meta-analysis. BMJ 327(7411): 361, 2003.

Huttemann E, Schelenz C, Kara F, Chatzinikolaou K, Reinhart K: The use and safety of transoesophageal echocardiography in the general ICU – a mini review. Acta Anaesthesiol Scand 48(7):827–836, 2004.

Iberti TJ, Fischer EP, Liebowitz AB et al: A multicenter study of physicians' knowledge of the pulmonary artery catheter. JAA 264:2928, 1990.

Knutstad K, Hager B, Hauser M: Radiologic diagnosis and management of complications related to central venous access. Acta Radiol 44(5):508–516, 2003.

Mermel LA, Farr BM, Sherertz RJ et al; Infectious Diseases Society of America; American College of Critical Care Medicine; Society for Healthcare Epidemiology of America: Guidelines for the management of intravascular catheter-related infections. Clin Infect Dis 32(9):1249–1272, 2001.

Porembka DT, Hoit BD: Transesophageal echocardiography in the intensive care patient. Crit Care Med 19:826, 1991.

Taylor RW, Ahrens T, Bennet ED et al: Pulmonary artery catheter consensus conference: consensus statement. Crit Care Med 25:910–925, 1997.

Teichgraber UK, Gebauer B, Benter T, Wagner HJ: Central venous access catheters: radiological management of complications. Cardiovasc Intervent Radiol 26(4):321–333, 2003.

Williams G, Grounds M, Rhodes A: Pulmonary artery catheter. Curr Opin Crit Care 8(3):251–256, 2002.

Modern Acid–Base Physiology

JOHN A. KELLUM, M.D., F.A.C.P., F.C.C.P.

RINALDO BELLOMO, M.D., F.R.A.C.P., F.C.C.P.

DAVID STORY, M.D., F.A.N.Z.C.A.

Significant advances in medicine, like other fields of science, are the products of multiple individual discoveries, usually by many different people, often over many years. Furthermore, pivotal advances, those that alter the very way we look at a particular issue, occur only very rarely given the thousands of individual investigators who contribute to the collective literature of science and medicine. These paradigm shifts are often met with great resistance in part because they require us to unlearn the old way as much as they require us to learn something new. When it was first reported that peptic ulcer disease was due to *H. pylori* infection, the scientific community reacted slowly and then with skepticism.

Little more than 20 years ago Peter Stewart published his revolutionary physical chemical analysis of acid-base physiology. Stewart's approach to acid-base was praised by some and criticized by others, but mostly it was ignored. Indeed, there has been very little interest in this approach until quite recently. It would seem that the disinterest was due mainly to the fact that the approach, while conceptually simple and elegant, is operationally complicated and unwieldy. Most clinicians feel quite comfortable with the traditional approach to acid-base physiology and few can be easily convinced that "re-learning" this area is worthwhile. However, for patients in the intensive care unit (ICU), extreme derangements in physiology are common and traditional methods are often inadequate to explain the severe acid-base disorders present in some of these patients. Although the Stewart approach is based on the same physical chemical principles on which more traditional approaches are based, this new approach is vastly different. The most important difference is that, in this view of the biological universe, hydrogen ions and bicarbonate ions are not independent variables but are instead determined by other factors. Changes in pH are not the result of the generation or removal of these ions per se, but rather are the result of changes in other variables. In this universe, it is the Earth rather than the Sun that moves.

The Stewart approach has now been found very robust in a wide variety of patient types and experimental conditions. Recently, it has been shown that quantitatively this approach is compatible with the more traditional approaches; the difference lies in the understanding of the mechanisms involved. The observation that metabolic acidosis is associated with a decrease in plasma bicarbonate and base excess remains valid. However, the implication that these changes *cause* the acidosis is not. Some might argue that such a conceptual change makes little difference. If one can measure the size and origin (respiratory vs. metabolic) of a change in acid-base status, does the average clinician really need to understand how it occurs? Of course, this was the same argument facing Galileo when he insisted that the Earth was not the center of the universe. Even without

Copernicus's theory it was still quite possible to "understand" the universe and it is very unlikely that the life of the average person living in those times was altered in any way by this new knowledge. The argument obviously evaporates when considered in these terms. The understanding that bicarbonate (HCO_3^-) and hydrogen ions (H^+) are not at the center of the acid–base universe produces as violent a change in our concepts of physiology as did Copernicus change our concepts of astronomy.

At this point, the authors of this chapter find it intellectually impossible to continue to teach conventional acid–base physiology.

In this chapter we explain the fundamental aspects of the Stewart approach, review the implications for clinical medicine, particularly in the ICU, and consider some of the more practical aspects of acid–base management from this perspective.

HISTORICAL BACKGROUND OF THE ACID–BASE PHYSIOLOGY DEBATE

In the late 1800s Arrhenius, a Swedish physicist, developed two chemical concepts important to acid–base physiology. The first was a new approach to the dissociation of chemical salts into electrolytes; for this work Arrhenius almost failed his doctorate but was later awarded a Nobel prize. The second concept was a new definition of an acid: a substance that when added to a solution increases the hydrogen ion concentration. The next important development was the work of a Boston physician, Henderson, in the early 1900s. From in vitro work, Henderson rewrote the law of mass action equation to describe the role of weak acids in maintaining "neutrality regulation in the animal organism." The "Henderson" equation applies particularly to bicarbonate and carbonic acid:

$$\left[H^+\right] = k \times \frac{\left[H_2CO_3\right]}{\left[HCO_3^-\right]}$$

where k is a constant.

Over the next 20 years several developments came from Denmark. A new definition of an acid was developed by Brønsted: an acid is a substance that donates hydrogen ions in solution. Brønsted noted that an Englishman, Lowry, had developed a similar definition. This became the Brønsted–Lowry definition, still the dominant definition of an acid. *The operative and scientific superiority in the biological field of this later definition of acid over Arrhenius's concept is neither obvious nor proven.*

CURRENT CONTROVERSY

What is an acid? The definition of an acid is just that: a definition. It cannot be proved to be false or true. All that one can do is to see how, from an operative point of view, such a definition is internally consistent and able to fit into all observations that are made empirically. Which definition dominates at a particular time in history is not the product of science alone but also the product of the spirit of the times, politics, influence, and other non-scientific factors. If we add hydrochloric acid to saline, does the pH fall because we add the hydrogen ions of the acid or because the chloride lowers the strong ion difference or both? Is hydrochloric acid an acid because it donates hydrogen ions or because it increases the concentration of hydrogen ions in the solution?

Sorensen, a chemist, made two further major contributions. First he developed the concept of taking the negative logarithm to the base ten of the hydrogen ion concentration, which he called pH. Second he called chemicals that reduced pH changes in solutions "buffers" after the springs on the end of railway carriages. Hasselbalch, a physician-farmer, combined Sorensen's work with Henderson's to produce the Henderson-Hasselbalch equation:

$$pH = pKa + \log_{10} \times \frac{\left[HCO_3^-\right]}{\left[H_2CO_3\right]}$$

Whether concepts like "buffers" and the continued use of a logarithmic scale for changes in hydrogen ion activity serve modern medicine well remains doubtful.

CURRENT CONTROVERSY

What is a buffer? Why use pH? The same issues related to the definition of an acid pertain to the definition of a buffer. Sodium lactate is a "buffer" in conventional acid-base physiology. However, if enough sodium lactate is given fast enough, hyperlactatemia occurs and the base excess falls. Is this because lactate is not transformed into CO_2 (conventional explanation) by the liver or because the SID has decreased due to the rapid infusion of a solution with a SID of 0 (Stewart explanation)? It is not possible to tell. Equally, is the use of pH helpful to clinicians to appreciate changes in acid-base balance more than the actual hydrogen ion activity in nmol/l? We doubt it. In our opinion, the use of pH in modern medicine appears unnecessary and potentially misleading.

Over the next 50 years acid–base physiology centered on the Henderson-Hasselbalch equation. The partial pressure of carbon dioxide was substituted for carbonic acid. The non-volatile, or metabolic, component was interpreted as being due to the body controlling plasma bicarbonate concentration. One difficulty in clinical application was that changes in bicarbonate had to be interpreted while allowing for changes in the partial pressure of carbon dioxide. To deal with this problem, Schwartz and Relman, Boston physicians, produced "rules of thumb." The rules of thumb were equations to determine whether the simultaneous changes in bicarbonate and carbon dioxide were a single process, such as metabolic acidosis with compensation, or mixed processes.

In the 1960s Siggard-Anderson, a Danish physician, introduced "base excess" as a measure of the metabolic acid–base status. Using base excess did not require calculating the rules of thumb. Base excess assumes a partial pressure of carbon dioxide of 40 mmHg and includes the plasma bicarbonate concentration in the calculation. The subsequent controversy between Boston and Copenhagen over the merits of the rules of thumb versus base excess was known as the "Great Transatlantic Debate." It continues to this day.

In the late 1970s and early 1980s, in several papers and a book, Peter Stewart, a Canadian-American physiologist working at Brown University, introduced a new approach to acid–base physiology and disorders. While using the partial pressure of carbon dioxide, Stewart used two other variables, the strong ion difference and the total weak acid concentration, instead of bicarbonate. Stewart based his work on several chemical principles, particularly electroneutrality, conservation of mass, and dissociation of electrolytes. Unfortunately for the ongoing debate, Stewart died in 1993.

The main principles of Stewart's approach are that there are three important independent factors controlling the acid–base status of a physiological solution: the partial pressure of carbon dioxide, the strong ion difference, and the total weak acid concentration. The role of carbon dioxide, controlled by the lungs, is similar to that in the Henderson-Hasselbalch approach. Strong ions are ions that are completely dissociated in solution. The most important strong ions are sodium, potassium, and chloride. The important factor is the difference between the strong ions rather than the absolute concentrations of the ions. As the strong ion difference falls the hydrogen ion concentration increases. Lactate is treated as a strong ion because with a pKa of 3.4 it is almost completely dissociated at a pH of 7.40. The most important weak acids in plasma are albumin and, to a lesser extent, phosphate. Stewart emphasized that the three independent factors must be considered simultaneously. These independent factors will control dependent factors including bicarbonate, hydroxyl ions, and hydrogen ions. The source

of hydrogen ions in the Stewart approach is the dissociation of water molecules. Important underlying factors are the temperature-dependent dissociation constants of weak acids, including carbonic acid, and the dissociation constant of water.

CLINICAL CAVEAT

What is the source of hydrogen ions? The source of hydrogen ions is plasma water not "acid" generation by cells. One liter of water contains approximately $55 \times 6.022 \times 10^{23}$ hydrogen ions. The quantity of hydrogen ions that is released from water depends on the independent variables described by Stewart. Normally, at 25°C, one in 10^{14} molecules of water is dissociated. To put it another way, in a solution of distilled water, not all of the water is water. Some of it is dissociated into hydroxyl ions and hydrogen ions. The glass electrode measures free hydrogen ions and, of course, ignores free hydroxyl ions. The more water is dissociated, the greater the amount of free hydrogen ions and the lower the pH.

For several reasons Stewart's work provoked, and continues to provoke, strong adverse reaction from those committed to the Henderson-Hasselbalch approach. First, he rejected bicarbonate as a vital controlling factor. Second, he emphasized the vital role of strong ions; he saw hydrochloric acid as acidifying not because it has hydrogen ions but because it has strong anions, chloride, without strong cations. Third, he rejected the notion of buffers, and instead talked of weak acids. Fourth, he rejected pH in favor of a return to hydrogen ion concentration. Last, he returned to the acid definition of Arrhenius: a substance that when added to a solution increases the hydrogen ion concentration. This definition accommodates both carbon dioxide and strong anions.

Many groups have continued Stewart's work: in clinical work (particularly critical care), in exercise physiology, and in veterinary work.

FUNDAMENTAL PRINCIPLES OF HYDROGEN ION REGULATION

Before we examine this area it is first necessary to review the basic principles of H^+ regulation. Large living organisms seek to maintain plasma pH within strict tolerance limits. In fact, the free H^+ concentration is maintained within the nmol/l range (36–43 nmol/l). By contrast, most other ions are regulated in the mmol/l range. One reason H^+ concentration is so closely regulated is that these ions have very high charge densities and consequently very large electric fields. Furthermore, the strength of H^+ bonds (ubiquitous in biologic systems) is very sensitive to local H^+ concentration. Biochemical reactions as well as interactions of hormones and drugs with plasma proteins and cell surface receptors are also influenced by changes in H^+ concentration. In addition, fluctuations in intracellular H^+ concentration have major effects on cellular performance presumably by altering protein charge, thereby affecting structure and enzymatic function. Obviously then, in order to understand how the body regulates plasma H^+ concentration, we must first understand the physicochemical determinants of H^+ concentration.

Biochemistry of Aqueous Solutions

Virtually all solutions in human biology contain water and aqueous solutions provide a virtually inexhaustible source of H^+. In these solutions, H^+ concentration is determined by the dissociation of water into H^+ and OH^- ions. In other words, changes in H^+ concentration occur *not* as a result of how much H^+ is added or removed but as a consequence of water dissociation. The factors that determine the dissociation of water are the laws of physical chemistry. Two in particular apply here, *electroneutrality* (which dictates that, in aqueous solutions, the sum of all positively charged ions must equal the sum of all negatively charged ions) and *conservation of mass* (which means that the amount of a substance remains constant unless it is added or generated, or removed or destroyed). In pure water, according to the principle of electroneutrality, the concentration of H^+ must always equal the concentration of OH^-. In more complex solutions we have to consider other determinants of water dissociation, but still the source of H^+ remains *water*. Fortunately, even in a solution as complex as blood plasma, the determinants of H^+ concentration can be reduced to three. If we know the value of these three determinants, the H^+ concentration can be predicted under any conditions. These three determinants are the *strong ion difference* (SID), pCO_2, and *total weak acid concentration* (A_{TOT}).

Strong Ion Difference, pCO_2, and Total Weak Acid Concentration

The SID is the net charge balance of all strong ions present, where a "strong" ion is one that is completely (or near-completely) dissociated. For practical purposes this means $(Na^+ + K^+ + Ca^{2+} + Mg^{2+}) - (Cl^- + lactate^-)$. This is often referred to as the "apparent" SID (SIDa) with the understanding that some "unmeasured" ions might also be present. In healthy humans this value is 40–42 mEq/l, although it is often quite different in critically ill patients. Of note, neither H^+ nor HCO_3^- is a strong ion. The pCO_2 is an independent variable assuming that the system is open (i.e., ventilation is present). Finally, the weak acids (A^-), which are mostly proteins and phosphates, contribute the remaining charges to satisfy the principle of electroneutrality. A^-, however, is not an independent variable because it changes with alterations in SID and pCO_2. A_{TOT} ($AH + A^-$) is the third independent variable because its value is not determined by any other. The essence of the Stewart approach (and indeed what is revolutionary) is the understanding that only these three variables are important. Neither H^+ nor HCO_3^- can change unless one or more of these three variables change. The principle of conservation of mass makes this point more than semantics. Strong ions cannot be created or destroyed to satisfy electroneutrality but H^+ ions are generated or consumed by changes in water dissociation. Hence, in order to understand how the body regulates pH we need only ask how it regulates these three independent variables (SID, pCO_2, and A_{TOT}).

CLINICAL APPLICATIONS

This "new" approach changes nothing about the measurement or classification of acid–base disorders. All of the careful observations that have been made over the years are no less valid under this approach. What does change is the interpretation of these observations. The Sun still sets in the west and rises in the east, but now it is the Earth that moves.

Quantification of Acid–Base Disorders

While the understanding of how an acid–base disorder occurs is now quite different, it is important to emphasize that not only does the traditional approach to *quantifying* an acid–base disorder still "work," but that it is entirely complementary to this physical chemical analysis. In fact the standard base excess (SBE) can be used to quantify the amount of change in SID that has occurred from baseline. The SBE can be thought of as the amount of change in the SID that is required in order to restore the pH to 7.40, given a pCO_2 of 40 mmHg (a negative SBE refers to the amount the SID must *increase*). This is because the SID is essentially equal to the buffer base of Singer and Hastings and base excess (BE) quantifies the change in buffer base. SBE is superior to BE because the former has been "standardized" to account for the difference between CO_2 equilibration in vitro compared to in vivo. Although SBE is not strictly comparable to the change in SID because it deals with whole blood as opposed to plasma, the two are generally close enough for most clinical circumstances. Thus, SBE provides an estimate of the amount of strong anion that needs to be removed or strong cation added in order to normalize the pH. For example, in order to change the SBE from −20 to −10 mEq/l by adding $NaHCO_3$, the serum Na^+ concentration would need to be increased by 10 mEq/l.

Recently, Schlichtig and co-workers described the changes in SBE that occur with acute and chronic disorders of $PaCO_2$. The SBE does not change with acute changes in $PaCO_2$. During chronic respiratory acidosis or alkalosis the change in the SBE is equal to 0.4 × ($PaCO_2$ − 40). Similarly, the expected change in $PaCO_2$ for a given abnormality in SBE is as follows: for acidosis the decrease in $PaCO_2$ is equal to the change in SBE; for alkalosis the increase in $PaCO_2$ is equal to 0.6 × SBE.

Chloride: The "Forgotten Electrolyte"

One of the most important implications of the Stewart analysis is the role of chloride in acid–base homeostasis. If the body is to alter the SID, its primary tools are Na^+ and Cl^-. An increase in Na^+ relative to Cl^- (or a decrease in Cl^- relative to Na^+) increases the SID and hence the pH. The opposite effects, a decrease in the SID and a fall in the pH, occur when Na^+ and Cl^- concentrations move closer together. Since Na^+ concentration is tightly regulated by the body to control tonicity, Cl^- emerges as the body's foremost tool for adjusting the SID and hence the plasma pH. Furthermore, acid–base abnormalities are frequently the result of disorders in chloride homeostasis. For example, a common form of metabolic alkalosis seen in the ICU is caused by the loss of gastric secretions. The loss of HCl from the stomach results in a hypochloremic metabolic alkalosis sometimes severe enough to require therapy. Of course this is the loss of H^+, but H^+ is also lost with every molecule of water removed from the body. Moreover, gastric secretions may reach a pH of 1.0, or a H^+ concentration of 10^8 nmol/l. If one liter of gastric fluid is lost, this would mean that 10^8 nmol (0.1 mol!) of H^+ would be removed. If one considers that plasma H^+ concentration is 40 nmol/l (or 4 × 10^{-8} mol/l), and if the majority of body fluids are at or near this concentration, one sees that the amount of total body free H^+ is only about 1.6 × 10^{-7} mol. If physiology were just simple accounting, a patient with a 200 ml emesis would entirely deplete the H^+ stores of the body and die of severe alkalemia in minutes. Of course this is not what happens and in reality the H^+ concentration decreases by a much smaller amount. The reason it decreases at all is because the plasma SID is increased and this is because Cl^- (a strong anion) is lost without loss of a strong cation. This *increased* SID forces a *decrease* in the amount of water dissociation and hence a *decrease* in the plasma H^+ concentration. When H^+ is "lost" as water rather than HCl, there is virtually no change in the SID and hence no change in the plasma H^+ concentration.

Next, consider the treatment for a hypochloremic metabolic alkalosis. Aside from preventing further Cl^- loss, the therapy is to give back Cl^-. Saline works in this regard because even though one is giving equal amounts of Na^+ and Cl^-, the plasma Cl^- concentration is always much lower than the plasma Na^+ concentration and thus Cl^- increases more than Na^+ when large amounts of saline are administered. KCl works better for this indication because, with a metabolic alkalosis, much of the K^+ goes intracellular leaving much of the Cl^- in the plasma to decrease the SID.

From the example above, one can easily understand not only how administration of 0.9% saline can correct a hypochloremic metabolic alkalosis but also how massive amounts would lead to a decreased plasma SID and thus a *hyper*chloremic metabolic *acidosis*. This particular issue has been the focus of two recent studies, one in animals with experimental sepsis the other in humans undergoing surgery.

> **CURRENT CONTROVERSY**
>
> What is the cause of so-called dilutional acidosis? The conventional view of this phenomenon is that the "buffers" are diluted by the administration of fluids. The Stewart explanation is simple. If one adds solutions with a SID of 0, the SID of plasma will fall and water will be more dissociated with a greater release of hydrogen ions.

In the first study we administered *E. coli* endotoxin to dogs and then volume resuscitated with 0.9% saline. Over a 3 hour period, each animal received an average of 1.8 liters of saline and the pH decreased from 7.32 to 7.11 ($p < 0.01$) while CO_2 and lactate were unchanged. Using the SID it was possible to calculate the amount of acidosis that was attributable to saline. Although the serum Na^+ concentration did not change, the serum Cl^- concentration increased by almost 10 mmol/l. It was concluded that saline alone was responsible for 42% of the total acid load experienced by these animals. In the second study, Scheingraber and colleagues randomized patients undergoing major gynecologic surgery to receive either 0.9% saline or lactated Ringer's solution. Patients receiving saline exhibited a decrease in their arterial pH from 7.41 to 7.28 while no change occurred in the lactated Ringer's group. These investigators also used the SID to calculate the expected change in pH with saline and found that the acidosis was entirely explained by chloride administration.

Although dilutional acidosis was first described over 40 years ago, it has more recently been likened to Lewis

Carroll's Cheshire cat in that it is more imaginary than real. In healthy animals large doses of NaCl have been demonstrated to produce only a minor hyperchloremic acidosis. These studies have been interpreted to show that if dilutional acidosis occurs it is only in the extreme case and even then it is only mild. This line of reasoning cannot be applied to many critically ill patients for two reasons. First, large-volume resuscitation is commonly required in patients with sepsis and trauma. These patients may receive crystalloid infusions of 5–10 times their plasma volumes in a single day. The second problem with this line of reasoning is that it fails to consider the fact that critically ill patients are frequently not in normal acid–base balance to begin with. These patients may have lactic acidosis or renal insufficiency. Furthermore, critically ill patients might not be able to compensate normally by increasing ventilation and may have abnormal buffer capacity owing to hypoalbuminemia. In patients, as well as in animals with experimental sepsis, dilutional acidosis does occur and can produce significant acid–base derangements.

The clinical implication for management of patients in the ICU is that when large volumes of fluid are used for resuscitation they should be more physiologic than saline.

CLINICAL CAVEAT

How can one avoid "dilutional" acidosis? Dilutional acidosis can be avoided by administering "balanced solutions" which have a SID close to the normal SID of plasma. Lactate Ringer's solution is such a fluid. It is important to realize that if large amounts of this fluid are given to critically ill patients, hyperlactemia might be induced. Such hyperlactemia is usually mild to moderate and should not be misunderstood as a sign of clinical deterioration.

One alternative is lactated Ringer's solution. This fluid contains a more physiologic difference between Na^+ and Cl^- and thus the SID is closer to normal (roughly 28 mEq/l compared to saline which has an SID of 0 mEq/l). Of course this assumes that the lactate in lactated Ringer's is metabolized, which may take several minutes. Until the lactate is removed the effect of lactated Ringer's is identical to saline since one strong anion (i.e., lactate) is as good as another (i.e., Cl^-). Therefore, massive doses of sodium lactate, for example given as replacement fluid for hemofiltration, may transiently result in acidosis as the SID decreases.

Other Anions

When the SID decreases, metabolic acidosis ensues. When this occurs as a result of increased Cl^-, the anion gap (AG), which is a measure of missing charge, does not change. However, when other anions are present, the AG increases. Unfortunately, the accuracy of the AG is questionable in certain clinical situations, particularly in critically ill patients who are frequently hypoalbuminemic and acidotic. This has prompted some authors to adjust the "normal range" for the AG by the patient's albumin or even phosphate concentration. Each g/dl of albumin has a charge of 2.8 mEq/l at pH 7.4 (2.3 mEq/l at 7.0 and 3.0 mEq/l at 7.6) and each mg/dl of phosphate has a charge of 0.59 mEq/l at pH 7.4 (0.55 mEq/l at 7.0 and 0.61 mEq/l at 7.6). Except in cases of abnormal paraproteins, globulin does not contribute to the AG. Thus a convenient way to estimate the "normal range" of the AG for a given patient is by use of the following formula:

"Normal" AG = 2(albumin g/dl) + 0.5(phosphate mg/dl)

Or for international units:

"Normal" AG = 0.2(albumin g/l) + 1.5(phosphate mmol/l)

Figge et al. have shown that in the majority of critically ill patients the "normal" AG can be estimated by using 2.5 times the albumin concentration in g/dl (or 0.25 for albumin in g/l). However, if the serum phosphate concentration is significantly abnormal this estimate will be inaccurate.

CLINICAL CAVEAT

With regards albumin and the anion gap, the anion gap must always be adjusted for the effect of hypoalbuminemia. In a critically ill patient with an albumin of 1.5 g/dl a normal unadjusted anion gap can coexist with a lactate of 6 mmol/l!

The etiology of anions other than Cl^- varies depending on the population studied. Ketones, organic acids accumulating in renal failure, and toxins are important causes in appropriate patient groups. In critically ill patients lactate is a particularly important cause. Lactate is a strong ion by virtue of the fact that at pH within the physiologic range, it is almost completely dissociated (i.e., the pK of lactate is 3.9; at a pH of 7.4, 3162 ions are dissociated for every one that is not). Because the body can produce and dispose of lactate rapidly, it functions as one of the most dynamic components of the SID. Lactate therefore can produce significant acidemia. However, often critically ill patients have hyperlactatemia that is much greater than the amount of acidosis seen. Physical chemistry also allows us to understand how hyperlactatemia may exist without metabolic acidosis. First, acid is not being "generated" apart from lactate such as through "unreversed ATP hydrolysis" as some have suggested. Phosphate is a weak acid and does not contribute substantially to metabolic acidosis even under extreme circumstances. Furthermore, the H+ concentration is not determined by how much H+ is produced or removed from the plasma but rather by changes in one of the three independent variables (SID, pCO$_2$, or A$_{TOT}$). Virtually anywhere in the body, pH is above 6.0 and lactate behaves as a strong ion. Its generation will then decrease the SID and result in increased water dissociation and thus increased H+ concentration.

How then might the plasma lactate concentration be increased and the H+ concentration not? There are two possible answers. First, if lactate is added to the plasma, not as lactic acid but rather as the salt of a strong acid (i.e., sodium lactate), there will be little change in the SID. This is because a strong cation (Na+) is being added along with a strong anion. In fact, as lactate is then removed by metabolism, the remaining Na+ will increase the SID resulting in metabolic alkalosis. Hence it would be possible to give enough lactate to increase the plasma lactate concentration without any change in H+ concentration. However, the amount of exogenous lactate required would be very large. This is because normal metabolism results in the turnover of approximately 1500-4500 mmol of lactic acid per day. Thus, only very large amounts of lactate infused rapidly will result in appreciable increases in the plasma lactate concentration. In this setting, a mild acidosis may occur until the lactate is metabolized (usually within several minutes). Levraut et al. infused 1 mmol/kg of lactate over 15 minutes in 10 patients with acute renal failure on continuous renal replacement therapy. Their mean plasma lactate concentration increased from 1.4 to 4.8 mmol/l after the infusion but normalized rapidly. Under such conditions it is possible (if transiently) to produce hyperlactatemia without acidemia. Unfortunately, these authors do not report the acid–base status of their patients. However, in another recent study, Morgera et al. showed that lactate-based hemofiltration resulted in *increased* plasma HCO$_3^-$ concentration and pH as well as hyperlactatemia. A more important mechanism whereby hyperlactatemia exists without acidemia (or with less acidemia than expected) is where the SID is corrected by the elimination of another strong anion from the plasma. This was demonstrated by Madias et al. In the setting of sustained lactic acidosis induced by lactic acid infusion, these investigators found that Cl- moves out of the plasma space to normalize pH. Under these conditions hyperlactatemia may persist but BE may be normalized by compensatory mechanisms to restore the SID.

The meaning of hyperlactatemia is very different depending on the patient population being considered. Healthy humans can achieve plasma lactate concentrations with exercise in excess of 25 mmol/l without any

long-term sequelae. By contrast, hyperlactatemia in the critically ill is an important predictor of mortality. One of the major controversies associated with hyperlactatemia and associated acidosis or indeed acidemia concerns its treatment.

Treatment of Acidosis and/or Acidemia

Whether induced by the accumulation of the lactate anion or by the accumulation of other anions (chloride, ketones, exogenous acids, acids associated with renal failure), severe acidosis may be associated with inadequate physiological compensation and lead to acidemia. Although it is agreed by all that treatment of such acidemia/acidosis should first and foremost involve correction of its cause, it is controversial whether some or all of these patients should also receive alkalinizing solutions such as sodium bicarbonate. The biologic rationale for administering sodium bicarbonate rests on three major considerations: (1) a low pH impairs myocardial contractility, (2) IV sodium bicarbonate can increase pH, and (3) any adverse effects of sodium bicarbonate are outweighed by its benefits. However, concerning point (1), evidence that a low pH decreases myocardial contractility is mostly based on data from isolated animal heart muscle preparations. In whole-animal preparations the effects of acidosis on contractility are much more difficult to document. In humans data from patients with permissive hypercapnia or with diabetic ketoacidosis support the view that there is marked tolerance to a low pH without major adverse effects. Furthermore, there is a body of data to suggest that acidosis may protect cells from anoxia, chemical hypoxia, and reperfusion injury. With regard to point (2), clinical studies show that the effect of up to 2 mmol/kg of sodium bicarbonate on pH is small with increments in the range 0.05-0.014 in humans. In addition, sodium bicarbonate fails to predictably increase intracellular pH and often appears to induce a decrease instead. Changes in blood pH may also decrease oxygen delivery to tissues by changing the dissociation curve of hemoglobin. Thus the efficacy of sodium bicarbonate in lowering pH where it matters is unclear. The hemodynamic effects of IV sodium bicarbonate have been studied in humans. They were indistinguishable from those of an equivalent amount of sodium delivered as saline. In uncontrolled studies of patients with diabetic ketoacidosis no benefits could be seen and delayed clearance of ketones and lactate were documented. Bicarbonate also lowers ionized calcium concentrations and PaO$_2$ in animals and non-acidemic patients with congestive cardiac failure. Thus the safety of IV bicarbonate remains untested. Other alkalinizing preparations exist:

1. Carbicarb (equimolar mixture of sodium carbonate and sodium bicarbonate)

2. Dichloroacetate (an agent that stimulates pyruvate dehydrogenase and lowers lactate levels)

3. Tris-hydroxymethyl aminomethane (THAM)

Carbicarb has also undergone limited studies in humans and its role is unclear. Dichloroacetate has been tested in a large randomized controlled trial in patients with lactic acidosis. In this trial it was found efficacious in lowering lactate levels and increasing bicarbonate concentration and pH. However, it did not achieve any changes in hemodynamics or clinical outcomes. THAM appears to improve contractility in isolated rabbit heart preparations. However, no controlled studies are available to support its use in humans with acidemia and the side effects of hyperkalemia, hypoglycemia, extravasation-related tissue necrosis, and neonatal hepatic necrosis demand great caution in its utilization.

CURRENT CONTROVERSY

The administration of IV sodium bicarbonate in patients with acidemia remains one of the most passion-laden areas of anesthetic and critical care practice. Like other similar areas of controversy, the intensity of opinion is inversely proportional to the quality and amount of evidence available. There are insufficient data to support the use of IV sodium bicarbonate in patients with acidemia. There are also insufficient data to proscribe the use of sodium bicarbonate in these patients. If a decision is made to administer IV sodium bicarbonate, we recommend that it should occur with close hemodynamic and biochemical monitoring and that the agent be administered in the presence of a physician.

Other Mechanisms of Lactic Acidosis

Although lactic acidosis is associated with major physiological stress in all patients and with shock in most, some particular situations occur where neither may be at work. A unique situation that requires separate discussion is that of the patient receiving artificial kidney support.

The Artificial Kidney and Lactate

The use of the artificial kidney also has a clinically significant impact on lactate balance and on plasma lactate concentrations. This impact may derive from lactate removal as well as lactate administration. Lactate clearance during intermittent hemodialysis or intermittent hemofiltration has not been formally studied but is likely to be similar to that of other small molecules given the molecular weight of lactate. Assuming a small molecular clearance of 200 ml/minute, lactate clearance during dialysis would reach approximately 20% of endogenous clearance. The impact of such clearance on lactate levels, however, has not been studied. Lactate has not been traditionally used as a buffer for intermittent hemodialysis, and therefore there is little specific information on the use of lactate-buffered dialysate on lactate levels and acid–base balance in dialysis patients.

When intermittent hemofiltration is used, however, and lactate-based replacement fluid is administered at high rates (approximately 200 mmol/hour), a significant increase in plasma lactate levels can be easily demonstrated. Although the clinical significance of such increases in lactate levels is unknown, this iatrogenic phenomenon needs to be appreciated in order to avoid misdiagnosis. Also, the magnitude of this phenomenon (average peak increase of 3 mmol/l at 3 hours) needs to be understood to separate it from other factors, which may simultaneously be operative in determining the patient's lactate levels.

A similar phenomenon has been described during continuous renal replacement therapy (CRRT), but the increment in lactate levels was less due to the lower rate of lactate administration. However, it is important to note that increments in lactate levels in patients on CRRT are not simply dependent on the rate of lactate administration but also on the body's ability to handle a given lactate load. Thus, the administration of up to 200 mmol/hour of lactate may lead to modest changes in lactate levels and pH. However, the administration of the same amount or even less in a patient with pre-treatment lactate intolerance (liver failure, severe septic shock) will induce a dramatic increase in lactate concentration and a profound acidosis. Under such circumstances, lactate-buffered replacement solutions should be avoided. Furthermore, in patients with lactic acidosis and acute renal failure receiving CRRT, the administration of bicarbonate-based replacement fluids is an effective way of avoiding any exacerbation of hyperlactatemia and of restoring acid–base homeostasis. Some investigators have suggested that lactate removal during CRRT may lower plasma lactate levels and participate in the correction of acidosis seen during bicarbonate-based CRRT. In response to this hypothesis, Levraut and colleagues conducted a careful analysis of lactate clearance during CRRT and compared it to endogenous clearance. They found that the median endogenous lactate clearance was 1379 ml/minute, while the median filter lactate clearance was 24.2 ml/minute. Thus, CRRT-based lactate clearance accounted for <3% of total lactate removal.

It may appear surprising that increases in plasma lactate concentration of up to 8 mmol/l would not induce a pronounced degree of acidification. It should do so by increasing the concentration of anions in plasma and thus decreasing the SID and its effect on the dissociation of plasma water into hydrogen ion. In fact some preliminary observations suggest that several complex events occur during the onset of such rapid iatrogenic hyperlactatemia. In particular, a marked decrease in chloride appears to occur despite the administration of chloride-rich replacement fluid. This change in chloride is likely to be secondary to a shift into cells similar to that seen in venous blood when the CO_2 rises (Hamburger shift). Such a shift in chloride rapidly attenuates the impact of hyperlactatemia on pH and prevents the development of a progressive and sustained acidemia.

Finally, it must be emphasized that the view of lactate as representative of so-called "anaerobic glycolysis" is not supported by the data available. The hyperlactatemia of septic shock, for example, appears most likely secondary to accelerated glycolytic flux, where glucose breakdown into pyruvate is proceeding faster than pyruvate can be channeled into the citric acid cycle via acetyl coenzyme A.

CURRENT CONTROVERSY

What is the meaning of hyperlactatemia? There is no evidence to indicate that hyperlactatemia is due to anaerobic glycolysis in critically ill patients and much evidence to suggest that it occurs in the setting of full intracellular oxygenation and in the presence of elevated levels of pyruvate. As fast glycolysis occurs in the liver and glucose is the preferred fuel of stress, it appears likely that peripheral lactate generation allows rapid fuel supply for glycolysis (lactate from muscle to liver, in liver to pyruvate for gluconeogenesis (Cori cycle), then glucose use for energy generation: the lactate shuttle). Alternatively, glucose breakdown is so fast under stress that pyruvate is generated faster than it can be taken up by mitochondria, and thus it becomes lactate and is recycled.

It is important to note that not all anions appearing in the blood of the critically ill can be explained. The SID can be used to detect unexplained anions because the apparent SID (SIDa) calculated from the measurable ions should be equal to the effective SID (SIDe) derived from the remaining charges attributable to CO_2 and A^-. If a difference exists between the SIDa and SIDe, then unmeasured anions must be present. This difference has been termed the strong ion gap (SIG) to distinguish it from the AG. Unlike the AG, the SIG is normally zero and does not change with changes in pH or albumin concentration as does the AG. However, it should be noted that this "gap" need not be filled by strong ions. Weak acids may also play a role.

In recent years unmeasured anions have been reported in the blood of patients with sepsis and liver disease. These anions may be the source of much of the unexplained

acidosis seen in patients with critical illness. The presence of unexplained anions in the blood of both patients with sepsis and liver disease was investigated further in an animal model of sepsis using endotoxemia. In this study it was found that during control conditions the liver cleared unmeasured anions from the circulation (mean flux −0.34 mEq/minute). With early endotoxemia, however, the liver switched to release of anions (0.12 mEq/minute, $p < 0.005$). These data suggest that the liver has a role in systemic acid-base balance by way of regulating anion fluxes apart from metabolism of lactate.

EFFECTS OF PLASMA PROTEINS

Considerable controversy has developed over the past decade as to how to classify acid-base derangements occurring as a result of abnormalities in the weak acids, A_{TOT}. A sudden decrease in A_{TOT} produces alkalosis while an increase is acidifying. Some have advocated a third classification for this effect, perhaps termed "proteinaceous acidosis or alkalosis," to be added to "metabolic" (SID) and "respiratory" (pCO_2). Others have strenuously objected. The debate may actually prove moot in light of more recent evidence. When the SID of critically ill patients was compared to SBE the intercept for SBE = 0 was found to be 30-35 mEq/l rather than 40-42 mEq/l as for healthy individuals. Thus, in these critically ill patients, many of whom had a decreased A_{TOT} secondary to hypoalbuminemia, the SID was reduced even when there was no apparent acid-base disorder. The reason for this is obvious from a physical chemical perspective. As a patient's albumin decreases so does A_{TOT} and thus A^-. This decrease in weak acid has a slightly alkalinizing effect. The body could adapt to this change by retaining CO_2 but it appears to reserve this adaptation for changes in SID. Instead, the body adapts to a decreased A_{TOT} by decreasing the SID. While one might be tempted classify this adaptation as a mixed acid-base disorder, a hypoalbuminemic alkalosis with a compensatory metabolic acidosis, it does not appear to be a disorder at all. Indeed, a patient who failed to reduce their SID in response to a decreased A_{TOT} should be considered to have a metabolic alkalosis as consequence of failed renal homeostatic mechanisms (e.g., secondary to hypovolemia), not a proteinacious alkalosis secondary to hypoalbuminemia. The findings of Wilkes in critically ill patients and Wooten in mathematical simulations appear to support this assertion. Both authors have demonstrated that the "set point" for the SID to achieve a normal pH given a normal pCO_2 changes with changes in A_{TOT}. Furthermore, although the loss of weak acid from the plasma space is an alkalinizing process, there is no evidence that the body regulates A_{TOT} to maintain acid-base balance and there is no evidence that clinicians should treat hypoalbumin-emia as an acid-base disorder.

CASE STUDY

A 77-year-old man has cardiopulmonary bypass (CPB). On admission to the ICU he has a pH of 7.24, CO_2 of 47, bicarbonate of 19 mmol/l, and BE of −7 mEq/l. He is receiving a low-dose epinephrine infusion at 3 μg/minute for a poor cardiac output following separation from the pump. His urea and electrolytes show a sodium of 140 mmol/l, chloride of 110 mmol/l, potassium of 6 mmol/l, and urea of 6 mmol/l (BUN of 16.5 mg/dl). His anion gap is 11 (normal). Does this man have a lactic acidosis? What acid-base disorders does this man have? A normal anion gap would suggest that this man does not have a lactic acidosis. However, the anion gap is not corrected for the serum albumin. This man had a crystalloid pump prime, which was saline based. He now has iatrogenic hyperchloremia with a low SID which is responsible for a degree of acidosis. The acidemia might have contributed to hyperkalemia which will have an alkalinizing effect on the SID. But he is also likely to have dilutional hypoalbuminemia, which would cause an alkalosis. When measured, the albumin concentration was in fact 1.5 g/dl. Thus the normal anion gap (assuming a normal phosphate) should actually be about 4.5-5 mEq/l. The fact that it is 11 mEq/l indicates that there are approximately 6-7 mEq/l of unmeasured anions, which of course could be due to lactate. The lactate was indeed measured. It was 6.3 mmol/l. This man had iatrogenic hyperchloremic acidosis, iatrogenic hypoalbuminemic alkalosis, a mild hyperkalemic alkalosis, a mild respiratory acidosis, and a moderate lactic acidosis. No obvious cause for his lactic acidosis was found. Epinephrine was suspected as being responsible for it. His epinephrine was changed to milrinone. Within 6 hours his lactate level was down to 2.3 mmol/l and his cardiac index was preserved at 2.4 l/m²/minute.

CONCLUSION

In order to understand the causes of the acid-base derangements, many of which are common in the ICU, we need only look at three independent variables (SID, pCO_2, and A_{TOT}). Metabolic acidemia results from a decrease in the plasma SID usually brought about by the addition of strong anions (lactate, Cl^-, other "unknown" anions). Conversely, metabolic alkalemia occurs when the plasma SID is increased either as a result of the addition of strong cations without strong anions (e.g., $NaHCO_3$) or by the removal of strong anions without strong cations (e.g., gastric suctioning).

This "new" understanding has considerable impact on how we think about gastric suction alkalosis, dilutional acidosis, and lactic acidosis as well as how we approach the treatment of these disorders. Our understanding of many other medical conditions (e.g., renal tubular acidosis) relies on a paradigm of acid-base regulation that is inconsistent with established physical chemistry principles. In this "post-Copernican" era, we will need to rethink our approach to these areas in the light of this fact.

SELECTED READING

Figge J, Jabor A, Kazda A, Fencl V: Anion gap and hypoalbuminemia. Crit Care Med. 26:1807-1810, 1998.

Figge J, Mydosh T, Fencl V: Serum proteins and acid-base equilibria: a follow-up. J Lab Clin Med 120:713-719, 1992.

Kellum JA, Bellomo R, Kramer DJ, Pinsky MR: Etiology of metabolic acidosis during saline resuscitation in endotoxemia. Shock 9:364-368, 1998.

Kellum JA, Bellomo R, Kramer DJ, Pinksy MR: Hepatic anion flux during acute endotoxemia. J Appl Physiol 78: 2212-2217, 1995.

Kellum JA, Bellomo R, Kramer DJ, Pinsky MR: Splanchnic buffering of metabolic acid during early endotoxemia. J Crit Care 12:7-12, 1997.

Kellum JA, Kramer DJ, Pinsky MR: Strong ion gap: a methodology for exploring unexplained anions. J Crit Care 10:51-55, 1995.

Leblanc M, Kellum JA: Biochemical and biophysical principles of hydrogen ion regulation. In Ronco C, Bellomo R, editors: *Critical Care Nephrology*, Dordrecht, The Netherlands: Kluwer Academic, 1998, pp 261-277.

Levraut J, Ciebiera JP, Jambou P, Ichai C, Labib Y, Grimaud D: Effect of continuous venovenous hemofiltration with dialysis on lactate clearance in critically ill patients. Crit Care Med 25:58-62, 1997.

Madias NE, Homer SM, Johns CA, Cohen JJ: Hypochloremia as a consequence of anion gap metabolic acidosis. J Lab Clin Med 104:15-23, 1984.

Magder S: Pathophysiology of metabolic acid-base disturbances in patients with critical illness. In Ronco C, Bellomo R, editors: *Critical Care Nephrology*, Dordrecht, The Netherlands: Kluwer Academic, 1998, pp 279-296.

Salem MM, Mujais SK: Gaps in the anion gap. Arch Intern Med 152:1625-1629, 1992.

Scheingraber S, Rehm M, Sehmisch C, Finsterer U: Rapid saline infusion produces hyperchloremic acidosis in patients undergoing gynecologic surgery. Anesthesiology 90: 1265-1270, 1999.

Stewart PA: Modern quantitative acid-base chemistry. Can J Physiol Pharmacol 61:1444-1461, 1983.

CHAPTER 5

Metabolic Derangements

CARLOS J. LOPEZ III, M.D.

JUDIT SZOLNOKI, M.D.

Metabolic derangements can present with mild alterations in signs and symptoms or as life-threatening situations. Rapid recognition and understanding of the physiology involved allows a more directed approach to their management. In this chapter we review some common abnormalities in electrolyte homeostasis and briefly explore derangements in temperature regulation.

SODIUM DERANGEMENTS

Hyponatremia

Hyponatremia is defined as a $[Na^+] < 135$ mEq/l. Symptoms and signs are a factor of sodium concentration and rapidity of onset. They typically begin to occur at levels <130 mEq/l, primarily with neurologic symptoms such as headache, lethargy, and confusion. The more severe symptoms such as stupor, seizures, and coma generally do not occur until $[Na^+] < 120$ mEq/l. The biggest danger is the brain edema that occurs from movement of water from the extracellular fluid (ECF) to the intracellular fluid (ICF) compartments. The rapidity at which hyponatremia occurs will also play a role in development of the clinical picture. Patients with chronic hyponatremia will often be asymptomatic in spite of having remarkably low levels. There are dangers to an overly rapid correction of hyponatremia. Approaches to treating the hyponatremic patient must be tempered by the level, associated symptoms, and chronicity.

Causes of hyponatremia can be described by the osmolality of the ECF. The osmolality is the solute or particle concentration of a fluid. Box 5-1 presents the osmolality calculation for plasma.

The differential diagnosis includes (1) hypo-osmolar hyponatremia, (2) normo-osmolar hyponatremia, and (3) hyperosmolar hyponatremia.

Hypo-osmolar hyponatremia is the most common. In general it is caused by either sodium loss or primary water gain. Because the ECF volume reflects total body sodium, the volume status of the patient is used to further subdivide hypo-osmolar hyponatremia into decreased, normal, and increased ECF volume.

Box 5-1 Calculation of Osmolality

Osmolality = 2[Na$^+$] + glucose/18 + BUN/2.8, where normal = 282 – 292 mOsm/KG.

Decreased ECF volume is due to renal or extrarenal losses of sodium such as sodium wasting nephropathies, hypoaldosteronism, diuretics, and vomiting. These losses are often replaced with hypotonic fluids. The decreased arterial volume can also contribute by stimulating thirst and vasopressin release and impairing the ability of the kidneys to excrete a dilute urine. Diuretics and vomiting can also result in a large potassium loss which through transcellular ion exchange causes further hyponatremia. A $U_{Na+} > 20$ mmol/l in the face of a hyponatremic, hypovolemic state suggests a renal cause, while $U_{Na+} < 10$ mmol/l is consistent with extrarenal losses.

Normal ECF volume can present with SIADH which is the most common cause of normovolemic hyponatremia. It is associated with an impaired excretion of renal free water due to nonphysiologic release of antidiuretic hormone (ADH) or vasopressin. Malignant tumors, pulmonary diseases, central nervous system (CNS) disorders, and drugs are causes of SIADH. It is characterized by (1) hypo-osmotic, hyponatremia, (2) euvolemia, (3) no renal, adrenal thyroid dysfunction, or diuretic use, (4) $U_{Na+} > 20$ mmol/l, and (5) a less than maximally dilute urine UOSM > 300 mOsm/l. These patients are treated with water restriction, democycline, and treatment of underlying disorders. Other causes not related to SIADH are glucocorticoid deficiency, hypothyroidism, chronic renal failure, drugs, and primary polydipsia.

Increased ECF volume tends to have an increased total body sodium, but there is a much larger increase in total body water. It is usually a consequence of conditions associated with edema, congestive heart failure (CHF), cirrhosis, nephrotic syndrome, and acute renal failure. These conditions result in a decrease in arterial blood volume, which leads to increased thirst and vasopressin levels. Diagnosis is made by a $U_{Na+} \leq 20$ mmol/l for CHF and cirrhosis, and $U_{Na+} > 20$ mmol/l for acute renal failure.

Normo-osmolar hyponatremia is commonly due to a pseudohyponatremia resulting from hyperlipidemia and hyperproteinemia. Plasma is composed of water and nonaqueous plasma proteins and lipid. If proteins or lipids are elevated, the sodium concentration measured is less than its true concentration. These patients have both a normal plasma sodium and plasma osmolality. Elevations in solutes other than sodium, like glucose and mannitol, can also result in a similar picture.

Hyperosmolar hyponatremia is usually due to increases in nonsodium solutes that remain mostly in the ECF. Hyperglycemia and mannitol use are common causes of this condition. The sodium in hyperglycemia is corrected by adding 1.6 mmol/l to the sodium for every 100 mg/dl rise in glucose. Other solutes such as ethanol, methanol, and ethylene glycol which occur from intoxications may also be implicated.

CLINICAL CAVEAT

Hyponatremia
Hypo-osmolar: most common – sodium loss or primary water gain
- Decreased ECF – nephropathies, hypoaldosteronism, diuretics, and vomiting
- Normal ECF – SIADH, steroids, hypothyroidism, CRF, drugs, and primary polydipsia
- Increased ECF – CHF, cirrhosis, nephritic syndrome, and ARF

Normo-osmolar: most commonly pseudohyponatremia
- Hyperlipidemia and hyperproteinemia

Hyperosmolar: excess nonsodium solutes
- Hyperglycemia and mannitol

Treatment of hyponatremia depends on the sodium concentration, symptoms, and the ECF volume status. Mild asymptomatic hyponatremia requires no treatment. Patients with underlying chronic hyponatremia that have mild symptoms are treated gently with the goal of returning sodium levels to 125 mEq/l. Those patients with stupor, seizures, and coma, however, are treated aggressively with 3% NS in order to reach a sodium goal of 125–130 mEq/l. This must not be done too rapidly because of the risk of an osmotic demyelination syndrome called central pontine demyelination (CPM). These patients may develop flaccid paralysis, dysarthria, and dysphagia. The diagnosis is confirmed by magnetic resonance imaging (MRI). To avoid this one does not correct sodium at greater than 0.5 mEq/l/hour and one corrects to a sodium of 125–130 mEq/l. Mild symptomatic hyponatremia is treated with NS and occasionally 3% NS, while avoiding too rapid a correction. Patients with normal ECF volume may have pseudohyponatremia and not require treatment. Those with mild symptoms are treated with furosemide diuresis or isotonic saline.

In patients with increased ECF volume, fluid restriction and hypertonic saline are useful. Fluid restriction is particularly useful in patients with SIADH, renal failure, or primary polydipsia.

Hypernatremia

Hypernatremia is defined as a $[Na^+] > 145$ mEq/l. Symptoms and signs are typically seen with levels > 150 mEq/l. Neurologically these patients may present at first with neuromuscular irritability, ataxia, lethargy and progress to confusion, coma, and seizures as the sodium approaches 180 mEq/l. They may complain of increased thirst and have evidence of hypovolemia. They may have evidence of decreased urinary concentrating ability, renal insufficiency, and occasionally progress to acute renal failure.

Hypernatremia is typically caused by either a water loss or a primary sodium gain. Hypernatremia due to water losses is due to either renal or nonrenal causes. Renal losses are the most common and are either from diabetes insipidus or osmotic diuresis. Nonrenal losses are from the gastrointestinal (GI) tract and from insensible losses. Hypernatremia due to sodium gain occurs much less frequently. Hypertonic saline, sodium bicarbonate, and iatrogenic causes of sodium administration account for the majority of these patients. Less commonly hypernatremia can occur because of a decreased ability to take in PO fluids. Infants, patients with an altered mental status, and intubated patients may develop hypernatremia.

The treatment of hypernatremia requires the assessment of water deficit and ECF volume status. Box 5-2 presents the calculation for water deficit. Although useful in initiating therapy, this assessment tends to underestimate the free water loss in those patients with hypotonic fluid losses. Half the deficit is replaced over the first 24 hours and the remainder over the next 24–48 hours. Overly rapid correction of $[Na^+]$, however, can result in seizures, coma, and brain edema. Therefore a reasonable goal should be to limit the decline in $[Na^+]$ to 1–2 mEq/l/hour.

The specific therapy will depend on ECF volume status. Hypovolemic patients should be treated first with volume resuscitation using NS. The hypernatremia can subsequently be corrected with hypotonic fluid administration either PO or intravenously. Euvolemic patients are treated with hypotonic fluids to replace water deficits. This group also includes those with DI. Specific treatment using DDAVP along with water deficit replacement is used for central DI. In nephrogenic DI the concentrating defect may be reversed by removing the offending drug, restricting sodium and water intake, and administering thiazides. This strategy results in increased fluid reabsorption in the proximal tubules by decreasing ECF volume. Hypervolemic patients are sodium overloaded. They respond to increasing sodium excretion with loop diuretics and replacement of water deficit with hypotonic fluids.

POTASSIUM DERANGEMENTS

Potassium is the major intracellular cation. While normal plasma potassium is 3.5–5.0 mEq/l, normal intracellular concentration is 150 mEq/l. The concentration gradient between ICF and ECF is kept fairly constant. Since the ICF volume is much greater than ECF volume, the vast majority of potassium stores are intracellular. Therefore plasma potassium is a poor indicator of total potassium stores. Potassium concentrations are maintained by the Na-K-ATPase pump, which actively transports potassium into the cell and sodium out of the cell. It is the quantitative passive diffusion of potassium out of the cell that helps establish a resting membrane potential and generates action potentials. Therefore keeping potassium concentrations within normal range is important for the proper functioning of skeletal and smooth muscle, and for CNS function.

CLINICAL CAVEAT

Potassium
- An intracellular cation – serum levels do not reflect stores
- Requires repeated dosing to correct low levels

Hypokalemia

Symptoms and signs include myalgias, fatigue, ileus, constipation, and weakness which can progress to paralysis in severe cases. EKG changes with T-wave flattening,

---

Box 5-2   Calculation of Free Water Deficit

Free water deficit (liters) = (TBW) × [(plasma $[Na^+]$ − 140)/140], where TBW = 0.6 × BW in kilograms.

U waves, ST-segment depression; and cardiac arrhythmias such as APCs, PVCs, ventricular tachycardia, and ventricular fibrillation can occur. Severe hypokalemia can also result in decreased renal concentrating activity with polyuria and development of alkalosis.

Hypokalemia results from either a shift of potassium into the cells or by potassium depletion. The shifts can occur due to the increased activity of Na-K-ATPase pump by β-agonists, insulin, carbohydrate loading, or by alkalosis which causes a potassium–hydrogen exchange across the cellular membrane. Potassium depletion is due predominantly to renal losses but extrarenal losses can occur. Renal losses have $U_{K+} > 30$ mEq/l. They can be categorized on the basis of their acid–base status. They can have a serum bicarbonate less than 24 mEq/l such as in patients with renal tubular acidosis type I (distal) and type II (proximal). Others with metabolic acidosis include patients with diarrhea, chronic laxative abuse, and diabetic ketoacidosis (DKA). Patients with serum bicarbonate greater than 24 mEq/l can be differentiated by their urine [Cl$^+$] levels. For those with [Cl$^+$] > 10 mEq/l the etiology may be due to diuretics, hyperaldosteronism, steroids, and low magnesium levels. Cases with [Cl$^+$] < 10 mEq/l are caused by vomiting, nasogastric suctioning, and hyperventilation. Extrarenal causes of potassium depletion include diarrhea, villous adenoma, vasoactive intestinal peptide tumors, chronic laxative abuse, and profuse sweating. Inadequate intake of potassium by itself is rarely a cause of hypokalemia because the kidneys can effectively reduce potassium excretion.

The treatment depends on the potassium level and the clinical picture. Although a serum potassium level greater than 3.5 mEq/l is considered normal, one aims for a level of 4.0 mEq/l in the critically ill patient. A [K$^+$] of 3.0 mEq/l in a patient with a normal acid–base status correlates with a 200–400 mEq deficit. For nonlife-threatening hypokalemia oral KCl is given at 10–40 mEq PO qd to bid depending on the level. In patients who are critically ill or who are not eating, KCl IV at 10 mEq/l peripherally or 20 mEq/l centrally is administered at a rate no more than 10–20 mEq/hour to avoid hyperkalemic complications. If more rapid replacement is required because of very low plasma levels and signs of hypokalemia, continuous EKG monitoring and frequent [K$^+$] checks should be used. One should avoid glucose-containing solutions, insulin, β-agonists, and other agents that may shift potassium intracellularly. The underlying cause of hypokalemia should be diagnosed and treated. Potassium-sparing diuretics should be considered for those with continuing losses.

Hyperkalemia

Hyperkalemia is typically defined as a [K$^+$] > 5.0 mEq/l, although patients are generally asymptomatic at [K$^+$] < 6.0 mEq/l. EKG changes and cardiac arrhythmias account for the most severe presentations. When the plasma potassium is above 6.0 mEq/l the patient's EKG begins to show tall narrow T waves, blunted P waves, prolonged PR intervals, which progress until the P wave disappears and eventually QRS widening and cardiac asystole. Neuromuscular symptoms and signs can occur at plasma levels of [K$^+$] around 7.0 mEq/l, with proximal muscle weakness, flaccid paralysis, and even respiratory failure occurring in severe cases.

Hyperkalemia can result from pseudohyperkalemia due to hemolysis during venipuncture, prolonged tourniquet use, and marked leukocytosis. Hyperkalemia can also occur due to redistribution of potassium from ICF to ECF and increased total body potassium stores. Redistribution of potassium is seen in acidosis, hypoinsulinemia, and digoxin toxicity. Destruction of cellular membranes due to rhabdomyolysis and hemolysis also results in the release of potassium into the ECF. Reduced renal excretion and exogenous administration account for the rest of the causes. Reduced renal excretion occurs in severe renal failure with a GFR less than 10 ml/min, adrenal insufficiency, potassium-sparing diuretics, angiotensin-converting enzyme (ACE) inhibitors, and nonsteroidal anti-inflammatory drugs (NSAIDs). These patients have a reduced urine [K$^+$] < 30 mEq/l. Exogenous causes include diets rich in potassium, iatrogenic administration and blood transfusions. These patients have urine [K$^+$] > 30 mEq/l.

DRUG INTERACTIONS

Exogenous Potassium
- Examine closely medication list for exogenous sources of potassium
- Do not forget diet as a contributor

Treatment depends on the level. Removal of all exogenous causes is the first step in mild hyperkalemia. Kayexelate (polystyrene sulfonate), a cation-exchange resin, removes potassium through the GI tract and is given as 30 g in 100 cm³ 20% sorbitol every 3 to 4 hours orally or 50 g in 200 cm³ 20% sorbitol as a retention enema. Lasix by enhancing renal excretion is also useful. Life-threatening cases, however, require more aggressive therapy. Treatment to minimize membrane repolarization, to decrease quickly plasma potassium levels, and to decrease total body stores needs to be instituted. Calcium gluconate 10% at 10 cm³ over 3 minutes is given to antagonize membrane hyperexcitability. Glucose as 50 cm³ D50 and regular insulin at 10 units is given to promote an intracellular shift of potassium. This effect lasts approximately 15 to 30 minutes and can be repeated.

Sodium bicarbonate by alkalinizing the plasma will also cause a transcellular shift and is given either as one 50 cm³ ampule over 5 minutes and repeated in 10 minutes as needed, or as a drip by placing 3 ampules in 1 liter of D₅W. Patients with chronic renal failure respond poorly to this intervention. Nebulized albuterol at 2.5 mg can also be used and lasts approximately 2 to 4 hours. Care in patients with tachycardia needs to be observed. Decrease in potassium stores, however, does not occur unless kayexelate and lasix are used. Hemodialysis which removes 70-150mEq of potassium is usually reserved for very severe cases which are complicated by unresponsiveness to treatment, volume overload, and acidosis.

CALCIUM DERANGEMENTS

Normal total serum calcium in plasma is 8.5-10.2 mg/dl, while normal ionized calcium is 4.8-7.2 mg/dl or 1.1-1.3 mmol/l. Ionized calcium is the physiologically active form of calcium. The total serum calcium as commonly measured is not. Therefore ionized calcium should be measured instead. Total serum calcium is dependent on albumin level, acid-base status, and chelators. A low total serum calcium, which commonly occurs in critically ill patients due to a low albumin, is generally associated with a normal ionized calcium level. These patients may not truly be hypocalcemic. If ionized calcium cannot be measured, the total serum calcium is often adjusted upward by 0.8 mg/dl for every 1 mg/dl decrease in albumin below 4.0 mg/dl. Calcium is responsible for normal neuromuscular function and bone formation. Alterations in calcium levels will affect normal muscle, cardiac, respiratory, neurologic, and psychiatric function.

CLINICAL CAVEAT

Calcium
- Ionized calcium is a more accurate measure of calcium homeostasis
- Ionized calcium is the physiologically active form of calcium
- Ionized calcium is affected by albumin level, acid-base status, and chelators

---

Hypocalcemia

Manifestations of hypocalcemia include neuromuscular excitability such as paresthesia, cramps, hyperreflexia, spasms, tetany, and Chvostek's and Trousseau's signs; cardiovascular signs such as peripheral vasodilatation, hypotension, ventricular tachycardia, and prolonged QT interval; respiratory signs including laryngospasm and apnea; and psychiatric presentations with anxiety, irritability, and depression.

The causes of hypocalcemia are varied. Decreased parathyroid hormone (PTH) secretion due to hypoparathyroidism, hypomagnesemia, hypermagnesemia, or surgical damage can result in hypocalcemia. Hypocalcemia will occur 24-36 hours postoperatively following surgery on the parathyroid glands and on the thyroid gland if all four parathyroid glands are removed. Alkalosis which results in increased calcium binding to albumin can cause a precipitous fall in plasma calcium. Massive blood transfusions, especially in patients with hepatic and renal failure where citrate clearance is reduced, can develop hemodynamically significant hypocalcemia due to the chelation effect of citrate. Other causes include reduced intestinal absorption of calcium from vitamin D deficiency, renal insufficiency, hyperphosphatemia, and liver disease; drugs such as lasix and aminoglycosides; sepsis; and pancreatitis.

Aggressive treatment should be limited to ionized calcium levels below 0.8 mmol/l or to symptomatic patients. Replacement should be initiated with 1 amp IV calcium chloride and continued with an IV infusion to keep the level between 0.8 and 1.0 mmol/l. A drip at 1 mg/kg/hour can be used to keep levels replaced as calcium diffuses into tissues and is eliminated in the urine. Special attention needs to be given to certain conditions. For instance rhabdomyolysis and tumor lysis syndrome can result in a hyperphosphatemic hypocalcemia. Treating these patients with calcium may cause calcium precipitation, which can lead to organ injury. These patients are treated by lowering phosphorus levels. This can be accomplished with phosphorus binders, dialysis, and diuresis. Severe hypomagnesemia can inhibit PTH production and action. Replacement of magnesium generally corrects the ionized calcium level by stimulating PTH secretion.

DRUG INTERACTIONS

Calcium
- Rhabdomyolysis and tumor lysis syndrome can result in hyperphosphatemic hypocalcemia
- Treatment with calcium may cause calcium precipitation with organ injury
- Treat by lowering phosphorus with phosphorus binders, dialysis, and diuresis

---

Hypercalcemia

The signs and symptoms of hypercalcemia are often described by the constellation of symptoms referred to as "bones, stones, psychic moans, and abdominal groans." The symptoms and signs include weakness, hypotonia, hyporeflexia, and seizures; confusion, psychosis, and coma; anorexia, vomiting, and constipation; polyuria and nephrocalcinosis; fractures, osteopenia, and ectopic calcification; hypovolemia and hypotension; and QT shortening, cardiac arrhythmias, and heart block. Causes of hypercalcemia include primary hyperparathyroidism, the most common cause in outpatient setting. However, malignancies such as squamous cell cancer of the lung, head and neck tumors, metastatic disease from breast cancer, multiple myeloma, and lymphoma are the most common in hospitalized patients. Other etiologies include sarcoidosis, hyperthyroidism, immobilization, thiazide diuretics, aluminum intoxification in renal failure patients, and vitamin A and D intoxication.

CLINICAL CAVEAT

Hypercalcemia
- "Bones, stones, psychic moans, and abdominal groans"
- Hyperparathyroidism most common cause in outpatient setting
- Malignancies most common cause in hospitalized patients

Hypercalcemia is defined as a $[Ca^+] > 1.3$ mmol/l, or serum calcium level > 10.5 mg/dl. Patients are asymptomatic or with mild symptoms until the serum calcium levels are above 11.5 mg/dl. Moderate symptoms then occur with the more severe presentations occurring at levels of greater than 13 mg/dl. Management requires efforts to lower directly the calcium and treatment of the underlying disease. Drugs that may elevate calcium levels are removed. Normal saline at 250-500 cm³/hour is given to correct volume depletion, dilute the ionized calcium, and inhibit calcium reabsorption by increasing sodium excretion by the kidneys. After volume replacement is complete, a loop diuretic such as furosemide 40-100 mg IV every 2 hours is given to further enhance calcium excretion. Calcitonin, 4-8 IU/kg IM or SC q12 hours × 2, inhibits bone resorption and increases calcium excretion. It is most effective in patients with increased bone resorption. It begins to lower calcium within 2 hours, with a peak effect at 6 to 10 hours. Due to tachyphylaxis it lasts only a few days. An added benefit appears to be its potent analgesic activity in patients with bone metastasis. It is associated with allergic reactions and skin testing should be done before its use. Pamidronate, a biphosphonate, is used at 60 mg IV over 4 hours for mild cases of hypercalcemia and 90 mg IV over 24 hours for severe cases. Bone resorption is decreased because of its inhibitory effect on osteoclasts. Another biphosphonate, etidronate disodium, 7.5 mg/kg over 4 hours for 3-7 days, is also useful. Its use is limited because of diarrhea and nephrotoxicity. Mithramycin (Plicamycin),

25 μg/kg over 6 hours, is a cytotoxic agent that inhibits bone resorption. Due to its side effects of thrombocytopenia, coagulopathy, and hepatic and renal failure it is rarely used.

Hydrocortisone, 200-300 mg qd for 3 days, lowers plasma calcium by lowering cytokine release, inhibiting intestinal reabsorption, and increasing urinary calcium excretion. It is particularly effective in patients with lymphatic malignancies, multiple myeloma, granulomas, and vitamin D intoxication. Hyperparathyroidism and other tumors causing metastasis rarely respond. Phosphorus administration with Neutraphos at 0.5-1.0 g bid to qid may be useful because it inhibits calcium absorption and increases calcium deposition in bone. Use should be limited to patients with low phosphate levels because of the potential for soft tissue calcification. Dialysis can be done as a last resort prior to surgery. In patients with hyperparathyroidism due to an adenoma or hyperplastic thyroid tissue surgical removal is undertaken. Malignancies may require chemotherapy, radiation therapy, and surgery.

MAGNESIUM DERANGEMENTS

Magnesium is important for neuromuscular function, cardiac conduction, and many metabolic pathways. The physiologically active form of magnesium is ionized and normal levels are generally expressed as 1.6-2.6 mEq/l. In the critically ill patient, however, the goal for replacement is 2.0 mEq/l. Only 1% of total magnesium stores are in the ECF, the majority is in bone, muscles, and cells. Serum magnesium levels are therefore a poor reflection of total body stores.

Hypomagnesemia

Hypomagnesemia can present with neurologic manifestations such as parathesias, fasciculations, spasms, tetany, hyperreflexia, and seizures; cardiac signs such as APCs, PVCs, prolonged PR and QT intervals, atrial fibrillation, SVTs, and ventricular arrhythmias including torsades de pointes; CNS symptoms such as confusion, ataxia, and coma; and metabolic abnormalities such as refractory hypokalemia and hypocalcemia. Digoxin toxicity is exacerbated by hypomagnesemia.

CLINICAL CAVEAT

Magnesium
- Serum magnesium is a poor indicator of total body stores
- Optimal level in critically ill patients is 2.0 mEq/l
- Check $[Mg^+]$ and $[K^+]$ in the critically ill patient with arrhythmias
- Consider digoxin toxicity with arrhythmias

Etiologies are decreased intestinal absorption or increased renal excretion. Malabsorption, malnutrition, alcoholism, diarrhea, and gastric aspiration are common for decreased absorption. Renal losses result from osmotic diuresis, hypercalcemia, aminoglycosides, amphotericin B, and cyclosporin.

Treatment depends on the level and clinical signs. Because magnesium is essentially only eliminated by the kidneys, replacement in patients with renal insufficiency is done carefully. Chronic or mild hypomagnesemia is treated with magnesium oxide, 400 mg PO qid to bid. Magnesium sulfate IV is used in critically ill patients with symptoms or low levels. One gram of magnesium sulfate is approximately 4 mmol or 8.0 mEq of elemental magnesium. Generally 2 g are given over 1 hour and repeated several times depending on the level. Severe hypomagnesemia with serum levels less than 1.0 mEq/l can be treated with magnesium sulfate, 2 g IV over 30 minutes, followed by 6 g in 250 cm^3 NS over 6 hours. In life-threatening hypomagnesemia with seizures and arrhythmias, 2 g IV over 2 minutes is given, and followed with 6 g in 250 cm^3 NS infused over 3 hours. These patients will require further aggressive replacement over the next several days due to the large body deficits.

Hypermagnesemia

The manifestations of hypermagnesemia occur when serum magnesium is greater than 4 mEq/l. Neurologic and cardiac dysfunction predominates. Weakness, lethargy, and paralysis can occur, with progressive areflexia often present as the magnesium concentration increases. Cardiac signs include hypotension, bradycardia, prolonged PR, QRS, and QT, complete heart block, and asystole. The loss of tendon reflexes occurs as the level approaches 6 mEq/l, with respiratory paralysis at 12-15 mEq/l, then cardiac block and subsequently cardiac arrest at levels above 15 mEq/l.

The causes are few, because any excess magnesium is rapidly excreted by the kidneys. Acute renal insufficiency or renal failure especially when combined with magnesium-containing antacids, laxatives, and IV magnesium is the most common cause of hypermagnesemia. It can occur with the large amounts of exogenous magnesium used in patients with pre-eclampsia and eclampsia. Patients with rhabdomyolysis and hemolysis can also develop hypermagnesemia.

Treatment involves eliminating exogenous administration, antagonizing the chemical-electrical effects, and removing magnesium from the body. Calcium gluconate 10%, 10-20 cm^3 IV (1-2 g) over 10 minutes, temporarily antagonizes the effects. If renal function is not impaired severely and the patient makes urine, excretion of magnesium can be enhanced by providing 2 g of calcium gluconate 10% in 1 liter NS at 150-200 cm^3/hour.

Elimination of magnesium may require hemodialysis in patients with acute renal failure. Supportive care with mechanical ventilation or temporary pacemaker may be needed.

PHOSPHORUS

Phosphorus is important for cellular energy metabolism, the maintenance of acid-base balance, and bone formation. It is difficult to assess exactly the ion concentration and so it is measured in mg/dl with a normal range of 2.5-4.5 mg/dl. Bone accounts for 85% of total body stores, followed by cells with 14% and ECF at 1%. Serum phosphorus levels like potassium and magnesium are poor indicators of total deficit.

Hypophosphatemia

Symptoms and signs do not usually present unless the level is less than 1.0 mg/dl. There can be muscular, respiratory, cardiac, neurologic, hematologic, and bone involvement. Patients may complain of weakness; develop impaired diaphragmatic function, and respiratory and cardiac failure; progress to rhabdomyolysis; manifest confusion, stupor, and seizures; show hemolysis and thrombocytopenia; and develop osteomalacia and rickets.

Hypophosphatemia results from decreased intestinal absorption, increased urinary excretion, and redistribution into the intracellular space. Decreased absorption is seen in malabsorption, malnutrition, starvation, and administration of phosphate binders. Increased urinary excretion can result from hyperparathyroidism, diuretics, polyuric phase of ATN, postobstructive diuresis, DKA, RTAs, and renal transplantation. Redistribution occurs with glucose, insulin, β-agonists, respiratory alkalosis, alcohol withdrawal, and recovery phase of starvation. Patients with aggressive overfeeding poststarvation, alcohol abuse and withdrawal, hyperalimentation, DKA, and burns are at high risk for very low phosphate levels of less than 1.0 mg/dl.

Treatment depends on the level and clinical picture. Mild hypophosphatemia, in healthy patients tolerating PO, can be replaced with Neutraphos, 250-500 mg PO q 6 hours. In moderate hypophosphatemia, 1.0-2.0 mg/dl, elemental phosphate 0.08-0.16 mmol/kg in 100 NS IV over 6 hours can be used safely. Elemental phosphate comes as potassium phosphate which contains 3 mmol PO$_4$ with 4.4 mEq potassium per cm^3, and sodium phosphate which is 3 mmol PO$_4$ with 4 mEq sodium per cm^3. Severe hypophosphatemia is treated aggressively with elemental phosphate, 0.16-0.25 mmol/kg over 4-8 hours. Continued phosphate replacement will be required for several days due to depleted phosphate stores. Hypomagnesemia and hypokalemia often occur concurrently and must be addressed. Extreme care should be taken in treating patients with DKA, as the level often improves significantly with treatment of acidosis.

Hyperphosphatemia

Patients are generally asymptomatic until the level is >5.0 mg/dl. The clinical picture is due to hypocalcemia and ectopic calcification. Ectopic calcification occurs as the calcium × phosphorus product goes over 60. Heart block is a life-threatening complication for which one should monitor.

A common etiology is renal failure, but it also occurs due to cellular damage caused by trauma, acidosis, rhabdomyolysis, and tumor lysis syndrome. Hypoparathyroidism and exogenous phosphate syndrome are also frequently implicated as causes of hyperphosphatemia.

Management requires eliminating the cause; restricting dietary phosphate; increasing urinary excretion with normal saline and acetazolamide, 500 mg q 6 hours; and increasing GI losses with phosphate binders such as aluminum hydroxide, 30–45 cm³ q 6 hours. Patients with renal failure or ectopic calcification will benefit from dialysis. Associated hypocalcemia may also need to be treated, but care must be taken to keep the calcium × phosphorus product less than 60.

THERMAL DERANGEMENTS

Maintaining a normal body temperature despite environmental variations creates a stable milieu for the hundreds of heat-sensitive enzymes to function and to maintain homeostasis within normal ranges. There exists a 24-hour circadian temperature rhythm with a morning nadir and an afternoon peak that can be as much as 0.5–1°C. In ovulating women there is an additional increase in the baseline body temperature of approximately 0.5°C in the second half of the menstruating cycle. Other physiologic states that can affect baseline temperatures are postprandial state, pregnancy, and age.

HYPERTHERMIA

Hyperthermia describes the state when body temperature is above normal. Normothermia is generally accepted to exist between 36 and 37.5°C measured at the body surface. When an elevated body temperature exists because of a change that occurs in the thermoregulatory center at the anterior hypothalamus we talk about fever. Substances that cause fever are called pyrogens. Pyrogens can be further divided to endogenous and exogenous pyrogens.

When the elevation in the body temperature occurs without alteration in the hypothalamic set point we talk about hyperthermia. In this case the underlying process is either excessive heat production or inadequate heat dissipation or both. Hyperthermic syndromes include heat stroke and endocrinopathies, which are described elsewhere, and the drug-induced hyperthermias. The drug-induced hyperthermias are malignant hyperthermia, neuroleptic malignant syndrome, serotonin syndrome, sympathomimetic poisoning syndrome, and anticholinergic syndrome.

Heat Stroke

Heat stroke is an acute breakdown of the body's thermoregulatory mechanism in warm environments resulting in severe hyperthermia with core temperatures >40°C. There are actually two forms of heat stroke. Exertional heat stroke occurs typically in young individuals who engage in strenuous physical activity for a prolonged period in a hot environment, while classic nonexertional heat stroke occurs in sedentary elderly individuals, in persons who are chronically ill, and in the very young. This latter form is more prevalent during environmental heat waves. Both types are associated with high morbidity and mortality especially when diagnosis is delayed.

Increased heat production, impaired heat loss, and decreased ability to sweat effectively are important in the pathogenesis of the syndrome. High-risk groups include the elderly, patients with schizophrenia, Parkinson's disease, alcoholics, and paraplegics and quadriplegics. The pathophysiology involves muscle degeneration and necrosis resulting in rhabdomyolysis; increased cardiac output, with decreased systemic vascular resistance; direct thermal injury to brain and spinal cord resulting in edema and hemorrhage; acute renal failure due to dehydration and myoglobinuria; hepatic necrosis leading to death; coagulopathy; and multiple electrolyte abnormalities. The diagnostic criteria include a compatible history, core temperature >40°C, anhidrosis, elevated creatine kinase level, and depressed mental status.

Treatment with aggressive cooling is initiated by using evaporative cooling techniques such as wetting skin, cool water spray, and electric fans; direct careful external cooling by ice packs or cold water immersion; and occasionally when very severe hyperthermia is present by performing gastric lavage or peritoneal lavage with iced saline, or even hemodialysis. Aggressive hemodynamic monitoring and supportive care is instituted in an intensive care unit (ICU). Hypotension is common and is treated with warm IV fluids initially.

Dopaminergic and alpha agents should be avoided because they may enhance vasoconstriction and instead

CURRENT CONTROVERSY

Cooling Blankets

Traditionally cooling is initiated with cooling blankets; however, aside from inefficiency these blankets may cause localized areas of hypothermic injury. Evaporative cooling techniques using misted cool water spray with fans are more effective.

isoproterenol should be used if needed. Seizures are common and are treated with benzodiazepines. Liver failure and DIC may occur and are poor prognosticators.

DRUG-INDUCED HYPERTHERMIAS

Malignant Hyperthermia

Malignant hyperthermia (MH) is a life-threatening emergency with very high mortality rate if left undiagnosed. It has an autosomal dominant hereditary basis with reduced penetrance. Its prevalence is estimated to be 1 in 15,000 children and 1 in 50,000–100,000 adults treated with anesthetics. The suspected derangement is related to abnormal ryanodine receptors on the T tubules of the striated muscles. To date more than 20 different mutations of the ryanodine receptor have been reported worldwide.

In individuals susceptible to develop MH an increased and exaggerated calcium response exists to volatile anesthetics and succinylcholine (triggering agents) which leads to increased muscle metabolism, rigidity, rhabdomyolysis, hyperthermia, and metabolic and respiratory acidosis, and eventually cardiovascular collapse develops rapidly if prompt treatment is delayed. This abnormal metabolic response does not necessarily occur after each exposure to the triggering agents.

Although the syndrome's name carries the hyperthermia term, the elevated body temperature tends to be a relatively late sign preceded by increased carbon dioxide production and tachycardia. Prevention is based upon previous anesthetic and family history, but one needs to keep in mind that negative history for both of those does not exclude the future possibility of an MH event. The gold standard treatment consists of immediate cessation of any triggering agent still in use, hyperventilation with 100% oxygen, intravenous Dantrolene sodium, and intense supportive measures. Dantrolene is given at 2.5 mg/kg IV bolus q15 minutes up to a total dose of 10 mg/kg. A maintenance dose is continued at 1–2 mg/kg PO for 3 days. Intense supportive measures include close hemodynamic and acid–base balance monitoring, mechanical ventilation to correct respiratory acidosis, forced diuresis with alkalinization of the urine to prevent renal damage secondary to myoglobinuria, and cooling the patient. Getting in contact with the North American MH Group and the MH Association of the US provides not only up-to-date information for the practitioner but supplies data for these organizations for epidemiologic purposes. Definitive diagnosis of MH can be established on the results of caffeine-halothane contracture testing of fresh muscle biopsy samples taken from the suspected individual.

CLINICAL CAVEAT

Malignant Hyperthermia

- Autosomal dominant distribution with reduced penetrance
- Triggering agents are succinylcholine and inhalation agents
- Multiple exposures may occur before clinical presentation
- Tachycardia and increased CO_2 production occur before hyperthermia
- Rapid recognition is crucial
- Treatment requires immediate Dantrolene and supportive care
- MH hotline number 1-800-MH-HYPER (800-644-9737)

Neuroleptic Malignant Syndrome

Neuroleptic malignant syndrome (NMS) is a potentially life-threatening idiosyncratic reaction, resulting from the blockade of central dopamine receptors. Although the blockade may cause a disruption of the thermoregulatory role of the hypothalamus, it is the generalized muscle activity and rigidity that are thought to be the main contributors to the hyperthermia. Antipsychotic agents, especially Haldol, are generally implicated. A history of rapid upward titration or depot preparations is common. Other associated predisposing factors are a prior episode of NMS, organic brain syndrome, psychomotor agitation, and dehydration.

Although there are no widely accepted criteria for diagnosing NMS, there is a characteristic presentation. Most patients present within 30 days of initiating therapy. The initial presentation is of a psychiatric patient with an altered mental status, who is found to have fever and muscle rigidity. The constellation of signs and symptoms typically develop over 24 to 72 hours. Hyperthermia which is not universal can range between 38 and 42°C. Patients develop a generalized "lead-pipe" muscle rigidity which may result in involvement of the chest wall muscles. Motor abnormalities that are typical of parkinsonian-type extrapyradimal reactions occur. Autonomic instability with hypotension, hypertension, diaphoresis, bladder and bowel incontinence, and nausea and vomiting are frequently seen. Laboratory tests are generally nonspecific and reflect organ involvement. Elevations in creatine kinase due to rhabdomyolysis from hyperthermia and muscle rigidity, elevations in blood urea nitrogen and creatinine due to pre-renal azotemia and myoglobinuria, leukocytosis from the stress response, and multiple electrolyte and acid–base abnormalities are frequently seen.

Treatment includes discontinuation of the neuroleptic agent. General measures to lower body temperature such as removal of excess clothing and cool water spray with air circulation should start immediately. In mild cases supportive care may be sufficient. In moderate to severe NMS aggressive monitoring and support in an ICU setting is necessary. Dantrolene which reduces thermogenesis by reducing muscle contraction is given at 1.0–2.5 mg/kg IV q6 hours until a dose of 100–300 mg/day PO can be given. Neuromuscular blockade may be useful initially to reduce the metabolic rate and muscle contraction. Specific drug therapy to lower core temperature and reduce extrapyramidal side effects is initiated. Dopamine agonists such as bromocryptine, amantadine, and levo-carbidopa combination are recommended. Bromocryptine 5–20 mg/day given in divided doses has been shown to decrease the course of NMS. It is continued at 2.5 mg PO tid for 1 week or longer depending on the rate of elimination of the offending drug. Recurrence can occur if dopamine agonists are prematurely discontinued. Mean recovery time is approximately 9 days.

Serotonin Syndrome

Serotonin syndrome results from increased central serotonin receptor activity which produces a clinical picture of encephalopathy, neuromuscular hyperactivity, and autonomic dysfunction. Initially described in association with monoamine oxidase inhibitors, serotonin uptake inhibitors are more commonly implicated reflecting their increased use. It typically occurs from the use of two or more drugs with serotonergic activity, or from the overdose of a single agent. Increased serotonin synthesis from L-tryptophan; decreased metabolism of serotonin due to MAOIs; serotonin receptor agonists busripone, lithium, LSD; increased serotonin release caused by amphetamines, amphetamine derivatives, and cocaine; nonselective serotonin reuptake inhibitors like TCAs, cocaine, amphetamines, meperidine, dextromethorphan, and selective inhibitors such as sertaline, fluoxetine, and nefazodone are all mechanisms that can interact to cause a serotonin overload.

Signs and symptoms are acute, within 24 hours of a precipitating event. Altered sensorium with hyperactivity, agitation, delirium, and occasionally seizures occur.

Neuromuscular irritability is reflected mostly in the lower extremities with tremors, myoclonus, and muscle rigidity. The autonomic instability is characterized by diaphoresis, dilated reactive pupils, labile blood pressure, arrhythmias, and vomiting. Hyperthermia is common and can reach 40°C. Laboratory abnormalities are minimal and nonspecific, but in severe cases leukocytosis, metabolic acidosis, renal failure, rhabdomyolysis, and DIC may occur.

Treatment includes immediate withdrawal of the offending drug, aggressive supportive care and monitoring in an ICU, rapid cooling, and the use of benzodiazepines for the treatment of neuromuscular irritability. The serotonin antagonist cyproheptadine, at 4–8 mg repeated every 4 hours to a total daily dose of 32 mg, has been reported to shorten the course of serotonin syndrome. Methysergide, another nonspecific serotonin receptor blocker, has had mixed results. Fatalities do occur, but recovery is expected in most patients.

Sympathomimetic Poisoning Syndrome

Sympathomimetic poisoning syndrome results from an increase central sympathetic activity due to both therapeutic and recreational drugs. Over the counter cold remedies, appetite suppressants, and frequently abused drugs such as cocaine, amphetamines, LSD, and PCP are known causes. Increased ambient temperature is an associated predisposing factor.

Patients are usually referred to the emergency department because they are delirious, agitated, and combative. Tremors, hyperreflexia, rigidity, and occasionally seizures occur. On physical examination patients are diaphoretic with dilated but reactive pupils, and are hypertensive and tachycardic. Hyperthermia as a marker of moderate to severe poisoning is associated with many complications involving organ damage. Rhabdomyolysis, acute renal failure, metabolic acidosis, DIC, and liver failure similar to the other drug-induced hyperthermias may occur. The diagnosis is suggested in those patients with previous drug use and confirmed by a positive toxicology screen.

Treatment requires aggressive cooling including possibly neuromuscular blockade and benzodiazepines to treat delirium, agitation, and seizures. Nitroprusside or labetolol may be needed to treat the hypertensive manifestations of the syndrome. Aggressive monitoring and supportive care, including mechanical ventilation, may be needed for several days.

Anticholinergic Syndrome

Anticholinergic syndrome results from the blockade of central and peripheral muscarinic receptors. Many drugs including over the counter medications and some plants are known to precipitate this syndrome. Medications such as atropine, scopolamine, belladonna extracts, TCAs, oxybutynin, antihistamines including diphenhydramine and meclizine, phenothiazines, antiparkinsonian agents, and the antiarrhythmics quinidine, procanamide, and dispyramide can be causes of the syndrome.

Presentation is usually due to an altered fluctuating mental status. Patients can manifest a depressed sensorium including unresponsiveness and even coma, or an agitated, hyperactive, delirious state which may result in seizures. Dry mouth, dry skin, blurry vision with dilated unreactive or slightly reactive pupils, hypoactive bowel sounds, and hyperthermia characterize the syndrome. The hyperthermia is only seen in a quarter of patients, and can be mild to severe.

Treatment is mostly supportive. Aggressive cooling and monitoring are necessary. Physostigmine, an acetylcholinesterase inhibitor that increases the concentration of acetylcholine and overcomes the muscarinic block, is sometimes used. Physostigmine, however, is associated with serious adverse effects such as bradycardia, asystole, salivation, bronchorrhea, and seizures. Therefore it is reserved for severe cases presenting with seizures, severe delirium, cardiovascular collapse, or life-threatening hyperthermia in the absence of sweating. Physostigmine 1–4 mg IV is given slowly while monitoring the heart rate. The effect is quick, but lasts less than 60 minutes. The dose may need to be repeated.

HYPOTHERMIA

Hypothermia is characterized by a core body temperature < 35°C. It can be classified as mild hypothermia, 32–35°C; moderate hypothermia, 30–32°C, and severe, < 32°C. Predisposing factors are advanced age, exposure to cold, drug use (especially alcohol), trauma, CNS dysfunction, SCI, endocrine dysfunction, and iatrogenic causes. Signs and symptoms are characterized by a depressed level of consciousness. Mental status can range from stuporous or confused at temperatures < 35°C to coma when the temperature is < 27°C. Other physiologic affects of hypothermia include cardiac dysfunction with decreased cardiac output, bradycardia and cardiac irritability at < 33°C, ventricular fibrillation at < 28°C, and hypotension at < 25°C; hematologic abnormalities with coagulopathy, and decreased oxygen delivery; and endocrine dysfunction with decreased insulin release and insulin resistance.

Treatment with rewarming is initiated at 2°C/hour depending on the degree of hypothermia. Mild exposure requires passive external warming with blankets, clothing, and warm IV fluids. Moderate exposure requires active rewarming with hot blankets, circulating warm air blankets, and immersion in warm baths. Severe hypothermia requires active core rewarming with humidified warmed oxygen, gastric lavage, peritoneal or pleural lavage, and may include cardiopulmonary bypass. Cardiac medications are typically not effective. However, bretrylium for arrhythmias and dopamine for ionotropic support have been shown to be effective. Electrical defibrillation may be ineffective until the core temperature is >30°C. Although hypothermic patients may be brought into the emergency department without a blood pressure or rhythm, they cannot be pronounced dead until they are at 37°C.

PERIOPERATIVE HYPOTHERMIA

Anesthesia and surgery commonly cause substantial thermal perturbations. Hypothermia, the typical alteration, results from a combination of anesthetic-induced impairment of thermoregulatory control, a cool operating room environment, and factors unique to surgery that promote excessive heat loss. Hypothermia develops with a characteristic pattern. An initial decrease of the core temperature by 1–1.5°C over the first hour is followed by a slower linear decrease, which finally leads to a plateau phase during which the temperature remains constant. Data suggest much more hypothermia results from altered distribution of body heat rather than from a systemic imbalance between metabolic heat production and heat loss.

Since intra- and postoperative hypothermia carries many disadvantages (including increased blood loss secondary to impaired coagulation and reduced platelet function, myocardial ischemia secondary to the increased oxygen consumption associated with shivering, decreased drug metabolism, and of course patient discomfort), all patients should be protected from it. Patients especially susceptible to hypothermia are those in extremes of age.

In neurosurgical procedures, however, mild systemic hypothermia carries the advantage of cerebral protection due to decreased cerebral metabolic rate. This neuroprotective effect of decreased body temperature also seems to be useful at the initial resuscitation phase in closed head injured trauma patients as long as the degree of hypothermia does not jeopardize other vital functions.

SUMMARY

Metabolic abnormalities are extremely common in the critically ill patient. Maintaining electrolytes at normal levels is important for the proper functioning of the electrochemical reactions of the body. Failure to do so will result in abnormalities in neuromuscular, cardiac, and metabolic pathways. For instance, calcium and phosphorus which are very closely interrelated are important in neuromuscular function, cellular metabolism, maintenance of acid–base balance, and bone formation. A poor understanding of this relationship may result in the inappropriate replacement of calcium in the hyperphosphatemic, hypocalcemia patient, rather than the correct treatment with phosphate binders and cause

calcium precipitation with organ injury. Similarly hypothermia and hyperthermia require an appreciation of the interrelationship between the physiology and the pharmacologic actions of both recreational and therapeutic drugs. Recognizing the syndrome, avoiding inadvertent interactions, selecting medications to counter the deleterious effects, and aggressive supportive care are essential for proper care.

SELECTED READING

Boucharma A, Knochel J: Heat stroke. N Engl J Med 346:1978–1988, 2002.

Braunwald E et al: *Harrison's Principles of Internal Medicine*, ed 15, McGraw Hill, 2001.

Carbone JR: The neuroleptic malignant and serotonin syndromes. Emerg Med Clin North Am 18:317–325, 2000.

Goldman L et al: *Cecil Textbook of Medicine*, ed 21, W.B. Saunders, 2000.

Hopkins PM: Malignant hyperthermia: advances in clinical management and diagnosis. B J Anesth 85(1):118–128, 2000.

Longnecker D et al: *Principles and Practice of Anesthesiology*, ed 2, Mosby, 1998.

MacLennan DH: Ca^{2+} signalling and muscle disease. Eur J Biochem 267:5291–5297, 2000.

Murray M et al; ASCCA: *Critical Care Medicine: Perioperative Management*, ed 2, Lippincott Williams and Wilkins, 2002.

Sambuughin N: North American malignant hyperthermia population. Anesth 95:594–599, 2001.

Sessler DI: Perioperative heat balance. Anesth 92(2):578–596, 2000.

Simon HB: Hyperthermia. N Engl J Med 329:483–487, 1993.

CASE STUDY

An 18-year-old male is admitted to the ICU early Monday morning after being brought to the ER because of delirium, tremors and high fever. According to his girlfriend who called 911, he had returned late Sunday evening after attending a weekend concert with his friends. He is agitated, confused, hallucinating, tremulous, and notably hot to touch. On exam, his blood pressure is 199/115, heart rate 160 and regular, respiratory rate 30–40, and his temperature is 40°C. Since arrival to the ER 4 hours before, he has made 10 cc of dark colored urine, and his lab work has returned with a K 6.9 meq/l, HCO_3 12 meq/l, BUN 65 mg/dl, creatinine 2.6 mg/dl and a PO_4 of 9.9 mg/dl.

QUESTIONS

1. What further information would you like from his girlfriend?
2. What is your differential diagnosis?
3. How would you explain the signs and symptoms?
4. What is your initial treatment plan?
5. What are the potential pitfalls during treatment?

CHAPTER 6

Fluid, Electrolyte, Blood, and Blood Product Management

JAMES E. SZALADOS, M.D., J.D., M.B.A.

Physiologically, intravenous fluid administration serves two purposes: (1) to replete or maintain intravascular fluid volume and (2) to maintain or replete free water, electrolyte, blood component, or protein concentration derangements. Ultimately, the purpose of fluid volume administration is to maintain cardiac preload and cardiac output, oxygen delivery, and tissue perfusion to maintain cellular homeostasis.

Intravascular volume is essential to maintain cardiac filling volume. Diastolic tension and cardiac sarcomere "stretch" imposes a preload which directly affects the development of muscular tension in the ventricular chambers. Preload, measured directly as end-diastolic volume or indirectly as end-diastolic pressure, then determines cardiac function, measured as cardiac output or ejection fraction (Figure 6-1). Cardiac output is a key determinant of tissue and organ perfusion. Diminished organ perfusion is associated with decreased oxygen and nutrient delivery, removal of metabolic by-products, and in the case of the kidneys decreased filtration pressure and waste elimination in urine output. Tissue hypoperfusion, and even transient ischemia, triggers metabolic alterations such as a shift from oxidative phosphorylation to anaerobic glycolysis with ensuing lactate and hydrogen ion production, and alterations in cellular water, sodium, and calcium flux. Cellular metabolic alterations are the trigger for activation of the cellular and humoral inflammatory response which perpetuates the cycle of ischemia, cell death, tissue necrosis, and systemic inflammatory response.

The electrolytes, water, and protein content of body fluids are regulated within a narrow range; however

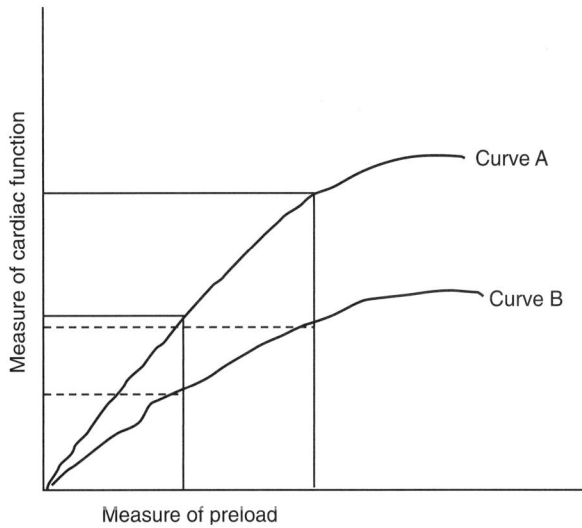

Figure 6-1 Starling curves.

physiologic and pathophysiologic processes result in continual transformation, redistribution, and loss of the various components. Under normal circumstances nutritional intake replenishes losses; the result is that the "homeostatic milieu" in which cells and tissues function is constant. Tissue perfusion with a nutrient-rich and electrolyte-balanced fluid to deliver fuel and extract waste is the basic function of body fluid.

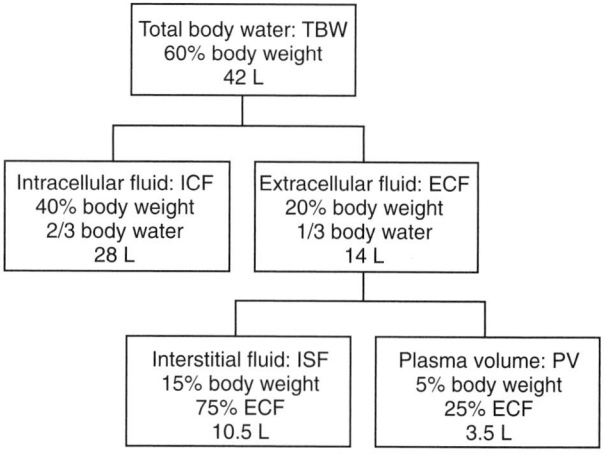

Figure 6-2   Distribution of body water.

body water and of body weight. The ECF is divided between blood volume (8% body weight), plasma (5% body weight), and interstitial fluid (ISF; 15% body weight). Intracellular fluid (ICF) comprises two-thirds of total body water and about 40% of body weight.

PEARLS

- Hypovolemia is decreased effective intravascular volume. Cardiac signs of hypovolemia are decreased preload (low CVP, pulmonary artery occlusion pressure, or diminished end-systolic ventricular chamber volumes on echocardiography), tachycardia, and decreased cardiac output (oliguria, vasoconstriction, acidosis, lactate accumulation, and altered mental status).
- The Starling curve depicts the effect of incremental changes in preload on cardiac function. See Figure 6-1.
- Decreased oxygen delivery to tissues resulting from diminished cardiac output defines the state known as "shock."
- Empiric therapy based on the clinical presentation may suffice; however, if there is no response or a continued deterioration, then invasive monitoring is necessary to determine intravascular volume and cardiac output, and to guide resuscitation.

NORMAL BODY FLUID AND ELECTROLYTE COMPOSITION (TABLE 6-1)

Fluid Compartments

Total body water is distributed across semipermeable membranes into fluid compartments as outlined in Figure 6-2.

For an average adult male, body weight is comprised of 60% water, 7% minerals, 18% protein, and 15% fat. Females have a slightly increased body fat content and a correspondingly decreased water content of 50%. Extracellular fluid (ECF) comprises one-third of total

---

PEARLS

- Total body water = $0.6 \times$ wt (kg) in males; and $0.5 \times$ wt (kg) in females
- Serum osmolarity = $(2 \times [Na]) + [glucose]/18 + [BUN]/2.8$. Normal serum osmolarity = 290 mOsm/kg H_2O.
- The fractional excretion of sodium (FEN) is extremely useful in the management of oliguria (FENa = $[Na_{Urine}/Na_{Serum}]/[Cr_{Urine}/Cr_{Serum}]$). A FENa of less than 1% is an excellent indicator of prerenal oliguria in the absence of diuretic therapy, renal failure, or osmotic load.
- The Starling-Landis equation (transcapillary fluid flux) is: $F = k[(P_H - P_{ISF}) - \delta (COP_V - COP_{ISF})]$, where k is the ultrafiltration coefficient of fluid; P_H is the intravascular hydrostatic pressure; P_{ISF} is the hydrostatic pressure of intravascular fluid; δ is the reflection coefficient; COP_V is the intravascular oncotic pressure; and COP_{ISF} is the oncotic pressure of the interstitial fluid.

Table 6-1   Average Electrolyte Content and Daily Volumes of Body Fluids and Secretions

Fluid	Na (mEq/l)	K (mEq/l)	H (mEq/l)	Cl (mEq/l)	HCO₃ (mEq/l)	Adult Volume (ml/day)
Saliva	60	20	0	15	50	1500
Gastric	20-120	15	60	130	0	2500
Pancreatic	140	5	0	70	70	1000
Biliary	140	5	0	140	44	600
Ileostomy	120	20	0	100	40	3000
Diarrhea	100	20	0	100	40	–

Electrolyte Distribution

Osmotic pressure is the tendency of fluid to equilibrate across membranes to maintain equivalent solute concentrations (Box 6-1).

Box 6-1   Definitions

- Cations are positively charged ions such as sodium and potassium. Anions are negatively charged ions such as chloride and bicarbonate.
- The mole is a standard unit of measurement defined as the gram-molecular weight of a substance consisting of 6×10^{23} molecules.
- The electrical equivalent is one mole of an ionized substance divided by its equivalence. The milliequivalent (mEq) is 1/1000 of 1 equivalent.
- The osmole (Osm) is the molecular weight of a substance in grams divided by the number of particles liberated in solution.
- Osmolarity pressure refers to the concentration of osmotically active particles (osmolarity; mOsm/l) in a solution. When solute concentrations differ across a semipermeable membrane the resulting tendency of a fluid to equalize the concentrations is the osmotic pressure. The differing solute concentration is also expressed as tonicity.
- Oncotic pressure, or colloid osmotic pressure (COP), is the pressure required to prevent net fluid movement between two solutions separated by a semipermeable membrane when there is net difference of colloid concentrations between them.

Hydrostatic pressure forces water and electrolytes from the intravascular into the interstitial space. Hydrostatic pressure is greatest at the arteriolar end of capillaries. Oncotic pressure, due mainly to serum albumin concentration, draws this ISF into the intravascular space. Oncotic pressure exerts its greater influence at the venular end of the tissue capillary beds.

Normal body fluid losses (urine, stool, tears) are from ISF space. A constant flux between the intravascular, interstitial, and intracellular spaces exists and normally is at equilibrium. Thus, when there is volume loss all fluid compartments will be affected.

FLUID AND ELECTROLYTE LOSS AND REDISTRIBUTION IN PATHOLOGIC STATES

Acute volume depletion represents almost exclusively ECF loss. A 2% body weight loss represents 10% ECF loss

and results in thirst and oliguria. A 4% body weight loss represents 20% ECF loss and results in tachycardia and postural hypotension. A 6% body weight loss represents 30% ECF loss and results in shock and acute tubular necrosis. Laboratory values suggestive of dehydration (prerenal oliguria) include a serum BUN/creatinine ratio > 20, a urine specific gravity ≥ 1.020, urine sodium < 20 mEq/l, a urine osmolarity > 500 mOsm/l, and a fractional excretion of sodium (FENa) < 1%.

Fluid balance is represented as interval and cumulative intake/output (I/O). Positive fluid balances occur when I > O and typically represent third space fluid sequestration, persistent vasodilation, or compromised elimination (renal failure).

I/O balances represented on intensive care unit (ICU) flowsheets do not include insensible losses (sweat, stool, respiratory evaporation, etc.). Insensible losses are normally approximately 1–1.5 l/day in adults but can be much greater in pathologic conditions such as loss of epithelial integrity (i.e., burns), fever, unhumidified respiratory gases, and diarrhea. I/O balances, as they appear on the ICU flow sheet, generally also fail to account for the differences in crystalloid, colloid, or blood component volumes infused; this is important because the relative contributions of these different fluids to volume expansion varies significantly.

PEARLS

- The initial approach to shock is restoration of circulating volume, cardiac output, and oxygen-carrying capacity.
- Cardiac output can be adversely affected by decreased preload, decreased cardiac contractility, or increased afterload.
- Hypovolemia has a dual adverse effect on cardiac output: a low preload decreases cardiac output as per the Starling curve, and compensatory vasoconstriction increases afterload and impedes cardiac output.
- Intravascular volume must always be corrected before diuretics are used in the treatment of oliguria. The use of diuretics in the ICU should always be questioned.
- It is easier to treat congestive heart failure, even pulmonary edema, than it is to treat renal failure.
- Optimum care of the patient is data driven. First there is a question: if it cannot be answered with the data at hand then there is a manifest need for more information. The ICU is an information-rich environment: there is examination, testing, analysis, and monitoring, all of which assist in decision-making. This feedback loop must be very tight in the ICU. Information gathering seldom occurs only once a day.

Plasma volume is the first ECF space. The normal ISF space is the second ECF space. A pathologically expanded ISF space is a third ECF space, increased primarily at the expense of plasma volume referred to as a "third space" loss. Tissue edema is one type of third space fluid loss. Third space losses can constitute tremendous plasma volume loss: 1 mm of diffuse peritoneal edema in an adult represents approximately 20 liters of fluid. Failure to replace lost intravascular fluid results in diminished cardiac output and tissue perfusion, and ischemic tissue injury. Third space losses occur in the setting of injury and inflammation and do not equilibrate with other fluid compartments. Third space fluid cannot be mobilized and removed by changing the volume of other fluid compartments. Third space fluid mobilizes spontaneously when inflammation subsides and the fluid moves from the abnormal interstitial compartment to the plasma volume.

Electrolyte Deficit and Excess

Glucose

Blood or serum glucose levels must be closely monitored in critically ill patients since both hyperglycemia and hypoglycemia have important therapeutic ramifications. Sources of glucose include endogenous synthetic processes, such as gluconeogenesis and glycogenolysis, and exogenous sources, such as enteral or parenteral nutrition and intravenous fluids. It is important to realize that glucose is present in intravenous fluids either to create a fluid which is isotonic for safe intravascular administration (without precipitating hemolysis), or with the specific intent of glucose administration. Glucose administered intravenously is rapidly metabolized and the fluid in which it was contained then becomes hypotonic and behaves as "free water." Thus, dextrose-containing solutions such as D_5W represent a major source of free water and should not be administered to patients with head injury or after recent neurosurgery where there is a risk for the development of cerebral edema, or in those patients with pre-existing hyponatremia. The administration of intravenous glucose does not have any measurable "protein-sparing effect" in catabolic states. Furthermore, the metabolism of glucose will typically result in some level of hypokalemia as glucose and potassium are co-transported into cells.

Hypoglycemia

Glucose is an important metabolic substrate. Hypoglycemia should be considered as a potential cause of any acute deterioration, such as mental status change or cardiac arrest, in critically ill patients. Hypoglycemia is an important cause of agitation, somnolence, or seizures. Early symptoms of hypoglycemia include tremulousness, diaphoresis, palpitations, and nausea; however, profound hypoglycemia can precipitate a myocardial infarction or encephalopathy. Tissues may be starved for glucose either due to absolute hypoglycemia (low serum glucose levels), or relative cellular hypoglycemia (insulin resistance, defective glycolysis or oxidative phosphorylation). Patients at risk for fasting hypoglycemia include those with depleted glycogen stores or impaired glycogenolysis, such as patients with malnutrition, cirrhosis, renal failure, alcoholic ketoacidosis, or patients with inborn errors of metabolism. Medications that can lead to hypoglycemia include ethanol, oral hypoglycemic agents, insulin, pentamidine, moxifloxacin, salicylates, haloperidol, and trimethoprim-sulfamethoxazole. Hypoglycemia of endocrine origin is seen with glucocorticoid deficiency, hypopituitarism, and glycogen storage diseases.

Hyperglycemia

Hyperglycemia is most often seen in the setting of diabetes, insulin resistance, diabetic ketoacidosis, or nonketotic hyperosmolar states. Hyperglycemia may also result from overfeeding, stress, or medications. Patients with renal failure typically have insulin resistance and hyperglycemia. Hyperglycemia in critically ill patients has been shown to increase morbidity due to hospital-acquired infections, and also increase overall mortality. Relative insulin resistance occurs in the setting of glucocorticoid or catecholamine administration. Hyperglycemia causes a relative hyperosmolar state and can thereby precipitate an osmotic diuresis, which can lead to dehydration and electrolyte imbalances (hypokalemia, hypernatremia) due to diuresis of a very dilute urine. Hyperglycemia has also been shown to detrimentally affect neurologic outcome after cardiac arrest, presumably by increasing the level of intraneural lactic acidosis in the setting of cerebral ischemia. Thus, insulin is an important adjunct therapy for most critically ill patients and is most appropriately administered intravenously, especially in instances where there is peripheral edema or anasarca which impairs the absorption of subcutaneous insulin.

CLINICAL CAVEAT

Infusion of Free Water

Free water should never be infused in patients with head injury or those undergoing neurosurgery because it exacerbates cerebral edema. Normal saline is the fluid of choice in these patients.

Sodium and Water

A minimal urine output of 500 cm³/24° is required for solute excretion in a normal adult. In the adult ICU patient, oliguria is defined as a urine output of < 0.5 cm³/kg/hour over two consecutive hours. Adult maintenance

Table 6-2   A Diagnostic and Therapeutic Approach to Hypernatremia

Low Total Body Na⁺ [Na⁺ and H₂O Loss]		Normal Total Body Na⁺ [H₂O Loss Only]		Increased Total Body Na⁺ [Exogenous Na⁺ Load]
Extrarenal loss	Renal loss	Extrarenal loss	Renal loss	Cushing's syndrome, hyperaldosteronism
Perspiration	Osmotic diuresis	Insensible losses (respiratory, skin)	Diabetes insipidus	$NaHCO_3^-$; NaCl dialysis
Hypertonic urine	Iso- or hypertonic urine	Hypertonic urine	Variable urine tonicity	Iso- or hypertonic urine
Urine Na⁺ < 10 mEq/l	Urine Na⁺ > 20 mEq/l	Variable urine Na⁺	Variable urine Na⁺	Urine Na⁺ mEq/l
Hypertonic saline		Water replacement		Diuretics + water

fluid requirements are approximately 2500 ml/day under normal conditions. Serial body weight and daily intake/output measurements are important to follow total body water status. Normal plasma or serum sodium concentration ranges from 135 to 145 mEq/l. Serum osmolarity (mOsm/kg) = total solute (mOsm)/ total body water (kg). Sodium is the main determinant of plasma (serum) osmolarity. The disorders of sodium balance are summarized in Tables 6-2 and 6-3.

Hypernatremia

Symptoms of hypernatremia include lethargy, irritability, seizures, and coma. The in-hospital mortality associated with severe hypernatremia exceeds 50%. The diagnosis of hypernatremia relies on the measurement of urine sodium and/or osmolarity.

Hypernatremia (plasma sodium > 145 mEq/l) may be a result either of hypertonic fluid gain (sodium infusion), or more commonly a relative free water deficit. The differential diagnosis and treatment of hypernatremia depends on the estimated total body sodium (Table 6-2). Thirst occurs when serum sodium rises by 3–4 mEq/l. Calculated

water deficit = 0.6(M) or 0.5(F) × Wt(kg) × ([Na⁺] − 140/140) *or* water deficit = 0.6(M) or 0.5(F) × Wt(kg) × [plasma Na⁺/140 − 1] × 10. Males (M) have slightly higher total body water content than do females (F).

CLINICAL CAVEAT

Correction of Hypernatremia
- Hypernatremia that is corrected too rapidly may result in acute cerebral edema.
- Urine osmolality less than that of plasma suggests central (antidiuretic hormone (ADH)-deficient) or nephrogenic (ADH-resistant) diabetes insipidus.
- Urine sodium is low in the setting of water loss and high with salt ingestion.
- The water restriction test is helpful in hypernatremic states to diagnose central diabetes insipidus: water intake is stopped to stimulate ADH release; if no response occurs then 1-deamino-8-D-arginine vasopressin (DDAVP) is administered. If the urine osmolality rises the patient has central diabetes insipidus.

Table 6-3   A Diagnostic and Therapeutic Approach to Hyponatremia

Deficit of Total Body Water and Sodium [ECF Depletion]		Excess Total Body Water [Minimal ECF Excess]		Excess of Total Body Sodium and Water [Significant ECF Volume Excess]
Extrarenal loss	Renal loss	Glucocorticoid deficiency, hypothyroidism, SIADH	Nephrotic syndrome, cirrhosis, heart failure (natriuretic peptide deficit)	Renal failure
Vomiting, diarrhea, third space losses, burns	Diuresis, nephritis, renal tubular acidosis, ketosis, osmotic diuresis			
Urine Na⁺ < 10 mmol/l	Urine Na⁺ > 20 mmol/l	Urine Na⁺ > 20 mmol/l	Urine Na⁺ < 10 mmol/l	Urine Na⁺ > 20 mmol/l
Isotonic saline		Water restriction		Water restriction

Hyponatremia

The assessment of volume status is essential to the diagnosis. If the measured plasma osmolality is elevated with respect to the calculated value, the diagnosis is pseudohyponatremia. Hyponatremia in the setting of a low urine sodium or high urine osmolality (>100 mOsm/kg) suggests defective urinary dilution, whereas lower urine sodium or osmolality suggest polydipsia. Equations that calculate excess body water are not reliable. Hyponatremia is classified based on estimated volume status and on urine sodium or osmolarity (Table 6-3). Pseudohyponatremia occurs in the setting of severe hyperlipidemia, hyperproteinemia, or hyperglycemia. Hyperglycemia does not cause hyponatremia until the plasma glucose exceeds 300 mg/dl. Sodium concentration decreases by approximately 1.6 mEq/l for every 100 mg/dl rise in serum glucose or change in sodium = $0.016 \times$ (glucose − 100). Hyponatremia is characterized clinically by central nervous system (CNS) changes such as nausea and vomiting, disorientation, seizures, coma, and respiratory arrest. SIADH is under-recognized in hospitalized patients. SIADH is a cause of isovolemic hypotonic hyponatremia and is associated with stress, drugs, tumors, or CNS and pulmonary infections. The rate of change of serum sodium may be more important clinically than the absolute value. Hypertonic (1.8 or 3%) saline is indicated for the treatment of severe symptoms of hyponatremia. Intravenous medication formulation and enteral free water load should be considered when treating hyponatremia. Free water restriction is a first-line therapy in hypervolemic hyponatremia.

CLINICAL CAVEAT

Correction of Hyponatremia

- The rate of serum sodium increase during the correction of hyponatremia should not exceed 0.5–2 mEq/l/hour (12–20 mEq/l) in the first 24 hours; and 0.3–0.5 mEq/l/hour thereafter. In extreme emergencies a maximum of 20 mEq/l/day may be tolerated but has significant associated risks which should not outweigh benefits.
- Hyponatremia corrected too rapidly can produce central pontine myelinolysis (osmotic demyelination) syndrome which is an irreversible CNS injury related to both rate and degree of Na^+ correction. Imaging studies may not be positive for up to weeks.

In the setting of hypervolemia, a hypo-osmolar serum and a urine sodium less than 10 mmol/l is usually associated with congestive heart failure, nephritic syndrome, hypothyroidism, malnutrition, and hypoalbuminemia, cirrhosis, or pregnancy. In the setting of hypovolemia, a hypo-osmolar serum is associated with gastrointestinal (GI) losses or pancreatitis, burns, or diaphoresis if the urine sodium is less than 20 mmol/l; and with renal disease (nonoliguric renal failure, renal tubular acidosis, interstitial nephritis), diuretic use, or cerebral salt wasting if the urine sodium is greater than 20 mmol/l. Volume status is measured clinically: heart rate, jugular venous distention, edema, central venous pressure (CVP), pulmonary capillary wedge pressure (PCWP), orthostasis, or pulse pressure. Adrenal insufficiency presents as hyperkalemia, hyponatremia, acidosis, and perhaps fever and leukocytosis.

PEARLS

- Whenever any laboratory value is inconsistent with the clinical picture it must be treated as suspect and reconfirmed immediately if the situation allows it.
- The diagnosis of the etiology of hyponatremia depends on an accurate determination of fluid status.
- The rate of correction of hyponatremia should be as slow as is safe given the patient's symptoms.
- Hypernatremia is usually due to a free water deficit and can be corrected by free water administration, enterally or intravenously.
- Rarely, hypernatremia is due to diabetes insipidus and may require treatment with antidiuretic hormone (ADH).

Potassium

Hyperkalemia

Normal plasma or serum potassium concentration ranges from 3.5 to 5.5 mEq/l. Body potassium stores are primarily intracellular and total body potassium is approximately 50 mEq/kg or 3500 mEq in a 70 kg person. Of this total, 2% (70 mEq) are found in the ECF. Hypokalemia (<3.5 mEq/l) signals total body depletion of potassium stores, a deficit of approximately 250–300 mEq in a 70 kg adult. This deficit must be replaced gradually. Hyperkalemia in the face of acidosis signals a significant total body potassium deficit. Untreated hypokalemia can be expected to worsen as the pH rises. Acidosis promotes an efflux of potassium from the ICF compartment. Sources of hyperkalemia include renal failure, hypo-adrenocorticalism (Addison's syndrome), hemolysis, rhabdomyolysis, potassium supplements, and medications such as penicillin-K, heparin, aldosterone antagonists, ACE inhibitors, and succinylcholine. Pseudohyperkalemia may result from leukocytosis (>100,000/mm³) or elevated platelet count (>600,000/mm³).

Hyperkalemia causes tall peaked T waves, widened QRS, and wide PR. These patients should be carefully monitored.

CLINICAL CAVEAT

Treatment of Hyperkalemia

- Plasma or serum hyperkalemia can be reduced by promoting alkalosis (hyperventilation, exogenous bicarbonate), or increasing intracellular glucose by the administration of glucose (0.5-1.0 g/kg) and insulin (0.1 unit regular insulin/kg); beta$_2$-agonist (albuterol); maneuvers that move potassium from the ECF to the ICF compartment. Ten percent calcium gluconate 50 mg/kg IV or 10% calcium chloride 10 mg/kg IV transiently antagonize the effects of hyperkalemia at excitable membranes.
- Sodium polystyrene sulfonate in 20% sorbitol by mouth, NG tube, or enema removes approximately 1 mEq/g of K^+, but simultaneously adds approximately 1.7 mEq of Na^+/g.
- Hyperkalemia decreases the transmembrane electrical potential and will arrest the heart in diastole. Intravenous calcium administration preserves cardiac contractility and transiently antagonizes symptomatic hyperkalemia.

Hypokalemia

Hypokalemia is defined as a serum potassium concentration of less than 3.5 mEq/l and is due to either intracellular potassium shift or total body potassium depletion (renal losses with diuresis, diarrhea). Urine potassium can help guide diagnosis. If urine potassium is less than 20 mmol/l one should consider inadequate intake, diarrhea, biliary loss, or diuresis. If the urine potassium is greater than 20 mmol/l in a normotensive patient one should consider renal tubular acidosis, diabetic ketoacidosis. If the urine potassium is greater than 20 mmol/l in a hypertensive patient one should consider malignant hypertension or renal artery stenosis if the plasma renin activity is elevated; otherwise one should consider mineralocorticoid use or Cushing's syndrome. Clinical manifestations of hypokalemia include muscle weakness, cardiac arrhythmias, cardiac U waves, flattened and inverted T waves, ileus, paresthesias, and prolongation of the QT interval. Severe hypokalemia can precipitate rhabdomyolysis. Hypokalemia will also increase renal ammonia production and worsen hepatic encephalopathy. Magnesium depletion impairs potassium reabsorption across the renal tubules; therefore effective treatment of hypokalemia is difficult in the setting of magnesium depletion.

CLINICAL CAVEAT

Treatment of Hypokalemia

- Potassium repletion can be accomplished using enteric or intravenous supplementation. Intravenous potassium repletion should never exceed 40 mEq/hour in adults and administration of more than 10 mEq/hour should be performed with telemetry monitoring.
- The average increase in serum potassium is 0.25 mmol/l per 20 mmol infused.

Chloride

Gastric secretions are a primary source of loss producing hypochloremic metabolic alkalosis. (See section on acid–base physiology below). Exogenous chloride and renal failure are the primary causes of hyperchloremic metabolic acidosis.

Magnesium

Since magnesium is primarily intracellular, serum magnesium levels can be normal while total body magnesium is severely depleted. Magnesium is a cofactor for many enzymatic reactions and therefore plays an important role in ATP mediated processes (N^+–K^+ ATPase) such as electrical membrane potentials, neurotransmitter release, and smooth muscle contraction. Magnesium deficiency predisposes to arrhythmias especially those arising from QT and PR interval prolongation; and intravenous magnesium is the treatment for torsades de pointes. Magnesium deficiency may also manifest as vertigo, dysarthria, psychosis, weakness, tremor, paresthesias, and seizures. Magnesium deficiency is extremely common and under-recognized. Losses are from the GI and renal systems. Predisposing conditions include chronic alcohol abuse, secretory diarrhea, diabetes mellitus, myocardial infarction, and drug therapy (furosemide, aminoglycosides, amphotericin, pentamidine, cyclosporine, digitalis). Gentamicin induces magnesuria. Alcoholics are particularly likely to have magnesium depletion. In addition, magnesium is a cofactor for thiamine action. There are no specific clinical manifestations of magnesium deficiency. However, reactive CNS magnesium deficiency can mimic a cerebrovascular accident (ataxia, dysarthria, seizures, obtundaton, and spasms).

CLINICAL CAVEAT

Magnesium Repletion

- Magnesium repletion can be accomplished using enteral or intravenous supplementation. Magnesium sulfate delivers 8 mEq/g and may be given intravenously over minutes to hours. A typical dose in a 70 kg adult with moderate magnesium depletion would be in the range 2–4 g IV. Magnesium oxide delivers 20 mEq, 10 mmol, or 241 mg of elemental magnesium per 400 mg tablet.
- Magnesium is administered in obstetric patients in large doses for severe eclampsia and pre-eclampsia where the dose is titrated to diminished deep tendon reflexes (DTRs). DTRs are abolished above serum levels of 4 mEq/l; somnolence accompanies levels of 7 mEq/l; and heart block and paralysis is likely at levels of 10 mEq/l or greater.

Magnesium has also been used as an adjunct bronchodilator in status asthmaticus. Magnesium accumulation occurs in patients with impaired renal function and supplementation should be with great care in these patients. Hypermagnesemia also occurs with adrenal insufficiency, hyperparathyroidism, and lithium intoxication. Clinical effects of hypermagnesemia include diminished neuromuscular function and paralysis, vasodilation and hypotension, bradycardia, heart block, respiratory depression, and coma. Hemolysis releases magnesium from lysed erythrocytes.

CLINICAL CAVEAT

Treatment of Elevated Magnesium
- Neuromuscular and cardiac toxicity from hypermagnesemia can be treated emergently but transiently with calcium, 100–200 mg slow IV push.
- Forced diuresis will decrease serum magnesium in patients with intact renal function.
- Magnesium can be removed by dialysis

Calcium

Calcium is the most abundant electrolyte in the human body but 99% is bound in bone. Calcium is mainly distributed in ECF where 50% is bound to plasma proteins. Albumin accounts for 80% of calcium binding in plasma. Some 5–10% is chelated to sulfates and phosphates. Calcium is important to blood clot formation, excitation–contraction coupling, neurotransmission, enzyme function, cell division and motility, and wound healing. Only unbound, or ionized, plasma calcium is physiologically active.

Normal total serum calcium ranges from 8.0 to 10.2 mg/dl or 2.2 to 2.5 mmol/l; and normal serum ionized calcium ranges from 4.0 to 4.6 mg/dl or 1.0 to 1.5 mmol/l.

Hypocalcemia

Calcium must be corrected for plasma albumin levels. Corrected total Ca = measured total Ca + 0.8 × (4.0 − albumin). The key clinical manifestations of hypocalcemia are enhanced neuromuscular excitability and reduced muscle contractility. Hypocalcemia is associated with decreased parathormone (PTH) levels following parathyroidectomy, tumor, or hemochromatosis. Pseudohyoparathyroidism is end-organ unresponsiveness to PTH and is often nephrogenic. Vitamin D deficiency due to inadequate dietary intake is rare. However, vitamin D deficiency due to malabsorption, hepatobiliary disease, renal disease, and alcoholism is a relatively common cause of hypocalcemia. Classic but insensitive clinical signs of hypocalcemia are Chvostek's (facial hyperreflexia) and Trousseau's (carpopedal spasm) signs. Ionized hypocalcemia (<1.0 mmol/l) occurs in the setting of alkalosis, magnesium depletion, renal insufficiency, and sepsis, and with the use of medications such as aminoglycosides, estrogen, dilantin, theophylline, and heparin. Hypocalcemia is refractory to

calcium administration in the presence of concomitant hypomagnesemia.

Ionized calcium levels can decrease rapidly in the presence of pancreatitis, where fat necrosis binds calcium in a process of saponification; and following massive red cell transfusion where the anticoagulant citrate in transfused red blood cells binds plasma ionized calcium (especially with coexisting liver disease which impairs citrate metabolism). Calcium is administered intravenously as either 10% (100 mg/ml calcium salt) calcium chloride (0.1–0.2 ml/kg) or 10% calcium gluconate (0.5–1.0 ml/kg). However, calcium chloride contains three times as much elemental calcium (1.36 mEq/ml) as calcium gluconate (0.46 mEq/ml). Ten milliliter amps contain 272 mg compared to 90 mg of elemental calcium, respectively. Intravenous calcium administration can precipitate ventricular arrhythmias in patients receiving digoxin because calcium antagonizes potassium at the cardiac muscle membrane. Calcium supplementation should be avoided in digoxin toxicity.

Hypercalcemia

Hypercalcemia (>10.5 mmol/l) or ionized hypercalcemia (>1.3 mmol/l) is relatively rare, most commonly due to hyperparathyroidism, sarcoidosis, milk-alkali syndrome, vitamin A or D intoxication, malignancy, thyrotoxicosis, or drugs (lithium, tamoxifen, thiazides). Hypercalcemia produces an osmotic diuresis resulting in symptoms of polyuria and polydipsia. Clinical manifestations of hypercalcemia are nonspecific and include ileus, pancreatitis, nephrocalcinosis, confusion, and coma. Electrocardiographic effects of hypercalcemia include PR prolongation, QRS widening, ST shortening, and flattened T waves. Management of hypercalcemia is with saline infusion and diuretics to maintain a brisk diuresis. Severe or symptomatic hypercalemia can be managed with calcitonin IM/SQ; hydrocortisone; pamidronate IV; and mithramycin or plicamycin IV. Calcium salts are deposited in tissues when a critical calcium–phosphate product is reached (>60). Administration of either salt in the presence of high concentrations of the other must be carried out with caution.

Phosphate

Phosphate is the most abundant intracellular anion and is essential for energy storage and transport (ATP, cAMP, cGTP, CPK, etc.). Normal dietary phosphate accounts for 1 g/day. Most body phosphorus is in the bony skeleton; the rest is bound in phospholipids and phosphoproteins. The remaining 15% exists as inorganic phosphorus which is primarily intracellular, mainly as high-energy phosphates. Normal serum phosphate ranges from 2.5 mg/dl (0.8 mmol/l) to 4.5 mg/dl (1.4 mmol/dl). Phosphorus is filtered at the glomerulus and reabsorbed in the proximal tubules, regulated by PTH and vitamin D. Hypophosphatemia (<3 mg/dl) is common in hypermetabolic states (diabetic ketoacidosis, alcohol withdrawal, refeeding syndrome, trauma, etc.). However, even severe hypophosphatemia is usually clinically silent. Phosphate depletion can also occur with medications such as aluminum- or calcium-containing antacids, sucralfate, diuretics, androgens, salicylates, aminoglycoside and acetaminophen toxicity, and cisplatin therapy. Clinical manifestations of hypophosphatemia may become evident with stress and include acute skeletal myopathy, respiratory muscle dysfunction, cardiomyopathy, decreased platelet adhesion and prolonged bleeding time, phagocytic impairment, and hemolysis.

CLINICAL CAVEAT

Treatment of Hypophosphatemia
- Intravenous replacement therapy for hypophosphatemia is with either sodium (4.0 mEq/l Na) or potassium (4.3 mEq/l K) phosphate. A dose of 0.02–0.04 mmol/kg (15–30 mmol in a 70 kg patient) over 1–4 hours is a typical starting dose. Phosphate replacement should be slow and cautious in patients with renal failure.
- Enteral phosphate replacement with Neutra-Phos or K-Phos is an alternative.

PEARLS

- A decrease in plasma albumin affects primarily protein-bound calcium. Measured serum calcium is low in hypoalbuminemia but the physiologically active ionized calcium fragment may be unaffected.
- Calcium chelates phosphorus; caution must be used when administering either when the concentration of the other is high.

Hyperphosphatemia (>4.5 mg/dl) is common in renal failure and widespread tissue or cell lysis syndrome (tumor lysis, rhabdomyolysis). Calcium acetate, sucralfate, or hemodialysis will lower serum phosphate.

ACID–BASE PHYSIOLOGY

In general, mild acidosis is better tolerated physiologically than alkalosis, because of improved oxygen kinetics in the setting of acidosis. With the exception of the pulmonary vasculature, all vascular beds vasodilate in response to acidosis. Acidosis causes pulmonary vasoconstriction and bronchodilation. Acidosis increases catecholamine release but severe acidosis impairs catecholamine responsiveness. Proper arterial blood collection technique is essential. If the specimen is not placed on ice $PaCO_2$ rises 3–10 mmHg/hour with a concomitant fall

in pH. Pseudohypoxemia and pseudoacidosis can occur when increased oxygen consumption and CO_2 production occurs in the sample due to active metabolism in the setting of temperature, leukocytosis (>10^5/mm³), or thrombocytosis (>10^6/mm³). Pseudohypocarbia and false oxygen PaO_2 can occur in the setting of trapped air bubbles. Air bubbles can increase PO_2 by >25 mmHg, but are unlikely to affect PCO_2. The oxygen saturation of a blood gas specimen is not measured but calculated from the PaO_2 using a normogram. The body temperature should be recorded at the time of ABG collection. Gas solubility decreases with warming and "temperature correction" of PaO_2 and PCO_2 may be necessary. Venous blood gases have a higher PCO_2 and lower PO_2 than arterial blood. Venous blood gases may be adequate indicators of acid–base and, when used with oximetry, approximate arterial blood gases. In the ICU the number of blood gas analyses correlates with the presence or absence of an arterial cannula. Normal arterial pH varies from 5.35 to 7.45. A pH less than 7.35 is a relative acidosis, whereas a pH greater than 7.45 is a relative alkalosis.

Acidosis

Metabolic acidosis represents excess unbuffered H^+ ion concentration. Metabolic acidosis is usually partially compensated by hyperventilation and a relative respiratory alkalosis. Bicarbonate is not measured during blood gas analysis; it is calculated from the pH and PCO_2 using a normogram derived from the Henderson–Hasselbach equation. Directed automated determination of HCO_3^- (PCO_2) is standard with electrolyte panels using the sequential multichannel analyzer (SMA). The bicarbonate (carbonic acid) buffer is quantitatively the most important plasma buffering system. In metabolic acidosis bicarbonate is consumed and depleted. Bicarbonate compensation occurs over 24–38 hours. Below a pH of 7.15 the conformation of catecholamine receptors is altered and there is a decreased responsiveness to endogenous and exogenous catecholamines. Acidemia also decreases conduction in excitable tissues. Hyperkalemia in acidosis increases cardiac depression and arrhythmias. Acidosis in the setting of excessive lactate production (Type A) usually occurs in the setting of anaerobic glycolysis in shock. Excess lactate production suggests an imbalance in oxygen delivery and extraction ($DO_2 < VO_2$).

Type B lactic acidosis is differentiated into subtypes: B1 is due to underlying diseases such as liver disease, malignancy, pheochromocytoma, and, most importantly, thiamine deficiency; B2 is associated with medications or toxins such as biguanides, ethanol, methanol, salicylates, acetaminophen, or propylene glycol; B3 occurs with inborn errors of metabolism such as glucose-6-phosphate dehydrogenase deficiency, pyruvate dehydrogenase deficiency, or fructose-1,6-diphosphatase deficiency. The anion gap is given by $(Na^+ + K^+) - (HCO_3^- + Cl^-)$.

Box 6-2 Acidosis Treatment

Identification and directed treatment of the underlying cause of metabolic acidosis is essential.

TRIS (Tromethamine, THAM) is an intravenous buffer solution with a buffering capacity of 1 mEq/ml at a concentration of 36 g/l. The advantage of THAM is a relatively low sodium load, which is beneficial in the setting of acidosis and pre-existing hypernatremia or sodium overload.

Normal anion gap is 15 mEq/l. K^+ is sometimes omitted and changes the normal value of the anion gap to 12 mEq/l. Anion gap acidotic states are due to excess lactate, salicylate intoxication, renal failure, penicillins, diabetic ketoacidosis, or methanol, ethylene glycol, or paraldehyde intoxication. Decreased serum unmeasured cations such as potassium, calcium, and magnesium will increase the anion gap. Increased unmeasured anions such as phosphate and sulfate will increase the anion gap. Bicarbonate loss is most often due to renal failure (renal tubular acidosis), diarrhea, hypersecretory states, or cholestyramine. Lost bicarbonate will be compensated by Cl^- reabsorption to maintain electrical neutrality (Box 6-2).

Patients with chronic respiratory acidosis who acutely receive mechanical ventilatory support are at risk of developing a relative state of acute metabolic acidosis, whereby the artificially imposed hyperventilation impairs the ability of their kidneys to retain bicarbonate. Thus, over-ventilation is a common iatrogenic cause of failure to wean from mechanical ventilation. Acute hyperventilation of patients with chronic respiratory failure will delay weaning because chronically retained HCO_3^- will be rapidly lost, and during weaning increased PCO_2 (which may be unavoidable because of abnormal respiratory mechanics) will cause an acutely uncompensated acidosis. Respiratory acidosis is usually well tolerated to a pH $\geq$ 7.25. Respiratory acid–base physiology is covered in Chapter 4. Bicarbonate administration may be used to correct metabolic acidosis. A pitfall of bicarbonate administration is the development of acute hypernatremia.

Alkalosis

Metabolic alkalosis is usually due to chloride loss (vomiting, nasogastric suction, cystic fibrosis, villous adenomas, post-hypercapneic alkalosis) or acute intravascular volume loss (volume contraction) which is accompanied by hyperaldosteronism. Chloride replacement (NaCl, HCl) will correct metabolic acidosis due to chloride loss. Urine chloride is a diagnostic aid: low urine chloride (<15 mEq/l) is seen in vomiting, nasogastric

suction, acute diuresis, post-hypercapnic syndrome, and alkali loading; high urine chloride (>20 mEq/l) is seen with mineralocorticoid excess, alkali loading, chronic diuresis, hypokalemia, and Bartter's syndrome. Metabolic alkalosis resistant to chloride replacement is frequently due to hyperaldosteronism, hyperreninism, severe potassium depletion, refeeding alkalosis, hypoparathyroidism, licorice ingestion, 11- or 17-adrenal hydroxylase deficiency, or Cushing's syndrome. It should be aggressively treated. Alkalosis causes bronchoconstriction, coronary artery vasoconstriction, and can cause shifts in potassium intracellularly which can affect cardiac pacemaker cells and lead to arrhythmias. Alkalosis also decreases ionized calcium levels and affects cardiac contractility. Hyperkalemia can precipitate intracellular acidosis in the renal tubules, which results in bicarbonate retention and metabolic alkalosis.

CLINICAL CAVEAT

Treatment of Alkalosis
- Acetazolamide is useful in those patients who have excess total body water but are alkalotic. Acetazolamide is a diuteric that inhibits carbonic anhydrase and leads to HCO_3^- (and K^+) loss.
- HCO_3^- excess = 0.5 × Wt (kg) × (HCO_3^- observed − HCO_3^- desired).
- Normal hydrochloric acid (HCl) is used to treat severe metabolic alkalosis; 0.1 or 0.2 N HCl has 100 mEq/l hydrogen and chloride ions.

PEARLS

- pH, PaO_2, $PaCO_2$, and saturation are measured. HCO_3^- is calculated. CO_2 is measured.
- An acute increase in PCO_2 of 10 mmHg will decrease pH by 0.05 unit.
- An acute decrease in PCO_2 of 10 mmHg will increase pH by 0.1 unit.
- An acute increase in PCO_2 of 10 mmHg will be buffered by 1 mEq/l increase in HCO_3^-.
- An acute decrease in PCO_2 of 10 mmHg will be buffered by a 2.5 mEq/l decrease in HCO_3^-.
- A chronic increase in PCO_2 of 10 mmHg will be buffered by 2.5–3.5 mEq/l increase in HCO_3^-.
- A chronic decrease in PCO_2 of 10 mmHg will be buffered by a 5 mEq/l decrease in HCO_3^-.

CRYSTALLOIDS

Crystalloids are electrolytes dissolved in sterile water. Normal saline (NS) is 0.9% saline. It is not electrically normal (1 gEq/l). NS is termed "normal" because it is isotonic (actually slightly hypertonic at 308 mOsm/l) with human ECF.

NS is acidic and unbuffered. Accumulation of chloride with NS administration results in hyperchloremic metabolic acidosis. Lactated Ringer's solution, or Hartman's solution, is a balanced-salt solution with a composition closely approximating human ECF. Under normal conditions the infused lactate is extracted (primarily in the liver) and converted to bicarbonate and water. Solutions containing dextrose, acetate, or lactate (RL, D_5W, $D_51/2NS$, $D_51/4NS$, Normosol, etc.) add to free water load. Free water is contraindicated in head injury patients and hyponatremia. Hypertonic saline (1.8%, 3%, or 5%) expands intravascular volume transiently primarily through its osmotic effects, drawing fluid from the interstitial and intracellular spaces (Table 6-4).

COLLOIDS

Colloids maintain or increase oncotic pressure (COP). Normal plasma COP is 25–30 mmHg. COP cannot be inferred from plasma protein concentrations – it must be measured. Albumin accounts for most of the COP of plasma. However, albumin also accounts for binding of electrolytes, drugs, and other molecules, free radical scavenging, toxin binding, and inhibition of platelet aggregation. If plasma COP remains above 20 mmHg it is likely that plasma albumin concentration, in itself, is of no significance in transmembrane fluid flux (Box 6-3).

In the absence of pathologic capillary leak syndrome, edema is favored by increased intravascular hydrostatic pressure, increased interstitial oncotic pressure, or decreased intravascular oncotic pressure. Tissue edema increases the diffusion distance for oxygen and can lead to widespread relative cellular hypoxia.

Volume for volume, colloids increase threefold the effect of crystalloids on preload. In the setting of inflammation "capillary leak" may allow colloids to leak from the vascular to the ISF space, diminishing volume expansion and contributing to "third space" losses and diffuse edema. The intravascular half-life of colloids depends on elimination and metabolism, molecular size, and the presence of capillary leak. Six percent Hetastarch in 0.9 normal saline (Hespan[R]) is implicated in coagulopathy (alteration of platelet rheology and adhesion) at volumes exceeding 1.5 liters in a 70 kg patient and in hyperchloremic acidosis due to the chloride load inherent in saline. Six percent Hetastarch in Ringer's lactate (Hextend[R]) is not presently implicated in either coagulopathy or hyperchloremic acidosis (Table 6-5).

BLOOD AND BLOOD PRODUCTS

Red Cell Transfusion

Anemia is frequently diagnosed in hospitalized patients, especially those with critical illness. Whereas acute anemia, most commonly due to blood loss, may be life-threatening, anemia of gradual onset is usually well-tolerated due to cardiovascular compensation (increased cardiac output). Causes of anemia which are often overlooked include hemodilution, phlebotomy, or drug-induced hemolysis. The primary function of red blood cell transfusion is to maintain oxygen carrying capacity. Red blood cell transfusion should never be used solely for intravascular volume expansion. Although the transfusion of red blood cells to maintain an arbitary hematocrit level has been a mainstay of ICU therapy, the practice of routine red blood cell transfusion is being increasingly challenged. Transfusions have been shown to impair immune function, to increase the risk of nosocomial infectious complications, and also to promote the spread of tumor emboli during cancer surgery. Moreover, critically ill patients are at risk of erythropoietin deficiency. Therefore, alternatives to transfusion such as therapeutic erythropoietin supplementation, vitamin and mineral supplementation, and appropriate caloric intake are important adjuncts in both acute and chronic care.

Patients at risk for hemorrhage should have at least one catheter placed into a large vein. The Poisseuille–Hagen formula defines flow through catheters. Flow is faster with short, wide-bore catheters, and with fluids of low viscosity. As much as 750 cm^3 of acute blood loss can be tolerated without hemodynamic derangements in a typical adult. The first sign of acute hemorrhage is a narrowing of pulse pressure which occurs with a Class II (750–1000 cm^3) hemorrhage. Tachycardia does not occur until late in Class II hemorrhage. Patients with cardiomyopathy, medications that decrease or limit heart rate (beta-blockers, calcium channel blockers, digitalis), or patients with dysautonomia due to diabetes mellitus may not show tachycardia despite severe hypovolemia.

Box 6-3   Starling–Landis Equation

The Starling-Landis equation defines transcapillary fluid flux:

$$F = k[(P_H - P_{ISF}) - \delta(COP_V - COP_{ISF})]$$

where k is the ultrafiltration coefficient of fluid; P_H is the intravascular hydrostatic pressure; P_{ISF} is the hydrostatic pressure of intravascular fluid; δ is the reflection coefficient; COP_V is the intravascular oncotic pressure; and COP_{ISF} is the oncotic pressure of the interstitial fluid.

Table 6-4 Electrolyte Composition and Characteristics of Crystalloid Solutions

Solution	Na (mEq/l)	Cl (mEq/l)	K (mEq/l)	Dextrose (g/l)	Lactate (mEq/l)	Gluconate (mEq/l)	Acetate (mEq/l)	Ca (mEq/l)	Mg (mEq/l)	pH	mOsm/l	Cal/l
0.45% saline	77	77	0	0	0	0	0	0	0	5.7	155	0
D₅ 0.45 NS	77	77	0	50	0	0	0	0	0	5.2	406	170
0.9% saline	154	154	0	0	0	0	0	0	0	5.7	308	0
D – 5 saline	154	154	0	50	0	0	0	0	0	4.0	560	170
Ringer's lactate	130	109	4	0	28	0	0	3	0	6.7	273	9
D – 5 LR	130	109	4	50	28	0	0	3	0	6.7	525	170
D – 5% water	0	0	0	50	0	0	0	0	0	5.0	253	170
D – 10% water	0	0	0	100	0	0	0	0	0	4.9	505	340
D – 5% 1/2 N saline	77	77	0	50	0	0	0	0	0	4.9	407	170
Normosol	140	98	5	0	0	23	27	0	3	7.4	295	0
3% NS	513	513									1025	
5% NS	855	855									1710	
Standard PPN	47	35	23	100	0	0	36	12.5	12.5		880*	
Standard TPN	35	53	40	250	0	0	25	12.5	12.5		1825*	

* Protein 4.25 g/l.

Table 6-5   Electrolyte Composition and Characteristics of Typical Colloid Solutions

Solution	Na (mEq/l)	Cl (mEq/l)	Lactate (mEq/l)	Albumin (g/l)	Dextran (g/l)	HES (g/l)	pH	COP (mmHg)	Osm
Albumin 5%	154	154	0	50	0	0	6.6	20	290
Albumin 25%	154	154	0	250	0	0	6.9	100	310
HES									
Hespan^R	154	154	0	0	0	60			310
Hextend^{R*}	130	109	28	0	0	60			310
Pentastarch									
Dextran 40									
Water	0	0	0	0	100	0	6.7	68	320
NS	154	154	0	0	100	0	6.7	68	320
Dextran 70	154	154	0	0	60	0	6.3	70	320

* Hextend also contains K^+ 4 mEq/l; and Ca^{2+} 3 mEq/l.

PEARLS

- Oxygen delivery is the product of arterial oxygen content and cardiac output: $DO_2 = CaO_2 \times CO$.
- Arterial oxygen content includes the oxygen bound to hemoglobin and the oxygen dissolved in blood: $CaO_2 = ([Hg] \times Sat \times 1.34) + (PaO_2 \times 0.0031)$.
- Note that dissolved arterial oxygen, which is based in the PaO_2, is negligible.
- The Pouiseille–Hagen formula defines flow in catheters: resistance = $(8 \, \mu l / \pi r^4)$.
- Flow = $1/R$.
- Flow is inversely proportional to catheter length. Flow is directly proportional to radius to the fourth power; hence small increases in catheter diameter increase flow significantly.
- A short peripheral IV will have better flow dynamics than a long central line (triple lumen or PICC).

The optimal hematocrit in ICU patients has not been well defined. A hematocrit as low as 21% is often well tolerated. Cardiac output increases in anemia to maintain oxygen delivery (DO_2). Where increased cardiac output is not possible (cardiomyopathy) or potentially detrimental (myocardial ischemia) a hematocrit closer to 30% may be better. Patients with severe COPD often have hematocrits of 45–50% prior to admission to compensate for chronic hypoxemia. These patients may need hematocrits closer to their normal values to wean successfully from mechanical ventilation. The typical ICU patient loses the equivalent of approximately 1 unit of packed red blood cells (PRBCs)/week to diagnostic phlebotomy. Where possible, phlebotomy should be limited and blood collected in pediatric phlebotomy tubes. Blood conservation strategies may decrease the need for transfusions significantly, especially in chronic ICU patients. Empiric transfusion triggers should be avoided. Risk and benefit must be considered. Informed consent should be obtained and documented for all transfusions whenever possible. At higher hematocrits, blood viscosity increases and may decrease cardiac output and impair microcapillary blood flow. Whole blood is no longer available unless it is an autologous donation.

Red blood cells are stored in a CPD solution (citrate, phosphate, dextrose). Citrate metabolism can contribute to metabolic alkalosis; citrate accumulation binds calcium and can contribute to hypocalcemia. PRBCs are used to restore oxygen-carrying capacity. Each unit of PRBCs will increase the plasma hemoglobin by about 1% and the hematocrit by 3%. There is no rate limit on the transfusion of blood or blood products. The rate is determined by the clinical situation and the patient's physiology. Normal erythrocyte destruction in banked blood causes banked blood to progressively increase in potassium content. The K^+ in PRBCs stored longer than three weeks can approximate 20 mEq/l. Transfusion of PRBCs through intravenous catheters smaller than 18 gauge will lead to increasing levels of mechanical hemolysis the smaller the catheter size.

Leukocyte-poor PRBCs are indicated for patients who have had prior white cell or leukoagglutinin reactions, or who are at risk for graft versus host (GVH) reactions. In immunosuppressed patients at high risk for GVH, the blood is usually also irradiated to further decrease the number of viable leukocytes. The hematocrit of transfused red blood cells ranges from 60 to 80%. Transfusion flow can be increased by diluting PRBCs with 0.9 NS, which decreases viscosity. Ringer's lactate contains calcium and should not be mixed with PRBCs since it can precipitate thrombosis in vitro. Transfusion of PRBCs in D_5W, an iso-osmotic but hypotonic solution, will cause red cell lysis.

Complications of transfusion are of major concern to the public. TRALI is transfusion-related acute lung injury and is a pulmonary manifestation of systemic inflammation in the setting of large-volume transfusions. Infectious complications of transfusion persist despite testing and include transmission of HIV, hepatitis A–E, cytomegalovirus (CMV), West Nile virus, and prions. Transfusions must be administered through filters which filter microaggregates of fibrin, platelets, and cells ranging in size from 20 to 170 μm. Hypothermia can complicate rapid infusion of unwarmed PRBCs stored at 4°C. Acute hemolytic reactions have an incidence of 1/6000 and are fatal in about 1/100,000 transfusions. The most common cause of transfusion reaction is clerical error and therefore autologous blood is not significantly safer than homologous blood transfusion. Acute hemolytic transfusion reactions are usually due to ABO erythrocyte surface antigen incompatibility between donor and recipient red cells. Acute hemolytic transfusion reactions are potentially life threatening. Morbidity is related to the volume of cells infused. Recipient blood should be examined for xanthochromia and free hemoglobin. A positive direct Coomb's test confirms a hemolytic reaction; however, a false negative direct Coomb's test is seen when the majority of donor cells are already lysed. Serum LDH is usually elevated and serum haptoglobin decreased.

Platelet Transfusion

Thrombocytopenia is variably defined as a platelet count less than 100,000–150,000/mm^3. In the absence of risk factors, platelet counts as low as 5000/mm^3 may be tolerated without bleeding. Platelet counts below 5000/mm^3 are associated with a high risk of spontaneous hemorrhage. Platelet counts ≥ 50,000/mm^3 are sufficient to provide hemostasis for surgical procedures, assuming the platelets are functional (absence of uremia, NSAID, or aspirin therapy). Causes of thrombocytopenia include sepsis, disseminated intravascular coagulation, thrombotic thrombocytopenic purpura, and heparin-associated thrombocytopenia (HAT). Thrombocytopenia may be the earliest hematologic abnormality in sepsis. Dilutional thrombocytopenia can occur with large fluid volume or multiple packed cell infusions. The major complication of HAT is thrombosis, not bleeding. Platelet dysfunction is most commonly due to renal insufficiency, cardiopulmonary bypass, or medications. Platelets are stored at room temperature. Hypothermia interferes with platelet thromboxane synthesis and clotting. Platelets are normally pooled from multiple donors, increasing the potential for infectious complications. Each unit of platelets transfused is expected to increase the platelet count by 5000–10,000/mm^3, unless destruction or sequestration is ongoing. Platelets are usually administered as six-packs, which raise the platelet count by 25,000–50,000/mm^3. ABO compatible platelets are less likely to form antiplatelet antibodies and therefore survive longer post-transfusion. Platelets do not contain Rh antigens. DDAVP (Desmopressin) 0.3–0.4 μg/kg transiently improves platelet function in the setting of von Willebrand's disease, uremia, aspirin ingestion, or post-cardiopulmonary bypass.

Fresh Frozen Plasma

Fresh frozen plasma (FFP) contains antithrombin III and can be used to treat heparin resistance. A corollary is that FFP can increase the anticoagulant effect of heparin. The main indication for FFP is the rapid reversal of coumadin-induced anticoagulation, replacement of vitamin K-dependent coagulation factors (cirrhosis). FFP is indicated for replacement of factors II, V, VII, VIII, IX, X, XI, and XIII, and von Willebrand's factor. Each milliliter of transfused plasma contains only about 1 unit of each factor, necessitating large volumes of plasma for effective factor replacement. Allergic reactions to FFP are common because of platelets and leukocytes. FFP should be compatible with the recipient's red blood cells, but need not be compatible with the recipient's plasma. FFP is not indicated for volume expansion and should not be used as a colloid substitute.

Cryoprecipitate

Cryoprecipitate is a plasma concentrate pooled from multiple donors and contains primarily factor VIII and fibrinogen. A unit of cryoprecipitate contains about 100 units of factor VIII and 250 mg of fibrinogen. A typical dose of cryoprecipitate is 8–10 units, which increases factor VIII levels by an average of 2%. A thromboelastograph is a useful guide to platelet, FFP, or cryoprecipitate replacement.

SELECTED READING

Adrogue HJ, Madias NE: Management of life-threatening acid–base disorders. N Engl J Med 338:26–34; 107–111, 1998.

Bugg NC, Jones JA: Hyposphosphatemia. Pathophysiology and management in the intensive care unit. Anaesthesia 3:895–902, 1998.

Fawcett WJ, Haxby EJ, Male DA: Magnesium: physiology and pharmacology. Br J Anaesth 83:302–320, 1999.

Gennari FJ: Hypokalemia. N Engl J Med 339:451, 1998.

Mizock BA, Falk JL: Lactic acidosis in critical illness. Crit Care Med 20:80–92, 1992.

Palevsky PM: Hypernatremia. Semin Nephrol 18:20–30, 1998.

Wagner BKJ, D'Amelio LF: Pharmacologic and clinical considerations in selecting crystalloid, colloidal, and oxygen-carrying resuscitation fluids. Part I. Clin Pharm 12:335–346, 1993.

Wagner BKJ, D'Amelio LF: Pharmacologic and clinical considerations in selecting crystalloid, colloidal, and oxygen-carrying resuscitation fluids. Part II. Clin Pharm 12:415–428, 1993.

CHAPTER 7

Arrhythmia Management

SANJEEV V. CHHANGANI, M.D., M.B.A.

Fueled by evidence-based medicine, the pharmacologic and nonpharmacologic approaches to the management of arrhythmias have significantly evolved over the last two decades. The perioperative and critical care physician must be cognizant of the diagnosis and management of arrhythmias in the perioperative period and critical illness. The optimal management of arrhythmias in the perioperative period and critical illness requires knowledge of the basic cardiac electrophysiology, underlying medical problems, risk factors precipitating arrhythmias, pharmacology of antiarrhythmic drugs, as well as drug interactions between anti-arrhythmic drugs and drugs used in anesthesia and intensive care. In addition, the perioperative and critical care physician should be familiar with implantable devices used in the treatment of arrhythmias. This review summarizes recent advances in our understanding of arrhythmia mechanisms and management.

ELECTROPHYSIOLOGIC MECHANISMS OF ARRHYTHMIA

Knowledge of the cardiac action potential is a prerequisite for a better understanding of the pathophysiologic mechanisms underlying arrhythmia formation.

The cardiac action potential represents the rapid flux of ions across the cardiomyocytes producing a wavefront of excitation. An electrocardiogram (ECG) is a recording of the electrical activity of the heart from surface electrodes. Figure 7-1 summarizes the action potential and ECG. The ventricular cell at baseline maintains a resting potential of −80 to −90 mV (polarized state) as a result of a high level of potassium conductance across the cell membrane. The action potential is divided into four phases depending upon the channel activation and changes in membrane potential. Phase 0 is the result of activation of fast sodium channels producing an overshoot in membrane potential, phase 1 results from the transient outward potassium currents and results in a slight fall in membrane potential, phase 2 (plateau) results from a balance of inward (sodium and calcium)

and outward (potassium) currents, phase 3 results from the delayed activation of potassium channels, and in some pacemaker cells (sinoatrial and atrioventricular) phase 4 results in slow spontaneous depolarization leading to another action potential. This explains the automaticity of the pacemaker cells. Phases 0 to 2 represent *depolarization* and phase 3 *repolarization* of the cardiac myocyes. The ECG records the electrical activity of the heart that triggers heart muscle to contract (Figure 7-2). The sinoatrial (S-A) node signals the beginning of the cardiac cycle with the P wave on the ECG due to atrial depolarization. Atrial repolarization is usually too small in amplitude to be detected on the ECG. Next, the electrical impulse travels through the atrioventricular (A-V) node to reach the ventricular muscle cells. The QRS complex represents ventricular depolarization, and the ST-T complex represents ventricular repolarization. The J point is the junction between the end of the QRS complex and the beginning of the ST segment. The rapid upstroke (phase 0) of the action potential corresponds to the onset of QRS. The plateau (phase 2) corresponds to the isoelectric ST segment, and active repolarization (phase 3) to the beginning of the T wave.

There are three fundamental electrophysiologic mechanisms that are responsible for arrhythmia formation.

Reentry

Reentry is the most common mechanism underlying arrhythmia formation. Three conditions must be met for the reentry mechanism to result in an arrhythmia: the presence of a central area of inexcitable tissue separating two pathways for conduction, unidirectional block in one of the two pathways, and slow conduction permitting delay and recovery of excitability in the previously blocked area. Pathologic substrate, as in the tissue surrounding an infarct zone, or altered milieu, as in functional alterations in conduction secondary to electrolyte disturbance, or ischemia can predispose to reentry-induced arrhythmia.

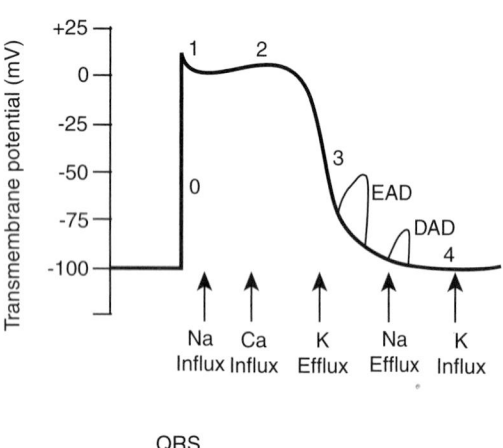

Figure 7-1 Phases of ventricular action potential and ECG. *Phase 0,* overshoot is caused by rapid inward Na current; *Phase 1,* transient potassium efflux; *phase 2 (plateau),* slow inward Ca current; *phase 3 (repolarization),* outward K current; *phase 4,* resting potential maintained by Na–K–ATPase pump. Specialized conduction system tissue has spontaneous depolarization during phase 4. EAD, early after-depolarization; DAD, delayed after-depolarization.

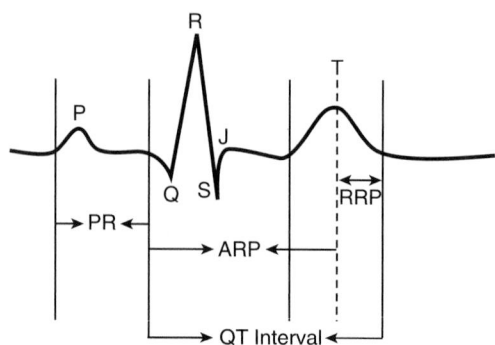

Figure 7-2 ECG cardiac cycle. ARP, absolute refractory period; RRP, relative refractory period; J, J-point.

Abnormal Automaticity

Abnormal automaticity refers to the development of slow, spontaneous phase 4 depolarization in the cells that otherwise do not exhibit automatic pacemaker activity. Under certain conditions ventricular myocytes may develop a "leakage current" during phase 4, resulting in impulse formation. Abnormal automaticity causes repetitive depolarization at rates faster than that found in normally automatic tissues, resulting in overdrive suppression of the S-A node. Ischemic and diseased cardiac tissue is susceptible to arrhythmias due to abnormal automaticity, especially under increased sympathetic activity and metabolic disturbances.

Triggered Activity

Triggered activity refers to abnormal impulse formation from after-depolarizations. Early or delayed after-depolarizations are oscillations of membrane potential occurring during or immediately after repolarization. The early after-depolarization appears to be related to delayed reactivation of ion channels that carry inward depolarizing currents. These channels are responsible for the plateau phase of the action potential (phase 3). With prolonged duration of the action potential, these channels may reopen, resulting in a net inward flow of ions. Once early after-depolarization reaches a sufficient threshold, abnormal impulse propagation is triggered. Certain conditions are associated with prolonged action potential (a prolonged QT interval), such as bradycardia, certain antiarrhythmic drugs (quinine, procainamide, and sotalol), and electrolyte disturbances, such as hypokalemia, hypocalcemia, and hypomagnesemia. Torsades de pointes is an example of triggered arrhythmia due to early after-depolarization. Delayed after-depolarization results from increased intracellular calcium levels. Catecholamines, ischemia, and digitalis-induced arrhythmias are examples of triggered arrhythmias due to delayed after-depolarization. The common finding among these causes is intracellular calcium overload.

RISK FACTORS FOR ARRHYTHMIAS IN ANESTHESIA AND CRITICAL ILLNESS

Anesthesia and critical illness are associated with significant perturbations that, in a susceptible patient, can precipitate cardiac arrhythmias. The risk of developing atrial fibrillation increases substantially with age. Arrhythmia formation is multifactorial. In the perioperative period the interaction between structural heart disease, altered milieu, and drugs often leads to the formation of arrhythmias (Box 7-1). Table 7-1 summarizes the triad of risk factors for arrhythmias. In addition, the type of surgery (cardiac vs. noncardiac) carries specific risk for certain types of arrhythmias. For example, atrial fibrillation is more common following cardiac surgery.

Box 7-1   Risk Factors for Arrhythmias
Structural heart disease, altered milieu, and drugs represent the triad of risk factors for arrhythmias.

Table 7-1   Risk Triad for Arrhythmias

1. Structural Heart Disease	2. Altered Milieu	3. Drugs
Coronary artery disease	Metabolic disturbances	Catecholamines
Valvular heart disease	Electrolyte abnormalities	Volatile anesthetics
Congenital heart disease	Hyperkalemia	QT interval-prolonging drugs
Cardiomyopathy	Hypokalemia	Beta-blocker withdrawal
Sick sinus syndrome	Hypomagnesemia	
Long QT interval syndromes	Hypocalcemia	
Wolff–Parkinson–White syndrome	Acid–base imbalance	
	Severe acidemia or alkalemia	
	Myocardial ischemia, CAD, hypotension, hypoxia	
	Neurohumoral stress response, hypoxia, hypercarbia, laryngoscopy and intubation pain, systemic inflammatory response, hypovolemia and fluid overload	
	Miscellaneous intravascular and intracardiac catheters, device malfunction and microshock	

Structural Heart Disease

Perioperative arrhythmias are more likely to occur in the presence of structural heart disease. Patients with chronic coronary artery disease (ischemia and infarction) have areas of normal, slow, or absent conduction interacting with nonuniform myocardial refractoriness. Valvular heart disease can be associated with myocardial fiber stretch (increased volume or wall stress). Cardiomyopathies of various etiologies, such as hypertrophic, dilated, infiltrative, or due to metabolic disorders (uremia, diabetes), usually lead to ventricular arrhythmias. Other examples of structural heart disease associated with increased risk of arrhythmia include congenital heart disease, sick sinus syndrome, long QT interval syndrome, and Wolff–Parkinson–White syndrome.

Altered Milieu

Anesthesia, perioperative period, and critical illness with its associated metabolic, ischemic, and neurohumoral stressors produce altered milieu surrounding cardiomyocytes and result in changes in refractoriness or conduction of impulses. Thus, in the patient with underlying structural heart disease, altered milieu can precipitate cardiac arrhythmias.

Metabolic Disturbances

Specific electrolyte abnormalities, such as potassium, magnesium, and calcium, are well known to produce arrhythmias.

Potassium

Hypokalemia hyperpolarizes the resting membrane potential to a more negative value, and may cause slowing of conduction. In addition, hypokalemia decreases potassium conductance producing delayed repolarization and early after-depolarization (enhanced automaticity). Hyperkalemia increases the permeability to potassium and shifts the resting membrane potential to a less negative value. This results in shortening of the action potential and suppressed automaticity, and slowing of conduction. QRS is markedly widened with severe hyperkalemia. Therefore, treatment of hyperkalemia demands immediate attention.

Calcium

Hypocalcemia causes prolongation of QT interval and may result in early after-depolarization and triggered arrhythmias, e.g., Torsade de pointes. Hypercalcemia produces shortening of QT interval and usually does not produce triggered arrhythmias.

Magnesium

Hypomagnesemia is also associated with prolongation of QT interval and torsades de pointes. Hypermagnesemia can lead to slowing of A-V nodal and ventricular conduction. Conditions associated with hypomagnesemia include cachexia and malnutrition, critical illness, cardiopulmonary bypass, hemodialysis, alcoholism, cancer and chemotherapy, and potassium-wasting diuretics. It is important to emphasize that magnesium, calcium, and potassium deficits often coexist and that magnesium repletion must be undertaken at the same time as repletion of potassium and calcium.

Acid–Base Imbalance

Acid-base homeostasis plays a critical role in tissue and organ performance. Management of arrhythmias in the presence of serious acid–base disorders demands precise diagnosis and treatment of the underlying disease. Severe acidemia can cause sensitization of the myocardium to reentrant arrhythmias and reduction in threshold for ventricular fibrillation. Severe alkalemia can sensitize the myocardium to refractory supraventricular and ventricular arrhythmias. Severe acid–base disorders are also associated with electrolyte abnormalities. Hyperkalemia is not uncommon with severe acidemia. Hypokalemia and hypocalcemia are frequently seen with severe alkalemia.

Ischemia

Myocardial ischemia in the perioperative period and critical illness can occur as a consequence of underlying coronary artery disease or from hemodynamic and hypoxic stress. Electrophysiologic effects of myocardial ischemia include partial depolarization of the resting membrane potential resulting in inactivation of fast sodium channels and slowing of conduction, increased intracellular calcium load, elevation of extracellular potassium, and prolongation of refractoriness. Ischemia-induced arrhythmias are mediated by abnormal automaticity, triggered activity, and reentry.

Neurohumoral Stressors

In addition to the above, many events in anesthesia and critical illness can invoke the neurohumoral stress response and precipitate arrhythmias. The result is increased sympathetic activity and catecholamine response. Examples of these events include hypoxia and hypercarbia, laryngoscopy and tracheal intubation, hypovolemia and fluid overload, pain, and systemic inflammatory response.

Miscellaneous

Diagnostic and therapeutic interventions involving intravascular and intracardiac catheters, device malfunction, or microschock can also predispose to mechanically induced arrhythmias.

Drugs

A multitude of drugs used in anesthesia and critical illness have effects on cardiac electrophysiology and can cause arrhythmias either by themselves or acting in concert with the two risk factors discussed above (structural heart disease and altered milieu).

Catecholamines

Through stimulation of β-adrenergic receptors, endogenous (sympathetic activation) or exogenous catecholamines can result in enhanced automaticity or triggered activity. Reentry may also be facilitated in the presence of ischemia.

Volatile Anesthetics

There is increasing evidence that volatile anesthetics have potent electrophysiologic influences on arrhythmias due to both altered impulse initiation and conduction. Depression of inward Ca^{2+} currents by the volatile anesthetics contributes to largely antiarrhythmic actions on mechanisms generating abnormal impulses as a result of intracellular Ca^{2+} "overload" resulting from catecholamine exposure, digitalis intoxication, and ischemia. On the other hand, the actions of volatile anesthetics in combination with catecholamines depressing conduction and altering refractoriness of the myocardium may potentially facilitate the induction of reentrant arrhythmias. The adverse interaction between volatile anesthetics and catecholamines remains a clinically relevant problem.

QT Interval-Prolonging Drugs

Prolongation of QT interval on the ECG can predispose to a potentially lethal arrhythmia known as torsades de pointes. QT interval-prolonging drugs have been implicated in torsades de pointes. Some patients have genetic predisposition for QT prolongation and manifest with overt QT prolongation only with exposure to QT-prolonging drugs. The presence of the triad of factors in association with QT interval-prolonging drugs can result in torsades de pointes. Table 7-2 lists commonly used QT interval-prolonging drugs. It is also very important to understand drug interactions between cardiac and noncardiac QT interval-prolonging drugs. These interactions can be pharmacodynamic (both drugs affect cardiac electrophysiology), pharmacokinetic (one drug affects clearance of the other), or mixed in nature. Therefore, combination of QT interval-prolonging drugs should be avoided.

Drug Withdrawal

Beta-blockers are commonly used in the prophylaxis and treatment of arrhythmias in the high-risk patient. Beta-blocker withdrawal has been associated with postoperative supraventricular arrhythmias. A state of increased catecholamine effect occurs because of chronic β-blocker associated up-regulation (higher density) of β-adrenergic receptors.

CLASSIFICATION, DIAGNOSIS, AND MANAGEMENT OF ARRHYTHMIAS

Cardiac arrhythmias may be simply classified as (1) those resulting in cardiac arrest, (2) bradyarrhythmias, (3) ventricular arrhythmias, and (4) supraventricular arrhythmias. This classification places an emphasis on the urgency of diagnosis and management. Table 7-3 summarizes the classification of cardiac arrhythmias.

Table 7-3   Classification of Cardiac Arrhythmias

Cardiac Arrhythmia	Examples
Cardiac arrest arrhythmias	Ventricular fibrillation
	Pulseless ventricular tachycardia
	Pulseless electrical activity (PEA)
	Asystole
Supraventricular arrhythmias	Paroxysmal supraventricular tachycardia
	A-V nodal reentry tachycardia (AVNRT)
	Atrioventricular reentry tachycardia (AVRT)
	Intraatrial reentry tachycardia
	Automatic atrial tachycardia
	A-V junctional tachycardia
	Atrial fibrillation/atrial flutter
	Multifocal atrial tachycardia
	Wolff–Parkinson–White syndrome
Ventricular arrhythmias	Nonsustained ventricular tachycardia
	Sustained ventricular tachycardia
	Monomorphic
	Polymorphic (Torsades de pointes)
	Ventricular fibrillation
Bradyarrhythmias	Sinus bradycardia
	First-degree heart block
	Second-degree heart block
	Type I (Mobitz I – Wanckebach)
	Type II (Mobitz II – non-Wanckebach)
	Third-degree heart block
	(A-V dissociation)

Table 7-2   QT Interval-Prolonging Drugs

Antiarrhythmics	Amiodarone, Disopyramide, Ibutilide, Dofitilide, Procainamide, Quinidine, Sotalol
Antipsychotics	Thioridazine, Pimozide, Ziprasidone, Haloperidol, Risperidone
Anti-infectives	Erythromycin, Clarithromycin, Pentamidine, Sparfloxacin
Antiemetics	Droperidol
Antifungals	Ketoconazole, fluconazole, itraconazole
Others	Cisapride, Bepridil

General Approach to the Diagnosis and Management of Arrhythmias

Basic Principles

The following basic principles must be followed in managing arrhythmias.

Treat the patient and not the ECG. One must first decide if the arrhythmia is real or an artifact and whether the arrhythmia is sufficient to account for the patient's symptoms and signs. A simply detached ECG lead can display as asystole on the cardiac monitor. Similarly, shivering can be associated with ECG artifacts, which can be misinterpreted as ventricular or supraventricular arrhythmias.

Establish the urgency of treatment. Clinical assessment of the patient will establish the urgency of treatment. Clinical assessment includes assessment of responsiveness (or lack of) and a quick ABCD survey. A defibrillator and help must be summoned for all unresponsive patients. The ABCD survey consists of assessment of **A**irway by opening the airway using head tilt–chin lift or jaw-thrust maneuver for effective spontaneous breathing; **B**reathing by securing and confirming airway device in an apneic patient and assuring oxygenation and ventilation; **C**irculation by checking for a pulse and blood pressure, evaluation of peripheral perfusion, presence of myocardial ischemia and congestive heart failure, and initiation of CPR in the pulseless patient or defibrillation of identified ventricular fibrillation using a defibrillator; and **D**ifferential **D**iagnosis and treatment of reversible causes, such as hypoventilation, hypoxia, hypovolemia, metabolic disorders, etc.

Establish hemodynamic stability. Following the initial ABCD survey and treatment, the goal must always be to establish hemodynamic stability. Slowing the ventricular response in the case of tachyarrhythmia or increase in ventricular rate in bradyarrhythmia, or maintaining adequate blood pressure using fluids or vasoactive agents may achieve this goal.

Specific antiarrhythmic therapy. Next, antiarrhythmic therapy is initiated based on arrhythmia diagnosis and specifically targeted against the subcellular units. The goal is to prevent recurrence of hemodynamic instability. Knowledge of ventricular function is also helpful in the choice of antiarrhythmic therapy.

Restoration of sinus rhythm. Restoration of sinus rhythm is always desirable, but may not be achievable under specific circumstances, such as a heightened state of sympathetic activity.

Prevention of complications. In patients in whom sinus rhythm cannot be achieved, measures must be taken to prevent complications related to specific arrhythmia, e.g., thromboembolic complications due to atrial fibrillation.

Approach to Arrhythmia Diagnosis

A 12-lead ECG must be obtained for complete interpretation of arrhythmia. In the absence of a 12-lead ECG, a long rhythm strip of a lead in which P waves are visible is preferred. Mere observation of ECG rhythm on the monitor may be misleading. A systemic approach to ECG diagnosis of arrhythmia includes the following.

Rate and regularity of rhythm. The rate of normal sinus rhythm in adults is between 60 and 100 beats/minute. Sinus tachycardia usually occurs at a rate between 100 and 180 beats/minute. The definition of clinically significant bradycardia or tachycardia must be individualized. Atrial tachycardia and A-V nodal reentrant usually present with rates from 140 to 220 beats/minute. Rates between 240 and 320 are most likely to represent atrial flutter. PP and RR cycles, and relation of P wave to QRS will suggest regularity of rhythm.

Location of P waves. Leads II, III, aVF, or V1 are best used to ascertain P waves. If no P waves are present and RR intervals are irregular, the rhythm is most likely atrial fibrillation. A narrow QRS complex tachycardia without discernible P waves is most likely caused by A-V nodal reentry. When the atria and ventricles are controlled by independent pacemaker foci with similar rates, P waves appear to "march in and out" of the QRS complex. This is termed isorhythmic A-V dissociation. P waves of two or more morphologies are characteristic of multifocal atrial tachycardia.

Relationship between P waves and QRS complexes. If there are more P waves than QRS complexes, then A-V block is present. If there are more QRS complexes than P waves, the rhythm is junctional or ventricular in origin.

QRS morphology. A narrow QRS complex (<0.12 ms) indicates supraventricular arrhythmia. A wide QRS complex (>0.12 ms) can be present with either ventricular tachycardia or supraventricular tachycardia with aberrant ventricular conduction.

Treatment of Specific Arrhythmias

Antiarrhythmic drug classification and agents are summarized in Table 7-4.

Cardiac Arrest Arrhythmias

Early defibrillation, CPR, airway management, and advanced cardiac life support are essential for neurologic outcome in patients after cardiac arrest.

Ventricular Fibrillation and Pulseless Ventricular Tachycardia

Pathophysiology. There are areas of normal myocardium alternating with areas of ischemic, injured, or infarcted myocardium, leading to chaotic pattern of ventricular depolarization.

Table 7-4	Classification of Antiarrhythmic Agents Based on Receptor Targets	
Receptor Target	**ECG Changes (Class)**	**Drugs**
Na and K channels	QRS and QT prolongation (IA)	Procainamide, Amiodarone, disopyramide, quinidine
Na channels	QRS prolongation (IB)	Lidocaine, phenytoin, mexiletine
Beta-receptors	PR prolongation (II)	Esmolol, Amiodarone, propranolol, atenolol, labetolol, sodalol
K channels	QT prolongation (III)	Bretylium, ibutilide, sotalol, dofetilide
Ca channels	PR prolongation (IV)	Verapamil, deltiazem, Amiodarone

ECG criteria (Figure 7-3). There are no recognizable P, QRS, or T waves. The rate is difficult to determine. The rhythm is indeterminate with patterns of upstrokes and downstrokes. Ventricular fibrillation (VF) can be fine (amplitude 1 to 5 mm) or coarse (amplitude 10 to 15 mm).

Clinical features. The patient becomes unconscious without pulse. Respirations become agonal and apnea quickly ensues. This can result in sudden death.

Etiology. Common etiologies of VF/pulseless ventricular tachycardia (VT) include acute myocardial infarction leading to areas of ischemic myocardium, untreated VT, primary or secondary QT interval prolongation, PVCs with R on T phenomenon, electrocution, and hypoxemia.

Therapy. Early defibrillation (asynchronous DC countershock) is the hallmark of treatment. Time to defibrillation is the most important determinant of survival from cardiac arrest. Probability of successful resuscitation declines by 2% to 10% per minute from the onset of symptoms. In this respect the use of automatic external defibrillators (AEDs) has gained popularity in a variety of settings, public and healthcare alike. After a sequence of three rapid defibrillation shocks (200, 220, 360 J),

pharmacologic therapy is considered. Current pharmacologic therapy consists of intravenous epinephrine 1 mg every 3 to 5 minutes as an adrenergic stimulant to improve perfusion pressure of vital organs. Vasopressin, administered as 40 units intravenous push single dose, may be used as an alternative to epinephrine and is associated with less risk of postresuscitation tachyarrhythmias. Amiodarone (300 mg intravenous push) is considered next to prevent refibrillation after a shock causes defibrillation. If VF/VT recurs, administration of a second dose of Amiodarone 150 mg IV should be considered, with a maximum cumulative dose of 2.2 g over 24 hours. Lidocaine and procainamide are considered of indeterminate class benefit for persistent VF/VT. Correction of hypomagnesemia and acidosis is considered using magnesium and sodium bicarbonate in prolonged arrest situations.

Pulseless Electrical Activity

Pathophysiology. In this condition there is electrical activity in the form of cardiac conduction impulses, but this fails to produce myocardial contraction or ejection.

ECG criteria (Figure 7-4). There is organized electrical activity with narrow (QRS < 0.10 ms) or wide (>0.10 ms) waves, and at a fast or slow heart rate.

Clinical features. Clinical manifestations are the same as those of pulseless VT/VF.

Etiologies. Common causes of pulseless electrical activity are often reversible and can be grouped under "five H's": hypovolemia, hypoxia, acidosis (increased hydrogen ion), hyperkalemia/hypokalemia, hypothermia; and "five T's": tablets (drug overdose, ingestions),

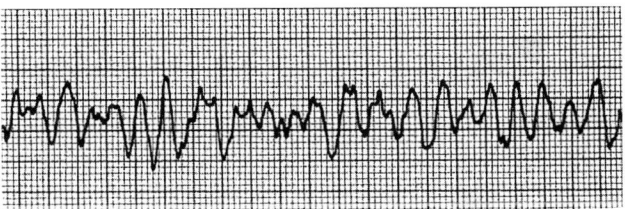

Figure 7-3   Ventricular fibrillation.

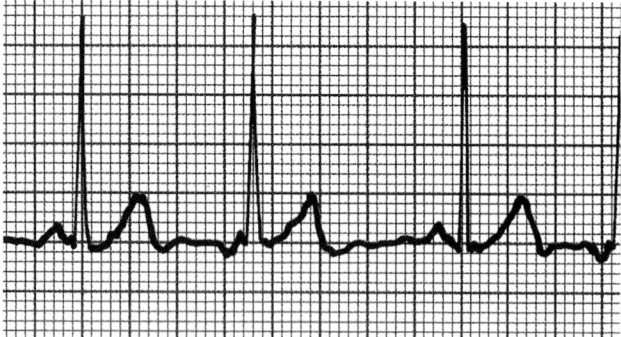

Figure 7-4 Pulseless electrical activity (PEA). Organized rhythm without detectable pulse.

tamponade (cardiac), tension pneumothorax, thrombus (coronary), thromboembolism (pulmonary).

Therapy. Identification and treatment of reversible causes is the mainstay of therapy. After establishment of airway, ventilation, and basic CPR, intravenous epinephrine 1 mg or atropine 1 mg can be administered if heart rate is <60 beats per minute.

Asystole

Pathophysiology. It usually represents a terminal rhythm.

ECG criteria (Figure 7-5). Classically asystole presents as a flat line. Asystole can be verified by checking the lead and cable connection, increasing monitor gain, and changing leads. There is no ventricular activity or at a rate of <6 beats per minute. Occasionally P waves are seen, but without R waves.

Clinical features. It presents as cardiac arrest with no pulse or blood pressure, and agonal respirations.

Etiology. Usually indicates end of life. Reversible causes such as the five H's and five T's should be sought and corrected. Asystole can also be seen after massive electrical shock or postdefibrillatory shock.

Therapy. After establishment of an airway, ventilation, and basic CPR, intravenous epinephrine 1 mg (every 3 to 5 minutes) and atropine 1 mg (total 2 mg) is administered. If considered, transcutaneous pacing is performed immediately. With respect to hospital admissions and discharge, a recent study found vasopressin (40 U) to be superior to epinephrine in patients with asystole.

Supraventricular Arrhythmias

Atrial Fibrillation/Atrial Flutter

Atrial fibrillation (AF) occurs in 0.5-1% of the general population, especially in patients older than 60 years. In postcardiac surgery patients AF is more frequent (10-65%). The frequency of AF in noncardiac surgery patients falls between the above two groups (2-10%). AF is the most common arrhythmia in the surgical intensive care unit (cardiac and noncardiac). Five independent risk factors were identified in a recent study of AF in surgical intensive care units. These were advanced age, withdrawal of calcium channel blockers, blunt thoracic trauma, shock, and use of a pulmonary artery catheter.

Pathophysiology. AF is an example of reentry tachyarrhythmia. In AF the atria contract in a chaotic fashion and impulses travel in a random pathway through the atria. The multiple wavelet theory is most common in explaining the erratic electrical conduction occurring in most AF. Alterations in the atrial electrophysiologic conditions, such as decreased repolarization time, decreased refractory periods, and variable refractory dispersion, are favorable conditions to stimulate and maintain AF. These conditions promote development of multiple reentry circuits that perpetuate throughout the atria and allow AF to sustain. Atrial flutter involves impulses traveling in a circular course around the atria.

ECG criteria (Figure 7-6). The classic pattern of AF is an irregular rhythm with varying RR interval. P wave and PR interval is not defined. In atrial flutter a "sawtooth" pattern is classic. Unlike AF, ECG rhythm and ventricular response is regular in atrial flutter with 2 to 1 or 3 to 1 ratio depending upon A-V node conduction block.

Clinical features. Signs and symptoms depend upon the rate of ventricular response, with dyspnea, chest pain, acute pulmonary edema, congestive heart failure, and

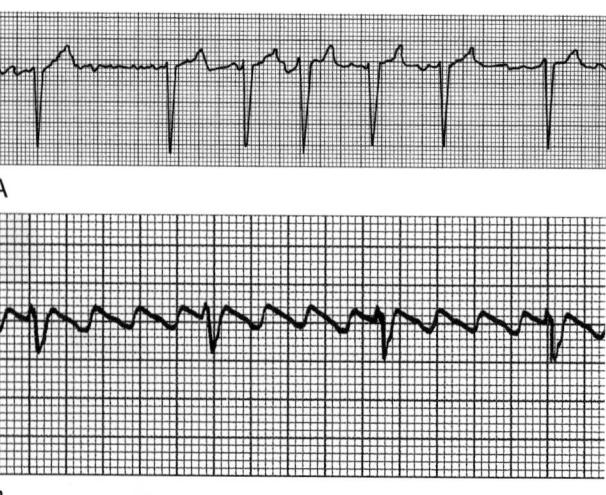

A

B

Figure 7-6 Atrial fibrillation (**A**) and atrial flutter (**B**).

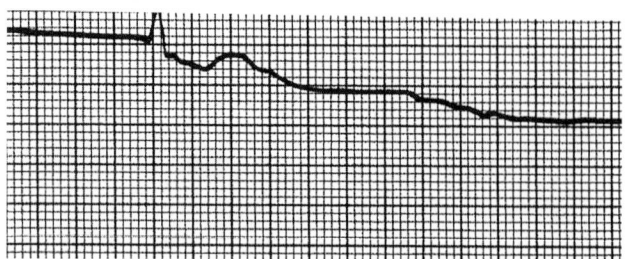

Figure 7-5 Asystole.

altered consciousness often occurring with rapid ventricular response. Loss of "atrial kick" may result in a drop in cardiac output and blood pressure in patients with ventricular hypertrophy and aortic stenosis.

Etiology. Common etiologies of atrial flutter/fibrillation include hypoxia (acute pulmonary embolism, chronic obstructive pulmonary disease), enlargement of atria (mitral or tricuspid valve disease, fluid overload), acute coronary syndromes, hyperthyroidism, and drugs such as digoxin and quinidine.

Therapy. The goals of AF/atrial flutter management are hemodynamic stabilization, restoration and maintenance of sinus rhythm, and prevention of thromboembolism. The therapeutic decisions are based on four factors: hemodynamic stability, cardiac function, presence of pre-excitation on ECG, and duration (two days or more).

Cardioversion

Electrical or pharmacologic cardioversion must be considered in patients with AF that presents with rapid ventricular rate with hemodynamic compromise. Early cardioversion increases both the success of cardioversion and reduces the rate of recurrence, as well as the need for anticoagulation. Current guidelines state that patients with AF of less than 2 days' duration can be cardioverted without anticoagulation. Direct current cardioversion usually is performed under sedation to minimize patient discomfort. Adequate oxygenation and ventilation must be ensured during the procedure. A standard defibrillator is used to deliver a *synchronized* shock at energies ranging from 100 to 300 J. The shock electrode position can be either anterior–anterior (right sternal border and left lateral chest wall) or anterior–posterior (precordial and interscapular). Atrial flutter requires a lower energy for cardioversion. Newer defibrillators with energy delivered in the form of biphasic waveforms require less energy and provide greater success with cardioversion. Several drugs, including ibutilide, Amiodarone, procainamide, flecainide and propafenone, have been used in the pharmacologic cardioversion of AF or atrial flutter. The caveats in the pharmacologic cardioversion of AF include avoiding multiple QT-prolonging drugs, close watch for torsades de pointes, and administration of magnesium.

CLINICAL CAVEAT

In pharmacologic cardioversion of atrial fibrillation/atrial flutter: avoid multiple QT-prolonging drugs, watch for torsades de pointes, and give magnesium.

Rate Control

For patients with AF or atrial flutter who present with rapid ventricular rate and stable condition, rate control can be achieved using pharmacologic means.

The rate-controlling drugs are A-V nodal blockers, which act by slowing down the rate. These include beta-blockers, calcium channel blockers, and digoxin. These drugs should be avoided in patients with AF in association with Wolff–Parkinson–White (WPW) syndrome. Pharmacologic agents used for heart rate control in AF are shown in Table 7-5.

Anticoagulation

Patients with AF lasting longer than two days or of unknown or intermittent duration should be anticoagulated with a therapeutic international normalized ratio (INR) of 2–3 for at least 2–3 weeks before and after cardioversion. Screening for left atrial thrombus by echocardiography is an acceptable alternative to routine pre-cardioversion anticoagulation. The risk of thromboembolic complications is higher in patients older than 65 years, with valvular heart disease, history of congestive heart failure, enlarged atrium, left ventricular dysfunction, and myocardial infarction.

Wolff–Parkinson–White Syndrome

Pathophysiology. A prototypical pre-excitation syndrome, WPW syndrome consists of an extra electrical connection (accessory pathway) between the atria and the ventricles that allows the atrial impulse to bypass the A-V node. The majority of arrhythmias associated with WPW syndrome are reciprocating tachycardias which may be narrow complex or wide complex.

ECG criteria (Figure 7-7). When the accessory pathways conduct impulses in an antegrade direction, there is a fusion of activation of the ventricles by the bypass tract and the A-V nodal His-Purkinje system. This is represented on the ECG by a short PR interval (<120 ms) and slurring of the initial component of the QRS complex (delta wave) giving it a widened appearance (>120 ms). Secondary ST-T wave changes generally are directed opposite to the major delta and QRS vector.

Clinical features. Patients with WPW syndrome may remain completely asymptomatic. Tachycardia may present as palpitation, dyspnea, chest pain, or congestive heart failure (CHF). Hereditary and male predisposition is common.

Etiology. The accessory pathway in WPW syndrome is a congenital malformation.

Therapy. Treatment of WPW syndrome is based on the presence of hemodynamic instability, cardiac function impairment, or duration of AF with WPW syndrome. AF with rapid ventricular response is the life-threatening arrhythmia in the patient with WPW syndrome and should be treated with electric cardioversion. In the patient with a normal heart the choice of antiarrhythmic drugs include Amiodarone, flecainide, procainamide, propafenone, or sotalol. In the patient with impaired cardiac function cardioversion or Amiodarone can be used. Anticoagulation is required for AF with WPW syndrome lasting more than two days.

Table 7-5   Pharmacologic Agents for Heart Rate Control in Atrial Fibrillation

Drug	Loading Dose	Infusion	Onset	Side Effects	Comment
Diltiazem	0.25 mg/kg IV over 5–10 minutes	5–15 mg/hour	2–7 minutes	Hypotension, heart block	May be considered in patients with low EF
Esmolol	0.5 mg/kg IV over 5–10 minutes	0.05–0.2 mg/kg/ minute	2 minutes	Hypotension, heart block, bradycardia, CHF	Caution in patients with asthma, low EF
Metoprolol	2.5–5 mg IV bolus over 2 minutes; repeat up to 4 doses	Not recommended	5 minutes	Hypotension, heart block, wheezing, bradycardia, CHF	Well tolerated in patients with normal EF and no history of asthma or COPD
Propranolol	0.15 mg/kg	Not recommended	5 minutes	Hypotension, heart block, bradycardia, CHF, wheezing	Avoid in patients with low EF and COPD
Verapamil	0.075–0.15 mg/kg IV over 5 minutes	Not recommended	3–5 minutes	Hypotension, heart block, CHF	Negative inotrope
Digoxin	0.25 mg IV every 2 hours, total 1 mg	Not recommended. Maintenance dose: 0.125– 0.25 mg daily	2 hours	Digitalis toxicity, heart block, bradycardia	May be considered in patients with low EF

CHF, congestive heart failure; COPD, chronic obstructive pulmonary disease.

Multifocal Atrial Tachycardia

Pathophysiology. Mutifocal atrial tachycardia (MAT) results from areas of increased automaticity arising irregularly and rapidly in different areas of the atrium.

ECG criteria (Figure 7-8A). Heart rate typically ranges from 120 to 130 beats/minute. The rhythm is usually irregular. There are three or more different morphologies of P waves and PR interval is variable. QRS complex is usually narrow.

Etiology. The common causes of MAT include chronic obstructive pulmonary disease (COPD), digoxin toxicity, and acute coronary syndrome.

Therapy. Adenosine or vagal stimulation may be helpful if ECG diagnosis is unclear. In patients with preserved heart function, beta-blockers can be used. In patients at risk for wheezing (COPD, asthma) or in patients with impaired heart function, calcium channel blockers

(diltiazem) and Amiodarone are effective. Direct current cardioversion is not effective in the treatment of MAT.

Paroxysmal Supraventricular Tachycardia

Pathophysiology. Paroxysmal supraventricular tachycardia (PSVT) is another example of reentry-mediated tachyarrhythmia. In patients with PSVT impulses arise and perpetuate repeatedly in the A-V node because of areas of unidirectional block in the Purkinje fibers.

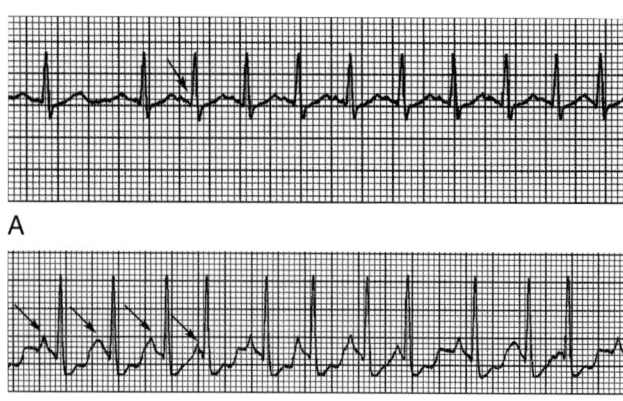

A

B

Figure 7-8   (A) Onset of supraventricular tachycardia (arrow). (B) Mutifocal atrial tachycardia (MAT). Arrows indicate multiple P wave morphologies.

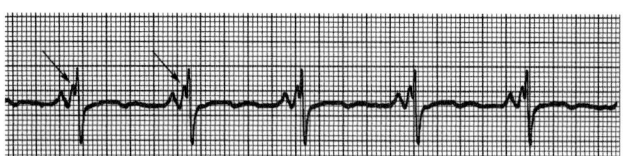

Figure 7-7   Wolff–Parkinson–White (WPW) syndrome. Arrows indicate delta waves.

ECG criteria (Figure 7-8B). The heart rate varies between 150 and 250 beats/minute and the rhythm is regular. P waves are absent or buried in T waves. QRS complex is usually narrow.

Clinical features. Palpitation, anxiety, low exercise tolerance, dyspnea, and light-headedness are common presenting features of PSVT.

Etiology. Many patients with PSVT have accessory conduction pathway. Factors that are known to precipitate PSVT include caffeine, hypoxia, smoking, stress, anxiety, and sleep deprivation.

Therapy. Vagal maneuver or adenosine may help differentiate between PSVT and AF. DC cardioversion should be considered in the hemodynamically unstable patient. The patient with preserved ventricular function will tolerate A-V nodal blockade using beta-blockers, calcium channel blockers, procainamide, or digoxin. In the patient with impaired ventricular function Amiodarone, diltiazem, or digoxin may be a better choice.

Junctional Tachycardia

Pathophysiology. This is an example of tachyarrythmia as a result of enhanced automatic impulse formation in the A-V node. Both antegrade and retrograde transmission of impulses occur.

ECG criteria. The rhythm is regular at a rate of 100–180 beats/minute. P waves are usually absent or inverted. QRS complexes are narrow in the absence of ventricular conduction delay.

Clinical features. CHF may occur as a result of loss of sinus (atrial) "kick." Symptoms of unstable tachycardia, dyspnea, chest pain, or light-headedness may occur.

Etiology. Acute coronary syndrome or digoxin toxicity are common causes of junctional tachycardia.

Therapy. DC cardioversion is usually not recommended. Beta-blockers, calcium channel blockers, or Amiodarone have been used with success.

Ventricular Arrhythmias

Ventricular arrhythmias are classified as benign or malignant based upon duration, absence or presence of hemodynamic consequences, or significant structural heart disease. Premature ventricular contractions (PVCs) and nonsustained ventricular tachycardia rarely require therapy in the absence of symptoms or structural heart disease.

Stable Monomorphic Ventricular Tachycardia

Pathophysiology. Sustained monomorphic VT is a reentry rhythm most commonly occurring after myocardial infarction or in the setting of cardiomyopathy. The area of injured myocardium serves as the source of ectopic impulses and the impulse conduction is slowed around this area, resulting in repetitive depolarizations.

ECG criteria (Figure 7-9A). Ventricular rate is typically 120–250 beats/minute, and the rhythm is regular without atrial activity. QRS complexes are wide and "bizarre" (>0.12 ms). The presence of three or more PVCs qualifies as VT. If the duration is <30 seconds, it is nonsustained VT.

Clinical features. Monomorphic VT can be asymptomatic. Symptoms of decreased cardiac output, such as orthostasis, hypotension, or syncope, are present. If left untreated it can deteriorate into VF or unstable VT.

Etiology. Acute myocardial ischemia or infarction, occurrence of PVC during the relative refractory period (R-on-T phenomenon), cardiomyopathy, or QT interval-prolonging drugs are some of the causes of monomorphic VT.

Therapy. In patients with normal ventricular function, drugs like procainamide, lidocaine, sotatol, or amiodarone can be used. Lidocaine, amiodarone, or DC cardioversion are recommended in patients with impaired ventricular function. Electrolyte abnormalities (hypokalemia and hypomagnesemia) must be corrected.

Polymorphic Ventricular Tachycardia

Pathophysiology. Polymorphic VT also results from reentry phenomenon, with multiple areas of ventricle serving as the source of ectopic impulse formation.

ECG criteria (Figure 7-9B). The ventricular rate is typically 120–250 beats/minute, and the rhythm is regular. P waves and PR interval are not seen. QRS complexes show marked variation and inconsistency. QT interval is classically prolonged in patients with Torsades de pointes.

Clinical features. The majority of patients show symptoms of decreased cardiac output. It tends to deteriorate rapidly into VF.

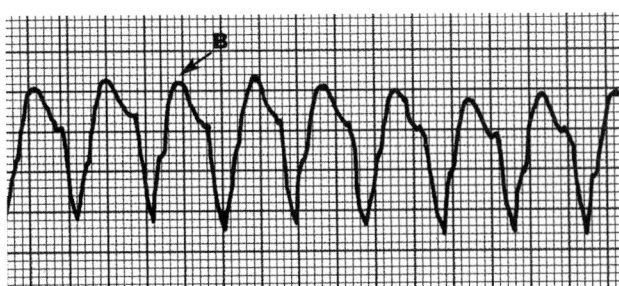

A

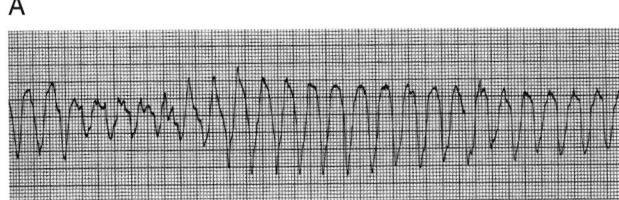

B

Figure 7-9 **(A)** Monomorphic ventricular tachycardia. **(B)** Polymorphic ventricular tachycardia (torsades de pointes).

Etiology. Myocardial ischemia and QT interval-prolonging drugs are common causes of polymorphic VT.

Therapy. In patients with normal QT interval, focus should be to treat ischemia and correct electrolyte abnormalities. Patients with normal heart tolerate well beta-blockers, lidocaine, procainamide, or sotalol. In the presence of impaired heart function, DC cardioversion or Amiodarone should be considered. In patients with prolonged QT interval and torsades de pointes, the therapeutic options include administration of magnesium, overdrive pacing, isoproterenol, phenytoin, or lidocaine. At the same time, cardiac ischemia and electrolyte abnormalities should be treated.

Bradyarrhythmias

Bradyarrhythmias are not uncommon in critical care settings and can be either an incidental finding or represent a potentially life-threatening problem. Sinus bradycardia (heart rate < 60 beats/minute) rarely requires treatment. Atropine or transcutaneous pacing may be used to treat symptomatic sinus bradycardia mediated by vagal stimulation. In addition to the oxygen, catecholamine infusions, such as dopamine, isoproterenol, or epinephrine, can be used as chronotropic agents (Box 7-2).

First-Degree Heart Block

Pathophysiology. In first-degree heart block each atrial impulse is successfully conducted to the ventricle but with a delay at the A-V node.

ECG criteria (Figure 7-10). Each P wave is followed by a QRS but with fixed and prolonged PR interval (>210 ms). QRS complex is most commonly narrow when the block occurs at the level of the A-V node. However, first-degree A-V block with a bundle-branch block and wide QRS represents delayed conduction in the infranodal conduction system.

Clinical features. First-degree heart block is usually asymptomatic at rest. Symptoms usually occur with the degree of bradycardia.

Etiology. The most common drugs associated with first-degree heart block include beta-blockers, calcium channel blockers, digoxin, clonidine, and amiodarone. Stimulation of vasovagal reflex (syncope), autonomic instability, and inferior wall myocardial infarction due to involvement of right coronary circulation are commonly associated with first-degree heart block.

Box 7-2 Common Causes of Bradycardia

Medications, electrolyte disturbances, and increased vagal tone are the most common causes of bradycardia in the critical care setting.

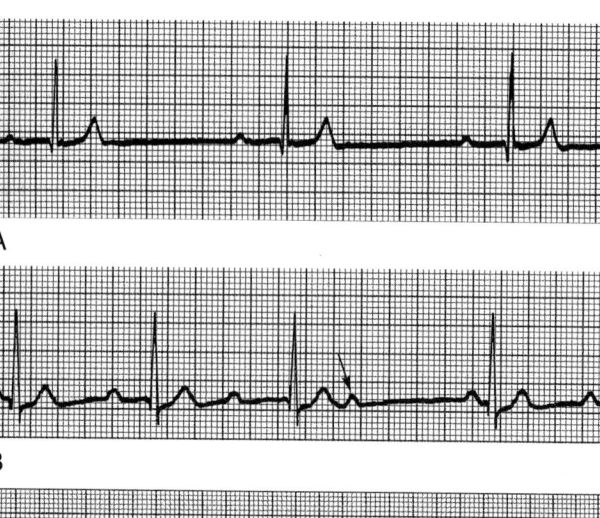

A

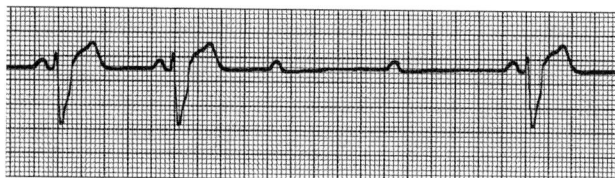

B

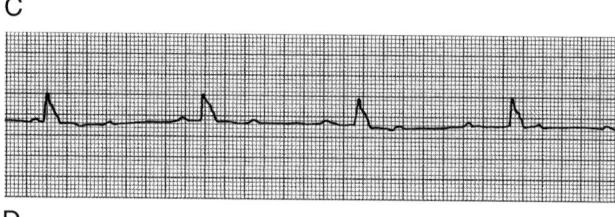

C

D

Figure 7-10   Heart blocks. (**A**) First-degree block (prolonged PR interval). (**B**) Second-degree, Mobitz type 1 (Wenkebach). (**C**) Second-degree type 2. (**D**) Third-degree (complete) heart block.

Therapy. In addition to oxygen, atropine, transcutaneous pacing, and catecholamine infusion may be used to treat symptomatic first-degree heart block.

Second-Degree Heart Block

Pathophysiology. Only some atrial impulses are conducted successfully in all types of second-degree heart block. In Mobitz type I (Wenkebach) block the site of block is at the level of the A-V node. However, in Mobitz type II block the site of the block is below the A-V node.

ECG criteria (Figure 7-10). The atrial rate is usually 60–100 beats/minute. The ventricular rate is slower than the atrial rate. In Mobitz type I block the PR interval progressively lengthens followed by absent QRS complex ("dropped beat"). The QRS is narrow (<0.120 ms). Mobitz type II block occurs without prolongation of the PR interval and the level of block is usually infranodal.

Etiology. A-V nodal blocking medications and vagal stimulation are common causes of second-degree heart block. Right coronary-associated infarction is commonly associated with Mobitz type I block and left coronary is associated infarction with Mobitz type II block.

Clinical features. Hypotension, shock, CHF, and syncope are seen with second-degree heart block.

Therapy. In addition to oxygen, atropine, and transcutaneous pacing, transvenous pacing is required with Mobitz type II block. Catecholamine infusions may be needed to treat hypotension.

Third-Degree Heart Block

Pathophysiology. No atrial impulses are conducted to the ventricles resulting in complete A-V dissociation. The level of block can be either in the A-V node or infranodal.

ECG criteria (Figure 7-10). Both atrial and ventricular rhythm are regular, but dissociated (independent). There is no relationship between P wave and R wave. QRS complex may be narrow (<0.10 s) or wide (>0.10 s) depending upon whether the block is above or below the A-V node.

Clinical features. Clinical manifestations are related to the heart rate. Bradycardia-related symptoms include chest pain, dyspnea, CHF, hypotension, and shock.

Etiology. Acute coronary syndrome involving branches of the left coronary artery (left anterior descending) or right coronary artery (inferior MI) can result in third-degree heart block.

Therapy. Medical therapy is only used until pacing can be initiated. Atropine and isoproterenol are the most commonly used medications and work by increasing the activity of the sinus node and improving block within the A-V node.

MANAGEMENT OF IMPLANTABLE CARDIAC DEVICES

Pacemakers and implantable cardioverter defibrillators (ICDs) are commonly utilized by cardio-electrophysiologists in the management of cardiac arrhythmias. Pacemakers are the mainstay of therapy for clinically symptomatic bradyarrhythmias. Temporary pacemakers are utilized for emergency treatment of patients with symptomatic bradycardia where arrhythmia is transient and reversible or as a bridge to a permanent pacemaker. ICDs are increasingly used in patients with known history of ventricular arrhythmias or those at high risk for ventricular arrhythmias. Perioperative and critical care practitioners must be cognizant of implantable cardiac devices and their management in the perioperative period and intensive care unit.

Pacemakers

General indications for cardiac pacing include symptomatic bradycardia due to sinus node dysfunction, A-V conduction abnormalities, cardiomyopathy, autonomic nervous system disorders, and as an adjunct in the treatment of AF.

Transcutaneous Pacing

Indications for transcutaneous pacing (TCP) include hemodynamically unstable bradycardia unresponsive to atropine, bradycardia with escape rhythm, cardiac arrest victims with profound bradycardia or PEA due to drug overdose, acidosis, or electrolyte abnormalities, and overdrive pacing of refractory tachycardia. TCP is achieved by direct stimulation of the myocardium using a single pair of electrodes (Zoll pads) placed anterior–posterior or sternal-apex on the chest wall. Electrical capture is characterized by wide QRS complex (resembling a PVC) with T wave opposite to the polarity of QRS complex. The hemodynamic response to pacing is assessed by motoring pulse, blood pressure, and return of consciousness. Advantages of TCP include convenience and speed, and no need for fluoroscopy. However, there are several limitations of TCP including pain with impulse delivery, skeletal muscle and diaphragm stimulation, failure to recognize the noncapture of pacing impulse or underlying VF, and skin burns with improper or prolonged pacing. Analgesia and sedation should be considered once the patient is hemodynamically stable.

Transvenous Pacing

Currently, transvenous pacing (TVP) is the method of choice for temporary pacing. TVP can be achieved by inserting a balloon-tipped pacing catheter into the right ventricle via a central vein, preferably the right internal jugular vein, or by passing a pacing wire via a central vein or a pulmonary artery catheter. Special pacing wires are also available for atrial pacing. Advantages of TVP include patient comfort, and relative ease, speed, and safety of insertion by skilled personnel. Potential complications of TVP include infection, bleeding, pneumothorax, perforation of cardiac chamber, ventricular ectopy/tachycardia, and pulmonary thromboembolism.

Permanent Pacemaker

Insertion of a permanent pacemaker (PPM) is considered for persistent, nonreversible symptomatic bradycardia. General indications for a PPM are mentioned above. A PPM is placed transvenously, preferably via the left subclavian vein. The PPM consists of a pulse generator and a lead system. The pulse generator contains a lithium battery, a silicon semiconductor chip, and electronic circuitry. Pacemaker leads can be unipolar or bipolar depending upon the presence of one or both electrodes within the heart. In a unipolar system the tip of the electrode is negatively charged (cathode) and the surface of the generator is positively charged (anode). For pacing to occur, the surface of the pulse generator must maintain contact with tissue. A bipolar lead houses both electrodes within the heart, the cathode being at the tip and the anode about 1-2 cm proximal to the tip of the electrode. The bipolar lead system is more commonly used and provides several advantages over unipolar leads. They are less susceptible to interference by electromagnetic current and skeletal myopotential, thereby there is less risk of inhibition by extraneous signals. A dual-chamber PPM (A-V) with rate-adaptive features allows preservation of A-V synchrony and "atrial kick," and an increase in the heart rate in response to exercise.

Implantable Cardioverter Defibrillator

Indications for an ICD are rapidly expanding. The ICD is indicated in patients with a known history of ventricular arrhythmias or those at high risk for ventricular arrhythmias, e.g., post-MI left ventricular ejection fraction (LV-EF) of 30–40% and inducible sustained ventricular tachycardia, LV-EF < 30% and QRS duration >120 ms, and patients with hereditary arrhythmias such as long-QT syndrome and the Brugada syndrome. The ICD consists of a generator, which houses a microprocessor, complex electronic circuitry, lithium battery and capacitor, and defibrillator electrodes. The maximal output from an ICD is about 30 J (45 J in "high-energy" devices), whereas external defibrillators deliver a maximal output of 360 J. Modern ICDs are also capable of functioning as pacemakers.

Clinical Management

In order to care safely for a patient with an implantable cardiac device in the perioperative and critical care setting, careful attention must be given to the following considerations.

Assessment of the Device

The routine history must include questions pertaining to the presence of an implanted cardiac device, its type, manufacturer, and model, and indication for insertion. A detailed cardiac history must be obtained. The patient's old medical record or wallet card may provide information about the type of the device as well as details on intrinsic rhythm, programming mode, and the rate. An ECG may be helpful to determine the type of pacemaker (atrial, ventricular, or dual chamber) and if the patient is completely dependent on the pacemaker. ECG must be obtained without applying a magnet on the device, as some ICDs may be permanently deactivated with magnet placement. A roentgenogram of the chest can identify if the pacemaker is single chamber vs. dual chamber, and with unipolar or bipolar leads. An ICD generator is usually larger than a pacemaker generator. Whenever feasible, a competent authority must interrogate the PPM or ICD and a copy of this report placed in the patient's chart.

Perioperative Care of the Patient

As a rule, a means of providing backup pacing or defibrillation must be immediately available.

An example of a perioperative guide for patients with PPMs or ICDs is shown in Figure 7-11.

Use of a Magnet

Contrary to the traditional belief, application of a magnet does not "turn-off" a PPM, but it allows the pacemaker circuitry to be switched to *asynchronous* mode and reveal remaining battery life and pacing threshold safety factors. At the same time, not all pacemakers switch to asynchronous mode when a magnet is placed on the generator. However, the response of an ICD to an externally applied magnet is different. ICDs will be prevented from delivering a shock when a magnet is placed over the generator for 20–30 seconds (Guidant devices signal a beeping tone). Placing the magnet over the generator again for 20–30 seconds can reactivate Guidant devices. The ICDs of other manufacturers will remain inactive as long as an external magnet remains over the generator. If the magnet is removed, the ICD becomes active. The pacemaker function of ICD generators is not affected by application of a magnet. When in doubt, one must contact the manufacturer to find each device's response to a magnet.

Monitoring

In addition to basic monitoring, a five-lead ECG system is helpful in analyzing the rhythm during periods of interference from cautery. A pulse oximeter or arterial catheter provides monitoring of beat-to-beat mechanical activity of the heart and ensures perfusion during periods of interference. If present, minute ventilation rate responsiveness is turned off before surgery.

Electrocautery

Electrocoagulation (repeated bursts of current) and electrocutting (sustained current) are commonly used during surgical procedures. Electrosurgical units (ESUs) may be unipolar or bipolar. With a unipolar ESU, current is passed over a large area before it is returned to the pad. However, a bipolar ESU allows limited dispersion of current due to housing of both cathode and anode within the tip of cautery. Therefore, most pacemaker-related complications are likely to occur with unipolar and cutting systems. When using the unipolar system, short bursts are recommended. The cautery pad should be in full contact with the patient's skin and placed as close as possible to the site of surgery and as far as possible from the generator. Potential adverse consequences of cautery device interference include bradycardia, asystole, tachyarrhythmia, and unintended delivery of shock, impaired cardiac output, and endocardial injury.

Effect of Drugs, Metabolic, and Electrolyte Imbalance

Common metabolic and electrolyte abnormalities such as acidosis, alkalosis, myocardial ischemia, hyperkalemia, and severe hyperglycemia may result in an increase in pacing threshold and failure to pace. Many antiarrhythmic drugs may potentially increase pacing threshold.

Perioperative care guide for patients with pacemakers or ICDs

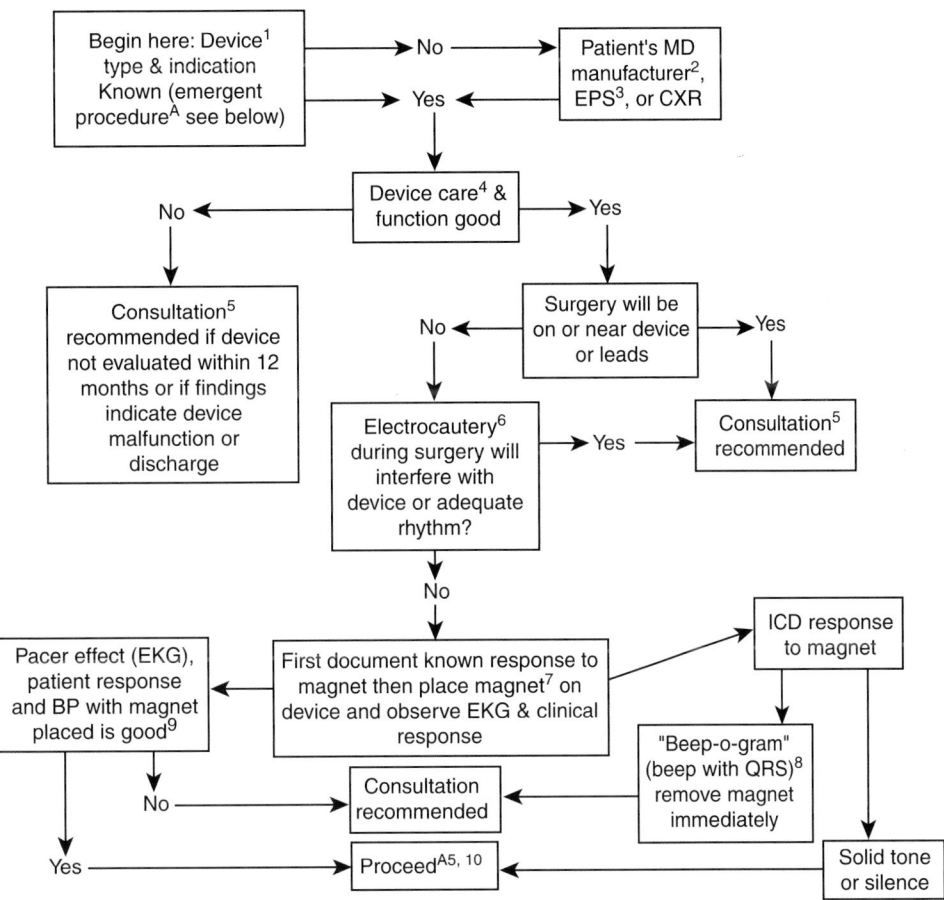

¹"DEVICE" = pacemaker or ICD (Internal Cardioverter Defibrillator). ICDs defibrillate but may also have pacing capabilities.
²MANUFACTURER CONTACTS: MEDTRONIC: 800-462-7775 or 800-551-5544 (after hours page rep at 800-MEDTRONIC): GUIDANT: 800-CARDIAC (medical records); ST JUDE: 888-756-2763 x 5802 (7-5 PST, after hours page rep at 800-PACE-ICD)
³EPS = Electrophysiology service of cardiology
⁴Proper care includes device assessment or interrogation at least once a year.
⁵CONSULTATION = Consultation with either the patient's cardiologist, the manufacturer of the device, or the EPS service
⁶ELECTROCAUTERY: You can minimize electrocautery impact on device function in most patients. Bipolar electrocautery is safest. Unipolar electrocautery is safest when short burst (<1 sec) and distant from the device and its leads (not abdominal or thoracic). Other electromagnetic sources (e.g. MRI, lithotripsy, ECT) can affect devices. The return pad (sometimes called grounding although it is not) should be placed furthest from the device and its leads.
⁷ MAGNET placement over a pacer results in an asynchronous pacing rate of 80-100 and is usually tolerated unless patient requires optimal pacing (e.g. atrial synchronization) for adequate hemodynamics. Electrocautery may reprogram a pacer to other rhythm which is usually safe. MAGNET on an ICD disables defibrillating capability (sometimes indicated by a tone of 20-30 sec) as long as the magnet is over the device. ICDs with pacing function do not have their pacing function disabled by a magnet, but can have their pacing function inhibited by electrocautery. Majority of patients are not pacer dependent; pacer dependent patients paced with an ICD may require consultation and reprogramming of their ICD pacing function if electrocautry will interfere with ICD pacing.
⁸Beep-o-gram indicates that defibrillating capability will be disabled after 30 sec of exposure to magnetic field. Reprogramming will be necessary to restore this function. Guidant beep may require stethoscope to be heard. No beep or beep-o-gram = consult recommended.
⁹Some patients may not tolerate asynchronous pacing (e.g. they require AV synchrony to optimize atrial "kick")
¹⁰All patients should have their devices interrogated after surgery.
ᴬEMERGENT PROCEDURE: No time for consultation, perform quick check of 1) current rhythm, 2) pacer type & function, 3) effect of magnet, 4) minimize electrocautery, 5) consider preparing alternate means of pacing &/or defibrillating.   Updated12 9 02
(Copyright pending Peter L Bailey, MD)

Figure 7-11   An example of a patient care guide for PPM or ICD. (Courtesy of Department of Anesthesiology, University of Rochester.)

Myopotentials resulting from skeletal muscle fasciculations secondary to succinylcholine may result in failure to pace due to pacemaker oversensing, especially of a unipolar system.

External Defibrillation

External synchronized cardioversion or defibrillation may potentially damage pacemaker circuitry and result in increased pacing threshold. Therefore, before elective cardioversion the pacemaker threshold must be increased and the pacemaker appropriately reprogrammed after shocks have been delivered. Minimally effective energy output is selected and paddles are positioned such that current is delivered perpendicular to the pacing system.

Special Circumstances

Magnetic resonance imaging (MRI) is known to cause serious derangements in pacemaker activity and should be avoided in pacemaker patients. When administered asynchronously, shock waves and electrical interference during lithotripsy can inhibit pacemaker output. Therefore, shock waves are synchronized with the QRS. The rate-responsive feature of the pacemaker and anti-tachycardia feature of the ICD must be deactivated during lithotripsy. Radiation therapy may potentially damage the silicon processor chip of the pacemaker. Cardiopulmonary resuscitation can be safely performed in patients with ICDs.

SUMMARY

There have been tremendous advances in the diagnosis and management of arrhythmias over the last two decades.

Optimal management of cardiac arrhythmias requires a basic understanding of cardiac electrophysiology and pharmacology of antiarrhythmic drugs. Perioperative period and critical illness present with unique metabolic, ischemic, and neurohumoral stressors that can result in arrhythmia formation. The basic approaches to arrhythmia management include airway support, correct diagnosis, establishing urgency of treatment and hemodynamic stability, and prevention of complications. It is important to remember that antiarrhythmic drugs can also be proarrhythmogenic. PPMs and ICDs require unique considerations. Using care guides for patients with PPMs or ICDs and a means of providing backup pacing or defibrillation will ensure safe patient care.

SELECTED READING

Al-Khatib SM, Allen LaPointe NM, Kramer JM, Califf RM: What clinicians should know about the QT interval. JAMA 289:2120–2127, 2003.

Amar D: Perioperative atrial tachyarrhythmias. Anesthesiology 97:1618–1623, 2002.

Chaudhry GM, Haffajee C: Antiarrhythmic agents and proarrhythmia. Crit Care Med 28(Suppl):N158–N164, 2000.

Guidelines 2000 for cardiopulmonary resuscitation and emergency cardiovascular care. International consensus on science. Circulation 102:1–376, 2000.

Seguin P, Signouret T, Laviolle B, Branger B, Malledant Y: Incidence and risk factors of atrial fibrillation in a surgical intensive care unit. Crit Care Med 32:722–726, 2004.

Stone KR, McPherson CA: Assessment and management of patients with pacemakers and implantable cardioverter defibrillator. Crit Care Med 32(Suppl):S155–S165, 2004.

Critical Care Pharmacologic Principles: Vasoactive Drugs

CURTIS E. HAAS, Pharm.D.

JACLYN M. LEBLANC, Pharm.D.

Hemodynamic resuscitation, management, and stabilization of medical, surgical, and trauma patients is a primary therapeutic indication for admission to the intensive care unit (ICU), and often involves the administration of vasoactive drugs. The term "vasoactive drugs" encompasses two major classes of compounds, vasopressors and vasodilators. The vasopressors include primarily the parenteral catecholamines, while the vasodilator class includes drugs from diverse pharmacologic categories that demonstrate variable effects on global hemodynamics. This chapter reviews the pharmacologic and clinical properties of vasoactive drugs commonly used in the critical care setting for the acute management of hemodynamic alterations in the adult patient.

VASOPRESSORS

Depending upon the underlying etiology and patient characteristics, the management of shock states involves three general therapeutic modalities: volume resuscitation, vasopressor therapy, and inotropic therapy. The most common indication for the administration of vasopressor agents in the critical care setting is septic shock refractory to adequate volume resuscitation, and therefore most of the literature has focused on the use of these agents for this indication. Other potential indications for vasopressors include the treatment of vasodilatory shock following cardiopulmonary bypass, anaphylaxis, vascular surgery (e.g., carotid endarterectomy), drug overdoses (e.g., tricyclic antidepressants), and spinal cord trauma. In the neurosurgical and trauma ICU vasopressors are often used to manipulate mean arterial pressure in an attempt to promote cerebral perfusion in patients with an elevated intracranial pressure.

Catecholamines

The most widely used class of drugs for vasopressor support is the parenterally available catecholamines. The four agents available for this indication are dopamine, norepinephrine, epinephrine, and phenylephrine. Although these drugs are grouped together as direct-acting catecholamines, their pharmacology is quite diverse and the pharmacodynamic response leading to an increase in mean arterial pressure (MAP) differs between agents (see Table 8-1). Although these differences in pharmacology are appreciated and may have an important impact on the appropriate clinical use of these agents, there is a paucity of information from controlled clinical trials concerning the relative merits of one drug versus another in the treatment of common shock states. Due to this lack of well controlled data, the updated Practice Parameters for Hemodynamic Support of Sepsis in Adult Patients published by the Society of Critical Care Medicine (SCCM) in 2004 based the recommendations on relatively low level scientific evidence (Levels C and D). Although there is on-going debate, there is currently inadequate evidence to declare definitively a drug

Table 8-1	Hemodynamic Response to Catecholamines During Septic Shock			
	MAP	**CI**	**HR**	**SVR**
Dopamine	+++	+++	++	0/+
Norepinephrine	+++	0/+	+	+++
Epinephrine	+++	+++	++	+
Phenylephrine	+++	0/+	0/+	+++

MAP, mean arterial pressure; CI, cardiac index; HR, heart rate; SVR, systemic vascular resistance.

of choice among the available agents for the treatment of common shock states. Therefore, a complete understanding of the differences in pharmacology, pharmacodynamics, and safety among the available agents, and a discussion of the limited comparative data that are available, will permit the critical care clinician to make the best decision concerning the use of intravenous catecholamines.

Dopamine

The effects of dopamine (DA) are dose-dependent, although it should be appreciated that there is considerable overlap in the dose ranges for the effects of the drug. At low doses (<5 µg/kg/minute) DA has predominantly nonspecific agonist activity at DA_1 and DA_2 dopamine receptors, resulting in vasodilatation of renal, mesenteric, and coronary vessels, and inhibition of sodium reuptake by proximal tubular cells leading to a potent naturesis. This dose range has been referred to as "renal dose dopamine" with the expectation that the

---

CURRENT CONTROVERSY

Low-Dose Dopamine
- Traditional teaching: low-dose dopamine (LDD) has beneficial effects on renal blood flow and glomerular filtration rate in critically ill patients.
- Current evidence:
  - No evidence that LDD prevents the development of acute renal failure (ARF) in high-risk ICU patients.
  - No evidence that LDD has a beneficial effect on established ARF.
  - The increase in urine output with LDD is secondary to DA-induced naturesis, which may contribute to or mask hypovolemia.
  - LDD may have important noncardiovascular adverse effects secondary to alterations in the neurohormonal response to critical illness.
- Conclusion: the evidence does not support a role for LDD in the routine management of ICU patients.

---

increase in renal blood flow, glomerular filtration rate (GFR), and urine output will have beneficial effects on renal function in critically ill patients. The data from clinical trials over the past decade have generally concluded that low-dose DA does not result in beneficial effects on renal function in critically ill patients and may have some detrimental effects, and therefore its routine use for this indication has fallen into disfavor among most experts.

At slightly higher doses (5–10 µg/kg/minute) the β_1-adrenergic effects of DA are more prominent resulting in a positive inotropic and chronotropic effect. DA also has indirect pharmacologic activity resulting in the release of endogenous norepinephrine from sympathetic nerve terminals, which may also contribute to its inotropic and vasopressor effects. At doses exceeding 10 µg/kg/minute α_1-adrenergic effects become increasingly important leading to arterial vasoconstriction contributing to an increase in blood pressure. Similar to the other catecholamines, DA has a rapid onset of effect and short duration of action allowing careful titration of the infusion rate to clinical response. There is little further improvement in hemodynamic parameters when the DA dose exceeds 20–25 µg/kg/minute; however, the risk of tachyarrhythmias and other cardiovascular adverse effects does increase. Unlike other direct-acting catecholamines, DA does appear to have a ceiling effect, and doses above 20–25 µg/kg/minute are not recommended. An alternative agent should be used if a patient fails to respond to maximal doses of DA despite adequate fluid resuscitation. In addition, tachyphylaxis to the effects of DA has been reported, and if a patient requires prolonged vasopressor support, a direct-acting catecholamine may need to be substituted to maintain response.

Although relatively high-dose DA (10–20 mg/kg/minute) is commonly employed as a "vasopressor" in the management of refractory septic shock, the predominant hemodynamic response leading to improvement in blood pressure is an increase in left ventricular stroke volume and a modest increase in heart rate, with minimal effect on systemic vascular resistance. In most studies central venous, pulmonary, and pulmonary artery occlusion pressures and systemic and pulmonary resistance were unchanged. The evidence from clinical evaluations in sepsis therefore indicates that the predominant hemodynamic effect of DA is due to its cardiac inotropic effects, with arterial vasoconstriction being quantitatively unimportant.

DA increases cardiac contractility and heart rate when used for the treatment of common shock states. This contributes to left ventricular stroke work and myocardial oxygen demand, which may lead to the development of myocardial ischemia in patients with underlying coronary artery disease. However, improvements in diastolic blood pressure and subsequent coronary perfusion may offset the increased oxygen demand. Patients with a history of cardiovascular disease or evidence of on-going cardiac ischemia should be closely monitored or alternative vasopressors should be considered.

The most common reported adverse effects of DA are related to its cardiovascular effects and include sinus tachycardia, arrhythmias, cardiac ischemia, and a risk of excessive peripheral vasoconstriction leading to tissue necrosis. Extravasation of DA at the injection site can cause local tissue necrosis and sloughing. The drug may also have adverse effects on pulmonary gas exchange. DA has been consistently shown to increase pulmonary shunt fraction, which may lead to a worsening of oxygenation in some patients. However, an increase in mixed venous oxygen saturation secondary to effects on cardiac output may offset the increased shunt fraction minimizing effects on arterial P_aO_2. The drug may also inhibit the centrally mediated ventilatory response to hypercarbia.

With an increased emphasis in recent years on the effects of vasopressors on regional perfusion as a marker of comparative efficacy and safety, several investigators have evaluated the effects of DA on splanchnic perfusion and oxygen utilization with mixed results. The use of low-dose DA in combination with fluids and norepinephrine in patients with septic shock has been associated with variable effects on splanchnic perfusion. Splanchnic blood flow, O_2 delivery (DO_2), and O_2 consumption (VO_2) were increased in patients with a normal splanchnic DO_2 at baseline, but not in patients with an increased splanchnic DO_2. Despite increases in O_2 delivery and consumption, there was no change in gastric intramucosal pH (pHi) or hepatic vein lactate concentrations raising concerns about the relevance of the observed increases in DO_2 and VO_2 or the possibility of a direct metabolic effect of DA. In a randomized study comparing norepinephrine and DA in septic shock, the group randomized to DA experienced a significant reduction of gastric pHi despite improvement in global DO_2 and VO_2, suggesting that DA may increase splanchnic oxygen debt due to increased splanchnic oxygen utilization. Other investigators have found no important effects on splanchnic blood flow. The importance these variable effects on regional perfusion may have on clinical outcome is unknown and requires additional study.

An under-appreciated potential risk of DA in critically ill patients relates to its effects on anterior pituitary function. DA profoundly suppresses prolactin, thyroid-stimulating hormone (TSH), and luteinizing hormone (LH) secretion from the anterior pituitary. Prolonged hypoprolactinemia in critically ill patients receiving DA induces an impairment of the T-lymphocyte proliferative response, which may increase susceptibility to infectious complications. DA induces or aggravates the low-T3 syndrome of critical illness due to direct inhibition of TSH secretion. DA attenuates pulsatile growth hormone secretion, and prolonged infusions are associated with low insulin-like growth factor-I, without influencing cortisol or insulin secretion. These effects may contribute to the catabolic response of critical illness and interfere with protein anabolism. In addition, DA has been associated with suppression of dehydroepiandrosterone sulfate serum concentrations, an androgenic hormone with immune stimulatory effects. Lastly, DA aggravates the pituitary blunting of LH pulse amplitude observed in critically ill patients and may also decrease pulse frequency leading to iatrogenic suppression of the gonadal axis which delays the recovery of testosterone secretion in men. This may contribute to negative nitrogen balance, delayed anabolic response, and immune suppression. An appreciation of the complex effects DA may have on neuroendocrine response, and the increasing recognition of the importance of endocrine responses on outcome of critically ill patients raises several concerns about the routine use of DA for hemodynamic support in the ICU.

In summary, DA effectively improves MAP in patients with refractory septic shock primarily by increasing cardiac index. In the SCCM Practice Parameters updated in 2004 DA is recommended as a first line vasopressor for septic shock. In the absence of definitive data concerning the drug of choice for the management of refractory septic shock, DA remains a reasonable treatment alternative. For other indications for vasopressor therapy where the primary objective is to increase peripheral vascular resistance, DA should not be considered the first-line agent.

Norepinephrine

Over the past decade there has been a renewed interest in the use of norepinephrine (NE) for the treatment of common shock states, especially hyperdynamic septic shock. At pharmacologic doses used for the treatment of shock, NE has a predominant agonist effect at α_1-adrenergic receptors, with a lesser effect at β_1-receptors, and relatively little effect at β_2-receptors. The typical hemodynamic response to NE is an increase in diastolic, systolic, and pulse pressures, no change to a slight reduction in cardiac output, marked increases in peripheral vascular resistance, and a reduction in heart rate with an increase in left ventricular stroke volume. NE has minimal effects on measures of preload and pulmonary vascular resistance. In the setting of septic shock the major contribution to the increase in MAP is vasoconstriction with a rise in vascular resistance, while the β_1 agonist effect appears to result in maintenance of cardiac output. Unlike DA, NE behaves as a vasoconstrictor in the treatment of septic shock. Although sinus tachycardia and other tachyarrhythmias may be seen, especially at higher doses, it is usually less frequent than what is observed at equally effective doses of DA.

Due to early observations of renal failure, bowel ischemia, metabolic acidosis, and severe peripheral vasoconstriction with tissue necrosis when NE was administered to patients with shock, for many years the drug was relegated to a second- or third-line role in the management of septic shock and was only used when the patient failed to respond to other agents. This has been referred to as a "pharmacologic extreme unction" and NE picked up the nickname "leave-em-dead," a play on the original trade name Levophed. Many textbooks still recommend maximal doses of 10–12 µg/minute in the treatment of adult patients with shock, primarily based upon these fears of potent vasoconstriction.

Multiple studies over the past 10–15 years have clearly demonstrated that NE can be safely used in the hemodynamic management of septic shock provided the patient has been adequately fluid resuscitated. The doses used in these trials have been higher by several orders of magnitude than the prior arbitrarily chosen maximal doses. Mean doses have been 0.2–1.3 µg/kg/minute, with doses as high as 3.3 µg/kg/minute being used. Despite these high doses, improvement in GFR, urine output, and renal blood flow have been reported, and patients have not experienced worsening of metabolic acidosis or complications from severe peripheral vasoconstriction. The primary difference between the current and historical experiences with NE appears to be the careful attention to adequate fluid resuscitation in the recent clinical reports, although there are no controlled data supporting this assumption.

In the setting of septic shock, high doses of NE are often required probably due to α-receptor downregulation and possibly other factors that reduce vascular smooth muscle response to catecholamines. For patients receiving NE for the treatment of shock or hypotension due to other causes, much lower NE infusion rates are typically required. NE should be started at rates of 0.03–0.05 µg/kg/minute (2–5 µg/minute in adults) and titrated to the desired hemodynamic response. In the management of septic shock the dose should be titrated to the goal MAP rather than a derived parameter like systemic vascular resistance. There is no apparent reason to dictate a maximal dose of NE in the treatment of septic shock provided the patient's intravascular volume status is adequately maintained and the patient has not developed intolerable adverse events (see later discussion of vasopressin in septic shock). Doses greater than ~3 µg/kg/minute have not been previously reported. All patients receiving intravenous infusions of NE should have their blood pressure and heart rate continuously monitored.

Several studies have evaluated the impact of NE, either alone or in combination with low-dose dobutamine, on measures of regional perfusion and oxygen utilization. Although the results have been somewhat variable, the overall conclusions are that if cardiac output is maintained, splanchnic perfusion and oxygen utilization are maintained or improved in patients with sepsis. Serum lactate concentrations are usually maintained or improved following the initiation of NE, and, as mentioned above, renal blood flow and renal function are improved in patients that have an adequate hemodynamic response to NE. Since all of the regional perfusion data come from patients with septic shock, it is possible that patients with hypotension due to other causes may experience decreases in renal and mesenteric blood flow similar to what has been observed in healthy volunteer studies, presumably due to a generalized vasoconstriction observed with NE.

Increases in afterload, combined with an increase in contractility and possibly heart rate, increase left ventricular stroke work and may precipitate myocardial ischemia and infarction. Like all catecholamines, NE should be cautiously administered to patients with known coronary artery disease or evidence of myocardial ischemia.

Other common adverse effects of NE are predictable extensions of its cardiovascular effects and include tachycardia, other tachyarrhythmias, marked increases in blood pressure, and severe peripheral vasoconstriction with tissue necrosis. Ensuring the patient has an adequate intravascular volume can minimize the risk of tachyarrhythmias and peripheral vasoconstriction. NE has fewer "hormonal" effects than epinephrine, but at high doses may cause hyperglycemia. Extravasation at the site of injection may cause local tissue necrosis and sloughing.

NE has emerged as a drug of choice for the management of refractory septic shock in the opinion of many experts. Recent clinical experience and published reports have dispelled many of the myths and fears surrounding the use of this drug; however, a strong bias against the routine use of NE persists in the minds and practices of many critical care practitioners. If NE is going to be used for the treatment of severe septic shock, it should be used early in combination with aggressive volume resuscitation and inotropic support as indicated, and not reserved as a second-line or late salvage therapy.

Epinephrine

Epinephrine (EPI) has potent agonist effects at both α- and β-adrenergic receptors. Due to its complex pharmacologic effects, the overall hemodynamic response to an infusion of EPI is dose-dependent. At relatively low doses, the β-receptor-mediated effects predominate leading to an increase in cardiac output due to an increased stroke volume and heart rate, and a reduction in afterload. The net vasodilation and reduction in afterload is primarily due to stimulation of β_2-receptors, which are predominantly present on the resistance arterioles of skeletal muscle. The overall effects on MAP at low dose are variable and dependent upon the patient's baseline hemodynamic state and the net effects on cardiac output and vascular resistance.

At higher infusion rates typically administered for the treatment of shock or hypotension, the balance shifts towards increased α-adrenergic effects leading to vasoconstriction and increased peripheral resistance. Cardiac effects will include an increase in heart rate and contractility. Cardiac output is typically increased, but may vary depending upon the effects on afterload. Due to the nature of the distribution of α- and β_2-receptors throughout the vasculature, the local effects of EPI on vascular tone and blood flow will depend upon the tissue. Vasoconstriction may predominate in the arterioles and precapillary sphincters of many tissues and organs including the parenchymous organs such as the kidney, liver, and lungs, the gut, cutaneous structures, and mucus membranes. A reduction in vascular resistance of the skeletal muscle vasculature is usually observed with the higher doses of EPI since the powerful β_2-receptor-mediated effects are only partially countered by α_1-receptor-mediated vasoconstriction. Understanding these variable local effects of EPI may explain the observed differences in regional perfusion and oxygen utilization between EPI and NE despite both agents being titrated to achieve a similar target MAP during the treatment of septic shock.

EPI effectively raises MAP in patients with septic shock that is refractory to volume resuscitation. The hemodynamic responses leading to the increase in MAP are an increase in cardiac output due primarily to increased stroke volume, combined with modest increases in vascular resistance and heart rate. Similar to DA, the predominant effect in septic shock is the increase in cardiac output. The increase in contractility and heart rate increases left ventricular stroke work and may precipitate cardiac ischemia and infarction.

Although EPI has shown consistent effects on improving global DO_2 and VO_2 in most clinical reports of patients being treated for refractory septic shock, recent studies have indicated that these global effects may not predict regional oxygen utilization. EPI has been shown to decrease splanchnic blood flow, increase arterial, venous, and hepatic venous lactate concentrations, and decrease pHi, especially in the first 12 to 24 hours of treatment. The importance of these regional effects on clinical outcome have not been evaluated; however, since the overall goal of resuscitation is to improve tissue perfusion and oxygen utilization these observations have raised significant concerns relative to the role of EPI in the treatment of refractory septic shock.

The most common adverse effects of EPI are predictable and similar to other catecholamines. These include tachycardia, other tachyarrhythmias, cardiac ischemia, excessive increases in blood pressure, and severe peripheral vasoconstriction. Reductions in renal blood flow appear to be more pronounced with EPI than

with other vasopressors. EPI also has important metabolic adverse effects. Hyperglycemia secondary to inhibition of insulin secretion, enhanced secretion of glucagon, inhibition of glucose uptake by skeletal muscle cells, and stimulation of glycogenolysis are commonly observed. EPI also stimulates K^+ uptake into cells due to activation of β_2-receptors. The resulting hypokalemia is often exacerbated by treatment of EPI-induced hyperglycemia with insulin. EPI increases triglyceride lipase activity, which increases the breakdown of triglycerides to free fatty acids and glycerol, increases circulating concentrations of free fatty acids, and has a significant calorigenic effect. Although some of these metabolic effects may be seen with high doses of NE, they are much more common during infusions of EPI.

In summary, EPI effectively increases MAP during the treatment of common shock states, but recent evidence suggesting that EPI may have more adverse effects on regional perfusion and metabolism have led to recommendations that EPI not be considered a drug of choice for the treatment of refractory septic shock. EPI has been commonly recommended for anaphylactic shock due to its combined effects on cardiovascular, pulmonary, and inflammatory systems during allergic responses. In most common shock states EPI is not considered a drug of choice and is often reserved as a second-line agent for patients failing to respond to NE or DA.

Phenylephrine

Despite several decades of clinical use for the treatment of shock, there is relatively little published data on the use of phenylephrine (PHE) and essentially no comparative studies with other catecholamines. PHE is a relatively selective α_1-adrenergic receptor agonist, although at high concentrations it may also stimulate β-receptors. When administered to patients with septic shock following fluid resuscitation there is typically an increase in MAP primarily due to peripheral vasoconstriction, an increase in stroke volume index, a small to no reduction in heart rate, and maintenance of cardiac output. The increase in stroke volume suggests a positive inotropic response to PHE, which may be due to stimulation of α-receptors present on the myocardium or some inherent β-adrenergic activity of PHE at the doses being used for septic shock. Unlike other catecholamines, heart rate typically remains relatively unchanged or decreased with the use of PHE as a vasopressor. In fact, sinus bradycardia and slowed atrioventricular (AV) nodal conduction may result from reflex vagal responses, although this is more likely in normotensive patients receiving PHE.

Limited data evaluating the effects of PHE on global oxygen utilization and regional perfusion during the treatment of septic patients indicate that DO_2 and VO_2 are maintained or increased, arterial lactate concentrations are decreased or unchanged, and urine output increases. There is no comparative data with other catecholamines for these parameters. In the treatment of sepsis and refractory septic shock PHE is usually initiated at a dose of 0.5 μg/kg/minute and titrated to goal MAP. The reported dose range has been 0.11–9.9 μg/kg/minute, which similar to NE is considerably higher than the traditionally quoted maximum dose of 200 μg/minute for adult patients. These higher doses have been well tolerated provided the patient is adequately volume resuscitated, suggesting that arbitrary maximum doses for PHE are not appropriate in the management of septic shock. For the treatment of hypotension secondary to causes other than sepsis, or for elevation of MAP in normotensive patients (e.g., head trauma), a much lower dose is typically required.

Adverse effects of PHE are predicted by its pharmacology and include excessive increases in blood pressure, severe peripheral vasoconstriction, bradycardia, cardiac ischemia, and local skin necrosis with extravasation at the injection site. The risk of adverse events appears to be reduced by ensuring the patient's intravascular volume status is optimized and maintained. PHE may be advantageous in patients with baseline tachycardia, intolerance to other catecholamines secondary to excessive increases in heart rate, or coexisting chronic or acute atrial fibrillation. Compared to other agents, the role of PHE in the management of common shock states requires further comparative studies.

CLINICAL CAVEAT

Catecholamine Safety
The safe use of catecholamines for the treatment of hypotension is improved by:
- Ensuring the patient is adequately fluid resuscitated based upon subtle clinical evidence of intravascular volume overload; PAOP = 14–18 mmHg; or CVP = 8–14 mmHg.
- Using the lowest effective dose for the shortest possible length of time – frequent and ongoing dose titration.
- Adding inotropic support (dobutamine) to NE or PHE with reduced cardiac output (CI < 3.0 l/minute/m²).

Choice of Catecholamine

Most of the literature and discussions on the choice of catecholamine therapy have focused on the treatment of hyperdynamic septic shock. There are no comparative clinical trials with patient outcome or survival as a primary or secondary endpoint. All of the comparative trials have relied upon various surrogate endpoints. Early trials looked primarily at differences in global hemodynamic responses, which were later followed by studies that included global DO_2 and VO_2 as primary endpoints or as components of a composite endpoint. As it became evident that these global surrogate endpoints were not predictive of survival, more recent studies have focused on measures of regional perfusion and oxygen utilization, most commonly focused on the splanchnic circulation. This attention to the splanchnic circulation has occurred for several reasons. First, it is thought that inadequate splanchnic perfusion and compromise of gastrointestinal mucosal integrity may play a central role in the pathogenesis of multiple organ failure in the setting of sepsis and septic shock. Secondly, due to the countercurrent flow in the splanchnic microcirculation the gut has a higher critical DO_2 than other organs and therefore may be more sensitive to changes in DO_2 and VO_2. Lastly, the gut is generally more easily accessible than other major organ systems, and therefore lends itself to study using relatively non-invasive means in the critical care setting. It is important to remember that despite the widespread attention to the effects of catecholamine therapy on splanchnic perfusion and metabolism there is no current evidence that differences in these intermediate endpoints translate directly into differences in clinical outcomes.

Table 8-2 summarizes the comparative studies that have evaluated catecholamine treatments in the management of patients with hyperdynamic septic shock. The overall trend in these comparative studies is that NE with or without concomitant dobutamine is superior to DA and EPI when evaluating either achievement of hemodynamic and oxygen transport goals, or effects on regional perfusion and oxygenation. There are no comparative studies involving PHE. Two recent reviews on the treatment of hyperdynamic septic shock have recommended NE as the drug of choice when vasopressor therapy is indicated (see Dellinger and Ruokonen et al. in Selected Reading), and the SCCM Practice Parameters consider NE

CURRENT CONTROVERSY

Norepinephrine is Drug of Choice for Septic Shock
- Surrogate endpoints of regional perfusion more consistently improved by NE compared to DA or EPI.
- Minimal tachycardia compared to DA and EPI.
- No alterations in neurohormonal response, unlike DA.
- More consistent achievement of global hemodynamic goals compared to DA.
- Contrary to traditional teaching, NE improves cardiac output, renal blood flow, and urine output in refractory septic shock.
- Potential survival advantage compared to other vasopressor choices.

Table 8-2 Comparative Studies of Catecholamines During Hyperdynamic Septic Shock

Author	Agents	Study Design	Study Endpoint(s)	Primary Findings
Martin[a]	DA 2.5–25 µg/kg/minute (n = 16) vs. NE 0.5–5 µg/kg/minute (n = 16)	Prospective, DB, R Refractory hyperdynamic septic shock patients Crossover allowed for treatment failures	Achieve and maintain goals for 6 hours: SVRI > 1100 dynes/s/cm⁵·m² or MAP > 80 mmHg CI > 4 l/minute/m² IDO₂ > 550 ml/minute/m² IVO₂ > 150 ml/minute/m²	DA group – 5/16 (31%) achieved goals NE group – 15/16 (93%) achieved goals 10/11 of DA failures responded to addition of NE
Marik[b]	DA (n = 10) vs. NE (n = 10)	Prospective, R, 3 hour study Hyperdynamic septic shock with MAP < 60 mmHg or SVRI < 1200 dynes/s/cm⁵·m² despite fluid resuscitation Infusions titrated to MAP > 75 mmHg No crossover permitted	Global hemodynamics Global oxygen utilization (IDO₂ and IVO₂) Gastric pHi Arterial lactate	No differences in global parameters except HR and CI (both greater with DA) Gastric pHi increased with NE, but decreased with DA ($p < 0.001$)
Day[c]	DA 2.5–10 µg/kg/minute vs. EPI 0.1–0.5 µg/kg/minute using stepped infusions	Open, R, crossover study Severe sepsis (n = 10) and severe malaria (n = 13)	Global hemodynamic response Acid-base balance	EPI – resulted in increased lactate (infusion stopped in 84%), decrease in arterial pH DA – small fall in arterial lactate and rise in arterial pH. Infusion not stopped in any patient. DO₂ and VO₂ increased with both drugs
Meier-Hellmann[d]	EPI vs. NE + DOB	Prospective, crossover study Refractory hyperdynamic septic shock (n = 8) 2 hour infusions titrated to achieve CI > 5.5 l/minute/m² or DO₂ > 650 ml/minute, and MAP ≥ 70 mmHg	Global hemodynamics and oxygen utilization Splanchnic perfusion, and oxygen utilization Gastric pHi	No difference in global parameters Splanchnic blood flow and VO₂ were lower, arterial, hepatic, and venous lactate were higher, and pHi was lower during EPI infusion
Levy[e]	EPI vs. NE + fixed dose DOB (5 µg/kg/minute)	Prospective, R study Hyperdynamic, DA-resistant septic shock (n = 30) Infusions titrated to MAP > 80 mmHg	Global hemodynamics and oxygen utilization Blood lactate and pyruvate Gastric tonometry – pHi and pCO₂ gap Measurements at 1, 6, 12, and 24 hours	No differences in global parameters At 6 hours, lactate, lactate/pyruvate ratio, and pCO₂ gap increased and arterial pH decreased in EPI group. Return to baseline by 24 hours. NE + DOB group had reduction in lactate, and normalization of tonometry values by 6 hours
Seguin[f]	EPI vs. NE + fixed dose DOB (5 µg/kg/minute)	Prospective, R study Hyperdynamic septic shock (n = 22) Infusions titrated to MAP of 70–80 mmHg	Global hemodynamics and oxygen utilization Gastric mucosal blood flow (Doppler flowmetry) Hepatic function (ICG clearance)	No difference in global hemodynamic parameters, except EPI had greater CI, DO₂, and gastric mucosal blood flow No difference in ICG clearance
Duranteau[g]	EPI vs. NE vs. NE + fixed dose DOB (5 µg/kg/minute)	Prospective, R, crossover study DA-resistant septic shock (n = 12) 60-minute infusions Infusions titrated to MAP 70–80 mmHg	Global hemodynamics Gastric mucosal perfusion (laser Doppler flowmetry) Gastric tonometry (pHi and pCO₂ gap)	EPI and NE + DOB increased CI and DO₂ compared to NE alone Increase in mucosal perfusion greater with EPI and NE + DOB than NE. pHi and pCO₂ gap better with NE + DOB compared to EPI or NE alone

Continued

Table 8-2   Comparative Studies of Catecholamines During Hyperdynamic Septic Shock—Cont'd

Author	Agents	Study Design	Study Endpoint(s)	Primary Findings
DeBacker[h]	DA vs. NE vs. EPI in moderate septic shock NE vs. EPI in severe septic shock	Prospective, R, crossover, open label Moderate shock (n = 10) Severe, DA-resistant shock (n = 10) All agents titrated to MAP > 65 mmHg	Evaluated effects on splanchnic circulation by: ICG clearance; hepatic vein oxygen saturation; gastric tonometry (pCO_2)	Moderate shock: NE and DA had similar HD effects, EPI had greater increase of CI. No differences in splanchnic blood flow or gastric pCO_2 Severe shock: EPI impaired splanchnic circulation compared to NE

CI, cardiac index; DA, dopamine; DB, double-blind; DOB, dobutamine; EPI, epinephrine; ICG, indocyanine green; IDO_2, oxygen delivery index; IVO_2, oxygen consumption index; MAP, mean arterial pressure; NE, norepinephrine; pCO_2 gap, difference between arterial pCO_2 and gastric mucosal pCO_2; pHi, intramucosal pH; R, randomized; SVRI, systemic vascular resistance index.

[a]Martin C, Papazian L, Perrin G et al: Norepinephrine or dopamine for treatment of hyperdynamic septic shock? Chest 103:1826–1831, 1993.

[b]Marik PE, Mohedin M: The contrasting effects of dopamine and norepinephrine on systemic and splanchnic oxygen utilization in hyperdynamic sepsis. JAMA 272:1354–1357, 1994.

[c]Day NPJ, Phu NH, Bethell DP et al: The effects of dopamine and adrenaline infusions on acid–base balance and systemic haemodynamics in severe infection. Lancet 348:219–223, 1996.

[d]Meier-Hellman A, Reinhart K, Bredle DL et al: Epinephrine impairs splanchnic perfusion in septic shock. Crit Care Med 25:399–404, 1997.

[e]Levy B, Bollaert PE, Charpentier C et al: Comparison of norepinephrine and dobutamine to epinephrine for hemodynamics, lactate metabolism, and gastric tonometric variables in septic shock: a prospective, randomized study. Intensive Care Med 23:282–287, 1997.

[f]Seguin P, Bellissant E, LeTulzo Y et al: Effects of epinephrine compared with the combination of dobutamine and norepinephrine on gastric perfusion in septic shock. Clin Pharmacol Ther 71:381–388, 2002.

[g]Duranteau J, Sitbon P, Teboul JL et al: Effects of epinephrine, norepinephrine, or the combination of norepinephrine and dobutamine on gastric mucosa in septic shock. Crit Care Med 27:893–900, 1999.

[h]DeBacker D, Creteu J, Silva E, Vincent JL: Effects of dopamine, norepinephrine and epinephrine on the splanchnic circulation in septic shock: which is better? Crit Care Med 31:1659–1667, 2003.

a first line agent. Dobutamine should be added if the cardiac index is < 3.0 l/minute/m². Although there are no randomized, prospective trials evaluating the effects of the choice of catecholamine therapy on outcome, a recently published prospective, observational, cohort study of 97 adult patients with septic shock concluded that NE was significantly associated with a lower overall hospital mortality rate than high-dose DA or EPI. Based upon these limited data, NE appears to be the vasopressor of choice for hyperdynamic septic shock at the current time.

The choice of vasopressor for other indications besides septic shock is less clear. If the primary desired effect is an increase in vascular resistance, then NE or PHE are preferred over DA or EPI. If the patient has baseline tachycardia, is at high risk for tachycardia, or is intolerant of other catecholamines due to tachycardia, then PHE may be considered. Due to the potential metabolic adverse effects and the risk of decreased organ perfusion, EPI should not be considered as a first-line vasopressor.

DRUG INTERACTIONS

Catecholamines

May potentiate pressor or cardiac effects of catecholamines:
- Tricyclic antidepressants.
- Antihistamines (e.g., diphenhydramine, tripelennamine, dexchlorpheniramine).
- Ergot alkaloids.
- MAO inhibitors (? clinical significance).
- Oxytocic drugs.
- Nonselective β-blockers ("unopposed α_1-stimulation").

May antagonize pressor or cardiac response:
- β-Blockers (decreased inotropic and chronotropic response).
- Haloperidol, phenothiazines (α_1-blocking effects).

May increase risk of cardiac arrhythmias:
- General anesthetics (halogenated hydrocarbons and cyclopropane).
- Digoxin.

Vasopressin

Recent evidence suggests that low-dose vasopressin may have a role in the hemodynamic support of hyperdynamic septic shock and possibly other causes of vasodilatory shock which are resistant or relatively refractory to catecholamines. Patients with septic shock have significantly lower plasma vasopressin concentrations than patients with cardiogenic shock, possibly due to exhaustion of neurohypophyseal stores during prolonged hypotension, blunting of baroreflex-mediated

stimulation of vasopressin release, and increased catabolism of circulating vasopressin. The administration of vasopressin at a rate of 0.01–0.04 Units/minute results in rapid and significant improvements in MAP, often allowing significant dosage reductions for concomitant catecholamines required for hemodynamic support. Although the initial studies are encouraging, the reports to date have involved relatively small numbers of patients, inadequate comparisons with conventional therapy, and inadequate safety assessments to justify recommendations for the routine use of vasopressin for septic shock, especially as a first-line agent. Vasopressin should be considered experimental and unproven until ongoing, large controlled studies are completed. Most clinicians recommend that the addition of vasopressin be reserved for patients that are refractory to or requiring high doses of catecholamines. This conservative approach is supported by the recent report of ischemic skin lesions developing in 30.2% of patients receiving vasopressin for catecholamine-resistant vasodilatory shock. Patients with pre-existing peripheral artery disease and septic shock appear to be at greatest risk for ischemic lesions.

If vasopressin is used for hemodynamic support of refractory vasodilatory shock, the dose should be limited to 0.01–0.04 Units/minute. Infusion rates greater than 0.04 Units/minute do not appear to increase the effectiveness, and may increase the risk of adverse events including myocardial and splanchnic ischemia. Once vasopressin is started the existing catecholamine infusion should be adjusted to the lowest dose necessary to maintain the desired MAP. The patient should be closely monitored for signs and symptoms of ischemic complications including myocardial ischemia and necrotic skin or mucus membrane lesions.

VASODILATORS

The most common indications for the use of parenterally administered vasodilators in the critical care setting include hypertensive crisis, cardiac ischemia, acute postoperative hypertension, cardiogenic shock, acute aortic dissection, and control of hypertension in a patient unable to take oral medications. Less common indications include pheochromocytoma and drug overdoses involving sympathomimetic agents or cocaine. The agents used for the acute management of MAP come from multiple pharmacologic categories including direct-acting vasodilators, nitrates, β-adrenergic antagonists, calcium channel blockers, angiotensin-converting enzyme inhibitors, and dopamine agonists. From the perspective of pharmacologic effects, the vasodilators can be divided into agents that have predominant effects on the arterial circulation, venous circulation, or mixed

Table 8-3 Predominant Site of Activity for Commonly Used Vasodilators

Venous Vasodilators	Mixed Vasodilators	Arterial Vasodilators
Nitroglycerin	Sodium nitroprusside	Hydralazine
	Enalaprilat	Labetalol
	Nesiritide	Nicardipine
		Fenoldopam

vasodilator activity (see Table 8-3). This chapter limits discussion to the vasodilators that are commonly administered intravenously in the ICU setting, and does not include orally administered drugs or agents of a more historical significance such as trimethaphan camsylate and diazoxide. Most prospective clinical trials comparing vasodilators for common indications, like hypertensive crises and acute postoperative hypertension, have not demonstrated important differences in efficacy or safety. Therefore, there is no clear agent of choice among the vasodilators for most indications, and the choice of an agent for the management of the individual patient is dictated by a thorough knowledge of the differences between agents, intensity of hemodynamic monitoring available, and individual patient characteristics.

Sodium Nitroprusside

Sodium nitroprusside (SNP) is a direct-acting, potent nitrovasodilator that affects both the venous and arterial vasculature. It is metabolized by the vascular endothelium to nitric oxide leading to vasodilation via the guanyl cyclase–cyclic-GMP pathway. This nitric oxide generation pathway is different than that of nitroglycerin, accounting for differences in hemodynamic effects and lack of tolerance. The advantages of SNP are its quick onset, short duration of action, minimal effects on heart rate, and no detrimental effects on cardiac function. It is considered the gold standard to which other parenteral antihypertensive agents are compared. Due to its short duration of action, SNP is administered by continuous infusion with the dose titrated to the desired hemodynamic response.

The hemodynamic effects of SNP include a reduction in peripheral resistance, MAP, pulmonary vascular resistance, and preload, with a maintenance or increase in cardiac output and stroke volume. Mild to moderate increases in heart rate (10–15%) commonly occur, but there is generally an improvement in myocardial oxygen balance provided excessive reductions in MAP are not achieved.

SNP is a highly effective vasodilator for most indications in the ICU. The usual starting dose is 0.25–0.5 μg/kg/minute with the dose increased by 0.5–1 μg/kg/minute every 5–10 minutes to achieve the desired response. For the treatment of decompensated heart failure, a lower starting dose of 0.125 μg/kg/minute is used with the dose adjusted every 5–10 minutes to achieve an improvement in stroke volume without precipitating hypotension or tachycardia. Although the maximum recommended dose is 10 μg/kg/minute, the dose should not exceed 5 μg/kg/minute for more than a few minutes to reduce the risk of acute cyanide toxicity. As a general rule, the lowest effective dose of SNP should be used for the shortest possible time. The most common reason for treatment failure with SNP is the development of adverse effects.

The most common or most concerning adverse events with SNP are hypotension, tachycardia, myocardial ischemia, cyanide and thiocyanate toxicity, and worsening of hypoxemia secondary to a reversal of hypoxic pulmonary vasoconstriction. Due to its potent and labile reduction in blood pressure, SNP should only be used in a well-monitored environment with continuous monitoring of blood pressure, preferably using an arterial catheter. Myocardial ischemia may occur secondary to excessive reductions in blood pressure with a loss of coronary perfusion pressure, reflex tachycardia with a resulting increase in myocardial oxygen demand, or a redistribution of coronary blood flow away from areas of ischemia ("coronary steal" syndrome). In the setting of documented or suspected myocardial ischemia, alternative agents are preferred.

One molecule of SNP is metabolized, by combining with hemoglobin, to produce one molecule of cyanmethemoglobin and four cyanide radicals. Cyanide radicals are detoxified by reacting with thiosulfate to form thiocyanate, which is then eliminated in the urine with a half-life of about 3 days. The detoxification of cyanide radicals is rate-limited by the availability of sulfur donors, especially thiosulfate, cystine, and cysteine. When cyanide production exceeds this capacity, excess cyanide can be buffered by combination with methemoglobin. Therefore, in a 70 kg patient with a normal red blood cell mass and methemoglobin level, cyanide accumulation will become significant after 2–2.5 hours of receiving SNP at a rate of 5 μg/kg/minute. In acutely ill patients the onset of cyanide accumulation and toxicity may occur earlier and at lower doses of SNP due to decreases in red blood cell mass and potential depletion of sulfur donors.

The signs and symptoms of acute cyanide toxicity include progressive central nervous system dysfunction with headache, anxiety, confusion, lethargy, and coma; cardiovascular instability with cardiac ischemia, dysrhythmias, AV block, and cardiovascular collapse; and changes in oxygenation and pH with venous hyperoxemia and lactic acidosis. Other manifestations may include nausea, vomiting, abdominal pain, increased salivation, and tachyphylaxis to the effects of SNP. The accumulation of cyanide and resulting toxicity can be prevented by co-administering sodium thiosulfate, typically in a 10:1 ratio in the same infusion. Sodium thiosulfate provides the necessary substrate to detoxify cyanide, does not interfere with the antihypertensive effects of SNP, and is inexpensive. Although this may increase thiocyanate accumulation and the risk of thiocyanate toxicity, this should not be a concern with short-term administration of SNP, and the adverse effects of thiocyanate are much less concerning than cyanide toxicity.

CLINICAL CAVEAT

Sodium Nitroprusside – Preventing Cyanide Toxicity

- Do not exceed infusion rates of 5 μg/kg/minute for more than a few minutes.
- Avoid prolonged infusions (>2 hours) using doses greater than 2.5 μg/kg/minute.
- Use alternative agents when high does of sodium nitroprusside are required.
- Add sodium thiosulfate injection (10:1 ratio) to infusions of sodium nitroprusside.
- Remain vigilant for common signs and symptoms of cyanide toxicity – mental status changes, venous hyperoxemia, lactic acidosis.

All institutions using sodium nitroprusside should have a cyanide antidote kit readily available.

SNP can result in the reversal of pulmonary hypoxic vasoconstriction and worsen ventilation:perfusion matching leading to increased hypoxemia. Potent vasodilators like SNP should be used cautiously in patients with compromised oxygenation due to chronic lung disease, acute respiratory distress syndrome, or severe pneumonia. Nitroprusside may also cause an abrupt increase in intracranial pressure (ICP) in patients with an elevated ICP and should be avoided in these patients. Abrupt discontinuation of SNP infusions carries a risk of rebound hypertension, and therefore should be tapered off slowly whenever possible.

Nitroglycerin

Nitroglycerin (NTG) is denitrated in vascular smooth muscle cells, releasing a free nitrite ion. A second enzymatic reaction releases nitric oxide, leading to vasodilation via the guanyl cyclase–cyclic-GMP pathway. NTG exerts its anti-ischemic and antihypertensive effects primarily through marked relaxation of the veins, resulting in decreased ventricular preload and increased venous capacitance. Although venodilation with resulting reduction in preload is the predominant anti-ischemic effect, NTG may also cause coronary vasodilation, reverse coronary vasospasm, improve myocardial collateral perfusion, and improve the epicardial to endocardial blood flow ratio. At higher doses, NTG also causes arterial vasodilation leading to a reduction in afterload. NTG is the vasodilator of choice for the management of cardiac ischemia, or for reducing MAP in a patient with underlying cardiac ischemia. NTG may also be used for rapid reduction of preload for patients with left ventricular dysfunction or cardiogenic shock who fail to respond to diuretics. However, the drug should be administered cautiously since excessive reductions in preload may lead to a reduction in cardiac output.

NTG is usually initiated at 5–10 μg/minute (0.075–0.15 μg/kg/minute) with the dose increased by 5–10 μg/minute every 3–5 minutes to achieve the desired clinical response. Like SNP, NTG has a rapid onset and short duration of action making it attractive for the management of acute elevations in blood pressure or cardiac ischemia in the ICU. Close monitoring of blood pressure and heart rate during the initiation and titration of the NTG infusion is recommended; however, invasive monitoring is not necessary.

Tolerance to the vasodilatory effects of NTG develops within 48–72 hours of starting an infusion. The development of tolerance is postulated to be secondary to baroreceptor- and hormonally mediated compensatory mechanisms evoked in response to reductions in arterial pressure, and from depletion of tissue sulfhydryl donors necessary for the metabolism of nitrates to nitric oxide. The most common side effects associated with NTG infusions are headache, hypotension, and reflex tachycardia. The free nitrite ion can react with hemoglobin to produce methemoglobinemia, which is of greatest concern with prolonged, high-dose infusions. When severe, methemoglobinemia can cause pseudocyanosis, tissue hypoxia, and death. Patients with critical aortic stenosis are preload-dependent and may tolerate NTG poorly; therefore NTG should be avoided or used very cautiously in these patients. NTG has less effect on hypoxic pulmonary vasoconstriction than SNP, and therefore may be better tolerated by the patient with hypoxemia.

Hydralazine

Hydralazine is a direct-acting arteriolar vasodilator leading to a reduction in systemic vascular resistance (SVR), with no effect on venous or epicardial coronary arteries.

Following intravenous administration, hydralazine reduces MAP, systolic and diastolic blood pressures, and increases heart rate, cardiac output, and myocardial contractility. An observed increase in sympathetic activity is predominantly a result of baroreceptor-mediated reflex, as well as a drug-induced release of NE from sympathetic nerve terminals. Hydralazine also directly increases cardiac contractility. Due to the effects on heart rate and contractility, no increase in epicardial blood flow, and the potential for "coronary steal" syndrome, hydralazine has negative effects on myocardial oxygen balance and may precipitate acute cardiac ischemia and infarction.

The initial dose of hydralazine should be 5–10 mg IV over 2 minutes, with additional doses used as needed. Single IV doses should not exceed 20 mg, and the dose is usually repeated every 6 hours due to its long duration of action. Intravenous hydralazine is contraindicated in patients with known coronary artery disease or evidence of cardiac ischemia, and should be used with caution in patients greater than 40 years of age. Although IV hydralazine has been widely used for many years in the treatment of hypertension and heart failure in the ICU, the drug should not be considered a first-line agent due to its potential for adverse effects, long duration of action, and the availability of safer options for achieving short-term hemodynamic goals.

Labetalol

Labetalol is a racemic mixture of four diastereomers that all have unique effects at α_1- and β-adrenergic receptors, with a net effect of nonselective β-receptor and α_1-receptor antagonism. The drug also demonstrates some β_2-receptor agonism, which may contribute to vasodilatation, and inhibition of the neuronal uptake of NE (a cocaine-like effect). Following intravenous administration, the potency for β-receptor blockade is about five to ten times that for α_1-receptor blockade. Labetalol is an attractive option for the management of acute hypertension since it potentially combines vasodilatation secondary to α_1-receptor antagonism, reversing the increases in afterload observed during common hypertensive syndromes, with β-receptor blockade to prevent reflex tachycardia. In the setting of acute aortic dissection, labetalol lowers MAP, decreases left ventricular contractility, and therefore the aortic wall is exposed to reduced shear forces, meeting the primary objectives of medical management for this condition.

A reduction in SVR is not universally observed with labetalol therapy. Hemodynamic studies of labetalol for acute postoperative hypertension have shown that the predominant effect of the drug is a reduction in systolic and mean arterial pressure, heart rate, and cardiac output, with no significant change in SVR. Right ventricular filling pressures remained unchanged or were slightly increased. This suggests that in some clinical settings the predominant effect on MAP is secondary to the nonselective β-blockade effects on the heart; however, the α_1-receptor antagonism appears to prevent an increase in SVR that is commonly observed following the administration of purely nonselective β-receptor antagonists. Differences in hemodynamic response may be due to differences in the severity of hypertension, or to the dose or method of administration of the drug.

Labetalol reduces indicators of myocardial oxygen demand while maintaining or improving indicators of myocardial oxygen supply. This apparent beneficial effect on myocardial metabolism may make labetalol a preferred agent in the setting of suspected or documented myocardial ischemia. In addition, labetalol does not affect ICP or cerebral blood flow, and is therefore an effective and safe agent for the control of blood pressure for neurosurgery and neurotrauma patients.

Onset of effect is within minutes following intravenous administration with peak effects observed within 5–10 minutes following a single intravenous injection. The drug has a long duration of action with an elimination half-life of up to 8 hours. Labetalol has been administered as individual bolus doses, by continuous infusion, or as a combination of bolus and infusion therapy for the management of acute hypertension. An initial dose of 10–20 mg administered over 2 minutes can be followed by increased doses of 20–80 mg every 10 minutes, until the desired blood pressure goal is achieved. The patient can receive subsequent bolus doses of labetalol if needed to maintain blood pressure within the desired range. Alternatively, the drug may be infused at a rate of 0.5–4 mg/minute until the goal blood pressure is achieved, and then should be stopped due to the long duration of action. Supplemental bolus doses of 10–20 mg may be given every 10 minutes during the early period of the infusion to achieve more rapid control of blood pressure. Blood pressure should be carefully monitored during dose titration; however, invasive monitoring is generally not required. The US FDA approved maximum dose is 300 mg over 24 hours; however, higher doses have been well tolerated provided the patient is properly monitored.

All of the usual precautions and contraindications for the use of a nonselective β-blocker should be observed. Patients with impaired left ventricular function, defined as an ejection fraction <40% or a cardiac index <2.5 l/minute/m^2, should receive alternative agents for the treatment of acute hypertension. In addition, patients with bronchospastic lung disease, impaired cardiac conduction, or resting bradycardia should not receive intravenous labetalol. The most common adverse effects associated with labetalol are hypotension, which can be precipitous, bradycardia, cardiac conduction delays, left ventricular dysfunction, bronchospasm, and rare skin rashes.

Nicardipine

Intravenous nicardipine, a dihydropyridine class calcium channel blocker, is the most widely studied calcium channel blocker for the treatment of hypertensive crises and acute postoperative hypertension. Like other dihydropyridines, nicardipine is relatively selective for vascular smooth muscle with little effect on cardiac conduction or inotropic activity in vivo. Therefore, the predominant hemodynamic effect of nicardipine is arterial vasodilation leading to a reduction in vascular resistance and MAP. There are typically small increases in cardiac output and heart rate with variable effects on preload. Nicardipine has beneficial effects on myocardial metabolism with increases in coronary blood flow and time to the development of angina or ECG evidence of ischemia during exercise.

Nicardipine has been shown to effectively lower blood pressure in multiple clinical trials involving patients with severe hypertension or postoperative hypertension. It has been found to be equally effective as SNP and NTG, and superior to placebo, with overall response rates of 86–98%. Compared to SNP, IV nicardipine demonstrated more consistent control of MAP necessitating fewer dose adjustments, and in some trials a shorter time to therapeutic response and fewer adverse effects necessitating discontinuation of the drug. The shorter time to therapeutic response and higher discontinuation rates may have been due to protocol design rather than true differences in efficacy or safety.

The recommended regimen for IV nicardipine is an initial infusion of 5 mg/hour with increases of 2.5 mg/hour every 15 minutes to a maximum of 15 mg/hour or until target MAP is achieved. The infusion should then be decreased to a maintenance rate of 3 mg/hour and adjusted by 1 to 2.5 mg/hour every 15 minutes to maintain target blood pressure. The controlled trials involving patients with acute postoperative hypertension started the infusion at 10 mg/hour, with increases of 2.5 mg/hour every 5 minutes to a maximum of 15 mg/hour or until target blood pressure was achieved. A similar maintenance infusion regimen was used. For acute postoperative hypertension the mean time to therapeutic response was approximately 10–15 minutes, and the time to offset of clinical effect after discontinuation of the infusion was approximately 15–20 minutes. Due to differences in dose titration, the mean time to therapeutic response in the severe hypertension trials was approximately 60 minutes. The recommendation for a loading infusion followed by a reduced dose maintenance infusion may create an opportunity for medication errors. Therefore, the clinical staff administering IV nicardipine should be properly instructed about the use of this drug, and orders should clearly indicate the need to reduce the infusion rate once blood pressure goals are achieved.

Adverse events have been reported in 7–38% of patients participating in controlled clinical trials of IV nicardipine. These were generally mild and transient, less common than with SNP, and usually did not require discontinuation of the drug. The most common adverse effects were headache, hypotension, sinus tachycardia, and nausea and vomiting.

Fenoldopam

Fenoldopam is a selective dopamine-1 (DA1) receptor agonist approved for the short-term treatment of severe hypertension. The stimulation of vascular DA1 receptors results in relaxation of vascular smooth muscle via a cyclic-AMP-dependent pathway. DA1 receptors are distributed throughout most arterial beds, but are present in highest density in renal and splanchnic arteries. Stimulation of DA1 receptors present on renal tubular cells produces a naturesis and increased urine flow rate. The naturetic effect may be augmented by an increase in renal blood flow and GFR associated with fenoldopam.

The predominant hemodynamic effect of fenoldopam is a reduction in SVR with decreases in MAP and systolic and diastolic blood pressure. Heart rate, cardiac output, and left ventricular stroke volumes are increased, and there is no significant effect on preload. Unlike SNP, fenoldopam does not significantly increase pulmonary shunt fraction.

Fenoldopam has been shown to be equivalent to SNP for the treatment of severe hypertension with a similar overall response rate and time to response. For the treatment of postoperative hypertension, fenoldopam has been shown to be superior to placebo and equivalent to SNP and IV nifedipine. The drug should be initiated at a rate of 0.1 µg/kg/minute, then titrated by increments of 0.05–0.1 µg/kg/minute at 15–20 minute intervals to achieve the goal blood pressure. The maximum recommended infusion rate is 1.6 µg/kg/minute. The mean time to therapeutic goal was 28 minutes in a placebo-controlled trial, and 70% of cardiac surgery patients had achieved goal blood pressure by 30 minutes after the start of treatment with fenoldopam. The time to therapeutic response may have been affected by the protocol design and rate of titration of the infusion. Due to its short half-life of approximately 5–10 minutes the effects of fenoldopam dissipate relatively quickly after cessation of an infusion, with about a 50% loss of effect by 15 minutes without evidence of rebound hypertension.

The effects of fenoldopam on renal blood flow and glomerular filtration pose a theoretical advantage for fenoldopam in the treatment of severe hypertension associated with compromised renal function. However, there are no clinical data to support the supposition that fenoldopam will improve the outcome of renal function when compared to other vasodilators. The most common adverse effects with fenoldopam are hypotension, tachycardia, headache, flushing, dizziness, and bradycardia. Fenoldopam increases intraocular pressure, and therefore should be avoided in patients with glaucoma or high intraocular pressure. Due to its potent naturetic effects, intravascular volume depletion may occur and urine output will not be a reliable clinical indicator of hypovolemia. Lastly, fenoldopam has been reported to cause changes in T-wave morphology on the surface ECG; however, these changes do not appear to represent myocardial ischemia. The major disadvantage of fenoldopam when compared to other therapeutic options is the high acquisition cost of this agent; however, the recent loss of patent protection for this compound is likely to lead to significant price erosion.

Enalaprilat

Enalaprilat is the only intravenous angiotensin converting enzyme inhibitor (ACEI) approved for clinical use, and has been evaluated for the treatment of severe hypertension, acute left ventricular failure, and perioperative hypertension. Enalaprilat is the active metabolite of the oral prodrug enalapril. ACEIs inhibit the enzyme responsible for the conversion of angiotensin I to angiotensin II, and the metabolism of bradykinin to its inactive form. The resultant pharmacodynamic effects include vasodilation, decreased sympathetic response, renal efferent arteriolar vasodilation, and decreased sodium retention. Bradykinin may also contribute to systemic vasodilation. Hemodynamic effects include reductions in MAP, systolic and diastolic blood pressure, and preload, with a variable effect on cardiac output. Reflex tachycardia is not observed, and arterial oxygenation is not affected.

Intravenous enalaprilat has been shown to effectively lower blood pressure in small studies involving patients with moderate to severe hypertension. The maximal decrease in blood pressure is usually observed within 30 minutes, and the duration of response has been variable depending upon the size of the dose administered. Intravenous enalaprilat has also been evaluated in a randomized, controlled trial for patients with hypertension following intracranial neurosurgery. Compared to the control group, enalaprilat effectively lowered blood pressure, with an average onset of approximately 15 minutes. The duration of response exceeded 4 hours in this study. The effect was primarily due to a reduction in vascular resistance with no significant change in cardiac output. There was a slight reduction in myocardial

perfusion pressure, which may be of some concern in patients with evidence of myocardial ischemia.

Patients with congestive heart failure (CHF) administered intravenous enalaprilat experience a reduction in blood pressure, SVR, preload, and heart rate, with an increase in stroke volume. These effects are similar to what has been observed following oral administration of an ACEI.

The initial adult dose of IV enalaprilat should be 0.625–1.25 mg, administered over 5 minutes. The dose can be repeated after 20–30 minutes if the patient has an inadequate response. The effective dose is typically repeated every 6 hours, and may be continued until the patient is able to transition to oral therapy. Since enalaprilat is cleared by the kidneys, the dose should be reduced in the setting of significant renal insufficiency.

The potential adverse effects from ACEI therapy include hypotension, which may be prolonged, acute decreases in renal function, hyperkalemia, and rare cases of angioedema. Patients with intravascular volume depletion are at greatest risk for hypotension and acute renal insufficiency, so careful attention should be paid to volume status. Bilateral renal artery stenosis or severe renal dysfunction are considered relative contraindications to treatment with ACEIs. The long duration of action of enalaprilat, while potentially advantageous from the perspective of dose frequency, may be a disadvantage if the patient experiences significant hypotension. For the treatment of severe hypertension in the critical care setting, enalaprilat should be considered a second-line agent.

Nesiritide

Nesiritide is a recombinant B-type naturetic peptide (BNP) approved for the management of acute, decompensated heart failure, and represents the first therapeutic advance in the treatment of severe CHF in over 10 years. Administration of nesiritide causes both arterial and venous vasodilation with a reduction in preload (pulmonary artery occlusion pressure (PAOP) and right atrial pressure) and SVR, with an increase in stroke volume and cardiac index. The peptide also has naturetic effects with increases in urinary sodium excretion and urine output, and may be associated with increases in GFR. Plasma aldosterone concentrations are also decreased following the administration of nesiritide.

Nesiritide is indicated for hospitalized patients with decompensated heart failure with signs and symptoms of volume overload over the past 72 hours. If a pulmonary artery catheter is inserted, the PAOP should be greater than 18 mmHg. Patients with a history of significant valvular stenosis; hypertrophic, restrictive, or obstructive cardiomyopathy; constrictive pericarditis; primary pulmonary hypertension; biopsy-proven active myocarditis;

or complex congenital heart disease were excluded from clinical trials and should not receive this drug until studies demonstrating safety in these conditions becomes available. In addition, patients receiving intravenous vasodilators (e.g., NTG, milrinone, amrinone, or nitroprusside), or patients with a systolic blood pressure consistently less than 90 mmHg, cardiogenic shock, or intravascular volume depletion are not candidates for nesiritide therapy.

Nesiritide has been compared to standard therapy (most commonly dobutamine and diuretics) and intravenous NTG in patients with decompensated heart failure. Global clinical status, dyspnea, and fatigue were improved by both standard therapy and nesiritide without significant differences between the groups. There is a suggestion from post hoc analysis of the data that long-term clinical outcomes were better in the nesiritide groups, but effects on long-term morbidity and mortality need to be further evaluated in larger properly designed clinical trials. Dobutamine was associated with a significant increase in cardiac ectopy, episodes of nonsustained ventricular tachycardia, and heart rate, while these endpoints were unchanged or decreased with nesiritide. Compared to NTG, nesiritide led to greater short-term reductions in preload and afterload, and greater increases in cardiac output. Measures of global clinical status and dyspnea were similar between the two groups; however, there were fewer adverse effects with nesiritide.

The recommended dose for nesiritide is an initial bolus dose of 2 µg/kg over 1 minute followed by an infusion of 0.01 µg/kg/minute. Time to onset of action is approximately 15 minutes, and the offset of effect is relatively rapid with an elimination half-life of 18 minutes. If the patient experiences hypotension or a systolic pressure <85 mmHg, the infusion should be stopped. It can be restarted at 50% of the previous dose once the systolic blood pressure is >90 mmHg. The infusion can be increased every 3 hours provided the systolic blood pressure is >100 mmHg and the PAOP is >20 mmHg (if available). The dose is titrated by administering a bolus dose of 1 µg/kg over 1 minute and increasing the infusion by 0.005 µg/kg/minute. The maximum infusion rate is 0.03 µg/kg/minute.

Nesiritide has been well tolerated with the most common adverse effects being hypotension and nausea. Despite beneficial effects on hemodynamic response, improvement in symptoms, and the novelty of its pharmacologic effects in heart failure, there is a need for clinical outcomes and economic data to justify the routine use of this expensive agent in the management of decompensated heart failure. Until these data become available, nesiritide should be considered a second-line agent reserved for patients refractory to traditional therapy.

Choice of Vasodilator Therapy

Table 8-4 summarizes some of the characteristics of the intravenously administered vasodilators. As mentioned above, there are no large controlled trials that support the use of one vasodilator over another for any of the common indications. Most of the small comparative trials demonstrate comparable efficacy with small differences in the incidence of adverse effects. Therefore the choice of a vasodilator is typically a bedside decision based upon the desired hemodynamic response, knowledge of the pharmacologic properties of the available options, clinical presentation of the patient, intensity of hemodynamic monitoring available, and clinician experience. There are, however, some general clinical caveats, which can be considered in the choice of a vasodilator.

For patients with evidence of cardiac ischemia or at high risk for developing cardiac ischemia, NTG, labetalol, and nicardipine are good choices while hydralazine is contraindicated. In the setting of acute left ventricular dysfunction, NTG, SNP, enalaprilat, and nicardipine are all reasonable choices; however, labetalol should generally be avoided. For patients with traumatic brain injury or other causes of an elevated ICP, labetalol is considered the vasodilator of choice and SNP and NTG should be avoided. Limited data suggest that nicardipine and enalaprilat may be safe alternatives to labetalol for patients with an elevated ICP. In the setting of acute aortic dissection, labetalol or SNP with β-blockade are considered the treatments of choice. Agents that may significantly increase aortic shear forces, like hydralazine, should be avoided. Fenoldopam may have some theoretical benefit in patients with severe hypertension and acute renal dysfunction although this is unproven and questioned by recent studies showing no renal protective effects of fenoldopam in other clinical settings. The place of relatively new or less well-studied agents like enalaprilat, fenoldopam, and nesiritide is currently uncertain.

SUMMARY

As reviewed in this chapter, there are many vasoactive drugs available for the acute management of hemodynamic response in the ICU, and despite many decades of experience there is still no clear-cut, definitive evidence of the superiority of any one agent for common clinical indications. Therefore, it is imperative that critical care practitioners have a thorough knowledge of the actions and adverse effects of these drugs, remain current with evolving clinical evidence relating to the optimal

Table 8-4 Parenteral Vasodilators

Agent	Typical Dose	Onset	Duration	Potential Adverse Events	Comments
Sodium nitroprusside	0.25-5 mg/kg/minute (max.10 µg/kg/minute)	<1 minute	1-3 minutes	Tachycardia, precipitous reductions in blood pressure, myocardial ischemia, cyanide and thiocyanate toxicity, pulmonary V/Q mismatch, rebound hypertension, restlessness, nausea, and vomiting	Requires continuous invasive monitoring; sodium thiosulfate (10:1) prevents cyanide toxicity
Nitroglycerin	5-300 µg/minute	<1 minute	5-10 minutes	Tachycardia, headache, hypotension, nausea, and vomiting	Tolerance develops; good choice with myocardial ischemia
Labetalol	Bolus: 10-20 mg, then 20-40 mg q 10 minutes; infusion: 0.5-4 mg/minute; maximum dose = 300 mg (?)	<5-10 minutes	3-5 hours	Bradycardia, bronchospasm LV dysfunction, prolonged hypotensive effect	Usual precautions for nonselective β-blocker; good choice with myocardial ischemia, aortic dissection, or ↑ ICP
Nicardipine	Initiate: 5 mg/hour, ↑ by 2.5 mg/h q5-15 minutes to maximum of 15 mg/hour. Maintenance: start at 3 mg/hour	10-15 minutes	15-20 minutes	Tachycardia, hypotension, nausea, and vomiting	Caution with loading infusion vs. maintenance infusion dose. Good choice with myocardial ischemia
Hydralazine	5-20 mg IV q6 hours	15-30 minutes	4-6 hours	Tachycardia, hypotension, headache, nausea, flushing, cardiac ischemia	Not routinely recommended. Contraindicated with cardiac ischemia
Enalaprilat	0.625-5 mg IV every 6 hours	15-20 minutes	>4 hours	Hypotension, renal dysfunction, hyperkalemia, angioedema	Contraindicated with bilateral renal artery stenosis. Good choice with congestive heart failure
Fenoldopam	Initial 0.1 µg/kg/minute, increase by 0.05-0.1 µg/kg/minute q15-20 minutes. Maximum of 1.6 µg/kg/minute	20-40 minutes	15-30 minutes	Hypotension, tachycardia, headache, flushing, dizziness, bradycardia, ECG changes, elevated IOP	Avoid in patients with glaucoma or high IOP. Theoretical good choice with acute renal failure

ICP, intracranial pressure; IOP, intraocular pressure; LV, left ventricle; V/Q, pulmonary ventilation:perfusion ratio.

use of vasoactive drugs, and not be inappropriately committed to their traditional approaches to therapy when new evidence from well-designed trials emerges to the contrary. While some questions relating to the use of vasoactive drugs are currently being addressed in large, multicenter trials, considerably more large studies focused on meaningful clinical outcomes are needed in this area of critical care pharmacotherapy.

SELECTED READING

Vasopressors

Dellinger RP: Cardiovascular management of septic shock. Crit Care Med 31:946-955, 2003.

Dünser MW, Mayr AJ, Tür A et al: Ischemic skin lesions as a complication of continuous vasopressin infusion in catecholamine-resistant vasodilatory shock: incidence and risk factors. Crit Care Med 31:1394-1398, 2003.

Dünser MW, Mayr AJ, Ulmer H et al: Arginine vasopressin in advanced vasodilatory shock. A prospective, randomized, controlled study. Circulation 107:2313-2319, 2003.

Hollenberg SM, Aherns TS, Annane D et al: Practice parameters for hemodynamic support of sepsis in adult patients: 2004 update. Crit Care Med 32:1928-1948, 2004.

Martin C, Viviand X, Leone M, Thirion X: Effect of norepinephrine on the outcome of septic shock. Crit Care Med 28:2758-2765, 2000.

Robin JK, Oliver JA, Landry DW: Vasopressin deficiency in the syndrome of irreversible shock. J Trauma 54:S149-S154, 2003.

Ruokonen E, Parviainen I, Uusaro A: Treatment of impaired perfusion in septic shock. Ann Med 34:590-597, 2002.

Vasodilators

Abdelwahab W, Frishman W, Landau A: Management of hypertensive urgencies and emergencies. J Clin Pharmacol 35:747-762, 1995.

Cherney D, Straus S: Management of patients with hypertensive urgencies and emergencies. A systematic review of the literature. J Gen Intern Med 17:937-945, 2002.

Goldberg ME, Larijani GE: Perioperative hypertension. Pharmacotherapy 18:911-914, 1998.

Keating GM, Goa KL: Nesiritide: a review of its use in acute decompensated heart failure. Drugs 63:47-70, 2003.

Murphy MB, Murray C, Shorten GD: Fenoldopam – a selective peripheral dopamine-receptor agonist for the treatment of severe hypertension. N Engl J Med 345:1548-1557, 2001.

CHAPTER 9

Nutrition in the Intensive Care Unit

IQBAL MUSTAFA, M.D., Ph.D.

XAVIER M. LEVERVE, M.D., Ph.D.

The comprehensive evaluation of nutritional status includes intake analysis, physical and anthropometric examination, laboratory examination, and radiology. Patient history is taken and physical examination is performed to identify the mechanisms underlying the occurrence of depletion or over-nutrition, such as inadequate intake or absorption, impeded utilization, and increasing nutrient loss.

Anthropometric examination provides information on the reserves of muscle mass and fat mass which describe the reserves of energy and protein mass. Normal examinations include body weight, body height, skin fold thickness, and the circumference of various body organs.

Energy balance can be determined by comparing direct energy with that obtained indirectly with calorimetry, or calculating the need using the Harris Benedict formula, which is compared with intake. Nitrogen balance can be determined by the balance between nitrogen intake from protein and nitrogen of urine urea (NUU), calculated by accommodating urine for 24 hours.

Visceral protein status is determined by albumin and transferin serum level. However, not all conditions correlate with nutritional status that affects albumin and transferin serum. Both these visceral proteins have a long half-life.

Retinol binding protein, transthretin, thyroxin binding prealbumin (TBPA), fibronectin, and somatomedin C can be used as nutrition markers during enteral nutrition in the critically ill. Visceral protein status can also be determined by an immune function test, such as total leukocyte count and skin hypersensitivity; however, the interpretation should be made carefully in patients with infection.

Somatic protein status can be determined by creatinine height index, because creatinine is released from muscle tissue at relatively constant speed, and so the amount of urine creatinine is proportional to muscle tissue. 3-Methyl histidine (3-MH) secretion through urine is another alternative for measuring somatic protein status. 3-MH is a metabolic result from muscles, and thus its value can be used to identify turnover from the muscle which is proportional to somatic protein reserves.

The nutrition risk index (NRI) takes into account body mass variation and serum albumin. NRI < 83.5 indicates severely malnourished patients for whom nutritional support is required.

ENERGY AND MACRONUTRIENTS USED IN NUTRITION

Energy

The energy expenditure of most hospitalized patients is often lower than values obtained from classic equations and textbook tables. The vast majority of patients, including those in the intensive care unit (ICU), have energy expenditures that do not exceed 2000 kcal/day.

The main objective is achieving a positive or zero nitrogen balance via hypercaloric support during the acute metabolic phase and preserving function, limiting major depletion of lean body mass by starting nutritional support at an early stage, but with limited amounts of energy substrates. Partial (under) feeding is acceptable during the hypermetabolic phase, while increased energy intakes may be useful in the recovery or anabolic phase of illness when tissue rebuilding is possible. Overfeeding should be avoided since it may be associated with major complications and side effects.

Carbohydrates

Glucose represents the major circulating carbohydrate fuel. Glucose may be used by most cells of the body, including the central and peripheral nervous system, as well as by blood cells and the ground substance of healing tissues. In resting patients consumption of glucose by the brain represents an important component of energy expenditure.

Glucose is stored as glycogen in the liver and skeletal muscles. The hepatic reserves are limited and exhausted after 24–36 hours of fasting. Glycogen in muscle is not available for utilization outside these cells. When hepatic reserves of glycogen are exhausted, glucose is produced via gluconeogenesis from amino acids (mainly alanine), glycerol, and lactate.

Glucose oxidation is associated with a higher production of CO_2, as shown by a higher respiratory quotient (RQ) for glucose than for long-chain fatty acids.

A large part of the glucose is recycled after anaerobic glycolysis into lactate (at the site of trauma, infection, or in cancer cells) which is then used for hepatic gluconeogenesis. That part of the glucose intake that is not immediately used as energy substrate is stored as glycogen in the liver and adipose tissues. Large glucose loads in hypermetabolic patients could result in hepatic accumulation of both glycogen and fat, and can be associated with severe dysfunction of the liver. The important insulin response to high glucose infusions markedly inhibits lipolysis and the mobilization of fatty acids from adipose stores as well as proteolysis and mobilization of amino acids from skeletal muscles. These effects prevent the mobilization of essential or conditionally essential substrates (e.g., glutamine, essential fatty acids, vitamins, and micronutrients) for maintaining key organ function. Despite elevated glucose turnover in conditions of stress, oxidative metabolism is not increased in the same proportion. Therefore, the maximal recommended infusion rate is 5 mg/kg/minute in adult patients.

Lipids

Lipids can be provided in enteral nutrition or as intravenous lipid emulsions. The major steps in lipid emulsion metabolism are hydrolysis of triglycerides, exchange of neutral lipids with endogenous cholesterol, and uptake of remnant particles. Each of these steps is largely influenced by the composition of the triglyceride and the phospholipid constituents.

Infusion of lipid calories allows a reduction of carbohydrate intake and a substantially decreased incidence and severity of side effects induced by high glucose loads. Apart from the advantages of balancing energy intake between carbohydrate and lipids, it is also important to consider the composition of fat intake with respect to the proportion of saturated, monounsaturated, and polyunsaturated fats and the ratio between omega-6 and omega-3 essential fatty acids and antioxidant content. Lipid intake may account for 30–50% of nonprotein calories, depending on the individual patient's tolerance to both carbohydrate and lipids. Lipid emulsions should not be given to those with marked hypertriglyceridemia.

During the first days of lipid emulsion supply, particularly in stressed patients, the prescribed lipid load should be infused as slowly as possible, e.g., at a rate lower than 0.1 g/kg/hour with LCT and lower than 0.15 g/kg/hour with a mixed MCT/LCT emulsion. Plasma triglyceride levels should be monitored during this initial period and the infusion rate adjusted to measured values.

Amino Acids

Amino acids are subjected within the body to a series of metabolic reactions. Part of the free amino acid pool is incorporated into tissue proteins. Because of protein breakdown, these amino acids return to the free pool after a variable period of time and thus become available for reutilization for protein synthesis or for catabolism.

Some of the free amino acid pool undergoes catabolic reactions. This process leads to the loss of the carbon skeleton as CO_2 or deposition as glycogen and fat while the nitrogen is eliminated as urea.

Finally some free amino acids are used for synthesis of new nitrogen-containing compounds, such as purine bases, creatine, epinephrine, etc. In general, these are subsequently degraded without return of end products to the free amino acid pool. The nonessential amino acids are made in the body using amino groups derived from other amino acids and carbon skeletons, formed by reactions common to intermediary metabolism.

The protein requirement for an average young adult is 0.75 g of protein/kg of body weight. This again presupposes a high proportion of first-class protein and an adequate energy supply.

During acute illness and convalescence intakes of 1.2–1.5 g/kg are desirable and have proved beneficial. In some diseases protein intake must be controlled, e.g., acute liver failure when the intake has to be restricted in order to avoid hepatic coma and uremia, during which the capacity to excrete nitrogenous end products is limited. In the dietary management of uremia, an intake of 0.5 g protein/kg allows the patient to resist inter-current infections better than for an earlier recommendation of 0.25 g/kg.

ENTERAL NUTRITION

Enteral nutrition is the preferred method of nutritional support in the critically ill with an intact functioning gastrointestinal tract. In general, enteral nutrition should be started within 48 hours of ICU admission with an aim of stimulating gut function and trophicity. There is some evidence that this goal can be attained with only minimal amounts of enteral nutrition.

Optimal timing of the onset of enteral nutrition is crucial. Unnecessary delay due to regurgitation caused by decreased gastroduodenal motility may prolong negative nitrogen balance.

The amounts of enteral nutrition are based on nutritional assessment, energy requirements, patient history, and medical condition. In patients with severe catabolic illness and/or poorly functioning gut, parenteral nutrition should be started concomitantly, in order to meet protein and energy requirements and minimize excessive muscle wasting. In patients with persistent gastroparesis and intolerance to gastric feeding despite adequate prokinetic treatment, endoscopic placement of a nasoduodenal tube should be the next step, while nasojejunal tubes should be used only as a last resort, since they are technically the most difficult to place, and do not protect from aspiration or duodenogastric reflux.

Percutaneous gastronomy has become a preferable route when long-term (≥4–6 weeks) enteral nutrition support is required. Although the risk of aspiration is decreased when the latter is administered in the jejunum, airway protective measures such as inclination of the torso 30° above the horizontal plane, endotracheal intubation, or tracheostomy should be considered.

The most comfortable tubes for patients are silicone or polyurethane small-diameter (6–12 F) tubes, the length of which depends on the location of feeding. When higher viscosity solutions such as fiber-enriched solutions are used, administration through smaller diameter tubes might be more difficult unless a constant infusion pump is applied. Since gastric aspiration is often required in ICU patients, it is preferable to use the latter in the early period of an ICU stay, and to switch to the smaller feeding tubes if enteral nutrition is well tolerated and expected to last for more than 10 days. After placement of the nasoenteric tube, an abdominal x-ray should be performed to verify its proper placement.

Hospital kitchen-prepared feeding solutions can cause numerous potential complications, such as nutritionally unbalanced solutions, water and electrolyte disorders, diarrhea, and severe nosocomial infection due to bacterial contamination. These problems have led to the development of standardized, industrially prepared feeding solutions. The most commonly used feeding solution is the iso-osmotic solution (±300 mOsm/l).

Standard feeding solutions are polymeric, being made up of substrates similar to those found in normal feeds. Recent studies suggest that polymeric solutions should be considered as the first line of enteral nutrition, while semi-elemental solutions should be considered in patients with severe small bowel disease or extensive intestinal resection.

Adding fibers to enteral feeding solutions is beneficial, as insoluble fibers (cellulose, lignin) absorb water, which leads to the improved regulation of intestinal transit and reduced incidence of diarrhea. Soluble fibers (pectin, gums, mucilages) are degraded into short-chain fatty acids, which enhance water and electrolyte absorption, and provide nutrition for colonicyte.

Enteral nutrition can be administered by gravity or with a constant delivery pump. The former is simple and cheaper, but less precise than the pump technique, and may cause accidental bolus administration, which increases the risk of gastroesophageal reflux and bronchoaspiration. Improved tolerance and a reduced incidence of diarrhea have been documented with continuous compared to bolus feeding.

Critically ill patients very often present with delayed gastric emptying and impaired gastroduodenal motility, which often cause incomplete delivery of the prescribed daily feed. Measuring gastric residuals by aspiration is often used as a monitoring tool.

An arbitrary value above which enteral nutrition is usually given at a slower rate or discontinued is 150 ml and may lead to underfeeding. Prokinetic drugs may be administered to help to lessen the gastric residuals.

Diarrhea is a frequent problem in ICU patients receiving enteral nutrition, and has often been associated with the osmolarity. Most standard polymeric industrial feeds have osmolarity of ≤380 mOsm/kg. There are many factors that determine the etiology of diarrhea in enterally fed patients, among which are factors related to the nutrition itself, antibiotics and other medications, *Clostridium difficile* colitis, hypoalbuminemia, sepsis, and fever.

Mild symptoms of intolerance are managed with observation by physical examination at the time of onset and within 6 hours, with the current rate of feeding being maintained. For moderate distention, tube feeds are stopped and the patient is assessed for evidence of small bowel obstruction. If distention remains moderate, an elemental formula is begun. Moderate diarrhea (3–4 times/shift) is managed by maintaining the current feeding rate and repeating the examination in 6 hours. Severe distention is managed by stopping all tube feeds, increasing IV fluid administration, and evaluating the possibility of nonocclusive bowel necrosis. For severe diarrhea, tube feeds are reduced by 50%, antidiarrheal medications are added, and the patient is evaluated for possible *Clostridium difficile* infection. Vomiting is managed by ensuring adequate gastric decompression and decreasing the infusion rate by half. High nasogastric output is treated by verifying postpyloric placement of the tube and checking the nasogastric aspirate.

PARENTERAL NUTRITION AND PERIOPERATIVE NUTRITION

Currently, total parenteral nutrition is used in a wide variety of patients when the enteral route cannot be used. Parenteral nutrition in the ICU is also being used commonly together with enteral nutrition.

Parenteral nutrition may be achieved using a peripheral venous catheter, but it is difficult to administer adequate caloric, protein, and electrolytes, and thus central venous access should be used. In the absence of a preexisting line, either the subclavian or internal jugular site is preferred. The former has lower infection risk and dressing care is easier, while the risk of pneumothorax or subclavian artery puncture is higher, both complications having potentially devastating effects in unstable ICU patients. In severely ill ICU patients a central venous line must be used solely for the purpose of parenteral nutrition.

Subcutaneously tunneled catheters should be reserved for long-term parenteral support (>3–4 weeks), such as in bone marrow transplantation associated with multiple intensive intravenous therapy.

A recent meta-analysis of perioperative feeding concluded that there was no benefit, and indeed possible harm, from the routine use of short periods of postoperative parenteral nutrition. There appeared to be some benefit when this was given perioperatively to patients with severe antecedent malnutrition.

Malnutrition in surgical patients is associated with delayed wound healing and increased risk of morbidity and mortality. The main goals of perioperative nutrition are to reduce the incidence of postoperative complications, the length of postoperative hospitalization, and operative mortality. An additional goal is to decrease the effects of disease and surgery-related malnutrition on body composition, organ function, and subsequent patient performance. Available trials concluded that the routine use of perioperative parenteral nutrition in unselected surgical patients was unjustified, but might be helpful in high-risk patients.

Approximately 40% of candidates to general and vascular surgery present with malnutrition. Postoperative outcome influenced by malnutrition may occur in major surgery and particularly in elderly patients. The severity of postoperative complications is related to the degree of preoperative malnutrition. Malnutrition most often reflects the severity of underlying disease and the occurrence of underlying disease complications.

Among anthropometric parameters, body weight loss is the most useful. A weight loss ≥20% clearly indicates poor postoperative outcome, while a weight loss ≥10% within a six-month period or a weight loss ≥5 kg during the three preoperative months indicates higher incidence of major postoperative complications.

Protein malnutrition is the best predictor of complications both in surgical and nonsurgical patients. Among 15 tested variables, it was shown that serum albumin <35 g/l, transferrin <1.74 g/l, and prealbumin <0.12 g/l had the highest predictive values of postoperative complications.

Nutrient metabolism during surgery depends on preoperative patient condition and surgery-induced metabolic changes. In normal subjects endocrine and metabolic adaptation will tolerate prolonged starvation without compromising survival. After 2 to 3 days of starvation, glucose needs are mainly satisfied by gluconeogenesis from amino acids released by protein degradation (approximately 75 g of protein/day, i.e., 300 g of muscle). Then, an increase in fat utilization and ketogenesis are associated with a decrease in gluconeogenesis, and proteolysis falls at 20 to 30 g/day. Surgical stress markedly impairs those adaptations and increases protein loss. Thus, tolerance to starvation depends on preoperative nutritional status, length of perioperative starvation, and intensity of aggression. Preoperative feeding can be altered by underlying disease, hospitalization, and preoperative investigations. In non-malnourished patients, during elective and noncomplicated surgery, starvation of 7 to 14 days will not affect the outcome.

Major surgery induces a systemic inflammatory response of varying intensity. Mobilization of fuel stores and gluconeogenesis are stimulated by the release of catecholamines, cortisol, glucagons, and growth hormone, as well as by insulin resistance. Interleukin-1 (IL-1) and tumor necrosis factor (TNF) are responsible for an increase in muscle protein catabolism and a decrease in protein synthesis, while IL-6 is responsible for acute-phase protein synthesis in the liver.

Endocrine changes in stress conditions are characterized by a downregulation of hypothalamus–pituitary–thyroid axis and low plasma T3 concentrations. Cytokines suppress prealbumin synthesis reducing retinol-binding protein. The subsequent release of increased amounts of thyroxine and retinol in free form strengthens the effect of cytokines. Thyroxine-binding globulin, corticosteroid-binding globulin, and IGF-binding protein-3 degradation allow the occurrence of peak endocrine and mitogenic influences at the site of inflammation. This mechanism is associated with hyperthermia, weight loss, and hypoalbuminemia. Increased protein catabolism and hypermetabolism vary with stress intensity and are responsible for a decreased response to nutritional support. The prolongation of such metabolic state results in severe protein depletion.

Enteral nutrition, using polymeric nutritive mixtures, is usually given through a nasogastric tube or by perendoscopic gastrostomy when long-term refeeding is expected. The association of enteral and parenteral nutrition is often necessary to achieve nutritional goals in the early postoperative period.

In malnourished patients preoperative nutrition should be given for 7 to 10 days. Longer preoperative nutrition support would increase the risk of nosocomial infection. Postoperative nutritional support should not be less than 7 days. In order to avoid overfeeding, it is recommended to ensure energy support equivalent to energy expenditure. Daily needs vary from 20 kcal/kg/day in non-malnourished patients to 35 kcal/kg/day in malnourished or severely stressed patients. Fat should not exceed 30% of nonprotein energy supply. Standard fat emulsions are usually given. Medium-chain triglycerides are well tolerated and may be useful in selected circumstances. According to the severity of the stress, nitrogen support should vary from 0.25 g/kg/day to 0.35 g/kg/day. No benefit is demonstrated for nutritional support higher than 0.35 g/kg/day. In severely ill patients glutamine-enriched parenteral nutrition can be proposed.

NUTRITION IN TRAUMA

Trauma patients are prone to develop acute protein malnutrition because of persistent hypermetabolism, which compromises the immune response and increases the risk of late MOF-associated nosocomial infection. Early administration of exogenous substrates to meet the increased metabolic demands would prevent or slow the development of acute protein malnutrition and improve patient outcome.

Although difficult for centers without experience, total enteral nutrition (TEN) is preferred over total parenteral nutrition (TPN) because it is safer, less expensive, and more convenient. Substrates delivered enterally appear to be better utilized and do not produce the hyperglycemia associated with TPN.

TEN prevents gut mucosal atrophy, attenuates the stress response, maintains immunocompetence, and preserves gut flora. In addition, to prevent acute protein malnutrition, early TEN with immune-enhancing diets also promote normal gut function and enhance systemic immune responses, thereby preventing nosocomial infections.

To achieve adequate amounts of early TEN, it is best delivered into the proximal small intestine. Enteral feeding access should be obtained at the time of initial laparotomy. If the patient undergoes an abbreviated laparotomy, the needle catheter jejunostomy (NCJ) can be placed during a subsequent operation while for those who do not undergo immediate laparotomy, the enteral nutrition can be delivered through a nasojejunal (NJ) tube for the first 24 hours after injury. A few patients may have contraindication to upper gastrointestinal endoscopy. In such patients a jejunostomy tube can be easily placed laparoscopically.

Immune-enhancing diets (IEDs) are indicated for patients with major torso trauma and who are at known risk for septic complications and MOF. Usage is limited up to 10 days, after which polymeric, high-protein formulas are used. Polymeric high-protein formulas are for patients who do not meet the criteria for IEDs, who have normal gut digestive and absorptive capacity, and are believed to have increased nitrogen requirements. Elemental formulas are given to those who are intolerant to polymeric formulas or who have not received enteral nutrition for the first week postinjury. Renal failure formulas (concentrated, reduced electrolyte) are for those who need intermittent hemodialysis.

Intolerance indicators of TEN are vomiting, abdominal distention or cramping/tenderness, diarrhea, high nasogastric tube output, and contraindications of specific medications. If enteral access is delayed or hemodynamic status prevents early enteral nutrition, early TPN is not indicated unless the patient is severely malnourished. Routine TPN may be associated with worse outcomes than no nutrition in patients with normal to moderate malnutrition.

For various reasons, trauma patients are at high risk for acute renal failure (ARF). This can be treated with CVVH/CVVHD, which allow TPN with high fluid volumes and high protein loads to be used. Alternatively standard isotonic, normal electrolyte solutions are used in enteral nutrition support initially (Box 9-1).

NUTRITION IN ACUTE RESPIRATORY FAILURE

Patients with trauma, burns, sepsis, acute respiratory distress syndrome (ARDS), and multiple organ dysfunction

Box 9-1   Enteral Nutrition

Enteral nutrition can be started with a rate of 10–15 cm³/hour of full-strength formula and advanced by 15 cm³/hour every 12 hours in the absence of moderate or severe intolerance symptoms until the rate of 60 cm³/hour is reached. The rate is maintained for 24 hours and then advanced by 15 cm³/hour every 12 hours. Early positive energy balance is not necessary and the initial goal could be lowered whenever necessary and only advanced to the patient-specific goal after 24 hours.

syndromes (MODS) present a hypermetabolic and catabolic state leading to extensive endogenous protein breakdown and major loss of muscle mass, including respiratory muscles. As a result, these patients are prone to respiratory muscle fatigue and/or failure, leading to unsuccessful weaning from a ventilator. In chronic obstructive pulmonary disease (COPD) with patients requiring mechanical ventilation, the weaning process can be extremely difficult due to the additive effects of chronic malnutrition, increased work of breathing, increased load on inspiratory muscles, hypoxia, and hypercapnia.

The association between respiratory failure and metabolic disturbances are complex and three groups of patients can be individualized. In the first group, the nutritional depletion is the result of COPD and the nutritional status is important to the patient's prognosis. The second group consists of acutely ill patients, with acquired malnutrition, among other factors (hypophosphatemia, hypocalcemia, hypomagnesemia, postsurgery pain, etc.), which could cause ventilator dependency or weaning difficulties. In the last group, an inadequate nutritional support containing too high calorie intakes might delay the weaning process.

Infection or inflammatory status is probably the most common feature of patients with respiratory failure and/or need for mechanical ventilation. It is now well recognized that acute or chronic inflammation results in a marked loss of lean body mass with nutritional consequences. Bronchial infection is known as the major cause of acute respiratory failure in COPD. Therefore, denutrition in these patients is the consequence of both pre-existing nutritional depletion and acute insult. Severe pneumonia due to bacteremia or virus infection is a very catabolic illness in which a prolonged ventilatory support is often associated with a significant denutrition.

A significant proportion of patients with chronic pulmonary diseases are malnourished and this nutritional depletion contributes to the deterioration of clinical

status and prognosis. The most severe nutritional deficits are observed in patients requiring mechanical ventilation. Nutritional depletion is predominant in patients with "pink puffer type" emphysema compared to those with "blue bloater type" chronic bronchitis. Muscle wasting is responsible for decreasing respiratory muscle function, which is significantly related to the patient's outcome as an independent parameter. Malnutrition and loss of body weight is the result of chronic negative energy balance related to decreased nutritional intakes, increased energy expenditure, or both. In most COPD patients, nutrient intake is largely adequate to meet their needs. Increased energy expenditure has been found in underweight COPD patients compared to those with normal weight or to underweight non-COPD patients. This finding may be attributed to the increased work of breathing due to obstructive disease and emphysema, which rises further during respiratory failure episodes. During acute episodes of respiratory tract infection, energy expenditure could further rise due to increased work of breathing. In addition, there is a decrease in nutritional intakes and intestinal absorption as a result of hypoxia and inflammatory status. In COPD patients, TNF was significantly higher in undernourished compared to obese patients. Prolonged hypermetabolism with a high level of protein catabolism will lead to severe consequences involving several organs and functions.

One of the key factors in prolonged ventilator dependency is respiratory muscle function. Although the underlying disease may have been controlled, weaning from the ventilator may cause tachypnea, rapid shallow breathing, and alterations in blood gases indicating insufficient spontaneous breathing, especially in patients with severe or prolonged hypermetabolic phase. Such impairment in respiratory muscle function is often the consequence of the severe skeletal muscle protein breakdown during the acute phase further amplified by muscle atrophy due to prolonged immobilization and the use of muscle relaxants. Acute myopathy or neuromyopathy can occur following the prolonged use of muscle relaxants, either alone or in association with corticosteroids. The impact of muscle loss on respiratory muscles, particularly the diaphragm, should not be ignored. The loss of diaphragmatic fat related to malnutrition is proportional to the atrophy of the nonrespiratory muscles.

The ability to maintain spontaneous breathing depends on three factors: the level of central respiratory drive, the capacity of the respiratory muscle pump, and the workload on the respiratory muscles. Other factors such as interstitial edema, reduced lung compliance, bronchoconstriction, left ventricular failure, hyperinflation, intrinsic positive end-expiratory pressure, and additional load due to endotracheal and ventilator circuit factors are often encountered in patients recovering from hypermetabolic conditions. All these factors participate in the increased load on respiratory muscles and therefore may worsen the weaning difficulties. Central respiratory drive is often elevated in patients during weaning trials. Therefore, the combination of increased load and central drive leads to a rise in the work of breathing when ventilatory support is withdrawn. The increased work of breathing can lead to fatigue of the respiratory muscles weakened by the prolonged catabolic phase.

Since the risk of nosocomial pneumonia increases by approximately 1–3% per day of mechanical ventilation, prolonged ventilator dependency can cause further muscle loss through hypermetabolic septic episodes and the ultimate chances of successful weaning become slimmer with each new episode.

Weaning difficulties are also often encountered in COPD patients with acute exacerbation. Pre-existing under-nutrition with the loss of diaphragmatic mass and strength adds to the problems described above. In these patients, inspiratory muscle workload is increased while the diaphragm is placed in adverse working conditions. The result is an increased work of breathing and muscle fatigue. This situation is worsened during weaning from the ventilator, due to the fact that the workload of the respiratory muscles increases.

NUTRITION IN SEPTIC PATIENTS

In septic patients the judicious use of substrate administration minimizes metabolic complications and overfeeding must be avoided.

The total energy expenditure (TEE) over the first week is approximately 25 kcal/kg/day but during the second week TEE can increase significantly.

Indirect calorimetry may currently be the best way to determine calorie needs and can provide improved knowledge on the proportion and quantity of substrates that should be used in septic patients.

Endogenous glucose production in sepsis is approximately 2.5 mg/kg/minute while exogenous glucose administration of 4–8 mg/kg/minute does not inhibit this process. It does, however, affect the respiratory quotient. Because of this, glucose should not be administered faster than 4 mg/kg/minute and should represent 50–60% of total calorie requirements or 60–70% of nonprotein calories. Overfeeding produces hypertriglyceridemia, hyperglycemia with potential hyperosmolar syndrome, osmotic diuresis, dehydration, increased CO_2 production (which can aggravate respiratory insufficiency and prolong ventilator dependency), hepatic steatosis, and cholestasis.

Hyperglycemia can glycosylate immunoglobulins and complement factors, and alter the respiratory burst of neutrophils and alveolar macrophage. It can also inhibit adhesions, chemotaxis, phagocytosis, and antimicrobial function of neutrophils and monocytes. Finally, and probably most importantly, hyperglycemia can induce oxidative stress. The general belief is that glucose levels should not exceed 220 mg%. However, a recent randomized study in a surgical ICU which also included septic patients showed a greater clinical benefit if the blood glucose could be maintained between 80 and 110 mg% with continuous drip of insulin.

Fat is efficiently used when it provides 25–30% of the total calorie requirement and 30–40% of nonprotein calories. A mixed fuel source reduces carbohydrate needs, improves glucose control, and reduces insulin needs. Excessive fat (ω-6) administration, however, results in neutrophil and lymphocyte dysfunction, blockades the mononuclear phagocytic system, induces hypoxemia due to ventilation-perfusion disorders and alveolocapillary membrane injury, induces hepatic steatosis, and increases PGE2 synthesis.

Fat composition in nutrition is important, since it is an essential compound of cellular membrane phospholipids. The proportion of polyunsaturated fatty acids (PUFA) of omega-6 and omega-3 series is responsible for membrane fluidity, ionic channel flow, activity of membrane receptors, and the mechanisms in cellular signal response. Both omega-3 and omega-6 compete for the same metabolic pathways. The omega-6 is a precursor of arachidonic acid from which eicosanoids-2 and leukotrienes-4 are synthesized. These products have intense inflammatory and immunosuppressive activity. The omega-3 is a precursor of docosahexaenoic (DHA) and eicosapentaenoic (EPA), which are synthesized to prostaglandins, thromboxanes-3, and leukotrienes-5. These cause inflammatory reaction and are less immunosuppressive. The exact proportion of essential fatty acids has not been defined. Usage of physiologic mixtures of long- and medium-chain triglycerides as well as omega-3 is currently under investigation.

During the catabolic state, muscular and visceral proteins are used as energy substrates in the muscle and for hepatic gluconeogenesis (alanine and glutamine) in the synthesis of acute-phase protein reactants. Protein needs exceed the normal requirement of 1 g/kg/protein/day and should be administered at 1.2 g/kg/day. Greater amounts of protein do not improve nitrogen balance but they increase blood urea. The quantity of protein should constitute 15–20% of total calories and be provided in a nonprotein calorie/nitrogen ratio of 80:1 to 110:1.

Branched-chain amino acids (BCAAs) are precursors of glutamine in skeletal muscle. In a study of septic patients given parenteral nutrition with 45% BCAAs, some positive benefits in mortality were noted with a highly branched-chain formula. Additional benefits have been noted through some nutritional parameters. The use of branched-chain amino acids in septic patients, however, still remains controversial.

Immunonutrition in Sepsis

This is covered in the section on immunonutrition.

NUTRITION IN ACUTE RENAL FAILURE

A negative nitrogen balance frequently characterizes ARF, and sometimes severe hypercatabolism can occur. Many factors are involved, such as endocrine abnormalities, metabolic acidosis, imbalance between protease and antiprotease, excessive cytokine activity (TNF, IL-1, IL-6), immobilization, and clinical conditions. Those factors can greatly affect the clinical course of the disease, e.g., entailing further accumulation of urea and other uremic toxins; promoting mineral and electrolyte problems (hyperkalemia, hyperphosphatemia); producing lean body mass depletion.

ARF per se is not generally associated with increased energy expenditure, which is lower than in patients affected by other acute conditions. However, coexisting acute traumatic conditions do increase resting energy expenditure (e.g., in sepsis the increase is approximately 30%). Generally, it suggests a higher energy intake in patients with higher urea nitrogen level and worse nitrogen balance, but energy supplies of more than 40 kcal/kg/day are seldom used and potentially dangerous. In most cases it does not exceed 1.3 basal energy expenditures, although it may reach 1.5–1.7 in some cases. To avoid the risk of overfeeding, calorie administration should be calculated on dry weight estimation.

The presence of reduced glucose tolerance and insulin resistance caused by acute uremia, acidosis, or increased gluconeogenesis needs careful monitoring of blood glucose levels and possible uses of insulin in glucose solutions for attaining euglycemic levels.

The utilization of exogenous lipids has decreased, while the utilization of medium-chain triglycerides does not offer more advantages than long-chain triglycerides. Lipid intake should be limited to 20–25% of total energy. However, lipids are very important because of the low osmolarity, source of energy, less CO_2 production, and essential fatty acids.

The total quantity of nitrogen to be administered to ARF patients depends on many factors mainly related to clinical conditions (degree of catabolism), renal dysfunction, delivery route of nutrients, and whether replacement therapy has been instituted.

The utilization of amino acids for protein synthesis might be impossible until uremia is controlled. Large quantities of glucose and amino acids during the "ebb phase" (first 48 hours after trauma) might increase renal oxygen consumption, and aggravate tubular damage and renal dysfunction. Patients with nonoliguric ARF are less catabolic; if they receive conservative therapy and are able to continue oral feeding, nitrogen provision should not exceed 0.55–0.6 g/kg/day of proteins of high biological value. Patients with anorexia and nausea who have a functional digestive tract may be given TEN, with a similar nitrogen intake. Protein intake gradually increases up to 0.8 g/kg/day if BUN levels are below 36 mmol/l; 0.6–1.0 g/kg/day of protein or essential amino acids (EAAs) and nonessential amino acids (NEAAs) has also been suggested. In ARF, NEAAs histidine, arginine, tyrosine, serine, and cysteine become indispensable, while others such as phenylalanine and methionine may accumulate. If more than 0.4–4.5 g/kg/day of amino acids are infused, NEAAs, and in particular those from the urea cycle (arginine, ornithine, or citrulline), must also be given. The use of EAAs alone must be avoided, as the occurrence of important amino acid imbalance could have severe clinical consequences.

Severely catabolic patients usually receive some sort of replacement therapy (hemodialysis, hemofiltration). This allows administration of a higher quantity of nitrogen, as well as a freer supply of fluid and electrolytes. Patients with such conditions are hardly able to feed themselves adequately by mouth and may therefore receive enteral nutrition or, more often, TPN or combined enteral nutrition and parenteral nutrition, because of the impaired gastrointestinal motility, vomiting, or diarrhea.

Protein and/or amino acids are given 1.0–1.5 g/kg/day, depending on the severity. This will result in better nitrogen balance, but it may promote nitrogen waste products. Protein/amino acid intake is higher (up to 1.5–2.5 g/kg/day) in more severe ARF patients treated with CVVH, CVVHD, CVVHDF, which have greater weekly urea clearances. In acute hypercatabolic patients, with superimposed ARF, positive nitrogen balance is achieved only if nitrogen intake is higher than 1 g/kg/day.

Replacement therapy also produces a considerable loss of amino acids and/or protein with dialysate, especially with high-flux dialysers. This loss should be integrated by artificial nutrition, so an additional amount of protein or amino acids is recommended. The amino acid solutions are delivered parenterally and contain both EAAs and NEAAs; the optimal ratio has not yet been established and can range from 2:1 to 4:1.

NUTRITION IN ACUTE PANCREATITIS

Most patients with acute pancreatitis have a mild disease with mortality rate below 1%. Almost all of these patients can be managed with standard supportive measures that do not need special nutritional treatment; most will resume a normal diet within 3–7 days.

During acute pancreatitis, specific and nonspecific metabolic changes occur. Under the influence of inflammatory mediators and pain, the basal metabolic rate may increase leading to higher energy consumption. If acute pancreatitis is complicated by sepsis, many patients are in a hypermetabolic state with an increase of resting energy expenditure (REE).

Gastric and duodenal perfusion of enteral diets is a powerful stimulant of exocrine pancreatic secretion, whereas jejunal administration induces minimal pancreatic secretion. Lipid, protein, and carbohydrate metabolism seems to be altered in acute pancreatitis. There is no evidence that infusion of exogenous fat could develop pancreatitis.

In severe acute pancreatitis, protein catabolism is increased. Parenteral administration of amino acids does not stimulate the exocrine pancreas directly, but through the stimulation of gastric acid. On the other hand, the anatomic site of protein and amino acid administration determines the degree and extent of pancreatic stimulation during enteral nutrition. Elemental diets are regarded as the most beneficial diets for patients with pancreatitis.

Glucose metabolism in acute pancreatitis is determined by an increase in energy demand. There is an increase of endogenous gluconeogenesis in patients with acute pancreatitis as the metabolic response to severe inflammation. Intravenous administration of high doses of glucose carries the risk of hyperglycemia, as the insulin response is often impaired. The insulin resistance can be corrected only in part by exogenous insulin administration.

Parenteral nutrition in acute pancreatitis is useful as an adjunct in patients' nutritional maintenance. A reduction in mortality has been claimed with improved nutritional status, especially in patients with moderate or severe acute pancreatitis. Patients with acute pancreatitis who receive parenteral nutrition have shown an increased rate of catheter-related sepsis and metabolic disturbances such as hyperglycemia. However, both catheter-related sepsis and hyperglycemia are often the consequence of overfeeding rather than of the mode of nutritional support.

The reduction in the ingestion of food together with an increased demand in patients with severe pancreatitis often results in negative energy balance with the potential development of malnutrition. Patients with severe acute pancreatitis are hypermetabolic, have a nonsuppressible gluconeogenesis despite sufficient calorie intake, an increased ureagenesis, and an accentuated net protein catabolism which can go up to 40 g of nitrogen/day.

In severely ill patients neither hypercaloric nor isocaloric nutritional support can prevent protein catabolism. In contrast, both enhance the metabolic burden as measured by energy expenditure, thermogenesis, urea production rate, and glucose and lactate levels. Therefore, a hypocaloric energy supply of ~15–20 kcal/kg/day is more suitable during the early catabolic stage

of nonsurgical patients with MOF. The goal of 1.2–1.5 g/kg/day of protein intake is optimal for most patients with acute pancreatitis. If an MOF syndrome complicates the course of the disease, the calorie and protein requirements have to be adapted; lower protein loads of ~1.2 g/kg/day should be given to patients with renal or hepatic failure.

It is important to deliver the caloric need by the enteral route. Enteral feeding is possible but prescribed intakes of nutrients are frequently not achieved. Nasojejunal tubes are feasible and desirable in the management of patients with acute pancreatitis but their placement is sometimes difficult without endoscopic help. There is some evidence that enteral feeding may improve disease severity and clinical outcome in patients with severe disease. The presence of complications (pancreatic ascites, fistula formation, or fluid collection) is not a contraindication to enteral feeding.

Oral refeeding can be started when pain is controlled and the pancreatic enzymes return to normal. Patients are re-fed with small amounts of carbohydrate–protein diet; the number of calories is gradually increased with careful supplementation of fat over a period of 3–6 days.

If the enteral supply is inadequate, then the rest should be given by the parenteral route. When enteral nutrition is impossible, TPN should be started.

IMMUNONUTRITION IN THE INTENSIVE CARE UNIT

Immune system changes/depression is a complicated factor in ICU patients. Recently, data from various experiments demonstrated the beneficial effects of immunonutrition supplementation to enhance or modulate the immune status in various group of specific patients, i.e., surgical, burn, and ARDS patients. Such nutrients include n-3 fatty acid, glutamine, arginine, and nucleotides. Many clinical trials have shown risk of infection, length of hospital stay, and medical cost are reduced by enriched nutritional support with immunonutrition. Nevertheless, this administration is not appropriate for every ICU patient; patients with severe sepsis, shock, and organ failure may actually be harmed.

N-3 Fatty Acid

Fatty acids are components of cell membranes, and influence cell functions and biological responses. Following stress, injury, or sepsis the demands of fatty acids are increased. N-3 fatty acid is an essential fatty acid, which is often found to be deficient in hospitalized patients. Although n-3 fatty acid is much needed, the ratio of n-3/n-6 fatty acid still has not been clarified, especially in the critically ill. Mechanisms by which n-3 and n-6 fatty acid may exert effects on the immune system are regulation of gene expression, signal transduction pathways, action of antioxidant enzymes, and production of eicosanoids and cytokines.

Glutamine

In the human body glutamine plays an important physiologic role in energy production, interorgan nitrogen and carbon transport, nucleotide synthesis, renal ammoniagenesis, glycogen synthesis, regulation of protein synthesis, and replication of cells. Glutamine is a NEAA in healthy people, but in catabolic patients, such as those suffering stress, injury, and sepsis, it becomes essential. Several studies proved that plasma glutamine declines in catabolic patients. Studies using stable isotopes in the critically ill demonstrate systemic demand of glutamine with large fluxes of glutamine from skeletal muscle. They show that the nutrient flow of glutamine is from muscle, where it is synthesized, and released to the tissues and not from the gut to the tissues. The human gut extracts 50-85% of enteral glutamine.

There is controversy as to the question of giving glutamine parenterally or enterally. Studies in experimental animals proved that gut villous height and thickness increased after appropriate doses of enteral glutamine. In other studies, enteral diets containing glutamine decreased bacterial translocation across the intestine. On the other hand, a randomized study with parenteral glutamine improved several clinical outcomes up to 6 months after administration.

The recommended dose of glutamine for less stressed patients is 12-15 g/day and for critically ill patients is >20 g/day up to 30 g/day. Recently, glutamine has become available as a dipeptide and enriched in certain solutions.

Arginine

Arginine is a semi-essential amino acid. In the body arginine participates in the urea cycle and the citric acid cycle, and stimulates the secretion of anabolic hormone. Arginine is also a precursor for polyamine synthesis and a nitrogen source for nitric oxide synthesis. This latter function is important; nitric oxide plays a role in hypertension, myocardial dysfunction, inflammation, cell death, and protection against oxidative damage. Enteral nutrition enriched with arginine leads to T-lymphocyte stimulation in critically ill patients. Doses of 15 g/day intravenous and 17-24 g/day of enteral arginine are adequate for improving immune system and wound healing. In ICU studies an amount between 16 and 19 g/day had a beneficial outcome. If the dose is too large it can induce lysine deficiency and could be harmful. Very high nitric oxide levels, produced from arginine, may mediate many of the effects of septic shock including vascular, myocardial, and hemodynamic instability.

Nucleotides

Nucleotides (purines and pyrimidines) are synthesized either de novo or salvaged from RNA turnover. If protein intake is adequate, the main source of nucleotide production is from de novo synthesis. Sufficient nucleotides promote restoration of intestinal function and immune status. The absence of nucleotides can cause loss of T-helper lymphocytes and suppression of IL-2 production.

SELECTED READING

ASPEN Board of Directors and The Clinical Guidelines Task Force: Guidelines for the use of parenteral and enteral nutrition in adult and pediatric patients. J Parenteral Enteral Nutrition 26(1; Suppl), 1-35, 2001.

Bertolini G, Iapichino G, Radrizzani D et al: Early enteral immunonutrition in patients with severe sepsis. Results of an interim analysis of a randomized multicentre clinical trial. Intensive Care Med 29:834-840, 2003.

Cano N: Perioperative nutrition. From nutrition support to pharmacologic nutrition in the ICU. Update in Intensive Care and Emergency Medicine. 34:220-231, 2000.

Cano N, Barnoud D, Leverne X: Nutritional management of acute renal failure and acute liver failure. Crit Care Shock 2:143-157, 1999.

Chioléro R, Tappy L, Berger MM: Timing of nutritional support. Clinical nutrition: early intervention. In Labadarios D, Pichard C, editors: Nestlé Nutrition Workshop Series. Clinical & Performance Program, vol 7, Nestle: Karger, 2002, p 151.

Consensus recommendations from the US summit on immune-enhancing enteral therapy. J Parenteral Enteral Nutrition 26(2; Suppl):S61-S62, 2001.

Griffiths RD: Specialized nutrition support in the critically ill: for whom and when? Clinical nutrition: early intervention. In Labadarios D, Pichard C, editors: Nestlé Nutrition Workshop Series. Clinical & Performance Program, vol 7, Nestle: Karger, 2002, p 199.

Jolliet P, Pichard C: A practical approach to feeding intensive care patients. From nutrition support to pharmacologic nutrition in the ICU. Update in Intensive Care and Emergency Medicine 34:1166-1178, 2000.

Kirby DF, Kudsk KA: Obtaining and maintaining access for nutrition support. From nutrition support to pharmacologic nutrition in the ICU. Update in Intensive Care and Emergency Medicine 34:125-137, 2000.

Kondrup J, Allison SP, Elia M et al: ESPEN guidelines for nutrition screening 2002. Clinical Nutrition 22(4):415-421, 2003.

Kudsk KA: Enteral versus parenteral feeding in critical illness. From nutrition support to pharmacologic nutrition in the ICU.

Update in Intensive Care and Emergency Medicine 34:115-124, 2000.

Leverve X, Barnoud D, Pichard C: Nutritional support in acute respiratory failure. From nutrition support to pharmacologic nutrition in the ICU. Update in Intensive Care and Emergency Medicine 34:303-315, 2000.

Meier R, Beglinger C, Layer P et al: ESPEN Consensus Group: Consensus statement. ESPEN guidelines on nutrition in acute pancreatitis. Critical Nutrition 21(2):173-183, 2002.

Sack GS, Genton L, Kudsk KA: Controversy of immunonutrition for surgical critical-illness patients. Curr Opin Crit Care 9:300-308, 2003.

Sobotka L, editor: Substrate used in parenteral and enteral nutrition. Basics in clinical nutrition. Galen 2:37-78, 2000.

Soeters PB, Dejong CHJ, von Meyenfeldt MF: Parenteral versus enteral nutrition: can we get rid of the myths? Clinical nutrition: early intervention. In Labadarios D, Pichard C, editors: Nestlé Nutrition Workshop Series. Clinical & Performance Program, vol 7, Nestle: Karger, 2002, p 183.

Stroud M, Duncan H, Nightingale J: Guidelines for enteral feeding in adult hospital patients. Gut 52(Suppl VII):vii1-vii12, 2003.

Tappy L, Chioléro R: Carbohydrate and fat as energetic fuels in intensive care unit patients. From nutrition support to pharmacologic nutrition in the ICU. Update in Intensive Care and Emergency Medicine 34:54-65, 2000.

CHAPTER 10

Catheter-Related Bloodstream Infections in the Intensive Care Unit

STEPHEN M. LUCZYCKI, M.D.

The majority of infections in the critically ill are associated with medical devices including the urinary catheter, the mechanical ventilator, and the central venous catheter. More than five million central venous catheters are utilized in the USA each year. These devices are associated with an infection rate of 3–8% with a concomitant attributable mortality of up to 35%. Bloodstream infections (BSIs) are up to seven times more frequent in the critically ill. Nationally, the central line-associated BSI rate averages from 2.9 per 1000 catheter days in cardiothoracic intensive care units to 10.6 per 1000 in the neonatal population. Approximately 80,000 central line-associated BSIs occur every year in the intensive care unit (ICU) in the USA. If entire hospital populations are assessed, approximately 250,000 central line-associated BSIs occur annually. These infections incur a significant cost to patient care not only in terms of potential morbidity and mortality but also in financial terms. The estimated costs are in excess of $25,000 per infection with a total annual cost from $300 million to more than $2 billion. With the improved understanding of the pathogenesis of catheter-related infections and the implementation of several strategies, the incidence of catheter-related infections can be reduced, thereby reducing the ultimate burden on the cost of patient care in terms of morbidity, mortality, and financial cost.

PATHOGENESIS

Catheter-related infection results from the interaction of the host, the catheter, and the microbial pathogen. The individual properties of the microbial pathogen are probably the most important in terms of the pathogenesis of catheter-related infections. An intimate understanding of these characteristics can potentially allow the modification of catheters to circumvent microbial adherence, thereby preventing infection. The interaction with the host cannot be ignored; with an emphasis toward optimizing the treatment of comorbidites and underlying illnesses to minimize immunosuppression, clinicians can optimize nutrition and ultimately augment immunity toward specific pathogens.

Central line-associated BSI begins with catheter colonization by the pathogen, although this may not necessarily lead to bacteremia. Extraluminal colonization is linked to the skin flora at the specific insertion site when the pathogen begins to adhere to and colonize the subcutaneous segments. This type of colonization can also occur by the hematogenous spread of a pathogen to an intravascular catheter tip from distant sites of infection where bacterial transmigration has occurred. Equally important is the intraluminal colonization that can potentially occur through catheter hubs, connections, and infusate, as these are accessed many times a day in the critically ill for blood draws and medications.

The development of thrombi associated with central venous catheters has been linked to the development of device-associated BSIs. Thrombus formation at the insertion site, along the subcutaneous segment, at the catheter tip, or intraluminally is likely a key event in microbial adherence and subsequent colonization that dramatically increases the risk of infection. The thrombus serves as both an excellent substrate for bacterial adherence and a medium for bacterial growth. Thrombus formation can be affected by the composition of the catheter material, the extent of damage to the vascular endothelium at the insertion site, and hematologic factors in the host affecting coagulation.

CLINICAL FACTORS

The patient's primary underlying disease and associated comorbidities play a potential role in the development of nosocomial infections, including catheter-related BSIs (see Box 10-1). An ICU admission alone increases this risk, as do interventions such as mechanical ventilation and invasive hemodynamic monitoring. A direct correlation is most notable in neutropenic patients, neonates, and in patients with severe burns, malignancies, and the presence of shock during the course of their ICU admission. Total parenteral nutrition has also been shown to increase the risk of catheter-related bacteremia. The risk of device-associated infection may be increased with the presence of additional nosocomial infections including active urinary tract infections, lower respiratory infections and colonizations, and intra-abdominal infections.

MICROBIOLOGY

In the USA the most common organisms associated with hospital-acquired BSI are coagulase-negative staphylococci (37%; see Box 10-2). *Staphylococcus aureus* and *Enterococcus* spp. each account for approximately 13% of these infections. Gram-negative bacilli (including

---

Box 10-1 Risk Factors for Catheter-Related Infections

Malignancy
Neutropenia
Patients receiving immunosuppression therapy
Use of parenteral nutrition
ICU admission
Mechanical ventilation
Use of multilumen catheters
Development of shock
The presence of additional nosocomial infections
Severe burns
Neonates

Box 10-2 Most Likely Pathogens in Central Line-Associated Infections

COAGULASE-NEGATIVE STAPHYLOCOCCI

Staphylococcus aureus
Enterococcus spp.
Enterobacter spp.
Pseudomonas aeruginosa
Klebsiella pneumoniae
Escherichia coli
Candida spp.

Escherichia coli (2%) and the Enterobacteriaceae *Klebsiella pneumoniae* (3%), *Pseudomonas aeruginosa* (4%), and *Enterobacter* spp. (5%)) account for 14% of catheter-related BSIs. *Candida* spp. are responsible for 8% of hospital-acquired BSIs.

The antimicrobial resistance patterns of these pathogens are continually evolving. Data from the National Nosocomial Infections Surveillance System indicate that 57% of the *S. aureus* isolates from ICU patients are resistant to methicillin. A full 89% of the coagulase-negative staphylococci are now resistant to methicillin. Over 27% of the enterococcal isolates are resistant to vancomycin. *P. aeruginosa* isolates in the ICU appear increasingly resistant to multiple antibiotics including imipenem (22%), quinolones (32%), and third-generation cephalosporins (30%). Other surveillance data indicate that 10% of the *C. albicans* isolates are now resistant to fluconazole. In addition, nearly half of the fungal isolates were non-*C. albicans* species which tend toward exhibiting resistance to multiple antifungals. While the national trends are alarming, ICU-specific antibiograms should be utilized to best guide empiric antimicrobial therapy in the treatment of catheter-related BSIs.

STRATEGIES FOR PREVENTION OF CATHETER-RELATED INFECTIONS

No single factor is reliably responsible for the development of BSIs associated with central venous catheters. Ultimately, there is an intimate relationship among many variables that can be potentially utilized for developing strategies to minimize or prevent catheter-associated BSIs (see Box 10-3).

CATHETER INSERTION SITE

The site at which a central venous catheter is placed can influence the subsequent risk of device-associated BSI.

Box 10-3 Strategies to Prevent Catheter-Related Infections

Education and training of personnel in catheter care and insertion

Use of specialized IV teams

Hand hygiene

Maintain strict aseptic techniques when manipulating the catheter

Use maximum sterile barrier precautions

Disinfect and clean the insertion site with chlorhexidine

Use sterile dressing at the insertion site and replace when soiled

Consider subclavian insertion site if possible

Remove unnecessary catheters as soon as possible

Replace administration sets, caps, hubs every 72 hours

Consider use of antibiotic-coated catheters in high-risk patients

It should be noted that no randomized trials have adequately assessed how variable placement sites affect the risk of infection. The potential relationship between catheter location and risk of infection can perhaps best be approached by ultimately understanding the pathogenesis of the infection. The bacterial colonization at any given site may ultimately play a role in providing the initial inoculum leading to infection. Not only does the bacterial colonization differ with each insertion site, but the potential for cross colonization and/or contamination with other bacterial sources (such as tracheal secretions, urine, and stool) also varies with the insertion site. There is some observational evidence that the internal jugular site may be associated with increased risk of infection when compared to the subclavian or femoral sites. In addition, the femoral site may be associated with increased catheter colonization potentially leading to BSI. The risk of deep vein thrombosis increases with the use of the femoral site versus the subclavian or internal jugular site. The development of thrombosis is a contributing factor to the development of BSI. These observations lead some authorities to recommend the subclavian site as the preferred site of venous access in the critically ill. The ultimate clinical decision may best be approached by weighing the potential for infection, the duration of access, and the potential for mechanical complications associated with each specific insertion site.

SITE PREPARATION

Intrinsic to the process of any catheter insertion is the ultimate decontamination of the skin at the insertion site.

Microbial colonization of the skin has been shown to be greatly influenced by the choice of the insertion site. For instance, the density of transient microflora appears to be greatest at the base of the neck when compared to the upper chest. Given the importance of the cutaneous microbial flora in the ultimate pathogenesis of catheter-related BSIs, the reduction of this microbial load at the insertion site can reduce the incidence of device-related infection. For years a povidone-iodine solution has been the standard skin antiseptic for catheter insertion. Several studies have shown that chlorhexidine reduces the incidence of microbial colonization when compared to other preparations including povidone-iodine and alcohol. Chlorhexidine has potent and broad-spectrum antimicrobial activity which persists on the skin surface even after a single application. It has been shown that the preparation of arterial and central venous sites with 2% chlorhexidine gluconate lowers catheter-related BSIs when compared to 10% povidone-iodine or 70% alcohol preparations. Additionally, a meta-analysis comparing chlorhexidine with povidone-iodine for vascular catheter site care revealed that skin sites prepared with chlorhexidine reduced the risk of infection by 49%. The majority of evidence now suggests that a 2% chlorhexidine solution is the agent of choice for skin preparation. Chlorhexidine has also been incorporated into a sponge for use as a catheter site dressing and has subsequently been shown to reduce the risk of catheter colonization and catheter-related BSI. If chlorhexidine is unavailable, tincture of iodine has been shown to be superior to povidone-iodine as a cutaneous antiseptic. The process of defatting the skin with acetone has not been shown to be of any value in the reduction of catheter-related BSIs.

ASEPTIC TECHNIQUE

The insertion of any medical device necessitates the adherence to good hand hygiene combined with proper aseptic technique. Hand hygiene can be achieved with either an antimicrobial soap and water or a waterless alcohol-based product. The insertion of short peripheral catheters can be accomplished aseptically with non-sterile gloves and a no touch technique. Central venous catheter insertion requires more stringent aseptic technique with full barrier precautions including cap, mask, long-sleeved sterile gown, sterile gloves, and a large sterile drape. Maintaining maximal barrier precautions during central venous catheter insertion has repeatedly been shown to reduce the incidence of catheter-related BSIs when compared to standard precautions. These precautions have not been well studied with regards peripherally inserted central venous catheters or midline catheters, but are nonetheless a prudent practice. One study showed that the use of full barrier precautions during the insertion of arterial catheters did not prevent arterial catheter colonization or infection.

CATHETER SITE DRESSING

Gauze or transparent semipermeable polyurethane dressings can both be utilized as there is no substantial clinical difference in the incidence or rate of catheter site colonization or phlebitis. The risk of development of catheter-related BSI when using gauze dressings has been compared to the use of transparent dressings with no difference in the risk of infection. As a result, the dressing used can be a matter of preference. Transparent dressings require less frequent changes and allow for the direct examination of the insertion site, but can also trap moisture and fluid collections, which could contribute to increased microbial colonization. Transparent dressings may be preferred in the presence of open wounds or tracheostomy near the insertion site.

The efficacy of the additional application of various antibiotic and antiseptic ointments to central venous catheter insertion sites is not clear. Studies have been carried out on the application of a povidone-iodine ointment to the insertion sites of subclavian hemodialysis catheters, which demonstrated a reduction in the incidence of catheter tip colonization, exit site infection, and associated BSIs. However, several randomized studies of the prophylactic use of povidone-iodine ointment applied to the insertion sites of short-term central venous catheters are indeterminate. In addition, there is some evidence that the use of some antibiotic ointments at insertion sites may increase the rates of catheter colonization by *Candida* spp., lead to the development of antibiotic resistance, and potentially compromise the integrity of the central venous catheter.

SYSTEMIC ANTIBIOTIC PROPHYLAXIS

The parenteral use of either vancomycin or teicoplanin during central venous catheter insertion does not reduce the incidence of subsequent BSI; in fact, one study revealed a higher incidence of BSI in the prophylaxis groups. Antibiotic solutions have also been utilized by flushing and filling the lumen of the catheter and leaving the solution to dwell as an "antibiotic lock" technique. Such prophylaxis has been shown to benefit neutropenic patients with long-term catheters. In addition, antibiotics such as vancomycin have been added to flush solutions, total parenteral solutions, and dialysate in attempts to reduce the incidence of BSIs. While some studies have revealed efficacy, the use of vancomycin has been shown to be an independent risk factor for the development of vancomycin-resistant enterococci. Prolonged use of

vancomycin may lead to the development of sub-populations of *S. aureus* with intermediate or reduced vancomycin sensitivity.

ANTICOAGULATION

The development of thrombin and fibrin deposits on central venous catheters can promote microbial adherence and is associated with catheter-related BSI. Although a meta-analysis has revealed that the routine use of prophylactic heparin reduced the risk of catheter-related central venous thrombosis, there appears to be no significant difference in the risk of development of catheter-related BSI. Warfarin has also been evaluated: while it reduces the incidence of catheter thrombus it does not reduce the incidence of catheter-related BSI.

IMPREGNATION OF CATHETER WITH ANTIBIOTICS AND ANTISEPTICS

Catheters coated with antimicrobial and antiseptic agents are now widely available. The use of these catheters can decrease the risk of developing catheter-related BSI. Catheters externally coated with chlorhexidine and silver sulfadiazine have been demonstrated in several studies to reduce the risk of catheter-related BSI when compared to uncoated catheters. The antimicrobial activity of these impregnated catheters decreases over time and the risk reduction is realized in the first 14 days. Although expensive, the cost reduction achieved in preventing a catheter-related BSI translates to net cost savings especially when used in high-risk patient groups such as burn patients and surgical ICU patients. It should be noted that patient allergy and medication sensitivity need to be taken into consideration as anaphylaxis has been reported with the use of these catheters.

Central venous catheters coated with minocycline and rifampin are also available. The use of these catheters is also associated with lower rates of catheter-related BSIs. The antimicrobial activity of this coating persists longer than the first-generation chlorhexidine/silver sulfadiazine catheters with a beneficial effect after day 6. The use of these antibiotics raises the potential issue of the development of minocycline and rifampin resistance among the pathogens responsible for catheter-related BSI.

Further study on the development of catheter coatings is ongoing. Catheters have been developed using ionic metals including platinum and silver, as well as coatings that extend the release of chlorhexidine and silver sulfadiazine. The efficacy of these catheters is not well known. Ionic silver has also been incorporated into a subcutaneous cuff to act as a mechanical barrier while providing antimicrobial activity against migrating pathogens along the subcutaneous portion of catheters. This strategy has failed to show a risk reduction in the development of catheter-related BSIs.

CATHETER CARE

Catheter access and use can be modified to help reduce the incidence of catheter infections. Excessive manipulation of catheters increases the risk of infection. Catheter ports and hubs require disinfection prior to use. In addition, the tubing and access hubs should be changed every 48–72 hours. Well-trained staff that adheres to strict aseptic principles can reduce the incidence of catheter infection. Institutions that utilize specialized IV teams can also reduce the infection rate. In addition, the reduction of nurse-to-patient ratios increases the risk of catheter infection. Routine replacement of central venous catheters does not reduce the infection rate. The use of guidewires to exchange catheters remains controversial. Several studies have shown trends toward increased colonization and infection, but these trends do not appear to be statistically significant. Therefore, guidewire exchange can probably safely be used, especially where access is difficult and the risks of insertion at a new site are thought to be high. Catheters should be removed as soon as they are no longer needed to eliminate a potential source of infection.

DIAGNOSIS

The diagnosis of catheter-related BSI cannot be made on clinical findings alone. Fever, leukocytosis, insertion site inflammation, and BSI alone are all unreliable in ultimately diagnosing catheter-related BSIs. Paired blood cultures (one from the catheter and one from a peripheral source) should be obtained when a catheter-related BSI is suspected. Negative cultures have been shown to have a high negative predictive value. When catheter removal is not desired, paired quantitative cultures can be obtained. If the colony count of a culture obtained from the catheter is 5–10 times greater than the colony count obtained from a peripheral sample, a catheter-related BSI is likely. One can also exploit the differential time to positive culture for blood sampled from the catheter and from the periphery to aid in the diagnosis of catheter-related infections. When blood cultured from the device has a positive result two hours before peripheral cultures, a diagnosis of device infection can be made with a sensitivity and specificity similar to that of quantitative blood cultures.

Samples of intravascular devices can also be cultured to aid in the diagnosis of catheter-related infection. Differences in the culture methods, the portion of the catheter cultured, and the source of the catheter

infection ultimately affect the sensitivity of the diagnostic method used. In general, semiquantitative and quantitative culture methods are thought to be the most reliable in the identification of catheter-related infection. Semiquantitative cultures are obtained by cutting open the desired portion of the catheter and rolling the device onto a culture medium. Quantitative cultures are obtained by either sonicating or vortexing the catheter sample in a broth and subsequently culturing the sample. A semiquantitative catheter culture with a yield of ≥15 cfu (colony forming units) or a quantitative yield of ≥100 cfu is considered indicative of a device-related infection. There is no definitive evidence to favor the culture of the catheter tip or the subcutaneous segment in the diagnosis of catheter-related infection. The increasing use of antiseptic- and antibiotic-coated catheters may affect the usefulness of these culture methods. Rapid diagnostic techniques such as the acridine orange stain may be useful diagnostic modalities in the future.

MANAGEMENT

Determining the etiology of fevers in the critically ill can be challenging. Once the central venous device is suspected, paired blood cultures (one peripheral and one central) should be obtained. Blood cultures from an arterial line could be used if peripheral blood cannot be obtained. However, a positive culture from the arterial line may indicate an infected arterial line. In the seriously ill or septic patient empiric antibiotic therapy should be instituted utilizing ICU-specific antibiograms. If no other source of fever is identified and the central line remains suspect, the line should be removed and cultured. A central line can then be inserted at a new site or exchanged over a wire provided that the insertion site does not appear to be infected. If both blood and device cultures are negative one must search elsewhere for the source of fever. If the blood cultures are negative and the catheter culture is positive, the clinician should consider a short course of antimicrobial therapy, follow closely for signs of ongoing infection, and repeat the blood cultures when necessary. If both blood and catheter cultures are positive, the catheter should be removed and the antimicrobial treatment is guided by the etiologic organism. Infusates such as total parenteral nutrition should also be cultured if contamination is expected.

Unfortunately there are few good data on the duration of antimicrobial therapy. In general *S. aureus*, *Candida* spp., and Gram-negative bacilli are treated for 10–14 days. Coagulase-negative *Staphylococcus* spp. can be treated for a shorter course of 3–7 days. Some clinicians approach coagulase-negative staphylococcus line infections with catheter removal only and no antimicrobial therapy. Persistent fevers and bacteremia despite catheter removal and appropriate antimicrobial therapy should raise the suspicion of entities such as bacterial endocarditis, septic thrombophlebitis, or other distant microbial metastasis. In these cases prolonged antimicrobial therapy for 4–8 weeks is indicated.

THE FUTURE

Future strategies aimed at preventing catheter-related BSIs will most certainly exploit both properties of the host and pathogen. The catheter design itself is constantly evolving to minimize bacterial adherence and colonization as well as thrombus formation with the ultimate goal of reducing associated BSI. Increasing abilities to affect the immunomodulation of the critically ill may one day allow the clinician to minimize the development of nosocomial infections. However, the importance of hand hygiene, maintenance of strict aseptic techniques, and continuing education and training of staff remain the cornerstones in preventing catheter-related infections in the critically ill.

SELECTED READING

Cook D et al: Central venous catheter replacement strategies: a systemic review of the literature. Critical Care Med 25(8):1417–1424, 1997.

Gowardman JR et al: Central venous catheter related bloodstream infections: an analysis of incidence and risk factors in a cohort of 400 patients. Intensive Care Med 24: 1034–1039, 1998.

Lane RK et al: Central line infections. Curr Opin Crit Care 8:441–448, 2002.

Maki DG et al: Prevention of central venous catheter related blood stream infection by use of an antiseptic-impregnated catheter: a randomized, controlled trial. Ann Intern Med 127(4):257–266, 1997.

Mermel LA et al: Guidelines for the management of intravascular catheter-related infections. Clin Infect Diseases 32:1249–1272, 2001.

National Nosocomial Infections Surveillance System report, data summary from January 1992–June 2003. Am J Infect Control 31:481–498, 2003.

O'Grady NP et al: Guidelines for the prevention of intravascular catheter related infections. Clin Infect Diseases 35: 1281–1307, 2002.

Polderman KH et al: Central venous catheter use: 2. Infectious complications. Intensive Care Med 28:18–28, 2002.

Raad II et al: The relationship between the thrombotic and infectious complications of central venous catheters. JAMA 271(13):1014–1016, 1994.

Safdar N et al: A review of risk factors for catheter-related bloodstream infection caused by percutaneously inserted, noncuffed central venous catheters. Medicine 81(6):466–479, 2002.

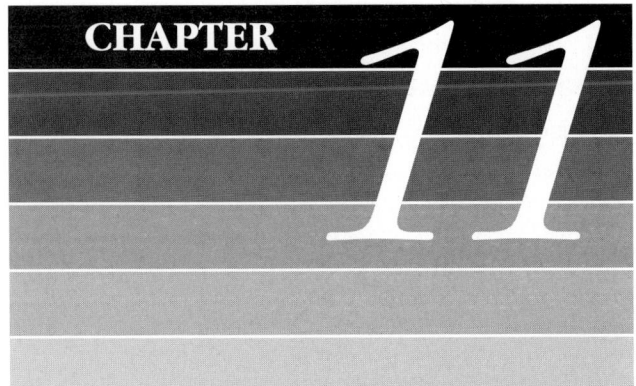

CHAPTER 11

Current Practices in Intensive Care Unit Sedation

TIMOTHY J. BARREIRO, D.O.

PETER J. PAPADAKOS M.D., F.C.C.P., F.C.C.M.

In publications from the late 1980s approximately half of the patients in intensive care units (ICUs) described their period of mechanical ventilation as unpleasant and stressful, and that their time requiring mechanical ventilation was associated with fear, agony, and panic. Some publications have suggested an association between the administration of large quantities of sedation and the development of post-traumatic stress disorders and memory problems while others have not found that association. In the past 5 years ICUs throughout the world have adopted the goal of maintaining an optimal level of comfort and safety for patients. The use and better understanding of newer sedatives and analgesics has given critical care practitioners the ability to titrate specific agents for different patient types allowing patients to be comfortable throughout their stay in the ICU.

As the customized care of patients continues to evolve, a common language is mandated for the titration and use of sedative agents. With this language also comes the development of protocols and guidelines to better use these drugs and to maximize each drug's unique pharmacodynamic profile for individual patients. No longer is it necessary to be trapped by the all-or-none effect of very long-acting compounds that depress respiration and prolong ICU stays.

AGITATION AND ANXIETY EVALUATION

There is no consensus as to what level of sedation is optimal for patients in the ICU; most likely the optimal level of sedation will vary according to patients' underlying mental and physical problems, along with the needed level sedation for patient safety. Agitation and anxiety are common in ICU patients of all ages, occurring at least once in most patients admitted to any ICU. Agitation can be caused by multiple factors such as extreme anxiety, delirium, adverse drug effects, and pain. Failure to provide adequate pain control is a significant factor in the development of agitation in critically ill patients. In most practices inadequate pain management is often a result of the dosing of opioids at suboptimal levels; this is because of concerns about respiratory depression and the development of dependence.

Hypoxemia has long been associated with agitation, despite the routine use of continuous plethmography. It is crucial for ICUs to monitor the oxygen levels in all patients. A partial pressure of oxygen (pO_2) of <60 mmHg (or oxygen saturation <90%) can contribute to agitation. Hypotension and transient myocardial ischemia can also lead to agitation.

One of the most common problems confronting the critical care physician is a patient's withdrawal from alcohol or other agents, including cocaine, opioids, and benzodiazepines.

In the ICU another common cause of agitation is ventilator dyssynchronization. This is frequently due to poorly set ventilator modes that delay in responding to patient's efforts and needs during spontaneous breathing. However, this problem is becoming less common due to computer-controlled ventilators and the use of graphic displays to titrate ventilation. Patients who undergo short- or long-term intubation also develop agitation because of the stimulus of the endotracheal tube itself. Patients who are alert and intubated can also become frustrated by the inability to communicate with staff and family and descend into a cycle of continued agitation. This along with the sounds, monitors, and continuous stimuli of the ICU itself can contribute to further agitation.

The consequences of numerous drug reactions, drug–drug interactions, and drug withdrawal all increase the incidence of agitation in the modern ICU (Table 11-1). The occurrence of undesirable drug interactions should always be considered when multiple agents are being used for pain, anxiety, infection, and cardiac disturbances. Even after the withdrawal of a pharmacologic compound suspected of increasing agitation, it may take several days for the drug and metabolites to clear a patient's system before a positive response can be seen.

The differential diagnosis of agitation begins with a review of the patient's current disease process, mechanism of injury, laboratory values, baseline medications, and a review of their past medical history. Only after this rapid evaluation can the process move toward proper treatment for agitation.

EVALUATION AND TITRATION OF SEDATIVE AGENTS

The disease state complexity of ICU patients typically demonstrates a rapidly changing spectrum of hemodynamic states, so the requirements to treat agitation fluctuate over time. Bedside clinicians must frequently reassess and redefine the goals of therapy. Tools and scales to monitor agitation in the ICU should be simple to apply, yet describe clearly graded changes between sedation levels to allow titration of both pharmacologic and nonpharmacologic interventions.

Table 11-1   Medications Associated with Agitation in the Intensive Care Unit

ANTIBIOTICS

Acyclovir
Amphotericin B
Cephalosporins
Ciprofloxin
Ketoconazole
Penicillin
Rifampin

ANTICONVULSANTS

Phenobarbital
Dilantin

MISCELLANEOUS

Theophylline
Hydroxycine
Ketamine
NSAIDs

CARDIAC DRUGS

Captopril
Clonidine
Digoxin
Dopamine
Labetalol
Nifedipine
Quinidine

CORTICOSTEROIDS

Dexamethasone
Methyl prednisone

NARCOTIC ANALGESICS

Codeine
Mereprine
Morphine sulfate

There are large numbers of scales and tools for evaluation described in the literature. Many of these evaluate the level of consciousness with described responses to interventions. There is no gold standard scale, but most ICUs use modification of those described in the literature. The development of customized unit-based scales, protocols, and guidelines is highly important for promoting their acceptance by all members of the health care team.

SEDATION SCALE(S)

The most commonly used sedation scale is the **Ramsey sedation scale** which identifies six levels of sedation ranging from severe agitation to deep coma (Table 11-2). Despite its frequent use the Ramsey scale has some shortcomings when applied at the bedside of

Table 11-2 Ramsey Scale for Assessing Sedation Levels

Level	Response/Description
1	Patient awake and anxious, agitated, and/or restless
2	Patient awake and cooperative, accepting ventilation, oriented, and tranquil
3	Patient wake; responds to commands only
4	Patient asleep; brisk response to light glabellar tap or loud auditory stimuli
5	Patient asleep; sluggish response to light glabellar tap or loud auditory stimulus but does respond to painful stimulus
6	Patient asleep; no response to light glabellar tap or loud auditory stimulus

Hansen-Flaschen J, Cowen J, Polomano RC: Beyond the Ramsay scale: need for a validated measure of sedating drug efficacy in the intensive care unit. *Crit Care Med* 22(5):732-733, 1994.

patients with complex problems. For example, a patient who appears to be asleep with a sluggish response to glabellar tap (Ramsey 5) may also be restless and anxious (Ramsey 1). The Ramsey scale is simple, however, and is widely used in many ICUs.

The **Riker Sedation–Agitation Scale** (SAS) was the first scale formally tested and developed for reliability in the ICU (Table 11-3). The SAS identifies seven symmetrical levels ranging from dangerous agitation to deep sedation. This scale provides a detailed description of a patient's behavior, allowing the bedside physician to adjust properly medications between agitation levels.

Table 11-3 Riker Sedation–Agitation Scale

Score	Diagnosis	Description
7	Dangerous agitation	Pulls at endotracheal tube; tries to remove catheters; climbs over bed rails; strikes at staff
6	Very agitated	Does not calm, despite frequent verbal reminding of limits; requires physical restraints; bites endotracheal tube
5	Agitated	Calm; awakens easily; follows commands
4	Calm and cooperative	Difficult to arouse; awakens to verbal stimuli or gentle asking but drifts off again; follows simple commands
3	Sedated	Arouses to physical stimuli but does not communicate or follow commands; may move spontaneously
2	Very sedated	
1	Unable to arouse	Minimal or no response to noxious stimuli; does not communicate or follow commands

Riker RR, Picard JT, Fraser GL: Prospective evaluation of the Sedation–Agitation Scale for adult critically ill patients. *Crit Care Med* 27(7):1325-1329, 1999.

Table 11-4 Motor Activity Assessment Scale

Score	Description	Definition
0	Unresponsive	Does not move with noxious stimulus
1	Responsive only to noxious stimuli	Opens eyes *or* raises eyebrows *or* turns head toward stimulus *or* moves limbs with noxious stimulus
2	Responsive to touch or name	Opens eyes *or* raises eyebrows *or* turns head toward stimulus *or* moves limbs when touched *or* name is loudly spoken
3	Calm and cooperative	Does not require external stimulus to elicit movement *and* adjusts sheets or clothes purposefully *and* follows commands
4	Restless and cooperative	Does not require external stimulus to elicit movement *and* picks at sheets or clothes *or* uncovers self *and* follows commands
5	Agitated	Does not require external stimulus to elicit movement *and* attempts to sit up or moves limbs out of bed *and* does not consistently follow commands
6	Dangerously agitated; uncooperative	Does not require external stimulus to elicit movement *and* pulls at tubes or catheters *or* thrashes side to side *or* strikes at staff or tries to climb out of bed and does not calm down when asked

Devlin JW, Boleski G, Mlynarek M et al: Motor Activity Assessment Scale: a valid and reliable sedation scale for use with mechanically ventilated patients in an adult surgical intensive care unit. *Crit Care Med* 27(7):1271-1275, 1999.

The **Motor Activity Assessment Scale** (MAAS) is similar in structure to the SAS because it also uses the patients' behavior to describe the different levels of agitation. The MAAS identifies seven levels, ranging from unresponsive to dangerously agitated (Table 11-4).

Ely and colleagues developed a new assessment tool, **Confusion Assessment Method for the ICU** (CAM-ICU), which has been well validated in the critically ill patient with delirium. It is used in combination with the Glasgow coma scale for highly complex agitated patients. The CAM-ICU is simple to apply at the bedside and has been found to have a high level of reliability, sensitivity, and specificity.

Current research is hoping that real-time computer base monitors of brain function will remove human variability in the evaluation of a patient with agitation. One such monitor popular in the operating room is the Bispectal index (BIS). This objective monitor is especially helpful for the deeply sedated patient receiving neuromuscular blockade. By incorporating several electroencephalograms, the BIS monitor provides a discrete value from 1000 (completely wake) to <60 (deep sedation) to <40 (deep hypnotic state or barbiturate coma). Although the technique has been shown to be useful in the operating room, it has *not* been studied to any great extent in the ICU.

ESTABLISHING AND IMPLEMENTING SEDATION GUIDELINES AND PROTOCOLS

One of the most important goals for any ICU is the development of protocols and guidelines for pain medication and sedative drugs. The development of such protocols requires multidisciplinary input and should be unit specific. All staff, including physicians and nurses, need to agree on which monitoring scales and tools to use and then ensure that these scales are used. It is important for staff to agree on documentation and assessment frequency, predefined end points of therapy, and evaluation of patient outcomes. Using these types of protocols and documenting their use in daily practice can foster communication between disciplines and shifts. Another important aspect of sedation guideline development is consultation with hospital pharmacists. Pharmacists can provide guidelines and educational input regarding specific pharmacodynamic profiles of individual agents. Participation of such professionals on rounds and as members of the ICU team can only improve the quality of care for complex cases. Each hospital should develop guidelines that foster current pharmacologic and pharmacokinetic recommendations that are supported by national standards.

CLINICAL CAVEAT

Protocol in the Intensive Care Unit
- Hospital- and unit-driven sedation/analgesic protocols improve patient care, decrease time on mechanical ventilation, and decrease hospital cost.
- Specific protocols should be supported by national standards.

REVIEW OF COMMON AGENTS USED IN SEDATION

All physicians have experienced and intuitively understand anxiety and pain. Analgesics and sedatives are the mainstay of supportive care in the ICU. Over the past few years several novel highly titratable agents have been introduced that have greatly enhanced patient care. The pharmacology of several of these widely used agents is reviewed (Table 11-5).

OPIOIDS

Opioids are the primary agents used for analgesia in the ICU. Traditionally they have been administered orally, intramuscularly, or intravenously; but more recently epidural, intrathecal, transdermal, and transmucosal delivery systems have been developed. Most opioids are lipid soluble and produce analgesia through their agonist effects on opiate receptors in the central nervous system (CNS) and peripheral nervous system. At low doses opioids provide analgesia but not anxiolysis, whereas at higher doses they act as sedatives. All the opioids share therapeutic properties but vary in potency and pharmacokinetics.

Even though opioids can be given via several routes, the intravenous (i.v.) method is the most common. When given in the intravenous form, in therapeutic doses, opioids cloud the sensorium but do not possess amnestic properties.

The removal of pain greatly affects the need for sedation and other therapies. Unrelieved pain evokes powerful stress responses, characterized by tachycardia, increased myocardial oxygen consumption, hypercoagulability, immunosuppression, and persistent catabolism. Effective analgesia has been shown to diminish pulmonary complications in postoperative patients.

Comparative trials of opioids have not been performed in critically ill patients. The selection of specific agents depends on the pharmacology and potential for

---

Table 11-5 Pharmacokinetics and Pharmacodynamics of Opioid Agents

Drug	Lipid Solubility	Half-life (hours)	Onset of Action (minutes)	Peak Effect (minutes)	Duration of Action (hours)
Morphine	Low	2-3	5	20-30	2-7
Fentanyl	High	4-10	1-2	5-15	0.5-1
Meperidine	Moderate	5-10	5	20-60	2-4
Hydromorphone	Low	2-3	10-15	15-30	2-4

adverse events. For opioids desirable attributes include rapid onset, ease of titration, lack of accumulation of metabolites, and low cost.

CLINICAL CAVEAT

Opioid and Pain Control
- Historically pain control has been poorly managed.
- Most physicians overestimate the risk of narcotic addiction in postoperative patients.
- Unrelieved pain evokes powerful stress responses.
- Unrelieved pain can result in pneumonia and atelectasis resulting from respiratory splinting, which decreases tidal volume, vital capacity, and functional residual capacity.
- Patient-controlled analgesia (PCA) produces adequate pain control and at the response of patients' needs.

Morphine Sulfate

Morphine sulfate, the prototypical opioid, is the preferred opioid analgesic in patients with stable hemodynamics. Morphine has a rapid initial redistribution phase of 1–1.5 minutes and an initial half-life of 10–20 minutes; the terminal elimination half-life is between 2 and 4.5 hours. Morphine has a lower lipid solubility which results in a slower onset of action when compared to fentanyl. This is important in that morphine slowly penetrates the blood–brain barrier. The liver primarily metabolizes morphine; however, the kidney eliminates approximately 40% of the drug. The major metabolite of morphine (morphine-6-glucuronide) is excreted in the urine and may accumulate in patients with renal failure. The opiate activity of the metabolite is several times greater than that of morphine and its accumulation in patients with renal failure has been reported to prolong narcosis. Morphine also induces the release of histamine, increasing the likelihood of causing hypotension secondary to vasodilation. The faster the rate of administration, the more pronounced the hypotension seen. Finally morphine can also slow the heart rate, by its stimulation of the vagus nerve and its depressant effects on the sinoatrial node. Despite its side effects, morphine is still very useful in the management of ICU patients.

Fentanyl

Fentanyl has the most rapid onset and shortest duration of the opioids. Fentanyl citrate is a synthetic narcotic analgesic that is 50 to 100 times more potent than morphine, it is highly lipid soluble, and has rapid onset of action because it quickly crosses the blood–brain barrier. Fentanyl onset of action is within 30 seconds, and its peak effect is within 5–15 minutes. The liver metabolizes fentanyl.

Fentanyl has no active metabolites. Fentanyl is not associated with histamine release and so it infrequently causes hypotension. Fentanyl, however, can cause bradycardia and decrease sympathic tone; these in turn can cause hypotension. Because of its rare hemodynamic side effects, it is an ideal drug for patients in the ICU.

Fentanyl should be administered by continuous infusion for sustained effect because of its short duration of action. Because of these characteristics, fentanyl has become one of the most widely used agents in the ICU. Caution should be used when fentanyl is administered at high doses for prolonged periods of time. Prolonged effects can be seen, because large amounts of the drug accumulate in the fatty tissues and then have to be metabolized in the liver. In these situations the terminal half-life of the drug can be as long as 16 hours.

Remifentanil

Remifentanil (Ultiva, Abbot), a newer agent, has not been widely studied in ICU patients. The drug has a very short half-life and may be best used in patients needing serial examinations or neurologic evaluation. Remifentanil is an ultrashort-acting narcotic that penetrates the blood–brain barrier within 1 minute, and its blood concentration decreases 50% by 6 minutes after a one-minute infusion. Because of its shortened duration of action, it requires continuous infusion for pain management. The novel aspect of remifentanil is its rapid hydrolysis by circulating and tissue nonspecific esterases (the beta-adrenergic blocker esmolol is metabolized by similar enzymes). There does not appear to be a cumulative effect seen with long infusions and organ dysfunction does not appear to alter the metabolism of the drug. Side effects of remifentanil include respiratory depression, hypotension, bradycardia, and *skeletal hypertonus*; this can make bag mask ventilation difficult or impossible. The administration of propofol or a paralytic agent prior to its administration can attenuate the skeletal rigidity seen with the drug.

CLINICAL CAVEAT

Opioid Reversal
- Narcan (naloxone hydrochloride) is an opioid antagonist.
- Narcan can prevent or reverse the effects of opioids.
- Narcan challenge test: inject 0.2 mg Narcan and observe for 30 seconds.
- Onset of action is usually within 2 minutes.
- Opioid dependence patients can have *acute withdrawal* if given Narcan.
- Smaller doses of 400 µg (dilute 9 cm³ saline with 1 mg of Narcan) can help reverse the effects of the opioid but prevent abrupt withdrawal.

Meperidine

Meperidine was once a standard drug used for pain control, *but is no longer recommended for repetitive use*, it has an active metabolite that causes neurotoxicity (apprehension, tremors, delirium, and seizures), and may interact with antidepressants, along with its well-documented *contraindication* with monoamine oxidative inhibitors (MAOIs) and is best avoided in patients taking selective serotonin reuptake inhibitors. Meperidine should not be used in the ICU due to risks from multiple interactions with other medication.

CLINICAL CAVEAT

Meperidine
- No longer recommended for use in ICU patients.
- Meperidine should *not* been given by the subcutaneous route; evidence that chemical irritation and necrosis may result.
- Meperidine is *contraindicated* in patients who are receiving monoamine oxidative inhibitors or those who have received such agents within 14 days.
  - Therapeutic doses of meperidine have inconsistently precipitated unpredictable, severe, and occasionally fatal reaction.
  - The mechanism of this reaction is unclear.

OPIOID ADVERSE EFFECTS

Certain adverse effects from opioid analgesics occur frequently in ICU patients. Of greatest concern is the respiratory, hemodynamic, CNS, and gastrointestinal effects. Respiratory depression is a concern in spontaneously breathing patients or in those receiving ventilatory support. Other common side effects include pruritus, urinary retention, and bradycardia. Opioids may also increase intracranial pressure in traumatic brain injury patients although the data are inconsistent and the clinical significance is unknown.

NONOPIOID ANALGESICS

The nonopioid analgesics include salicylates, acetaminophen, and other nonsteroidal anti-inflammatory drugs (NSAIDs). The uses of nonopioid agents are increasing in the ICU. The nociceptive stimuli caused by chemical as well as mechanical stimuli release prostaglandins and leukotrienes leading to inflammation and sensitization of nociceptors, resulting in hyperalgesia

that is characterized by a decrease in the pain threshold. The pain signal could be at the site of injury or the pain signal could also be amplified or modified in the spinal cord as a result of the action of prostaglandins. The NSAIDs provide analgesia via the nonselective competitive inhibition of cyclooxygenase, a critical enzyme in the inflammatory cascade. NSAIDs have many positive attributes, including reducing opioid requirements, but they also have many adverse effects. Unwanted effects include an increased incidence of gastrointestinal bleeding (secondary to platelets inhibition) and renal dysfunction. NSAIDs neither cause respiratory depression nor decrease level of consciousness. They also have no effect on intestinal and bile duct motility and thus compared with opioids they are less likely to cause nausea, vomiting, and ileus. Due to concerns of increased cardiovascular risks COX_2 agents have been withdrawn from use.

BENZODIAZEPINES

Benzodiazepines are the most widely used sedative drugs in medicine. They are sedative and hypnotic but not analgesic agents that block the acquisition and encoding of new information and potentially unpleasant experience (anterograde amnesia) but do not induce retrograde amnesia. They have an opioid sparing effect by moderating the anticipatory pain response. Benzodiazepines vary in their potency, onset, duration of action, uptake, and absence of active metabolites. The two predominant mechanisms of action of benzodiazepines involve activity at the gamma-aminobutyric acid (GABA) receptors. The potentiation of GABA-mediated transmission by benzodiazepines is responsible for the somnolent, anxiolytic, and anticonvulsant actions, whereas the amnestic property seems to correlate with GABA agonist activity in the limbic cortex.

Metabolism of benzodiazepines occurs in the liver, where they are extensively cleared. The effects of these drugs may be prolonged in critically ill patients. Accumulation of the parent drug or active metabolite may produce inadvertent and prolonged oversedation, as is seen in the elderly. It is therefore paramount that these drugs are titrated carefully and used in low doses or patients will be somnolent for several days after stopping the infusion.

Benzodiazepines should be titrated to a predefined end point, often using a series of loading (bolus) doses. Hemodynamically unstable patients may experience hypotension with initial sedation. Maintenance of sedation with intermittent or "as needed" doses of diazepam, lorazepam, or midazolam may be adequate to accomplish the goal of sedation secondary to the relative half-life of these drugs.

The new clinical practice guidelines of the Society of Critical Care Medicine (SCCM) currently recommend lorazepam for sedation in most patients either by intermittent intravenous dosing or continuous infusion. Lorazepam, an intermediate-acting benzodiazepine, is less lipophilic than diazepam and thus has less potential for accumulation. Lorazepam is associated with a stable hemodynamic profile even when opioids are concurrently administered. Lorazepam has no active metabolites and its metabolism is less affected by advanced age or liver dysfunction when compared with midazolam. Lorazepam should, however, be used with caution: *propylene glycol toxicity* marked by acidosis and renal failure has occurred with high cumulative doses or prolonged infusion of the drug.

CLINICAL CAVEAT

Lorazepam
- Sedative of choice.
- Prolonged use has been associated with acidosis and renal failure caused by accumulation of **propylene glycol**.

Midazolam

The other commonly used benzodiazepine is midazolam, used initially in the operating room and now widely accepted in the ICU. Midazolam is a slow-acting water-soluble benzodiazepine that is transformed to lipophilic compounds in the blood. Midazolam exhibits dose-related hypnotic, anxiolytic, amnestic, and anticonvulsant actions. The drug produces dose-related respiratory depression and larger doses may cause hypotension and vasodilation. Midazolam is metabolized in the liver to an active compound that is less potent and more transient than the parent compound. The new SCCM guidelines recommend midazolam for short-term use and rapid sedation of actively agitated patients. Midazolam produces unpredictable awakening and prolonged extubation times when infusions continue for longer than 48 to 72 hours.

Paradoxical agitation has been observed when using benzodiazepines: this may be the result of drug-induced amnesia or disorientation. The effect of these drugs can be reversed with a benzodiazepine receptors antagonist, flumazenil (Romazicon, Roche). However, the routine use of flumazenil is not recommended after prolonged benzodiazepine therapy because there is a risk of inducing withdrawal symptoms and increasing myocardial oxygen consumption, which can occur even with small doses.

CLINICAL CAVEAT

Flumazenil
- Romazicon (flumazenil) is a benzodiazepine receptor antagonist.
- Doses of 0.1 to 0.2 mg produce partial antagonism and 0.4 to 1 mg complete reversal.
  - Repeat doses of 0.5 mg at one-minute intervals to a maximum cumulative dose of 3–5 mg.
- Onset of reversal is usually evident within 1 to 2 minutes.
- The use of Romazicon has been associated with the occurrence of *seizures*; this is most frequent in patients who have been on long-term benzodiazepines or in overdose cases where patients are showing signs of serious cyclic antidepressant overdose.

Propofol

Propofol, 2,6-diisopropylphenol, is formulated as a 1% aqueous emulsion, containing 10% soybean oil, 2.25% glycerol, and 1.2% egg phosphatide. Although the mechanism of action of propofol is still not completely understood, the drug appears to activate the GABA receptors within the CNS. Propofol has a rapid onset of action, within 1 to 2 minutes after a single intravenous dose, and a short duration of action, only 10 to 15 minutes when discontinued. This short duration of action is due to its rapid penetration into the CNS and subsequent redistribution. Therefore, in the ICU propofol is used by continuous infusion. Propofol has *no* analgesic activity but has some antiemetic properties. The clearance of propofol cannot be explained by hepatic clearance alone; there appear to be extrahepatic sites of elimination. The clearance of propofol is rapid even after prolonged infusions, but accumulation of the drug in lipid stores can result in prolonged sedation.

Propofol alters the sensorium at an extremely rapid rate and in a dose-dependent manner, from light sedation to general anesthesia, making it a highly useful drug. Propofol is a respiratory depressant. Propofol also prophylactically attenuates induced bronchoconstriction but does not affect resting airway tone. The most commonly seen side effect of propofol, especially when it is given as a bolus, is hypotension. Propofol causes hypotension by reducing systemic vascular resistance and causing myocardial depression. These effects are attenuated in hypovolemic patients. Propofol decreases cerebral metabolism resulting in a decline in cerebral perfusion pressure. It has interesting effects on neurophysiology, causing disinhibition, dystonic or choreiform movements. Other side effects include phlebitis, hyperlipidemia, and pancreatitis.

One of the most important benefits associated with propofol is a decrease in weaning time from mechanical ventilation. A large Spanish study, using a cost-of-care approach, evaluated the impact of prolonged sedation of critically ill patients with midazolam or propofol, and weaning time from mechanical ventilation. Although both drugs provided equivalent sedation, the administration of propofol was associated with a shorter weaning time than midazolam resulting in a favorable economic profile. Due to its rapid wake-up time, propofol is considered the fundamental drug in many fast-track surgical procedures.

Within one year of its introduction in the USA, clusters of infections in surgical patients treated with propofol were reported. The majority of cases were due to contamination of the drug from poor aseptic techniques. This contamination resulted in the inclusion of an additive, ethylenediaminetetraacetic acid (EDTA), to help retard growth of microorganisms. EDTA at low concentrations has no effect on the physical or chemical stability of the emulsion compound. In the years following the introduction of the EDTA-containing formulations the incidence of fevers and infections were reduced to zero. EDTA is a chelator of various ions, including calcium. In a randomized multicenter trial, patients were treated with either the original propofol formulation or the formulation with EDTA. The EDTA-containing formulation had no effect on calcium or magnesium hemostasis, renal function, or sedative efficacy.

One of the interesting aspects of propofol with EDTA is it ability to modulate the system inflammatory response. In a study of surgical ICU patients, those receiving propofol with EDTA had significantly lower mortality rates at 7 days and 28 days compared to patients receiving the original formulation. This potential positive effect of propofol with EDTA may be related to the ability of EDTA to bind and increase the excretion of zinc; this, in turn, may diminish the inflammatory response to stress by decreasing the release of cytokines involved in inflammation and the generation of free radicals and other oxidases.

In the USA a generic formulation of propofol is available. The major difference with the generic product is the presence of sodium metabisulfite (0.025%) as a preservative. As a result of this additive, it carries an FDA warning about its use in patients sensitive to sulfite compounds and therefore should not be used in this group of patients. Thus it is highly important for clinical staff to know which propofol formulation is being used in their facility.

The use of propofol is *not currently recommended for pediatric patients*, due to reports of metabolic acidosis with accompanying lipemic serum, bradyarrhythmias, and fatal myocardial failure with excessively high doses; however, it should be noted that these occurred in highly complex patients with a high mortality index.

The SCCM guidelines recommend propofol as the agent of choice for rapid awakening and early extubation. Since propofol is formulated as a lipid emulsion, triglyceride concentrations should be monitored after two days of infusion. Also, the total caloric intake should be adjusted because the lipid emulsion adds calories to the nutritional prescription.

Haloperidol

Haloperidol, a butyrophenone neuroleptic drug, is the agent of choice for treatment of delirium in critically ill patients. Patients treated with haloperidol generally seem to be calmer and are better able to respond appropriately to commands. Haloperidol does not cause major respiratory depression.

The adverse effects associated with haloperidol include occasional hypotension resulting from the alpha blocking properties of the drug. Although rare with intravenous use, haloperidol may cause extrapyramidal effects such as drowsiness, lethargy and fixed stare rigidity and akathisia. A highly dangerous side effect is *neuroleptic malignant syndrome* (NMS) which has a mortality rate of up to 30%. NMS may develop slowly over 24 to 72 hours and can last up to 10 days after discontinuation of the drug.

CLINICAL CAVEAT

Side Effects of Haloperidol
- Neuroleptic malignant syndrome (NMS) can develop over 24 to 72 hours after administration of haloperidol.
  - NMS is characterized by hyperthermia, hypertonicity, and tachycardia.
  - TX: discontinue the drug, fluid resuscitation, cooling techniques, and intravenous **dantrolene sodium**, 2 mg/kg every 5 minutes to maximum dose of 10 mg/kg.
- Cardiac arrhythmias can occur. Most worrisome is torsade de pointes (polymorphic ventricular tachycardia).
  - Total daily doses should remain less than 50 mg.
  - Monitoring QT interval is recommended.
  - For corrected QT intervals exceeding 480 milliseconds the drug should be stopped.

Ketamine

Ketamine, a phencyclidine derivative, is unique among the intravenous agents in that it causes analgesia as well as amnesia. The drug does not necessarily cause a loss of consciousness, but patients lose their awareness; this unique anesthetic condition is described as a "*dissociative state.*" This is caused by electrophysiologic inhibition of the thalamocortical pathways and stimulation of the limbic system.

Ketamine and a benzodiazepine are frequently used for sedation in pediatric patients. In the ICU ketamine can be given before airway intubation in hypovolemic patients, dressing changes, laceration repair, abscess incision and drainage, and orthopedic manipulations. Ketamine can be given orally, rectally, intramuscularly, or intravenously. This drug is a racemic mixture, which is marketed in three concentrations so care is needed to avoid dosage error. The dose of ketamine is 0.5–1 mg/kg. Ketamine has an elimination half-life of 3 hours. Ketamine has no adverse effects on hepatic and renal function. The effects of a single injection of ketamine generally last less than 30 minutes, although coadministration of other drugs may prolong the effects.

There are well-described side effects of ketamine. General anesthesia with ketamine is characterized by a hyperdynamic circulatory response (tachycardia and increased blood pressure) caused by directly simulating the autonomic nervous system to release catecholamines and steroids. Despite this side effect, protective airway reflexes (coughing) and minute ventilation are maintained.

Although ketamine is a direct myocardial depressant, this drug inhibits reuptake of catecholamines and produces mild to moderate increases in blood pressure, heart rate, and cardiac output. These cardiostimulatory effects could be detrimental in patients with underlying cardiovascular disease.

Ketamine is useful in patients with airway disease in that it attenuates neurally induced bronchoconstriction. It also has a small direct effect on smooth muscle activation; however, it is unclear whether it can be utilized to improve asthma attacks.

During emergence from ketamine, patients may have vivid dreams (both pleasant and unpleasant) and hallucinations.

Etomidate

Etomidate is a nonbarbiturate, carboxylated, imidazole-containing compound. Etomidate is a hypnotic agent, commonly used to induce general anesthesia in the operating suite. It can also be used to facilitate rapid-sequence endotracheal intubation in the ICU. It is generally used in conjunction with neuromuscular blocking agents. For induction of anesthesia, the initial dose is 0.2–0.6 mg/kg over 1 minute. This drug, however, should not be given as an infusion. It is a favored drug because of its few cardiovascular side effects. Adverse effects are rare. Of particular importance are its neuromuscular and

skeletal muscle side effects, which include myoclonus (33%) and transient skeletal movements including uncontrolled eye movements; both effects are transient.

CLINICAL CAVEAT

Warning for Etomidate
- Etomidate inhibits **11-β-hydroxylase**, an enzyme important in adrenal steroid production.
- A single induction dose blocks the normal stress-induced increase in adrenal cortical production for 4–8 hours and up to 24 hours in the elderly.
- Continuous infusions of etomidate are *not* recommended.
  - Blunts the patient's ability to respond to stress.

Dexmedetomidine

Dexmedetomidine (Precedex, Abbot) is a newly approved selective α-2-adrenergic receptor agonist. It exhibits sympatholytic sedative and analgesics effects and is *eight times* more potent for the α-receptor than clonidine. Dexmedetomidine has been approved for short-term (24 hours) sedation and analgesia in the intensive care setting. Because of its short-term effects, dexmedetomidine is a highly promising therapy for ICU patients.

Dexmedetomidine works by presynaptic activation of the α-2-adrenoreceptor thereby inhibiting the release of norepinephrine and terminating the propagation of pain signals. It also affects postsynaptic activity resulting in a decrease in blood pressure and heart rate. Together these two effects can produce sedation, anxiolysis, and analgesia. Dexmedetomidine has several advantages for use as a sedative in the ICU. Because the drug does not cause respiratory depression, a patient can be extubated without prior discontinuation. This property also makes it ideal for patients being weaned from mechanical ventilation. The drug provides great flexibility. Since dexmedetomidine also lowers the requirement for narcotics it can decrease opioid effects. Because elimination is primarily hepatic, dexmedetomidine dosing should be lowered in patients with hepatic dysfunction. Also, inappropriate use of dexmedetomidine may induce or aggravate cardiac conduction defects. Dexmedetomidine should not be used in hypovolemic or bradycardic patients or in patients with low cardiac output or heart conduction blocks.

Dexmedetomidine is a promising agent with multiple actions that reduce analgesic and other sedative requirements and produce a cooperatively sedate patient. It may open a whole new arena in the sedation of extubated patients who have high levels of anxiety. Dexmedetomidine needs to be further studied to determine its role in the ICU.

INTRODUCTION TO MUSCLE RELAXANTS

Neuromuscular blocking agents (NMBAs) have the most fascinating history among the drugs used in anesthesiology and intensive care. Aborigines of South America used curare for centuries to hunt before Claude Bernard showed in 1850 that these drugs act peripherally, blocking conduction where motor nerves meet the muscle.

NMBAs are indeed a double-edged sword. They can be lifesaving in critical situations, such as airway management and respiratory failure, but they also can cause serious complications. NMBAs are divided by their chemical structure; by their duration of action – ultrashort, short, intermediate, and long acting; and by the type of block – depolarizing and nondepolarizing.

Neuromuscular blocking agents are utilized for many reasons (Box 11-1). Long-term use is not recommended and short-term use is considered less than two days. Few complications have been reported with administration for less than that time period. There are many complications associated with NMBAs including anaphylaxis and hyperkalemia associated with succinylcholine administration in selected patients with medical conditions like burns, muscle trauma, chronic renal disease, and long-term immobility.

Risk factors for prolonged weakness include vecuronium in female patients who have renal failure, high-dose steroids, more than two days' duration of relaxant administration, and administration of high doses of NMBAs. There appears to be several etiologies to the persistent weakness. One theory is that the persistent weakness may be due to muscle paralysis from NMBA metabolites. Vecuronium has an active metabolite, 3-desacetyl vecuronium, which persist particularly in women patients with renal failure. Pancuronium also forms active metabolites; therefore these drugs should not chronically be administered to patients who are in renal failure.

Another finding is in patients on corticosteroids who receive long-term muscle relaxants. They appear to develop a myopathic syndrome characterized by flaccid paralysis, increased creatine kinase (CK), and myonecrosis; these patients recover after many months. Plasma CK concentration appears to increase when the myopathy develops; therefore serum CK should be monitored in patients on corticosteroids and receiving muscle relaxants. All muscle relaxants have been associated with these syndromes.

A motor neuropathy has been reported after the administration of vecuronium or atracurium. The neuropathy affects all extremities and is associated with absent tendon reflexes. This syndrome also takes months to resolve. Another syndrome consisting of persistent motor weakness but with preservation of sensory sensations has been reported in patients receiving pancuronium and vecuronium. These patients do not have normal neuromuscular transmission and their symptoms also take months to resolve.

Patients can become tolerant to the effects of the NMBAs. This tolerance can develop in the first 48 hours. Tolerance appears to be due to the upregulation of acetylcholine receptors. Monitoring patients receiving NMBAs is critical. There are many ways to achieve this, but electrical stimulation is commonly used. Single twitch, tetany, and train-of-four (TOF) stimulation tests are commonly used. The most commonly used method of monitoring for appropriate muscle relaxation is the TOF responses. It is important to note that the TOF monitoring of patients does not ensure that persistent weakness will not occur. Table 11-6 lists commonly used muscle relaxants and their associated side effects.

CLINICAL CAVEAT

Train-of-Four Monitoring
- The most commonly used nerve/muscle combination for monitoring train-of-four (TOF) is ulnar nerve/adductor pollicis and facial nerve/orbicularis oculi.
- A sequence of four supramaximal stimuli with a frequency of 15–40 mA (four stimuli 0.5 seconds apart) is needed.
- Goal is keeping TOF at 2 out of 4.
- Combining clinical monitoring with the use of nerve stimulator is recommended in order to optimize patient care and minimize complications.

Box 11-1 Possible Indications for Neuromuscular Blocking Agents

Airway management
Decrease chest wall and/or pulmonary compliance (acute respiratory distress syndrome)
Respiratory asynchrony with mechanical ventilation
Elevated airway pressures
Muscular rigidity, such as in tetanus and status epilepticus
Control of intracranial hypertension
Minimizing metabolic demands and oxygen consumption
Severe agitation not controlled by sedatives
Maintenance of delicate surgical grafts until stable
Facilitation of certain procedures

Depolarizing Drugs

Succinylcholine

Succinylcholine is unique among the NMBAs. It is the *only* depolarizing drug in clinical use. Succinylcholine has the fastest onset of action and shortest duration of action. Succinylcholine binds to the nicotinic receptors mimicking the action of acetylcholine, this causing depolarization across the post-junctional membrane.

Table 11-6   Muscle Relaxant Properties

Drug	Initial Dose (mg/kg)	Duration (minutes)	Advantages	Complications
Pancuronium	0.07–0.1	Long acting; 6–120	Inexpensive	Tachycardia; accumulation in renal failure
Vecuronium	0.1	30–45	CVS stability	Active metabolite; accumulation in renal and hepatic insufficiency
Atracurium	0.5	30–45	Reliable recovery	Slow onset; no active metabolite
Rocuronium	0.6–1.2	30–90	Rapid onset	None
Cisatracurium	0.1–0.2	30–90	Reliable recovery	Slow onset
Succinylcholine	0.6–1	Ultrashort; 5–10	Fast onset and fast recovery	Hyperkalemia dysrhythmia

The main indication for use in the critically ill is rapid airway management. However, it is also associated with many cardiovascular side effects.

CLINICAL CAVEAT

Succinylcholine

- Reported cases of acute rhabdomyolysis with hyperkalemia followed by dysrhythmias, cardiac arrest, and death after the administration of succinylcholine in children. These children were subsequently found to have skeletal muscle myopathy, frequently Duchenne's muscular dystrophy.
- Relatively contraindicated in children and patients with burns, skeletal muscle injury, history of malignant hyperthermia, and renal failure because of the risk of hyperkalemia (the risk in these patients may last as long as 7 to 10 days).

Nondepolarizing Agents

Pancuronium

Pancuronium, one of the original NMBAs used in the ICU, is a long-acting, nondepolarizing compound that is effective after a bolus dose of 0.06 to 0.08 mg/kg for up to 90 minutes. It can be given as a bolus or continuous infusion. Pancuronium is vagolytic, which limits its use in patients who cannot tolerate an increase in heart rate. In patients with renal failure or cirrhosis pancuronium's neuromuscular blocking effects are prolonged by the increased metabolite 3-hydroxypancuronium.

Vecuronium

Vecuronium is an intermediate-acting NMBA that is a structural analog of pancuronium but is not vagolytic. It also can be given via bolus or continuous infusion. The bolus dose of 0.08 to 0.10 mg/kg produces effects within 3 minutes. Its neuromuscular blocking effects last approximately 30 minutes. A continuous infusion can be used at doses of 1–2 µg/kg/minute. Vecuronium also has

an active metabolite, 3-desacetylvecuronium, which can accumulate in patients with hepatic dysfunction. Also, up to 35% is renally excreted and dose adjustment and careful monitoring is needed in renal insufficient patients. Vecuronium is associated with *acute quadriparetic myopathy syndrome* (AQMS).

Rocuronium

Rocuronium is a newer nondepolarizing NMBA with a monoquaternary steroidal chemistry. It has intermediate duration of action and very rapid onset. When rocuronium is given as a bolus of 0.1–0.6 mg/kg, blockade occurs within 2 minutes. Continuous infusions, if needed, are usually started at 10 µg/kg/minute. Rocuronium is not affected by patients with renal failure and has little prolonged action in patients with liver dysfunction.

Atracurium

Atracurium is an intermediate-acting NMBA with minimal cardiovascular side effects but is associated with histamine release at higher doses. It is inactivated in plasma by ester hydrolysis and by Hoffmann elimination so renal and hepatic dysfunction does not affect the duration of blockade.

Cisatracurium

Cisatracurium, an isomer of atracurium, is an intermediate-acting benzylisoquinolinium NMBA that is increasingly used in lieu of atracurium. It produces few cardiovascular effects and has fewer tendencies to release histamine and mast cell degranulation. Bolus doses are with 0.1–0.2 mg/kg with a duration of action of 25 minutes. Infusion rates should be started at 2.0–3.0 µg/kg/minute. Cisatracurium is also eliminated by ester hydrolysis and by Hoffmann elimination so patients with renal or hepatic dysfunction do not have a prolonged duration of blockade.

Complications of Neuromuscular Blocking Agents

Multiple complications have been associated with the use of NMBAs, and the ICU physician should be familiar with their common side effects. There are many drug interactions with NMBAs that can prolong the neuromuscular blockade. Antibiotics such as neomycin, streptomycin, lincomycin, and tetracycline all have prolonged the effects of NMBAs. Electrolytes play an important role; hypermagnesemia, hypokalemia, hypocalcemia, and lithium all prolong neuromuscular blockade. Also, patients who are paralyzed are at risk for keratitis and corneal abrasions. The routine administration of ophthalmic ointment or drops is recommended. There is an increased risk for deep venous thrombosis and the most notable side effect is AQMS. AQMS is a serious complication of NMBAs, which significantly prolongs ICU and hospital stay. This is one of the reasons that NMBAs should be used with caution and only in experienced hands.

On examination, the paralyzed patient has significant motor deficits in the upper and lower extremities, along with depressed deep tendon reflexes. Sensory function and ocular muscle function are usually preserved. On electromyography (EMG), there are low-amplitude compound motor action potential and muscle fibrillations. Modest CK and lactate dehydrogenase increases are observed. This syndrome can be seen in patients receiving prolonged NMBAs for greater than 48 hours or with concomitant use of corticosteroids. Muscle biopsy shows Type II muscle fiber atrophy with vacuolization, disordered sarcomeric architecture, and extensive loss of myosin.

CONCLUSION

Critically ill patients frequently experience anxiety and pain and occasionally experience severe agitation. These factors have a significant effects on a patient's sense of well-being, and perhaps equally important, on patient outcomes. Health care providers are responsible for maintaining a stress-free and comfortable environment to minimize these perceptions. The most important aspect of ICU sedation is an understanding of the drugs used and their specific advantages and disadvantages. Each drug is ideal for a specific use. It is crucial for the clinician to develop guidelines and pathways for the use of these drugs within a specific environment. Newer drugs certainly will become available and more is being learnt about some of the new drugs and specific protocols that grade effect are being developed.

SELECTED READING

Arain SR, Ruehlow RM, Uhrich TD, Ebert TJ: The efficacy of dexmedetomidine versus morphine for postoperative analgesia after major inpatient surgery. Anesth Analg 98(1):153–158, 2004.

Barrientos-Vega R, Mar Sanchez-Soria M, Morales-Garcia C et al: Prolonged sedation of critically ill patients with midazolam or propofol: impact on weaning and costs. Crit Care Med 25(1):33–40, 1997.

Brook AD, Ahrens TS, Schaiff R et al: Effect of a nursing-implemented sedation protocol on the duration of mechanical ventilation. Crit Care Med 27(12):2609–2615, 1999.

Devlin JW, Boleski G, Mlynarek M et al: Motor Activity Assessment Scale: a valid and reliable sedation scale for use with mechanically ventilated patients in an adult surgical intensive care unit. Crit Care Med 27(7):1271–1275, 1999.

Devlin JW, Fraser GL, Kanji S, Riker RR: Sedation assessment in critically ill adults. Ann Pharmacother 35(12):1624–1632, 2001.

Devlin JW, Holbrook AM, Fuller HD: The effect of ICU sedation guidelines and pharmacist interventions on clinical outcomes and drug cost. Ann Pharmacother 31(6):689–695, 1997.

Ely EW, Truman B, Shintani A et al: Monitoring sedation status over time in ICU patients: reliability and validity of the Richmond Agitation-Sedation Scale (RASS). JAMA 289(22):2983–2991, 2003.

Hammond JJ: Protocols and guidelines in critical care: development and implementation. Curr Opin Crit Care 7(6):464–468, 2001.

Hansen-Flaschen J, Cowen J, Polomano RC: Beyond the Ramsay scale: need for a validated measure of sedating drug efficacy in the intensive care unit. Crit Care Med 22(5):732–733, 1994.

Jacobi J, Fraser GL, Coursin DB et al: Clinical practice guidelines for the sustained use of sedatives and analgesics in the critically ill adult. Crit Care Med 30(1):119–141, 2002.

Kress JP, Pohlman AS, Hall JB: Sedation and analgesia in the intensive care unit. Am J Respir Crit Care Med 166(8):1024–1028, 2002.

Mondello E, Siliotti R, Noto G et al: Bispectral Index in ICU: correlation with Ramsay score on assessment of sedation level. J Clin Monit Comput 17(5):271–277, 2002.

Murray MJ, Cowen J, DeBlock H et al: Clinical practice guidelines for sustained neuromuscular blockade in the adult critically ill patient. Crit Care Med 30(1):142–156, 2002.

Nasraway SA, Jr., Jacobi J, Murray MJ, Lumb PD: Sedation, analgesia, and neuromuscular blockade of the critically ill adult: revised clinical practice guidelines for 2002. Crit Care Med 30(1):117–118, 2002.

Riker RR, Fraser GL: Sedation in the intensive care unit: refining the models and defining the questions. Crit Care Med 30(7):1661–1663, 2002.

Riker RR, Picard JT, Fraser GL: Prospective evaluation of the Sedation-Agitation Scale for adult critically ill patients. Crit Care Med 27(7):1325–1329, 1999.

Szokol JW, Vender JS: Anxiety, delirium, and pain in the intensive care unit. Crit Care Clin 17(4):821–842, 2001.

Wheeler DS, Vaux KK, Ponaman ML, Poss BW: The safe and effective use of propofol sedation in children undergoing diagnostic and therapeutic procedures: experience in a pediatric ICU and a review of the literature. Pediatr Emerg Care 19(6):385–392, 2003.

ORGAN SYSTEMS

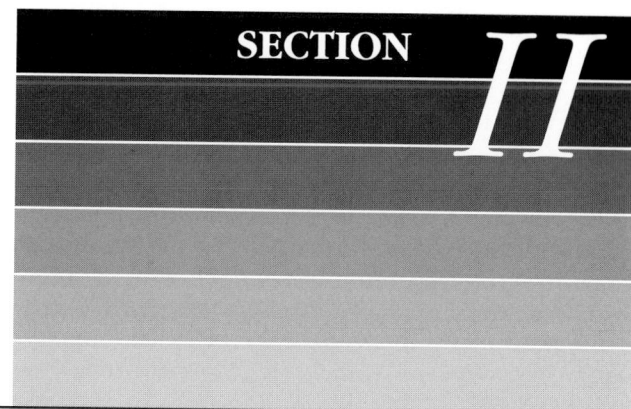

SECTION *II*

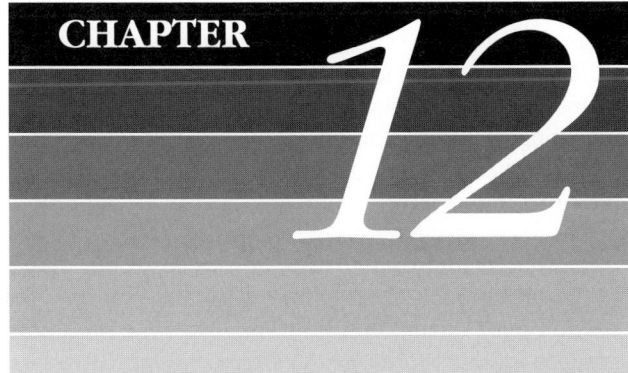

Hypertension

EWAN M. CAMERON, M.D.

HEIDI B. KUMMER, M.D., M.P.H.

In the general population hypertension is present in one in four adults in the USA. Among certain subgroups of the population, such as blacks and the elderly, the prevalence of hypertension is even higher. The importance of hypertension lies in its widespread effect on an individual's health including the potential for causing stroke, myocardial infarction, renal failure, congestive heart failure, progressive atherosclerosis, and dementia. More recently isolated systolic hypertension has been identified as a significant risk factor among the elderly for cardiovascular events. Both the duration and level of hypertension have a determining effect on outcome from cardiovascular disease in combination with other risk factors. There is no question that the treatment of hypertension reduces the risk of stroke and coronary artery disease as well as congestive heart failure. Importantly, it is also known that only 54% of patients with hypertension receive treatment and overall only 28% are adequately treated.

EVALUATION

The Joint National Committee on Prevention, Detection, Evaluation and Treatment of High Blood Pressure has classified hypertension as follows. High normal: 130–139 systolic, 85–59 diastolic; stage 1: 140–159 systolic or 90–99 diastolic; stage 2: 160–179 systolic or 100–109 diastolic; stage 3: >180 systolic or >110 diastolic. Blood pressure measurements should be accurate and should also be confirmed on at least three different occasions. So-called white coat hypertension can be excluded by obtaining ambulatory or at-home blood pressure monitoring. The latter is present in up to 20% of patients with elevated blood pressure but it may be a precursor of sustained hypertension and certainly warrants continued surveillance.

In addition to a history and physical examination, routine testing should include urinalysis, complete blood count, creatinine and urea, potassium, and 12-lead electrocardiography. Severe or resistant hypertension or clinical or laboratory findings indicative of underlying disease such as that originating in the kidney or adrenal gland should be further investigated. In 90% of patients the diagnosis is one of essential idiopathic hypertension.

PATHOGENESIS

In the majority of patients the cause of hypertension is unknown. Where no definable cause can be identified patients are said to have primary essential idiopathic hypertension. There are many systems involved in the regulation of blood pressure and the relations among these are also complex. Therefore it has been difficult to identify one single factor that is primarily responsible. While many different abnormalities have been described in the hypertensive patient, none has clearly been identified as primary. With the growth of new knowledge about hypertension in the last 20 years there has been some blurring between primary and secondary forms of hypertension.

Animal and population studies suggest that there is a genetic component although its influence is likely to vary among different patients. The genetic factor interacts with a number of environmental factors including salt intake, obesity, occupation, and family size and crowding. Overall these result in abnormal activity of the sympathetic nervous system. In the normal person changes in blood pressure are compensated by adaptive changes in activation of beta-adrenergic receptors and by secretion of renin by the juxtaglomerular apparatus of the kidney. Thus falls in blood pressure are accompanied by compensatory increases in heart rate, stroke volume, and systemic vascular resistance to maintain normal blood pressure. In patients with hypertension, by contrast, there are maladaptive compensatory mechanisms and therefore patients thus affected tend to exist in a chronic vasoconstrictive state. The kidney also contributes significantly to the development of hypertension. Normally the kidney secretes renin in response to hypertension-induced beta-adrenergic stimulation. In turn renin promotes the conversion of angiotensinogen to angiotensin I and angiotensin II. Angiotensin II increases blood pressure by causing vasoconstriction and by stimulating the release of aldosterone from the zona glomerulosa of the adrenal cortex. Aldosterone causes retention of sodium.

The course of hypertension is modified by a multitude of factors including race, gender, cholesterol, smoking, diabetes, and weight. The younger a patient is when hypertension is first diagnosed the greater the reduction in life expectancy. In the USA blacks have more than four times the morbidity associated with hypertension. At all ages and in both races females with hypertension fare better than males. Atherosclerosis is contributed to by many factors and so it is not surprising that the effect of hypertension on outcome may be enhanced by certain other conditions. Thus the probability of developing a morbid cardiovascular event with a given blood pressure will vary by many times. Hypertensive patients will develop further increases in blood pressure with time. From actuarial data and from the era prior to treatment it is clear that hypertension will significantly shorten life due presumably to the progression of the atherosclerotic process.

SECONDARY HYPERTENSION

Secondary hypertension accounts for 4–5% of all cases of hypertension. The major causes of secondary hypertension are renal or endocrine. Renal disease may cause hypertension either by an inability to excrete sodium and water, or by elaborating excess renin. In the former retention of sodium will result in an increased circulating volume leading to an increase in blood pressure. In the latter high levels of renin produce high levels of the vasoconstrictors angiotensin II and aldosterone. Another separate entity, renovascular hypertension, is due to atherosclerosis or fibrous dysplasia of one or both of the main arteries supplying the kidney. The resulting poor renal blood flow stimulates the secretion of higher levels of renin by the affected kidney. Patients known or suspected to have renovascular hypertension should not receive angiotensin converting enzyme (ACE) inhibitors as these may precipitate acute renal failure.

CLINICAL CAVEAT

Angiotensin Converting Enzyme Inhibitors and Renal Stenosis
   Patients known or suspected to have renovascular hypertension should not receive ACE inhibitors as they may precipitate acute renal failure.

The major endocrine causes of hypertension are hyperaldosteronism, Cushing's syndrome, and pheochromocytoma. Together these three causes account for 1% of all cases of hypertension. For example, patients with hypertension with profound hypokalemia in the absence of diuretics should be considered to have hyperaldosteronism. Cushing's syndrome should be suspected in those with a combination of truncal obesity, muscle weakness, and glucose intolerance.

Pheochromocytoma is characterized by diaphoresis and paroxysmal hypertension or orthostatic hypotension. The diagnosis is confirmed by showing increased presence of epinephrine and norepinephrine or their metabolites in a 24-hour urine sample. Other secondary causes include hypercalcemia, acromegaly, oral contraceptives, and coarctation of the aorta.

EFFECTS OF HYPERTENSION

The importance of hypertension lies in its deleterious effects on end organ function. The adverse effects of hypertension on the heart include changes in diastolic relaxation, impairment of coronary blood flow, progression of coronary artery disease, left ventricular hypertrophy, ventricular ectopy and sudden death, and congestive heart failure. The earliest change in the heart associated with hypertension appears to be loss of diastolic relaxation and the first manifestation of this abnormality is the sudden appearance of apparent cardiac failure often in the setting of stress or exercise.

Impairment of coronary blood flow reserve will manifest as angina in the absence of coronary artery disease. Thallium perfusion defects can be shown in those affected with hypertension and ambulatory recording has shown ischemia even in the absence of left ventricular hypertrophy. Animal studies of hypertension have shown that below certain regulatory thresholds the myocardium is at increased risk of subendocardial ischemia. In hypertensive patients blood pressure that would not be considered abnormally low in normotensive patients may lead to significant subendocardial ischemia and subsequent myocardial infarction. Treatment with antihypertensive therapy may reverse left ventricular hypertrophy. Patients with hypertensive cardiomyopathy are at increased risk of sudden death.

EFFECTS OF HYPERTENSION ON THE BRAIN

There is little question about the role of hypertension in the genesis of stroke. Conversely lowering blood pressure protects against cerebrovascular events. Strokes may be either hemorrhagic or ischemic in origin. The underlying pathological change is damage to the cerebral blood vessel wall. For example, high blood pressure induces damage to the vascular endothelium that in turn leads to thrombus formation and vessel narrowing. Hypertension also predisposes to hemorrhage as weakening of the wall occurs over time.

EFFECTS OF HYPERTENSION ON THE KIDNEY

Chronic hypertension induces permanent damage in the kidney characterized by atherosclerosis of afferent and efferent arterioles and glomerular tufts. Over time there is loss of glomeruli resulting in gradual deterioration in overall function as well as reserve. In addition, the autoregulatory curve is set higher so that lower levels of blood pressure are not well tolerated and may even produce acute renal failure.

ANESTHESIA AND HYPERTENSION

The two questions that have dominated this subject over the years are the following. Should antihypertensive medications be continued right up to and including the day of surgery? When should surgery be canceled in the hypertensive patient? Extensive studies performed in the past have demonstrated that hemodynamic stability in hypertensive patients is superior when antihypertensive therapy is continued into the operative period. Nowadays it is standard practice to continue antihypertensive therapy throughout the perioperative period. There are convincing data that the perioperative use of antihypertensive medication in those with known hypertension and in those with newly discovered hypertension results in significantly less ischemia in the postoperative period. This effect does not appear to be related primarily to better control of blood pressure so much as improved control of heart rate.

Patients with hypertension on the day of surgery should not have their surgery cancelled. In general, unless patients have diastolic blood pressure of >110 mmHg or hypertension is associated with evidence of compromised end organ function, elective surgery should proceed. In the case of emergency surgery blood pressure should be brought under control as soon as is practically possible and in any case blood pressure control can be continued in the operating room while surgery is proceeding. While it is well recognized that hypertension is a risk factor for poorer outcome there are no clear guidelines on when it is appropriate to intervene. Hypertension is just one of many factors that can determine outcome and so its presence and the amount of control that should be exercised cannot be considered in isolation. Interestingly, studies on hypertension have shown that the use of an antihypertensive such as atenolol when compared with a diuretic results in less ischemia that is clearly associated with tachycardia rather than changes in blood pressure.

In those patients with hypertension and diabetes the occurrence of hypotension or hypertension alternating with hypotension may increase the risk of postoperative renal failure. As was mentioned above, longstanding hypertension results in progressive loss of nephrons and therefore loss of functional reserve. In addition the autoregulatory mechanism operates at a higher level. These patients therefore cannot tolerate low blood pressure. These patients warrant close monitoring with an invasive blood pressure line. Similarly they have less coronary reserve, even in the absence of left ventricular hypertrophy.

The two most stressful periods in anesthesia are induction and extubation. These are the times when exaggerated responses are likely to be seen and precautions should be taken appropriately. Many drugs have been used. The preoperative use of atenolol will help as will intravenous lidocaine to blunt normal reflexes to laryngoscopy and intubation. The introduction of the ultra-short-acting intravenous beta$_1$-blocker esmolol has proved useful for rapid control of blood pressure and heart rate during the periods of induction, intubation, and extubation. One should also consider whether anesthesia can be accomplished without the need for endotracheal intubation; for example, the laryngeal mask airway does not stimulate as much hypertension or tachycardia when it is used. Many surgical procedures may be performed with regional anesthesia such as epidural or spinal techniques.

Special considerations attend those patients with aortic or cerebral aneurysm, as close blood pressure control is crucial to a favorable outcome. The control of blood pressure here is essential to prevent exacerbating the injured vessel or even causing outright rupture; on the other hand, too strict a control of blood pressure may result in ischemic hypotension.

Patients should be at ease preoperatively and should receive a mild sedative such as midazolam. As diuretics may render patients hypovolemic, these should probably be omitted on the day of surgery. The intensity of blood pressure monitoring should be decided after due consideration of the presence of comorbid disease, the type and duration of surgery, and the expected need for postoperative intensive care.

Before intervening with blood pressure control one should ensure that depth of anesthesia is appropriate, that adequate analgesia has been given, and that both hypercarbia and hypoxia have been excluded.

CLINICAL CAVEAT

Before using antihypertensive therapy intraoperatively, one should ensure that anesthesia and analgesia are effective and that there is no hypoxia or hypercarbia.

TREATMENT

Nitrates

These are time-honored drugs for control of intraoperative hypertension. These drugs work by increasing nitric oxide and thus causing smooth muscle relaxation. Thus they are direct-acting vasorelaxants. Nitroglycerin mainly works on the venous side and therefore is not as useful for control of high blood pressure. Sodium nitroprusside (SNP) works on both the venous and arterial sides of the circulation. One advantage of SNP is that it has rapid onset and offset. There are numerous side effects including profound hypotension, metabolic acidosis, tachyphylaxis, reflex tachycardia, cyanide toxicity, and thiocyanate accumulation in the presence of renal failure. Hydralazine is another direct-acting vasodilator. One must be aware of the possibility of reflex tachycardia.

Alpha$_2$-Adrenergic Agonists

These drugs have their greatest action at the central receptors and do so by decreasing sympathetic outflow. Clonidine is the best-known drug in this group. One may see unexpected falls in blood pressure with this drug as well as profound bradycardia. More recently dexmetomidine has been introduced but it has not been formally tested as an antihypertensive. The biggest drawback with clonidine is that it may cause rebound hypertension when withdrawn.

Beta$_1$-Adrenergic Antagonists

These are well tolerated and are recommended as first-line treatment. They act by blocking beta$_1$-receptors in the heart, decreasing heart rate and force of contraction, thereby causing a fall in cardiac output. As well as controlling blood pressure they are most valuable at slowing heart rate and thus avoiding the risk of ischemia associated with tachycardia. Both selective and nonselective beta$_1$-antagonists are available. In patients with significant bronchial disease it may be better to use a selective beta$_1$-antagonist. They should be used cautiously in patients with congestive heart failure as they depress myocardial function. The introduction of the short-acting agent esmolol has allowed more rapid control of blood pressure and tachycardia in the operating room. It also seems to be well tolerated by patients affected by bronchial smooth muscle disease.

Labetolol is useful for acute therapy of severe hypertension. It has both alpha- and beta-blocking activity and thus it brings about a concurrent decrease in contraction and vasodilatation. It is available for intravenous use.

DRUG INTERACTION

The preoperative use of a beta-blocker such as atenolol when combined with a spinal anesthetic can lead to profound bradycardia and possible cardiac asystole.

Alpha$_1$-adrenergic antagonists such as phentolamine and phenoxybenzamine are reserved for preoperative treatment of those patients with pheochromoctyoma.

Calcium Channel Blockers

These drugs – nicardipine, nefedipine, diltiazem, and verapamil – act by blocking the influx of calcium through calcium channels in smooth muscle and myocytes. As with beta$_1$-blockers they cause a decrease in the force of contraction of the heart and also peripheral vasorelaxation.

Nifedipine is the most potent vasodilator and it should probably not be used in the recovery room for control of postoperative hypertension as it may produce profound falls in blood pressure that result in stroke or myocardial ischemia.

CURRENT CONTROVERSY

The use of sublingual nifedipine for the treatment of postoperative hypertension may cause sudden severe falls in blood pressure.

Angiotensin Converting Enzyme Inhibitors

These drugs achieve their effect by inhibiting the conversion of angiotensinogen to angiotensin II thus limiting the constrictor effect of this compound on blood vessels and its ability to release aldosterone. They have many side effects including hypotension especially in patients who are hypovolemic. These agents are generally used in those patients who are unable to tolerate a beta$_1$-blocker. The only ACE inhibitor available for use in the USA as an intravenous preparation is enalaprilit.

ACE also causes the breakdown of bradykinin, a potent vasodilator. Bradykinin increases the presence of dilatory prostaglandins in tissues. Thus treatment with indomethacin reduces the effectiveness of these drugs. The hemodynamic actions of ACE inhibitors are unique. They depend on the level of renin. Blood pressure reduction depends on the level of initial renin. In those patients with normal or low levels of renin the response is more muted than in those with high levels. The initial response to ACE inhibitors is exaggerated in those with volume depletion; however, this excessive hypotension can be counteracted with an infusion of normal saline.

The use of ACE inhibitors is beneficial in those with diabetes as they provide some protection against decline in renal function and in those patients with heart failure ACE inhibitors have been shown to prolong life expectancy.

More recently angiotensin inhibitors such as losartin have been introduced. Whether these should be discontinued prior to surgery is controversial but if the patient is well hydrated there should not be a problem.

Diuretics

A whole host of diuretic agents are used for treating hypertension. They include thiazides, loop diuretics, and the potassium-sparing diuretic spironolactone. These control blood pressure by decreasing the volume of the circulation. They are often used as sole agents and as first-line treatment; when blood pressure becomes resistant to treatment these drugs are frequently combined with other agents such as beta$_1$-blockers or calcium antagonists. Diuretics have many metabolic side effects and preoperative preparation should include testing for changes in electrolytes and renal function.

HYPERTENSIVE CRISIS

This is defined as diastolic blood pressure > 130 mmHg. Malignant hypertension is marked by an increase in blood pressure with papilledema and presence of exudates in the optic fundus. Other signs and symptoms may include severe headache, vomiting, pulmonary edema, and visual disturbances. Only about 1% of hypertensive patients progress to the malignant phase. It can occur in either essential or secondary hypertension. This is a medical emergency and requires immediate treatment. These patients should be admitted to an intensive care unit (ICU) where close monitoring can be done preferably with a direct arterial pressure line. The aim of treatment is to lower blood pressure towards but not below 90 mmHg. Causes of hypertensive crises may be neurological, cardiovascular, or renal. The goal is to avoid rapid changes in blood pressure especially in the setting of acute stroke as this may precipitate ischemia.

The main cardiovascular event associated with hypertensive crisis is a dissecting thoracic aneurysm. Therapy should be aimed at decreasing blood pressure to 100 mmHg. The combination of SNP and a beta-blocker works well for this critical disease until definitive surgical correction can be achieved.

Renal causes include renal artery stenosis and parenchymal disease. In affected patients a pulmonary artery catheter should be used in order to assess the circulation with reasonable accuracy and avoid the risk of pulmonary edema.

Other causes of hypertensive crises are preeclampsia, recreational drug use, pheochromocytoma, and hyperautonomic syndromes such as tetanus.

SUMMARY

Hypertension is present in one-quarter to one-third of patients presenting for surgery. Therefore it is a disease that is commonly encountered in the perioperative setting. Many of these patients do not have adequate treatment of hypertension and therefore are likely to require some form of antihypertensive therapy while undergoing anesthesia and surgery. Unless confirmed blood pressure is very high (diastolic > 110 mmHg) or there is clear evidence of end organ compromise (e.g., myocardial ischemia) in association with high blood pressure surgery should not

CASE STUDY

A 55-year-old male presents for elective cystoscopy and transurethral resection of bladder tumor. He weighs 120 kg, he is 6 ft tall, has hypertension, diabetes, asthma, and a "bad back." He had two similar procedures done twice within the past year without any anesthetic or surgical problems. His usual medication includes glipizide, serevent inhaler, lisinipril, nifedipine, and ibuprofen. He confirms that he took all his medication as requested by his interviewer when he had his preoperative visit three weeks before. His blood pressure is 210/115 mmHg in the preoperative area.

QUESTIONS

1. What should the first action be on finishing an interview with this patient?
2. Are there any additional tests that should be done?
3. Should surgery be cancelled? If so, why?
4. If this patient presented emergently, what are the options (a) for treating the blood pressure and (b) for performing anesthesia safely?

be postponed. Patients on antihypertensive medication should continue with their usual medication right through the perioperative period. Those patients with newly diagnosed hypertension may best benefit from a $beta_1$-antagonist over the course of their surgical procedure.

There are many different antihypertensive medications available from which to choose and choice should be based on consideration of the individual patient, known side effects of medication, and goals of therapy. Certain conditions demand close and frequent monitoring of blood pressure in order to minimize morbidity. Hypertension is only one of many factors that determine surgical and anesthesia outcomes. It should be recognized that overtreatment of hypertension may be as detrimental as undertreatment.

SELECTED READING

August P: Initial treatment of hypertension. N Engl J Med 348:610–617, 2003.

Hulyalkar AR, Miller ED: Evaluation of the hypertensive patient. In Rogers MC et al, editors: *Principles and Practice of Anesthesiology*, Mosby Year Book, 1993.

Qureshi AI, Suri MF, Mohammed Y et al: Isolated and borderline systolic hypertension relative to long term risk and type of stroke: a 20 year follow-up of the national health and nutrition survey. Stroke 33:2781–2788, 2002.

Williams GH, Braunwald E: Hypertensive vascular disease. In Braunwald E et al, editors: *Harrison's Principles of Internal Medicine*, ed 11, McGraw-Hill, 1987.

Ziegler MG, Ruiz-Ramon P: Antihypertensive therapy. In *The Pharmacological Approach to the Critically Ill Patient*, ed 3, Williams and Wilkins.

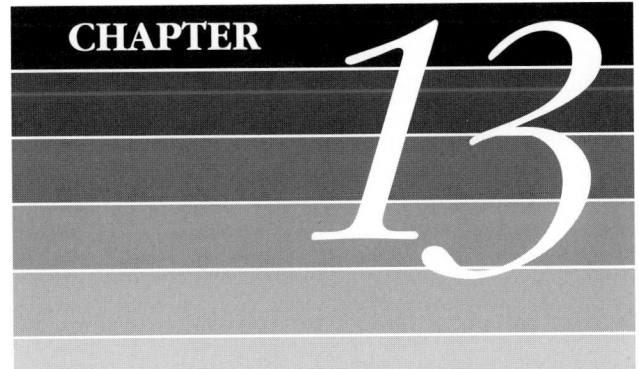

Myocardial Ischemia and Infarction in the Perioperative Period

HEIDI B. KUMMER, M.D., M.P.H.

EWAN M. CAMERON, M.D.

CHAPTER 13

Despite advances made in the area of risk stratification, risk reduction, and therapy, myocardial ischemia and infarction remain major sources of perioperative morbidity and mortality in patients presenting for noncardiac surgery. Each year an estimated 50,000 of these patients sustain a perioperative myocardial infarct and over one million will suffer some cardiac-related complication; all at an estimated cost of over $20 billion per year. It appears that patients with known coronary artery disease and patients with identifiable risk factors for coronary artery disease have a similar incidence of adverse advents; thus a comprehensive approach to prevention and treatment seems warranted.

PATHOPHYSIOLOGY

Myocardial ischemia and infarction occur when myocardial oxygen demand outweighs supply; in other words, there is too little pressure to perfuse normal coronaries (prolonged systemic hypotension), or blood flow is inadequate due to blockages/spasm in the coronary arteries, or shortened time for perfusion from a rapid heart rate (Box 13-1).

Clinically this imbalance manifests in a myriad of ways: from "silent" – the patient experiences no pain – to crushing substernal chest or arm pain; from symptoms of nausea, vomiting, diaphoresis to electrocardiographic changes and

arrhythmias; from mild shortness of breath to pulmonary edema and severe hemodynamic instability (Box 13-2).

Thus vigilance, a high index of suspicion, and early therapeutic interventions are required to minimize or prevent cell death. While high-grade stenoses and coronary plaques (with or without plaque rupture) are known to be associated with myocardial ischemia, more recent work has focused on hypercoagulable states and the inflammatory cascade as key components in the process leading to myocardial ischemia and infarction (Box 13-3).

RISK FACTORS AND RISK STRATIFICATION

Beyond a comprehensive history and physical examination, a thorough cardiac risk assessment has become an integral part of the preoperative evaluation of patients presenting for noncardiac surgery. These range from general criteria – age, gender, family history, life style choices (activity level, smoking, drug and alcohol consumption), work and family stressors, to more specific areas such as comorbid disease states – diabetes, renal insufficiency – and type of surgery – major, minor, elective, or emergent (Box 13-4).

In an attempt to synthesize the results of numerous studies that have examined risk factors and to present an evidence-based approach to therapeutic interventions, the American College of Cardiology (ACC) and the American Heart Association (AHA) published a set of guidelines for preoperative evaluation of patients undergoing noncardiac surgery in 1996. These guidelines were revised in 2000, and represent the most comprehensive step-wise approach to date; they are the guidelines most commonly used in preoperative centers across the USA. By combining clinical predictors with a patient's functional capacity and surgical risk, these guidelines provide a decision tree, outlining which patient warrants further cardiac testing preoperatively (Figure 13-1). The only

---

Box 13-1   Factors Contributing to Myocardial Oxygen Demand

- Preload
- Afterload/myocardial wall tension
- Heart rate
- Contractility

Box 13-3   Factors Contributing to Diminished Myocardial Supply

- Coronary stenosis due to atherosclerotic disease
- Coronary steal phenomenon
- Coronary vasospasm
- Acute plaque rupture
- Hypercoagulable states
- Inflammatory cascade

---

patients who seem to benefit from undergoing either coronary artery bypass grafting or percutaneous transluminal coronary angioplasty (PTCA) preoperatively are those in whom these procedures would have been indicated independently of the scheduled noncardiac surgery. Timing of such an intervention also makes a difference; a higher rate of complications, including stent thrombosis and severe bleeding, resulted when patients had their planned surgical procedure within two weeks of PTCA or stent placement. Adequate time must be given for the healing process and for a full course of aspirin/clopidogrel therapy to be complete; current recommendations are to wait at least two weeks, but preferably four weeks before proceeding with noncardiac surgery.

PREOPERATIVE PREPARATION

While there seems to be general agreement on the preparation of patients presenting for cardiac surgery – most of their usual medications are continued through the day of surgery, including heparin and nitrate infusions in urgent/emergent cases – variation exists in the perioperative care of the patient coming for noncardiac surgery (Box 13-5).

Many institutions prescribe antihypertensives, antianginals, and lipid-lowering agents right through the day of

surgery. Instructions to discontinue any aspirin or aspirin-related products up to two weeks and nonsteroidal anti-inflammatory agents for at least three days prior to surgery remain routine in most centers; however, there is no clear evidence that the approach is valid (Box 13-6).

Patients who have been on a regimen but omitted to take their cardiac medications on the morning of surgery should receive them either orally with a sip of water, or intravenously prior to the surgical procedure. There is good evidence that perioperative beta-blockade improves outcome beyond the immediate postoperative period. With the advent of more sensitive monitoring capabilities and results stemming from multicenter trials such as the McSPI group, target heart rates of

---

Box 13-2   Signs and Symptoms of Myocardial Ischemia

- "Silent" – no pain
- Pain or pressure – substernal or radiating to arms and neck
- Nausea and vomiting
- Diaphoresis
- Shortness of breath – pulmonary edema
- ECG changes – arrhythmias
- Hypotension – cardiovascular collapse

Box 13-4   Factors Associated with Perioperative Myocardial Ischemia

- Age > 65
- Male gender
- Type-A personality
- Family history of coronary artery disease
- Low activity level
- Smoking
- Drug (cocaine) and alcohol abuse
- Uncontrolled hypertension
- Hypercholesterolemia/hyperlipidemia
- Diabetes mellitus
- Renal insufficiency
- Obesity
- Known coronary artery disease, prior myocardial ischemia, angina
- Congestive heart failure
- Abnormal ECG/arrhythmias
- Significant valvular disease
- Emergency surgery
- Pain/anxiety

Figure 13-1   Stepwise approach to preoperative cardiac assessment. The steps are discussed in the text. *Subsequent care may include cancellation or delay of surgery, coronary revascularization followed by noncardiac surgery, or intensified care.
(Reprinted from Eagle KA, Berger PB, Calkins H et al: ACC/AHA guideline update for perioperative cardiovascular evaluation for noncardiac surgery – executive summary: a report of the American College of Cardiology/American Heart Association Task Force on Practice Guidelines (Committee to Update the 1996 Guidelines on Perioperative Cardiovascular Evaluation for Noncardiac Surgery). Anesth Analg 94:1052–1064, 2002.)

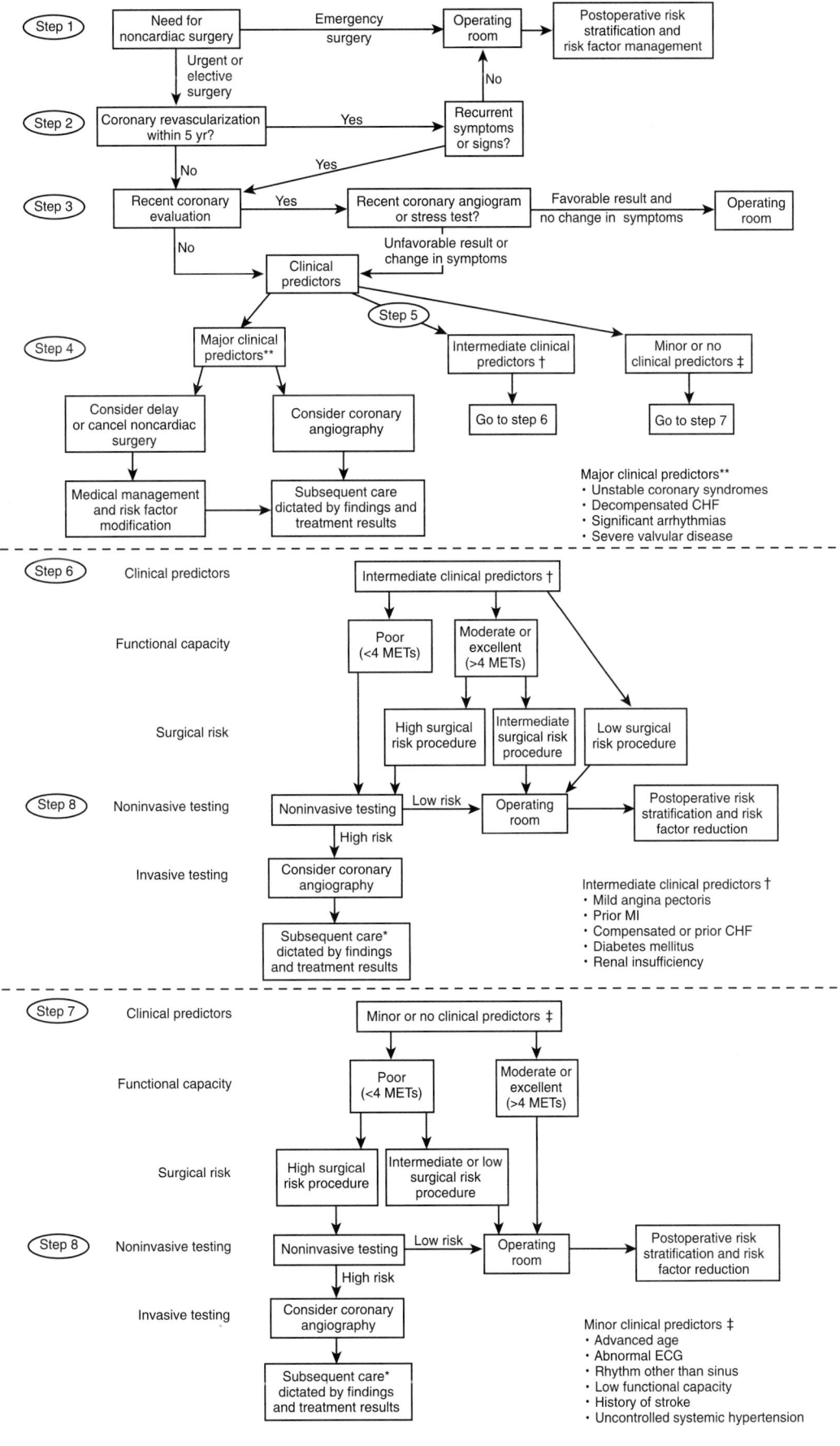

Step 1 — Need for noncardiac surgery → Emergency surgery → Operating room → Postoperative risk stratification and risk factor management

Urgent or elective surgery

Step 2 — Coronary revascularization within 5 yr? → Yes → Recurrent symptoms or signs? → No → Operating room

No ; Yes

Step 3 — Recent coronary evaluation → Yes → Recent coronary angiogram or stress test? → Favorable result and no change in symptoms → Operating room

Unfavorable result or change in symptoms

No

Clinical predictors

Step 5 — Clinical predictors

Step 4 — Major clinical predictors**   Intermediate clinical predictors †   Minor or no clinical predictors ‡

Intermediate clinical predictors † → Go to step 6
Minor or no clinical predictors ‡ → Go to step 7

Consider delay or cancel noncardiac surgery
Consider coronary angiography

Medical management and risk factor modification → Subsequent care dictated by findings and treatment results

Major clinical predictors**
- Unstable coronary syndromes
- Decompensated CHF
- Significant arrhythmias
- Severe valvular disease

Step 6 — Clinical predictors — Intermediate clinical predictors †

Functional capacity — Poor (<4 METs) ; Moderate or excellent (>4 METs)

Surgical risk — High surgical risk procedure ; Intermediate surgical risk procedure ; Low surgical risk procedure

Step 8 — Noninvasive testing — Noninvasive testing → Low risk → Operating room → Postoperative risk stratification and risk factor reduction

High risk

Invasive testing — Consider coronary angiography → Subsequent care* dictated by findings and treatment results

Intermediate clinical predictors †
- Mild angina pectoris
- Prior MI
- Compensated or prior CHF
- Diabetes mellitus
- Renal insufficiency

Step 7 — Clinical predictors — Minor or no clinical predictors ‡

Functional capacity — Poor (<4 METs) ; Moderate or excellent (>4 METs)

Surgical risk — High surgical risk procedure ; Intermediate or low surgical risk procedure

Step 8 — Noninvasive testing — Noninvasive testing → Low risk → Operating room → Postoperative risk stratification and risk factor reduction

High risk

Invasive testing — Consider coronary angiography → Subsequent care* dictated by findings and treatment results

Minor clinical predictors ‡
- Advanced age
- Abnormal ECG
- Rhythm other than sinus
- Low functional capacity
- History of stroke
- Uncontrolled systemic hypertension

Box 13-5 Medications to be Continued

- Antihypertensives
  - Beta-blockers
  - Calcium channel blockers
  - Angiotensin enzyme converting inhibitors
- Antianginals
  - Oral agents
  - Nitropatch and infusions
- Lipid-lowering agents/statins
- Antiglycemics
  - Oral intermediate acting
  - Subcutaneous short and intermediate acting
- Analgesics
  - Nonaspirin-containing agents
  - Narcotics

50–60 beats per minute are now recommended in high-risk patients.

Beta-adrenergic blockers remain the mainstay of therapy. However, alpha-2 agonists such as clonidine and more recently dexmedetomidine are gaining favor as agents; these drugs not only reduce the sympathetic stress response, but also have sedative and adjunctive analgesic properties.

All patients regardless of the type of surgery should receive anxiolysis. In addition to calming patients, sedatives such as benzodiazepines and analgesics such as morphine and fentanyl are the most commonly employed agents.

Whether or not to use invasive monitoring in these patients will depend largely on the proposed procedure and the patient's functional status. The threshold for placing an arterial line should be relatively low and is surely indicated once ischemia is suspected. Central venous monitoring is less helpful to look at absolute numbers, but good for following trends and useful for administration of vasoactive drugs. Where available transesophageal echo is preferred as a more sensitive monitor of cardiac function. This is common practice in

Box 13-6 Medications to be Considered Case by Case

- Diuretics
- Nitropatch and infusions
- Nonsteroidal anti-inflammatory drugs
- Antiplatelet agents
  - Aspirin, clopidogrel
- Thrombin inhibitors
  - Heparin, low molecular weight heparin
  - Hirudin
- Antiglycemics
- Long-acting oral and subcutaneous preparations

patients presenting for cardiac surgery in larger centers. Practices vary significantly regarding use of pulmonary artery catheters. In academic centers in patients undergoing major noncardiac surgery, the pulmonary artery catheter is still frequently used. It is most helpful in managing a patient's volume status postoperatively; ironically, if a patient does well, the catheter is discontinued on the first postoperative day, thereby losing whatever benefit one might have gained from following pressures on day three when most mobilization of fluids occurs. There are recent data to suggest that "who" monitors the patient may be of greater importance than with what: high-risk patients receiving postoperative care by dedicated, specialty trained intensivists appear to have better outcomes.

Despite a host of studies trying to show the benefit of regional over general, there is no one single best anesthetic technique. Therefore choice of anesthesia should take into account the type of procedure, patient's condition, and the anesthesiologist's experience. Using epidural analgesia adjunctively intraoperatively and postoperatively blunts the sympathetic response and provides optimal pain relief, thus reducing one of the major perioperative stress factors.

DIAGNOSIS OF MYOCARDIAL ISCHEMIA

In the absence of left bundle branch block, a properly calibrated, five-lead electrocardiogram (ECG) is still the gold standard for detecting myocardial ischemia in the operating room. Leads II and V5 are displayed for best rhythm and ischemia detection, respectively. A change in the ST segment of greater than 0.1 mV usually down sloping is considered diagnostic of ischemia. Monitors equipped with ST segment trending and analyses have made it much easier to follow and document such changes. Unfortunately there are still many factors in an operating room that may limit the effectiveness of ECG detection of ischemia: interference from electrocautery, a signal that is highly filtered, and leads placed to accommodate the surgical field not the specificity of the equipment. That is why such a change if observed must be correlated with the overall clinical picture and not used in isolation to direct therapy. We know now that ECG changes can be a relatively late sign in the progression of myocardial ischemia to infarction. Only through the more intensive use of echocardiography, specifically transesophageal echocardiography (TEE), have we learned how much later ECG changes appear in the early stages of diminished blood flow. Though not all wall motion abnormalities are caused by ischemia, once defined, ischemia-related regional wall motion abnormalities can be seen up to four times more often than ECG changes and are far more sensitive in the detection of myocardial ischemia than ECG. The fine points of TEE interpretation, especially concerning the septum, require skill and a lot of experience; it also requires considerable resources and as such is not as widely applicable as a routine intraoperative diagnostic tool. However, we have learned through the combined use of TEE and PA catheters how poorly pulmonary artery pressures correlate with a patient's true volume status. Furthermore regional ischemia can easily occur without an increase in pulmonary artery or wedge pressures. Thus, an invasive monitor previously considered essential in patients at high risk for cardiac events (the pulmonary artery catheter) has fallen out of favor. Furthermore, errors in data gathering and interpretation have led some to believe that therapies misguided by PA catheter readings may cause more harm than good.

Finally, documentation of a myocardial infarction still relies on 12-lead ECGs and blood testing for CK MB isoenzymes and troponin levels. No monitor can replace vigilance and sound clinical judgment (Box 13-7).

TREATMENT OF MYOCARDIAL ISCHEMIA

The goals of therapy are essentially the same, start with the ABCs: whether treating a patient with a recent MI +/– intervention presenting for an emergent procedure, or a high-risk patient for elective surgery, or a patient who develops signs and symptoms of myocardial ischemia postoperatively (Box 13-8).

Ensure airway, oxygenation, and ventilation are adequate; assess heart rate and blood pressure and treat to minimize myocardial oxygen demand while maintaining supply and coronary perfusion pressure; evaluate sympathetic response, is the patient in pain, anxious, is there an iatrogenic component, a reaction to a medication administered? While the overall goals are the same, the therapeutic options vary with the timing of the ischemic event within the perioperative period. Cooling or allowing a patient's temperature to drift with the purpose of

---

Box 13-8   Treatment of Myocardial Ischemia

- Determine etiology
- Ensure adequate oxygenation/ventilation
- Improve supply/demand balance
  - Control heart rate
  - Maintain coronary perfusion pressure
  - Augment coronary vasodilation
- Treat pain, anxiety
- Document 12-lead ECG
- Send blood for CK MB isoenzymes and/or troponins
- Consider use of aspirin
- If severe and persistent, consider cardiac cath lab intervention – time is of the essence!

---

decreasing oxygen demand and minimizing cell damage may be an option in the anesthetized patient, especially in cardiac surgery, but it is not applicable in the awake state as shivering would have the opposite effect.

Preoperative Angina

Preoperative therapy is designed to optimize a patient's condition prior to the surgical procedure. This includes effective pain control; for example, for patients with hip fractures who received epidural analgesia immediately in the emergency room to manage their perioperative pain, there was a dramatic decrease in preoperative cardiac events, including myocardial ischemia, infarction, and congestive heart failure compared with patients who received the usual regimen of intramuscular meperidine. Continuation or initiation of beta-adrenergic blockade is recommended and now widely accepted. With the development of newer, more selective agents they are increasingly being employed in patients in whom they were previously thought to be contraindicated – in cases of depressed left ventricular function and reactive airway disease. Although there is controversy over whether calcium channel blockers, antianginals, and angiotensin converting enzyme (ACE) inhibitors contribute to or exacerbate intraoperative hypotension, it is common practice to continue them throughout the perioperative period. With the additional beneficial effect that lipid-lowering agents/statins have on stabilizing plaques and decreasing C-reactive protein, their importance in preventive therapy is bound to increase and their administration should not be interrupted perioperatively. Finally, consideration should be given to continuing aspirin therapy in patients who are deemed at high risk for myocardial ischemia. Those who are not on aspirin, following discussion with the surgeon, may receive one ECASA immediately preoperatively or as soon as feasible (but within 48 hours) postoperatively. On rare occasion a patient who is not a candidate for

---

Box 13-7   Monitors for Detection of Myocardial Ischemia

- Physical markers
  - Angina or anginal equivalent in patients under MAC or regional anesthesia
  - Hemodynamic instability
  - Diaphoresis
- Technical markers
  - Five-lead ECG with ST segment trending and analysis
  - Pulmonary artery catheter
  - Transesophageal echocardiography
- Chemical markers
  - CK MBs isoenzymes
  - Troponins

cardiac revascularization or who requires an urgent noncardiac surgical procedure may warrant preoperative placement of an intra-aortic balloon pump in addition to optimizing medical therapy.

Intraoperative Myocardial Ischemia

Infusing nitroglycerin as prophylaxis intraoperatively has no evidence to support it; however, many practitioners believe in its effect and administer it routinely in high-risk patients. Others use it as a first-line agent when myocardial ischemia is detected. Identifying the etiology for the ischemia is key to successful therapy. Any intervention should only be employed after ensuring adequacy of anesthetic depth/management and hemodynamic profile. Control of heart rate with a selective beta-adrenergic blocking agent is imperative. If hypotension is due to volume or blood loss, blood pressure should be augmented with a vasoconstrictor such as phenylephrine while fluid or blood is being replaced. The controversy over the optimal hematocrit for a healthy patient in general and for the cardiac patient in particular persists; at this point clinical judgment about the risk/benefit ratio of a transfusion for the individual patient must guide transfusion therapy. If possible, coronary perfusion should be enhanced with nitroglycerin; if despite all therapies ischemic changes persist, the surgical procedure should be finished as quickly and safely as possible. Unless contraindicated, the administration of an anti-inflammatory/antiplatelet agent like aspirin or thrombin inhibitor like heparin is strongly encouraged. If ischemia persists despite all of these therapies, consultation with an interventional cardiologist for possible transfer from the operating room directly to the cardiac catheterization laboratory should be considered.

Postoperative Myocardial Ischemia

The focus of much anesthesia-based literature has been on preoperative and intraoperative myocardial ischemia. The fact that nearly half of all patients who experience perioperative myocardial ischemia do so in the postoperative period reminds us that our responsibility to protect a high-risk patient does not end in the recovery room with the end of surgery. Thus the same considerations mentioned above should be given to patients who develop signs and symptoms of myocardial ischemia postoperatively in the post anesthesia recovery unit (PACU) or on the ward. Unfortunately, postoperative ischemia is frequently asymptomatic; therefore during the early postoperative period these patients continue to be at very high risk of myocardial ischemia, infarction, or even sudden death. When ischemia is detected and does not readily respond to anti-ischemic therapies such as oxygen, nitrates, morphine, and beta-blockers urgent cardiologic consultation for potential intervention using TPA or angioplasty/stenting is indicated.

Recent studies looking at the effects of postoperative aspirin administration (in the cardiac surgical population) or use of beta-blockers for at least seven days postoperatively have shown promising results in terms of improved outcome.

Ideally any patient who suffers a perioperative event should undergo cardiac evaluation and further risk stratification prior to discharge.

CURRENT CONTROVERSY

- Continuation of aspirin in the perioperative period
- Pulmonary artery catheters do more harm than good
- Optimal hematocrit for patients at risk of myocardial ischemia
- Mild hypo- or normothermia for patients with myocardial ischemia

---

CLINICAL CAVEAT

- Continuation of aspirin in the perioperative period may increase bleeding
- Beta-adrenergic blockers may cause bronchospasm
- Beta-adrenergic blockers may cause significant bradycardia
- Alpha-2 agonists may cause bradycardia and hypotension
- ACE inhibitors may contribute to or exacerbate intraoperative hypotension
- Therapy with nitrates may contribute to intraoperative hypotension

---

DRUG INTERACTIONS

- Beta-adrenergic blockers may potentiate narcotic-induced bradycardia
- Alpha-2 agonists may potentiate anesthetic-related bradycardia and hypotension
- Angiotensin enzyme inhibitors may potentiate anesthetic-related hypotension

---

FUTURE PERSPECTIVES

With the advent of the electronic age and enhanced opportunity to perform large multicenter randomized controlled trials, some of the current controversies about appropriate monitoring and therapies for perioperative myocardial ischemia and infarction may be answered in the near future. Whether to transfuse or hemodilute, whether to keep patients cool or normothermic are all questions still being debated and investigated; until further evidence is available individual and institutional practice will vary. Dealing with the possibility of increased intraoperative bleeding as a result of continuation of aspirin therapy may turn out to be a small price to pay for the benefit of increased protection: not only the myocardium, but as a recent study of patients undergoing cardiac surgery suggested, also a multitude of perioperative complications, including stroke and renal failure. "Triple A" therapy with aspirin, atenolol, and alpha-adrenergic agonists may well become the optimum of care in this category of high-risk patients, and quantification of C-reactive protein levels may become part of routine preoperative blood testing to further evaluate patients at risk. Unfortunately despite our best care and therapies, a certain percentage of patients still go on to suffer perioperative events, for reasons still obscure. The goal remains to try to reduce morbidity and mortality to the best of our ability given our current state of knowledge. Over time we will improve the overall outcome of patients at risk and those who sustain a perioperative myocardial infarction.

CASE STUDY

A 63-year-old white male (77 kg, 70 in) presented for posterior C4-5, C5-6 facetectomies. He had experienced right arm weakness when trying to lift wood and now was unable to lift his right arm, but denied any pain. His blood pressure was 120/80, heart rate 62, sinus. Past medical history was significant for hypertension, high cholesterol, a 30-pack yr smoking history and daily alcohol intake. He denied any symptoms of chest pain or shortness of breath. His medications included Atenolol, HCTZ, Zocor, Elavil, and Prilosec. He was allergic to codeine. Only past surgical history was a tonsillectomy as a child. Preoperative studies showed a hematocrit of 46, a BUN of 28, and creatinine of 1.5; ECG: NSR, LAD, IMI, without significant change from 5 months prior.

He received midazolam 2 mg in the preoperative area, was brought to the operating room and induced on the stretcher using fentanyl 50 μg, propofol 150 mg, and rocuronium 50 mg. He was easily intubated and the first postinduction blood pressure of 84 systolic was treated with 5 mg of ephedrine with good effect. He was then positioned prone in Mayfield tongs and shortly after incision his blood pressure dropped again. At this time significant ST elevations were noted in lead II on the ECG. The hypotension was treated with phenylephrine and the ST segments normalized.

QUESTIONS

1. At what point would you consider aborting the procedure? Only if it happened again?
2. Should this patient receive aspirin in the PACU?
3. Should you check CK MBs/troponin levels? In the operating room or in the PACU?
4. How should this patient's risk be stratified postoperatively?

SELECTED READING

Bode RH, Lewis KP, Zarich SW et al: Cardiac outcome after peripheral vascular surgery: comparison of general and regional anesthesia. Anesthesiology 84:3-13, 1996.

Cahalan MK: *Detection and Treatment of Intraoperative Myocardial Ischemia*, IARS 2002 Review Course Lectures, pp 27-30.

Eagle KA, Berger PB, Calkins H et al: ACC/AHA guideline update for perioperative cardiovascular evaluation for noncardiac surgery - executive summary: a report of the American College of Cardiology/American Heart Association Task Force on Practice Guidelines (Committee to Update the 1996 Guidelines on Perioperative Cardiovascular Evaluation for Noncardiac Surgery). Anesth Analg 94:1052-1064, 2002.

Fleisher LA, Eagle KA: Lowering cardiac risk in noncardiac surgery. N Engl J Med 345:1677-1682, 2001.

Landesberg G, Mosseri M, Wolf Y, Vesselov Y, Weissman C: Perioperative myocardial ischemia and infarction - identification by continuous 12-lead electrocardiogram with online ST-segment monitoring. Anesthesiology 96:264-270, 2002.

Mangano DT, Layug EL, Wallace A, Tateo I: Effect of atenolol on mortality and cardiovascular morbidity after noncardiac surgery. N Engl J Med 335:1713-1720, 1996. [Erratum, N Engl J Med 336:1039, 1997.]

Mangano DT for the Multicenter Study of Perioperative Ischemia Research Group: Aspirin and mortality from coronary artery bypass surgery. N Engl J Med 347:1309-1317, 2002.

Matot I, Oppenheim-Eden A, Ratrot R et al: Preoperative cardiac events in elderly patients with hip fracture randomized to epidural or conventional analgesia. Anesthesiology 98:156-163, 2003.

Mosca L: C-reactive protein - to screen or not to screen? N Engl J Med 347:1615-1617, 2002.

Nishina K, Mikawa K, Uesugi T et al: Efficacy of clonidine for prevention of perioperative myocardial ischemia - a critical appraisal and meta-analysis of the literature. Anesthesiology 96:323-329, 2002.

Poldermans D, Boersma E, Bax JJ et al: The effect of bisoprolol on perioperative mortality and myocardial infarction in high risk patients undergoing vascular surgery. N Engl J Med 341:1789-1794, 1999.

Pronovost PJ, Jenckes MW, Dorman T et al: Organizational characteristics of intensive care units related to outcomes of abdominal aortic surgery. JAMA 281:1310-1317, 1999.

Raby K, Brull S, Timimi F et al: The effect of heart rate control on myocardial ischemia among high-risk patients after vascular surgery. Anesth Analg 88:477-482, 1999.

Ross AF, Tinker JH: Evaluation of the adult patient with cardiac problems. In Rogers MC, Tinker JH, Covino BG, Longnecker DE, editors: *Principles and Practice of Anesthesiology*, Mosby Year Book, 1993, vol 11, pp 168-194.

Sandham JD, Hull RD, Brant RF et al for the Canadian Critical Care Clinical Trials Group: A randomized, controlled trial of the use of pulmonary-artery catheters in high-risk surgical patients. N Engl J Med 348:5-14, 2003.

Valentine RJ, Duke ML, Inman MH et al: Effectiveness of pulmonary artery catheters in aortic surgery: a randomized trial. J Vasc Surg 27:203-212, 1998.

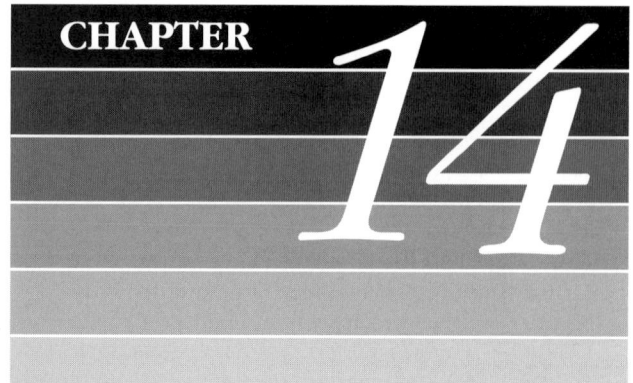

Adults with Congenital Heart Disease

JACEK A. WOJTCZAK, M.D., Ph.D.

Classification of Congenital Heart Defects
    Acyanotic Heart Defects
        Ventricular Septal Defect
        Atrial Septal Defect
        Patent Ductus Arteriosus
    Cyanotic Heart Defects
        Tetralogy of Fallot
        Transposition of the Great Arteries
        Tricuspid Atresia/Single Ventricle
    Obstructive Heart Defects
        Pulmonary Stenosis
        Coarctation of the Aorta
Noncardiac Complications of Congenital Heart Disease
    Pulmonary Complications
    Neurologic Complications
    Hematologic Complications
    Renal Complications
Management of Adult Patients with Congenital
    Heart Defects Requiring Critical Care and Anesthesia

Medical advances and refinement of surgical techniques have resulted in the survival of many children with congenital heart disease (CHD) to adulthood. However, for many adults with CHD further surgical interventions are necessary and the medical treatment and follow up are often life long. These patients may be assigned to different treatment categories such as a surgically cured group (e.g., an atrial septal defect repair), a surgically corrected group (anatomical correction with possible further surgery), or a surgically palliated group. There is also an "inoperable" group with conditions deemed inoperable except for organ transplantation and a medical group with no clinical indication for cardiac surgery.

Approximately 6–8% of CHD patients surviving to adulthood require hospitalization annually. Therefore, an increasing number of intensivists may be asked to care for these patients. This review is directed at the critical care specialists who will participate in their care.

CLASSIFICATION OF CONGENITAL HEART DEFECTS

Congenital heart defects can be classified as cyanotic, acyanotic, or obstructive (Table 14-1).

Acyanotic Heart Defects

Ventricular Septal Defect

Ventricular septal defect (VSD) is the most common congenital heart defect accounting for 25% of congenital heart lesions.

A small VSD, with a pulmonary/systolic flow ratio of less than 1.4, produces only a modest left-to-right shunt. Chest x-ray and ECG is usually normal as the left ventricle is not enlarged and there is no pulmonary hypertension. Clinical course is usually benign and the majority of these defects close spontaneously.

A moderate VSD results in a left-to-right shunt sufficient to produce significant pulmonary flow with a pulmonary/systemic flow ratio between 1.4 and 2.2. This flow will produce volume overload and enlargement of the left ventricle and left atrium.

These changes are even more pronounced with a large VSD which sometimes results in systemic pressure in the right ventricle. The pulmonary/systemic flow ratio is higher than 2.2. An infant with a large VSD and resulting severe pulmonary flow will eventually develop pulmonary vascular obstructive disease and chronic severe pulmonary hypertension (Eisenmenger's disease). Cyanosis will develop as the shunt reverses from left-to-right to right-to-left. Fixed high pulmonary vascular resistance precludes cardiac surgical correction.

A substantial percentage of VSDs undergo spontaneous regression in size or complete closure over time. Small VSDs have a higher risk of endocarditis but the life expectancy is normal. Moderate VSDs are unusual in the

Table 14-1 Classification of Congenital Heart Defects

ACYANOTIC (LEFT-TO-RIGHT SHUNT)
Ventricular septal defect
Atrial septal defect
Patent ductus arteriosus

CYANOTIC (RIGHT-TO-LEFT SHUNT)
Tetralogy of Fallot
Transposition of great arteries
Tricuspid atresia/single ventricle

OBSTRUCTIVE
Pulmonary stenosis
Coarctation of the aorta

adult but may occur if the defect is partially obstructed by a prolapsing leaflet of the aortic valve. Indications for surgical VSD closure include a pulmonary/systemic flow ratio higher than 2, pulmonary systolic pressure higher than 50 mmHg, and a progressive deterioration of ventricular function. Although this is a low-risk operation at any age, some of today's adults may have undergone surgery during an era when myocardial preservation and surgical techniques were not as good. Therefore, they may have some residual ventricular dysfunction, arrhythmias, and heart block. Aortic regurgitation may be present due to a prolapse of an aortic cusp or as a result of a suture placed through one of the aortic cusps during closure of a perimembranous VSD. Late ventricular arrhythmias and sudden cardiac death is a potential risk in patients repaired late in life. Heart block requiring pacemaker insertion may be seen occasionally, but is very rare.

Subacute bacterial endocarditis (SBE) antibiotic prophylaxis is recommended for 6 months following VSD closure and then is not necessary unless there is a residual defect.

Atrial Septal Defect

Atrial septal defect (ASD) accounts for about 7% of all cardiac anomalies. There are several types of ASD: primum, secundum, and sinus venosus. The *primum defects* (endocardial cushion defects) occur as large openings in the inferior atrial septum and often involve the mitral and tricuspid valves. Surgery carries slight risk of acquired heart block. Mitral valve rarely requires repair or replacement. The *secundum defects*, which are the most common ASD, occur in the center portion of the interatrial septum. Mitral valve prolapse is present in about 30% of patients. *Sinus venosus* defects are located at the posterosuperior atrial border adjacent to the superior vena cava. They are often associated with partial anomalous venous connection.

Unrepaired ASD allows asymptomatic survival to adulthood, but the death rate is about 6% over the age

of 40 years. Conditions that cause reduced left ventricular compliance during late adulthood (natural aging, systemic hypertension, or ischemic cardiomyopathy) will increase the left-to-right shunt through the ASD and the majority of patients over 60 years of age are symptomatic. Adult patients may develop moderate pulmonary hypertension, right ventricular overload, and late right heart failure (usually over the age of 40). The incidence of atrial fibrillation or flutter increases progressively after the age of 30.

Because of the preferential streaming of inferior vena caval flow towards the secundum ASD, uncorrected patients are at risk of paradoxical emboli from lower extremity thrombophlebitis or any other source. Incidents of air embolism into the left atrium have been reported with increases in intrathoracic pressure during a Valsalva maneuver or with high levels of positive end-expiratory pressure (PEEP).

Early closure of an ASD is recommended and there is no difference in survival between age- and sex-matched controls when surgery is carried out before the age of 24. Patients have an option of surgical or device closure. Early and intermediate outcome is excellent after device closure. Long-term outcome is unknown.

Supraventricular arrhythmias may persist after surgery in older patients. Atrial fibrillation may occur in about 30% of patients older than 40 years. Sick sinus syndrome may develop occasionally after the repair of a sinus venosus defect. A permanent pacemaker may be required for patients with sick sinus syndrome and symptomatic bradycardia.

SBE prophylaxis should be continued in patients with primum defects because of abnormalities of the mitral valve. The prophylaxis is not necessary for secundum and sinus venosus defects beyond 6 months after surgery.

Patent Ductus Arteriosus

Most patients with patent ductus arteriosus (PDA) are asymptomatic. When the magnitude of the left-to-right shunt is large, there may be evidence of left ventricular hypertrophy and increased pulmonary flow. A large PDA is rarely seen as a primary lesion in adults, but an occasional patient with a moderate-sized PDA may present in middle age in heart failure.

Adults with PDA and pulmonary vascular obstructive disease may have varying degrees of right-to-left shunting and symptoms related to pulmonary hypertension.

A large PDA is rare in adults but pulmonary hypertension is common and may not reverse with closure of the defect. Patients are symptomatic from dyspnea or palpitations.

It is generally recommended that a small or moderate PDA be closed by interventional catheterization techniques (coil closure). Surgical closure is reserved for the PDA too large for device closure. Postoperative complications may include recurrent laryngeal or phrenic nerve damage and thoracic duct damage. Residual ductal shunts may be encountered in patients who have had coil embolization procedures. If a small residual shunt remains, SBE prophylaxis is recommended, but when a PDA is eliminated SBE is not needed.

Cyanotic Heart Defects

Tetralogy of Fallot

This is a most common cyanotic lesion encountered in adults. Approximately 25% of unoperated patients will survive to adolescence but only 3% survive to the age of 40.

Tetralogy of Fallot (TOF) consists of the obstruction of the right ventricular outflow tract, VSD, right ventricular hypertrophy, and an aorta that overrides the pulmonary outflow tract. The clinical manifestations of TOF depend on the degree of stenosis of the right ventricular outflow tract and are due to right-to-left intracardiac shunts with reduced pulmonary outflow and arterial hypoxemia. About 35% of children with TOF develop hypercyanotic attacks or "tetralogy (tet) spells." They are due to a spasm of the infundibular cardiac muscle causing sudden reduction in pulmonary blood flow leading to severe hypoxemia, hypercapnia, and acidosis.

Surgical repair of TOF consists of closure of the VSD and enlargement of the right ventricular outflow tract. The majority of present-day adults who underwent a surgical TOF correction had the repair performed through a right ventriculotomy which may cause arrhythmias, decreased right ventricular function, and late right ventricular failure. Recently, the surgical technique has been changed and surgeons are using a transatrial approach.

Before the era of modern cardiac surgery, palliative procedures designed to increase pulmonary blood flow had been developed. They include Blalock–Taussig, Waterstone, and Potts shunts.

The Blalock–Taussig shunt consists of an anastomosis between the subclavian artery and ipsilateral pulmonary artery. The incidence of pulmonary hypertension is minimized with this shunt; however, complications include thrombosis of the shunt and the development of subclavian steal syndrome. A modified Blalock procedure employs a synthetic graft between the vessels and preserves the continuity of the subclavian artery.

The Waterstone shunt is a direct anastomosis between the ascending aorta and the right pulmonary artery. As the proper sizing of the anastomosis is difficult, an excessive pulmonary flow may lead to pulmonary hypertension.

The Potts shunt is a direct anastomosis between the descending thoracic aorta and the left pulmonary artery. This operation has been abandoned because of the resulting pulmonary hypertension and congestive heart failure.

The patient with a corrected TOF should be acyanotic and should not have any residual VSD. Pulmonary insufficiency is often present postoperatively but is usually well tolerated by patients. Only some patients develop significant pulmonary and tricuspid insufficiency with severe right ventricular dilatation and dysfunction.

The long-term prognosis for patients with repaired TOF is excellent, with nearly 90% survival at 30 years. Late sudden death due to ventricular arrhythmias is a recognized sequela of TOF repair with an overall prevalence of 3–6%. A sustained monomorphic ventricular tachycardia could be induced by programmed stimulation in 15–30% of patients and half had frequent and complex ECG. Sinus node dysfunction and intra-atrial re-entrant tachycardia occurred in 20–30% of patients with repaired TOF. In patients who have developed sustained ventricular tachycardia treatment options include antiarrhythmic drug therapy, map-guided ablation, surgery, and an implantable defibrillator.

Transposition of the Great Arteries

Transposition of the great arteries (TGA) results from failure of the truncus arteriosus to spiral. As a result, the aorta arises from the right ventricle and the pulmonary artery arises from the left ventricle. Complete TGA is a common congenital heart lesion accounting for about 7% of all congenital cardiac defects. To survive a patient with TGA must have communications between the left and right heart to allow mixing of the blood. Early survival at birth is possible when prostaglandin E1 is used to maintain ductal patency or a Rashkind balloon septostomy is performed to allow mixing. Patients with TGA never reach adulthood without having corrective surgery. The majority of patients who reach adulthood have undergone Mustard or Senning atrial switch procedures that create discordant atrioventricular connections in the presence of the preexisting discordant ventriculo-arterial connections. In the Mustard procedure the atrial septum is excised and a baffle made of native pericardium or synthetic material is used to redirect pulmonary and systemic venous blood. Systemic venous blood is routed to the left ventricle, which is connected to the pulmonary artery. Pulmonary venous blood is routed to the right ventricle, which is connected to the aorta. Baffle obstruction is one of the late complications after the Mustard procedure and may occur within months or a few years after the original operation. It has to be considered in any patient with otherwise unexplained peripheral edema, ascites, hepatomegaly, or pulmonary symptoms. However, late cardiac arrhythmias are the major problem after atrial switch procedures. Twenty percent of neonates have abnormal sinus node function or junctional rhythm when discharged from the hospital after atrial switch procedures. An increasing number of these patients gradually develop signs of sick sinus syndrome over the years. About 20% of these patients have had a pacemaker inserted because of severe bradyarrhythmias. Rapid atrial flutter and ventricular tachyarrhythmias are responsible for late sudden death in these patients. However, the majority of patient deaths are due to right ventricular dysfunction when the right ventricle, which becomes a systemic chamber, fails when subjected to abnormal afterload or preload.

Over the past ten years atrial switch operations have been replaced by the arterial switch operation (Jatene procedure). The arterial switch operation results in anatomic correction of the discordant ventriculoarterial connections. In this procedure the great arteries are transected distal to their respective valves and reconnected to their anatomically correct ventricles. A successful primary arterial switch must be performed within the first 10 days of life. The major issue in those patients who survive to adulthood is the status of the transferred coronary arteries; however, the incidence of coronary insufficiency is low. Supravalvular pulmonary stenosis is probably the most common complication of the arterial switch procedure. In contrast to the atrial switch procedures, electrophysiologic abnormalities are uncommon after the arterial switch procedure.

Tricuspid Atresia/Single Ventricle

Tricuspid atresia is characterized by a small right ventricle, a large left ventricle, tricuspid valve agenesis, and markedly reduced pulmonary blood flow. Therefore, it is a unique form of single ventricle, a term used to describe a group of CHDs in which there is abnormal development of both chambers, resulting in a single functioning ventricular chamber. All the blood from the right atrium is diverted across an atrial septal defect into the left atrium, mixes with oxygenated blood, and enters the left ventricle for ejection into the systemic circulation. Survival is possible if there is pulmonary flow through a ventricular septal defect or patent ductus arteriosus. To correct tricuspid atresia, the original Fontan operation was performed. Pulmonary flow was achieved by a right atrial to pulmonary artery connection. However, this direct connection leads to marked right atrial enlargement and the development of arrhythmias. The operation has undergone several modifications aimed at reducing the incidence of atrial arrhythmias. In one of the modifications inferior and superior vena caval blood flow is directed to the pulmonary arteries. Some surgeons have further modified this procedure by using an extracardiac conduit to connect the inferior vena cava to the pulmonary arteries. Therefore, patients who underwent Fontan procedures have circulation in series without the

ventricle driving the pulmonary flow and their survival depends on low pulmonary vascular resistance, low left ventricular filling pressure, and adequately high central venous pressure. Hypoxemia, hypercarbia, metabolic acidosis, high positive airway pressure, and hypovolemia may be detrimental in these patients.

Obstructive Heart Defects

Pulmonary Stenosis

Pulmonary stenosis accounts for as many as 8–10% of all congenital heart defects. It can be valvular (most common), supravalvular, or subpulmonary. Valvular pulmonary stenosis is often associated with a probe-patent foramen ovale and atrial septal defect.

Clinical manifestations will depend on the degree of obstruction to ejection of the right ventricle. Mild to moderate degrees of stenosis are often asymptomatic. Severe stenosis (gradient greater than 80 mmHg) causes right ventricular hypertrophy and failure. The surgical management of severe pulmonary stenosis with intact intraventricular septum has changed over the years from closed (no cardiopulmonary bypass) to open valvotomy (on bypass), and in the past few years balloon pulmonary valvulotomy became the preferred treatment method. However, if balloon pulmonary valvulotomy is ineffective in reducing the gradient, open valvotomy may be performed. Adult patients after these procedures are usually asymptomatic. Occasionally, an adult may require pulmonary valve replacement as a result of significant valvular obstruction and calcifications.

Coarctation of the Aorta

Coarctation is a discrete narrowing of the aorta either proximal to the ductus arteriosus (preductal, infantile) or distal to the left subclavian artery (postductal, adult). Infants with preductal coarctation of the aorta often have associated defects including patent ductus arteriosus, ventricular septal defect, and bicuspid aortic valve. They usually develop severe congestive heart failure as a result of this defect. After infancy coarctation is rarely associated with significant symptoms and is often diagnosed during routine physical examination when systolic murmur is detected in the second space at the left sternal border. Upper extremity hypertension and reduced pressure in the lower extremities is present. In older patients coarctation usually presents as an isolated lesion. Complications of unoperated coarctation include left ventricular hypertrophy and heart failure, cerebral hemorrhage or thrombosis, rupture of the aorta, and necrotizing arteritis. Surgical corrections include the removal of the coarcted region and end-to-end anastomosis, subclavian artery flap procedure, or patch angioplasty. The prognosis after repair of isolated coarctation is very good; however, complications include restenosis, late hypertension, and aneurysmal dilatation of the aorta.

NONCARDIAC COMPLICATIONS OF CONGENITAL HEART DISEASE

Pulmonary Complications

Dynamic lung compliance is decreased in patients with increased pulmonary blood flow (left-to-right shunt) and is unchanged in patients with decreased pulmonary blood flow. The mechanism for this change is not clear. However, it is possible that the increase in pulmonary artery pressure may result in an increase in the tension of the walls of the pulmonary vascular system. This "stiffer" vasculature may then oppose pulmonary expansion resulting in decreased lung compliance, which in turn increases the work of breathing. Enlarged pulmonary vessels may compress bronchi or cause a congestion and swelling of the bronchial wall, an increase in small airway resistance, chronic atelectasis, pneumonia, or focal emphysema. The likely site of compression by the enlarged left pulmonary artery is the left mainstem and upper lobe bronchi and the right middle lobe bronchus may be compressed by the right lower lobe pulmonary artery. An enlarged pulmonary artery can also compress the recurrent laryngeal nerve.

Patients with high pulmonary blood flow secondary to a large VSD or ASD, if not treated, will develop a pulmonary arteriolar injury secondary to sheer stress, leading to muscular hypertrophy, intimal proliferation, and obliteration of arterioles. As the vascular disease progresses and the pulmonary vascular resistance approaches systemic resistance, a right-to-left shunt develops, and the patient becomes cyanotic and polycythemic. This pathophysiologic sequence is described as Eisenmenger's syndrome. The presence of this syndrome precludes surgical correction of the defects, as pulmonary resistance is irreversibly elevated. These patients may have upper lobe pulmonary artery thrombosis and hemoptysis in end-stage disease.

Patients with CHD have blunted responses to hypoxemia but normal ventilatory response to hypercarbia. The oxygen–hemoglobin dissociation curve is normal or slightly right shifted. In cyanotic patients arterial pCO_2 is underestimated by capnometry (end-tidal pCO_2). In these patients even moderate hypercarbia and hypoxemia will increase pulmonary vascular resistance and right-to-left shunting.

Chronic pleural effusions are fairly common in adult patients who have had a Fontan procedure.

Neurologic Complications

Major neurologic complications of CHD include brain abscesses and paradoxical cerebral embolization. Paradoxical emboli originating in the lower part of the body in poorly mobile or postoperative adult patients might reach the brain in cyanotic patients with a right-to-left shunt or during a reversal of the shunt in patients with left-to-right shunt. The emboli may also originate from the intravenous lines and especially during placement and use of central venous and Swan-Ganz catheters. Air filters should be used in all venous lines in patients with CHD. Hyperviscosity and reduction in cerebral blood flow in patients with very high hematocrits may also play a role in increasing the risk of cerebrovascular accidents in patients with CHD.

Patients with atrial fibrillation after late closure of an ASD have a high risk of TIA or stroke and may be anticoagulated for the first six postoperative months. Anticoagulation may be later discontinued, if patients remain arrhythmia-free.

Adults with cyanotic CHD have a decreased risk of thrombotic intracranial events but a higher risk of intracranial bleeding. A cerebral hemorrhage can occur in patients with a history of aortic coarctation repair even if blood pressure is not elevated.

Patients who have already undergone successful correction or palliation of CHD may have residual neurologic deficits related to the preoperative pathology as well as to intraoperative (e.g., hypothermic circulatory arrest) or postoperative events. These significant symptomatic hyperviscosity neurologic sequelae may include seizures, dyskinesia, hypotonia, or choreoathetosis.

Patients with CHD may have an injury of the recurrent laryngeal nerve from prior surgery or compression by the pulmonary artery. They may also have diaphragmatic paresis or paralysis secondary to phrenic nerve injury.

Hematologic Complications

Patients with cyanotic CHD are usually polycythemic or erythrocytotic (an increase only in red cell number). Polycythemia is an adaptive response to chronic hypoxemia. Hypoxia triggers the release of erythropoietin by the kidneys. Erythropoietin stimulates bone marrow production of red cells and causes an increase in the circulating blood volume. As the hematocrit increases, there is a marked increase in viscosity. The increased viscosity and erythrocytosis is associated with the risk thrombosis in children under the age of 5 years, especially when they are febrile or dehydrated. Due to high hematocrits and limited pulmonary and systemic blood flows some patients will complain of fatigue, faintness, headache, dizziness, blurred vision or diplopia, myalgias and muscle weakness, paresthesias of fingers, toes and lips, and depressed mentation. Isovolemic phlebotomies are indicated in these patients based more on the development of significant symptoms of hyperviscosity rather than for a given hematocrit. Dehydration must be first ruled out before any decision to phlebotomize is made.

Patients with current or even corrected cyanotic heart disease have a higher incidence of bilirubin gallstones and billiary colic.

About 20% of patients with CHD, both cyanotic and acyanotic, have a variety of hemostatic abnormalities. They include platelet dysfunction, thrombocytopenia, hypofibrinogenemia, fibrinolysis, and abnormalities of the intrinsic and extrinsic coagulation systems with deficiencies of specific clotting factors. Patients may be very symptomatic with complaints of easy bruising, epistaxis, or excessive menstrual bleeding.

Prothrombin and partial thromboplastin time may be prolonged. The risk of spontaneous bleeding is low but the risk of excessive perioperative bleeding is fairly high, especially in patients who are maintained on platelet inhibitors (aspirin) due to their vascular anastomoses from Goretex (e.g., modified Blalock–Taussig anastomosis). Moreover, excessive bleeding may be caused by an increased tissue vascularity in cyanotic patients, increased venous pressure, and collateral vessels in obstructive defects (e.g., coarctation).

Renal Complications

Patients with CHD have a variety of renal abnormalities. They may be related to renal hypoperfusion hypoxia and hyperviscosity. These patients usually have high plasma uric levels, due to low fractional uric acid excretion rather than to urate overproduction. Hyperuricemia in CHD patients may be a marker of abnormal intrarenal hemodynamics, as the enhanced uric acid reabsorption is a result of renal hypoperfusion and high filtration fraction.

Glomerular enlargement and alteration in the glomerular capillary basement membrane have been described in patients with CHD and appear to be a result of hypoxia at an early age. These changes are associated with benign proteinuria and contribute to the higher incidence of nephrotic syndrome in these patients. Renal plasma flow is reduced in patients with cyanotic and acyanotic lesions and is due to the changes in the outer cortical flow. Successful surgical correction of CHD may not result in a return of the renal plasma flow to normal.

MANAGEMENT OF ADULT PATIENTS WITH CONGENITAL HEART DEFECTS REQUIRING CRITICAL CARE AND ANESTHESIA

Evaluation of patients with known CHD should be directed toward obtaining a complete description of anatomy of the defect and a description of all previous surgical procedures and detection of possible residual defects, sequelae, or late complications. For example, a history of continued postoperative hypoxemia indicates inadequate palliation and the existence of residual abnormalities. However, distinguishing between cardiac and pulmonary causes of hypoxemia may be extremely difficult.

A minimal workup should include a thorough clinical assessment, ECG, chest x-ray, and transthoracic (TTE) or transesophageal echocardiographic (TEE) examination. TTE and TEE may help to prove the existence of the lesion or residual shunt, better define its location, and rule out chamber enlargement, baffle obstruction, valvular insufficiency, or ventricular outflow obstruction.

Confirmed existence of an intracardiac shunt has several implications in the acute management of the critically ill or anesthetized patient.

Left-to-right shunts will result in pulmonary vascular overperfusion; however, initially ventilation and gas exchange are usually unaffected. These patients may have a history of pulmonary banding to control the pulmonary flow. In unrepaired patients one may expect marked pulmonary hypertension. The presence of pulmonary hypertension can be inferred from the marked right ventricular hypertrophy on the ECG and prominent main pulmonary artery on the chest x-ray. It can be confirmed either noninvasively by Doppler echocardiography or by Swan-Ganz catheterization. However, placement of a flow-directed catheter may be very difficult due to the flow through the intracardiac shunt. Left atrial pressure may be elevated due to increased pulmonary venous return. Increased volume workload may cause reduced myocardial contractility. These patients might require treatment with intravenous pulmonary vasodilators (e.g., milrinone, prostaglandin E_1) as well as the use of inhaled nitric oxide (NO). Some patients are at risk of pulmonary hypertensive crisis, which is easier to prevent than to reverse. Therefore, not only are vasodilators needed but patients should be hyperventilated ($PaCO_2 = 25-30$) and well sedated (fentanyl and propofol infusions).

As discussed above, enlargement of pulmonary vessels may result in extrinsic compression of the airways or congestion of the bronchial wall and an increase in small airway resistance as well as alveolar edema. An increased resistance to airflow combined with noncompliant lungs will increase the inspiratory pressure needed for adequate positive-pressure ventilation.

Anesthetics that may induce myocardial depression should be avoided. The uptake of inhaled anesthetic agents and therefore their cardiodepressive effects may be increased.

Right-to-left shunts will result in low PaO_2, only minimally improved by increasing the FIO_2. The ventilatory support and gas exchange will be less efficient. Capnometry (end-tidal pCO_2 measurements) will underestimate the arterial pCO_2 due to the large physiologic dead space. As the pulmonary flow is decreased management should be centered on the prevention of further reduction in flow. Therefore, excessive positive inspiratory pressure should be avoided and PEEP maintained at the lowest possible level. Adequate intravascular volume and ventricular function should be maintained.

Patients with right-to-left shunts are at high risk of systemic emboli from lower extremity thrombophlebitis and venous air embolism. They are also at risk of overdose with intravenous drugs. However, if inhalational anesthetics are used during anesthesia, one may expect a delayed uptake of inhaled agents.

Polycythemia may be present in cyanotic patients and should be carefully controlled either with phlebotomy or hemodilution, but the hematocrit should not be taken below 50. Despite the dangers of polycythemia, these patients are very dependent on high hematocrit to ensure adequate oxygen transport.

Obstructive defects will result in fixed stroke volume and dependence on heart rate to compensate for changes in metabolic demand and peripheral vascular resistance. Left or right ventricular hypertrophy and congestive heart failure will develop without corrective surgery. Therefore, optimal myocardial perfusion should be maintained in those patients by increasing the duration of diastole and the diastolic pressure. Tachycardia, which shortens diastole, should be avoided. Blood pressure should be maintained with pressors and volume.

Management of *arrhythmias* secondary to repaired, unrepaired, or palliated CHD may be extremely difficult. History of early postoperative arrhythmias is associated with a greater risk for development arrhythmias late in life. The spectrum of clinical consequences of arrhythmia in adults with CHD ranges from clinically occult arrhythmia to sudden death. Atrial arrhythmias are most common and are usually due to intra-atrial re-entrant tachycardia that may respond to class 1A and class 3 antiarrhythmic drugs. Automatic antitachycardia pacing has also been of value in some patients. Patients with unrepaired heart disease or residual obstructive lesions are more prone to atrial fibrillation. Sinus rhythm is hemodynamically preferred in CHD; therefore, cardioversion, antiarrhythmic drugs (e.g., amiodarone), and atrial pacing should be used to treat or prevent establishment of atrial fibrillation.

Gradual loss of sinus rhythm occurs after the Mustard, Senning, and all varieties of Fontan procedures. Interventricular conduction abnormalities, particularly right bundle branch block, are very common after surgery for CHD. Cardiac pacing in adults with CHD presents a variety of challenges. Anatomical abnormalities and shunting may not allow endocardial lead placement and require transthoracic pacing.

Ventricular arrhythmias are reported in about 2% of patients with repaired TOF. Although patients with Mustard, Senning, and Fontan experience atrial tachycardias, they are not prone to ventricular tachycardias. Class 1C and class 3 antiarrhythmic drugs should be used to suppress symptomatic ventricular arrhythmias.

Automatic implantable cardioverter and defibrillator therapy is feasible in many patients with CHD.

SELECTED READING

Bancalari E, Jesse M, Gelband H et al: Lung mechanics in congenital heart disease with increased and decreased pulmonary flow. J Pediatr 90:192-195, 1977.

Baum V: The adult with congenital heart disease. J Cardiothor Vasc Anesthesia 10:261-282, 1996.

Gersony W, Rosenbaum M: *Congenital Heart Disease in the Adult*, New York: McGraw-Hill, 2002.

Lake C: *Pediatric Cardiac Anesthesia*, Stamford, CA: Appleton & Lange, 1997.

Nollert G, Fishlein T, Bouterwek S et al: Long-term survival in patients with repair of tetralogy of Fallot: 36-year follow-up of 490 survivors of the first year after surgical repair. J Am Coll Cardiol 30:1374-1383, 1997.

Perloff J, Rosove M, Child J et al: Adults with cyanotic congenital heart disease: hematologic management. Ann Intern Med 109:406-413, 1988.

Perloff J, Warnes C: Challenges posed by adults with repaired congenital heart disease. Circulation 103:2637-2643, 2001.

CHAPTER 15

Pneumonia in Adults

JAMES E. SZALADOS, M.D., J.D., M.B.A.

The incidence of pneumonia is increasing. The exact annual incidence of pneumonia is difficult to determine because it is not a notifiable disease. The incidence varies with geography, population demographics, comorbid conditions, and the severity of the flu season. There are approximately 4 million cases of community-acquired pneumonia and at least 300,000 cases of hospital-acquired pneumonia reported annually. Pneumonia accounts for the largest mortality of any common infectious disease. Pneumonia ranks in the top seven among the major leading causes of death in adults in the USA. It is the fourth leading cause of death in the US elderly population. A large variety of organisms cause pneumonia (Table 15-1). The important complications of pneumonia include abscess formation, pleural effusion and empyema formation, bacteremia and sepsis, septic shock, acute respiratory distress syndrome (ARDS), meningitis, endocarditis, and multiple organ dysfunction or failure.

The rapid initiation of broad-spectrum empirical antibiotic therapy correlates with long-term morbidity and mortality from pneumonia. The earlier the specific infectious agent is appropriately treated the better the outcome is likely to be.

CLINICAL CAVEAT

Treatment of Serious Infection

Serious infection should be treated as a medical emergency and antibiotics must be initiated as soon as possible; there should be no delay in obtaining cultures or awaiting culture and sensitivity data.

The Centers for Disease Control (CDC) defines pneumonia to be present when the chest radiograph reveals a new or progressive infiltrate, pleural effusion, or cavitation, *and any one* of the following: (1) a change in the character, quantity, or consistency of the sputum, (2) the pathogen is isolated from the lower respiratory tract, by cultures, or by lung biopsy, (3) a virus or viral antigen is isolated in respiratory secretions, (4) a diagnostic serum IgM antibody titer or a fourfold rise in IgG antibody titers can be demonstrated in paired serum samples, (5) histologic evidence of pneumonia can be demonstrated in tissue biopsy. Note that these general criteria do not include sputum Gram stain or culture.

Pneumonia treatment is simplified by numerous guidelines which are described below. The standard of medical care for the management of pneumonia has evolved considerably over the last decade based on large multicenter outcome studies. The present evidence-based

Table 15-1 Pneumonia Pathogens

TYPICAL PATHOGENS

Gram-positive cocci: *Streptococcus pneumoniae, Staphylococcus aureus* and VISA, GISA, and VRSA, *Enterococcus faecalis, Enterobacter faecium* and VRE/VREF

Gram-positive bacilli: *Bacillus anthracis, Corynebacterium diphtheriae*

Gram-negative diplococci: *Moraxella catarralis*

Gram-negative bacilli: *Haemophilus influenzae, Klebsiella pneumoniae, Pseudomonas aeruginosa, Proteus mirabilis, Proteus morgagnii, Serratia marcescens,* Enterobacteriaceae

ATYPICAL PATHOGENS

Legionella pneumophilia (Legionnaire's disease)
Mycoplasma pneumoniae ("walking pneumonia")
Chlamydia pneumonia (previously "TWAR" agent)
Coxiella burnettii (Q fever)
Francisella tularensis (tularemia)
Bacillus anthracis (anthrax)
Yersinia pestis (pneumonic plague)
Mycoplasma tuberculosis (tuberculosis)
M. avium-intracellulare
Chlamydia psittaci (psittacosis or "parrot fever")
Pneumocystis carinii (PCP)

VIRUSES

Influenza A, B, others
Parainfluenza 1, 2, 3
Respiratory syncytial virus (RSV)
Epstein–Barr virus (EBV)
Hantavirus
Herpes virus (HSV I and II)
Varicella zoster
Respiratory syncytial virus
Cytomegalovirus (CMV)
SARS

MYCOSES

Cryptococcus
Histoplasmosis
Coccidiomycosis
Blastomycosis
Aspergillus spp.
Candida spp.

approach is based on best-practice data regarding diagnosis, risk stratification, and antibiotic management protocols. However, evolving patterns of antibiotic resistance, emerging pathogens, and new antibiotics require continual reassessment of existing guidelines. There is also sufficient variability between hospitals to require individualization of therapy based on local or institutional antibiogram data.

There is a clear genetic component to the risk of pneumonia and sepsis. Genetic polymorphism for molecules important in antigen recognition and binding such

as mannose-binding lectin, CD-14, and toll-like receptors as well as for inflammatory mediators such as tumor necrosis factor, the interleukin-1 family, interleukin-10, and angiotensin converting enzyme are likely to have pharmacologic significance.

There are a great many noninfectious diseases that cause febrile pneumonitis and mimic pneumonia. These include eosinophilic pneumonia, interstitial lung disease associated with connective tissue disorders or vasculitis or pulmonary airway disease, neoplasms, sarcoidosis, ARDS, exposure to inhaled gases or toxins, radiation pneumonitis, cytotoxin therapy, and pulmonary infarction.

Noncytotoxic pharmacologic agents which can mimic a pneumonia include antimicrobial agents, phenytoin, amiodarone, and narcotics. Aspiration pneumonitis, Mendelson's syndrome, occurs following aspiration of acidic gastric content and may present the lobar infiltrate progressing to a generalized pneumonitis (Figure 15-1). Antibiotic therapy is not indicated in the initial treatment of aspiration pneumonitis.

The general typical presentation of a pneumonia is that of a systemic inflammatory response syndrome (SIRS) with evidence of a widened arteriolar-alveolar oxygen diffusion gradient. History and physical examination and microbiologic or serologic studies help confirm the diagnosis.

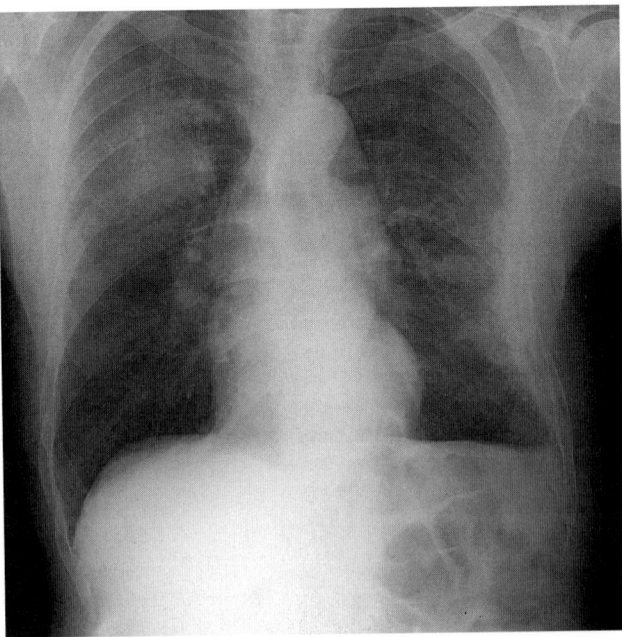

Figure 15-1 Aspiration pneumonitis. There is pseudolobar consolidation of the right upper and left lung fields. The accentuated interstitial markings with early alveolar changes reflect evolving local inflammation. Notably, the distribution of early aspiration pneumonitis findings depends on the patient's position at the time of aspiration and need not be localized to lower lung fields.

RISK FACTORS FOR AND MECHANISMS OF PNEUMONIA DEVELOPMENT

The risk factors that determine the virulence and severity of pneumonia are related to both pathogen and host characteristics. Characteristics of the pathogen include the organism, its resistance characteristics, its virulence, and the dose of the inoculum. Host factors are commonly divided into alterations of mucosal integrity or impaired immunity. Mucosal integrity can be compromised by epithelial injury ("viral priming"), mechanical injury such as endotracheal tubes or repetitive mucosal trauma resulting from vigorous tracheal suctioning, chemical injury from aspiration of gastric contents, tobacco abuse, and malnutrition. Impaired host immunity may be due to systemic immunosuppression due to infection, malignancy, malnutrition, liver or renal failure, diabetes mellitus; or the exposure to immunosuppressant agents such as steroids, chemotherapeutic agents, toxins, or pharmaceuticals with immunosuppressant side effects. Notably, blood transfusions have been demonstrated to suppress systemic immunity and to increase the risk of nosocomial infections including pneumonia.

CLINICAL CAVEAT

Aspiration
- Aspiration of oropharyngeal secretions is especially common in patients with depressed levels of consciousness due to intoxication, sedation, or central nervous system dysfunction.
- Disorders of deglutition due to neuromuscular disorders, gastroesophageal reflux, esophageal dysmotility, or prolonged nasogastric intubation also predispose to the aspiration of pooled secretions.

The lung is the body organ with the largest epithelial surface area in continuous contact with the external environment and therefore it is vulnerable. An area of approximately 70 m^2 participates in gas exchange and is continually exposed to airborne inorganic and organic particles, as well as microorganisms. Pulmonary infection can be caused by inhalation of aerosolized inoculate, aspiration of secretions or particulate matter, hematogenous spread, or direct inoculation. The most common mechanism of pneumonia development is by contamination of the naso-oropharynx or upper airway, and subsequent aspiration of infected secretions into the distal respiratory tree. In otherwise healthy patients, pharyngeal secretions have a bacterial concentration of approximately 10^{10} organisms/ml. Therefore, aspiration of exceedingly small volumes (<0.1 ml) introduces a high-titer bacterial inoculum into the respiratory tract. In patients with incapacitating or coexisting disease, decreased salivary flow, decreased cough reflexes, or poor oral hygiene (such as occurs in intubated and mechanically ventilated patients) the bacterial, viral, and fungal load of pharyngeal secretions is both greater and more virulent, and therefore a significant risk factor to the development of pneumonia.

Patients with chronic or acute sinusitis and postnasal drip are at risk for the aspiration of contaminated nasopharyngeal secretions. Rarely, in patients with pharyngeal pouches or esophageal (Zenker's) diverticuli, sequestered secretions and food particles may be aspirated during sleep.

One of the causes of contamination of the lung with organisms is the ventilator. The ventilator circuit regularly develops stagnant water as condensate which becomes rapidly colonized with pathogenic bacteria. If this water is inadvertently washed into the endotracheal tube, pneumonia results. Patients who undergo elective surgical tracheostomy must have their oropharynx well suctioned and preferably also decontaminated prior to deflation of the endotracheal tube cuff. A large number of ventilator-associated pneumonias inadvertently result from aspiration of pooled oropharyngeal secretions during the tracheostomy procedure.

Epithelial damage predisposes to successful pathogen colonization and the development of an infective nidus. Such epithelial injury can be caused by chronic or acute lung diseases such as environmental toxins, tobacco abuse, genetic predisposition such as alpha-1 antitrypsin deficiency, or chronic aspiration syndromes. Notably, mucociliary clearance is diminished in smokers and prior infections with *Mycoplasma pneumoniae*, viruses, and *Haemophilus influenza* have been shown to both destroy cilia and impair ciliary function. Additionally, the SIRS alters epithelial structure and function.

The presence of the endotracheal tube has been demonstrated in itself to inhibit synchronized ciliary motility. Therefore mucociliary clearance is impaired in intubated patients. Cytologic studies demonstrate structural changes in epithelial glycoprotein binding characteristics, mucus production, ciliary function, surfactant protein composition and concentration, and extracellular enzymatic profiles during severe systemic illness and which are thought to provide a critical initial link to bacterial adhesion, colonization, and infection. Fibronectin is an epithelial coating found on normal mucosa which prevents Gram-negative pathogens from adhering to respiratory epithelium. Loss of fibronectin facilitates bacterial pneumonia development after viral infections, for example. Hematogenous seeding of the lung from other infected sites is another possibility for the development of pneumonia. Infected prostheses, intravascular devices, or endocarditis and even possibly bacterial translocation from the lumen of ischemic abdominal viscus are potential sources of secondary or metastatic infection. Tumors compromise tissue integrity and suppress immunity. Tumors both predispose to colonization and local invasion but also are an important cause of postobstructive inspissation of mucus and secretions.

There is also a hypothesis whereby bacteria are thought to translocate from the gut lumen into the surrounding venous and lymphatic plexuses and induce generalized inflammation or bacteremia and this has been termed the "gut motor hypothesis."

DIAGNOSIS OF PNEUMONIA

Radiologic Diagnosis of Pneumonia

The chest radiograph is the mainstay of radiologic diagnosis and follow-up of pneumonia. The radiologic picture may lag behind the clinical condition. Interobserver variability remains a limitation to radiologic diagnosis. The radiologic appearance of hospital- and ventilator-acquired pneumonias is difficult to distinguish from atelectasis. However, serial radiographs may reveal atelectasis to resolve more rapidly. It is widely believed but unproven that a patient's hydration status affects the radiologic appearance of an underlying pneumonia. Therefore, the contention that a chest radiograph of a dehydrated patient is less likely to reveal a pneumonia-related infiltrate is an unreliable although attractive hypothesis.

Radiologic infiltrates may be more difficult to identify in patients with hyperexpanded lung fields (COPD), fibrosis and scars, atelectasis, and pulmonary edema. The radiologic appearance of pneumonia has traditionally resulted in a general classification based on appearance and distribution. Alveolar consolidation may occur as a result of inflammatory edema in alveolar segments. When the consolidation involves the entire lobe, it is called lobar pneumonia. Characteristics of lobar pneumonia include air bronchograms, volume loss, and mediastinal shift toward the side of consolidation. Consolidated pneumonias frequently occur with *S. pneumoniae* and *Klebsiella pneumoniae* (Figure 15-2). Air bronchograms demonstrate an air–soft tissue interface; they are especially helpful in the indirect delineation of consolidation posterior to the heart in the left hemithorax.

Bronchopneumonia, or lobular pneumonia, involves an inflammatory response primarily at the site of the bronchi and surrounding parenchyma tissue. Bronchopneumonia is usually seen as segmental or patchy infiltrates consistent with partial segmental consolidation. Consolidation is more likely to be locally segmental and involvement of the parenchyma more patchy with bronchopneumonia than with lobar pneumonia.

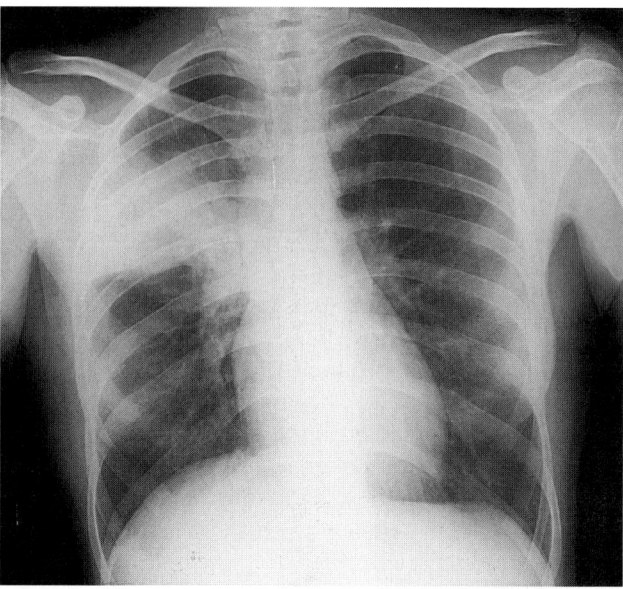

Figure 15-2 Lobar pneumonia. Pneumococcal pneumonia. Anterior segment of the right upper lobe is densely consolidated but there is little, if any, mediastinal shift. No effusion is present.

Bronchopneumonia is especially common when a pneumonic process is superimposed on underlying chronic bronchitis or bronchiectasis. Bronchopneumonias are commonly seen with *H. influenzae*, *S. aureus*, and *C. pneumoniae* (Figure 15-3).

Interstitial pneumonias, also known as peribronchovascular infiltrates, typically appear as reticular or reticulonodular patterns reflecting inflammation primarily localized to the interstitial tissue. Interstitial prominence resembles the early stages of pulmonary edema and is also associated with noninfectious causes of interstitial lung disease which must be included in the differential diagnosis. This interstitial picture is especially common with *M. pneumoniae*, *P. carinii*, other atypical organisms, and viruses. The radiologic appearance of *Mycoplasma* pneumonia is a unilateral or bilateral lobar or segmental infiltrate that shows a patchy or confluent air space disease. More severe cases reveal a diffuse bilateral reticulonodular pattern in both lung fields (Figure 15-4).

Nodular infiltrates are typically well-defined focal lesions greater than 1 cm^2 on chest radiographs. Nodular infiltrates may be abscesses, fungal or tuberculous granulomas, malignancy, Wegener's granulomatosis, or the necrotic vascular lesions that accompany severe *P. aeruginosa* infection. Nodular infiltrates may suggest histoplasmosis or tuberculosis. Cavitation is often associated with staphylococcal pneumonia or infection with *Aspergillus*. There is no good correlation between the radiologic appearance and the causative pathogen.

Pneumonia may be accompanied by pleural fluid collections known as parapneumonic infiltrates (Figure 15-5).

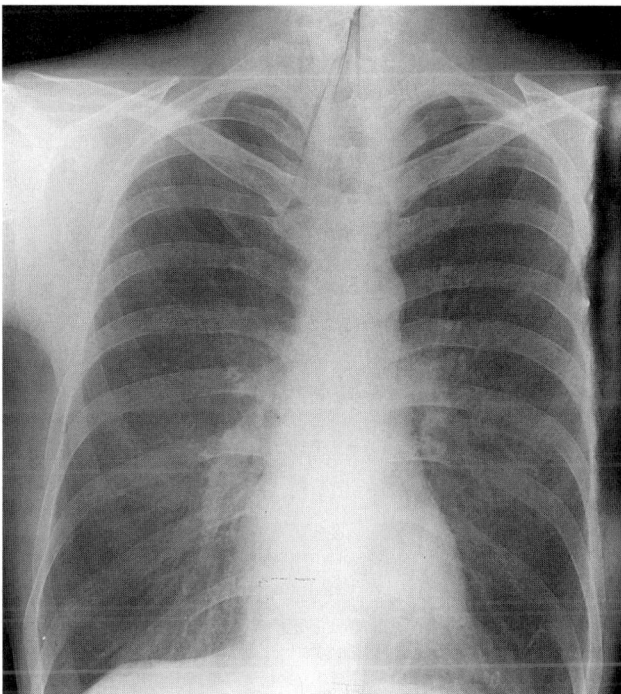

Figure 15-3   Bilateral bronchopneumonia. Radiograph reveals bilateral confluent infiltrates in pulmonary lobules (lobular pneumonia). The inflammation involves the terminal respiratory bronchioles.

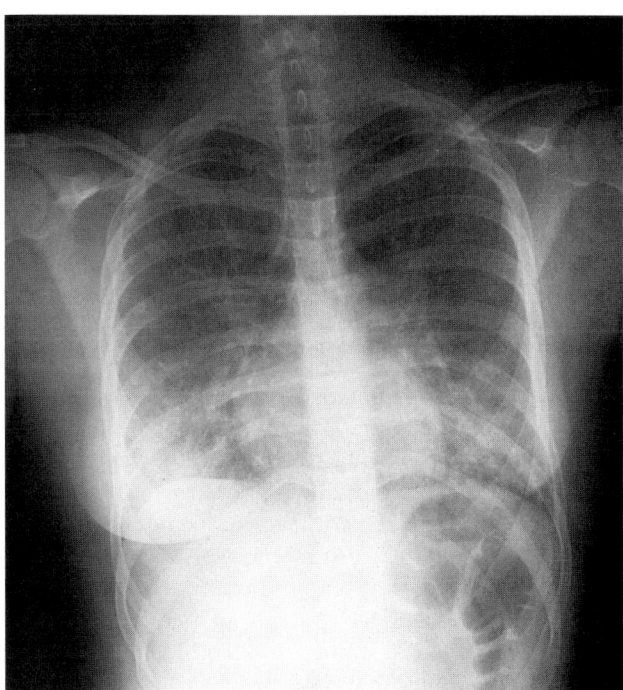

Figure 15-4   Mycoplasma pneumonia. Bilateral lower lobe infiltrates with prominent interstitial markings. The classic radiographic interstitial of "atypical pneumonia" process reveals accentuated reticular markings within the lung parenchyma as well as septal (Kerly A and B) lines. Air bronchograms are clearly visible bilaterally indicating lung consolidation which accentuates the air–tissue interface. There is no hilar prominence.

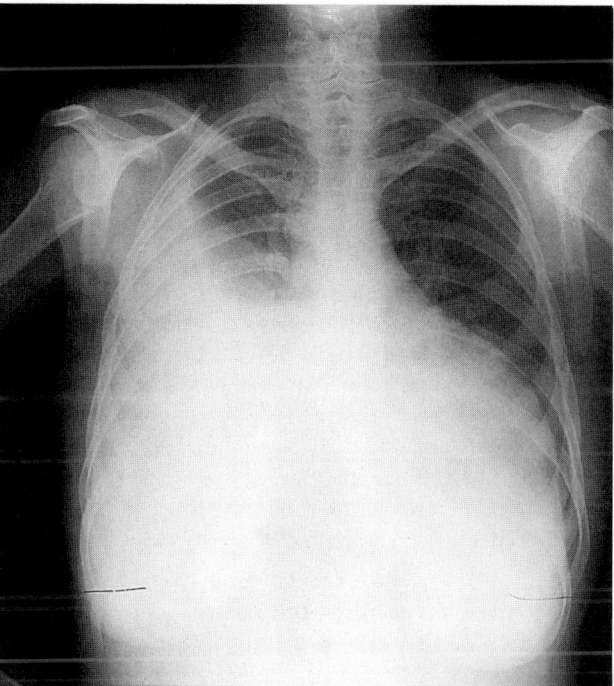

Figure 15-5   Right pleural effusion. There is a characteristic fluid meniscus on the right and there is evidence of some aeration within the right lower lobe. The underlying pneumonia is not apparent in this view but could be defined in a lateral decubitus view after the surrounding fluid layers away from the pulmonary tissue.

These may resolve or progress to organized empyemas which may be generalized or loculated.

Nonradiologic Diagnosis of Pneumonia

Direct microscopic examination of the Gram-stained sputum has major diagnostic value. The Gram stain is inexpensive, easily available, and has the advantage of immediacy. The sputum Gram stain can help guide antibiotic therapy based on the prevalence of Gram-positive or Gram-negative organisms. The false negative rate for sputum cultures obtained by expectoration is greater than 50%. The quality of sputum is determined by the presence of epithelial cells which indicate oropharyngeal contamination. The presence of >25 squamous epithelial cells per low-power field (×100) is indicative of specimen contamination with oropharyngeal secretions. The presence of one or more macrophages indicates that the sputum sample has been obtained from the lower respiratory tract. The presence of elastin fibers in a sputum sample smear prepared with 40% potassium hydroxide indicates that the specimen has been obtained from the lower respiratory tract and also indicates the presence of a necrotizing pulmonary process. The presence of ≥25 neutrophils per low-power field indicates infection such as pneumonia or tracheobronchitis. Sputum is plated on

Table 15-2	Serologic Testing for Pneumonia Diagnosis
S. pneumoniae	Serum, urine, or sputum counter-immunoelectrophoresis
	Latex agglutination
	Coagglutination
	Enzyme immunoassay
Legionella spp.	Urine or sputum direct fluorescent antigen detection test (DFA)
	Sputum polymerase chain reaction test
	Sputum indirect immunofluorescence antibody
	Serum enzyme immunoassay
Chlamydia	Serum polymerase chain reaction
	Serum complement fixation
	Serum micro immunofluorescence
	Serum enzyme immunoassay
Mycoplasma	Serum immunoglobulin IgM ("cold agglutinin")
	Serum polymerase chain reaction
	Serum complement fixation
Coxiella	Serum indirect immunofluorescence

culture media to determine innoculum density (colony forming units or cfu), definitive identification of colony types, and antibiotic susceptibility profiles.

CLINICAL CAVEAT

Sputum Cultures

Sputum cultures that are obtained after the initiation of empiric antibiotic therapy will yield a lower incidence of true positives but a greater incidence of false negatives.

Fever in the critically ill patient is a nonspecific sign of inflammation and does not always reflect the presence of underlying infection. Also, elevated liver function tests may occur with any infection and reflect a nonspecific finding but is often associated with *Legionella*, tuberculosis, *Mycoplasma*, Q fever, tularemia, and psittacosis.

Serologic testing is one of the most important diagnostic modalities to identify organisms that are not easily cultured (Table 15-2).

CLASSIFICATION AND TREATMENT OF PNEUMONIA

Community-Acquired Pneumonia

Community-acquired pneumonia (CAP) accounts for 10% of all medical intensive care unit (ICU) admissions. Approximately 50% of ICU patients with CAP will require mechanical ventilation. The incidence of CAP is

approximately 12 cases per 1000 adults per year in the USA, accounting for almost one million hospital admissions per year. The cost of treating CAP exceeds $10 billion per year in the USA. Although approximately three-quarters of patients with CAP are successfully managed as outpatients, those that require hospitalization account disproportionately for pneumonia-related health care costs. Since the cost of inpatient management of pneumonia exceeds the cost of outpatient care by at least a factor of 15, it is estimated that 90% of the total costs of treating CAP are hospital-related. The mean duration of hospitalization for CAP is 9 days, which includes both routine hospitalization as well as intensive care stay. The average mortality from CAP averages 40%. When CAP is complicated by ARDS, which occurs in approximately 5% of patients with CAP, the mortality rate approaches 70%.

Risk factors for CAP include chronic respiratory or cardiac disease, institutionalization, advanced age, and alcoholism. Additionally, dysphagia and sedation increase the risk for both aspiration and nonaspiration pneumonia in the elderly population. Risk factors for mortality from CAP include multi-lobar infiltrates, positive blood cultures, rapidly progressive infiltrates, polymicrobial infection, hypoalbuminemia, renal insufficiency, respiratory failure, serious comorbidities or advanced age, immunosuppression, altered mental status or coma, and prolonged mechanical ventilation.

Prevention may be an important strategy to reduce the impact of CAP, especially in vulnerable populations such as the elderly. Tobacco and alcohol abuse cessation programs may improve pulmonary function, mucus clearance, and decrease the risk of aspiration. Nutritional status is an under-recognized risk factor for pneumonia development. Additionally, the use of a polyvalent pneumococcal vaccine and annual influenza vaccinations many controversially decrease hospitalization, complications, and death.

Typical Community-Acquired Pneumonias

Streptococcal pneumonia is the *single most important cause of CAP* but may also be responsible for a significant number of hospital-acquired pneumonias. *S. pneumoniae* case mortality approaches 40%. Among patients admitted to the ICU with pneumococcal pneumonia with bacteremia, the case mortality rate approaches 80%. Penicillin-resistant *S. pneumoniae* (PRSP) is the result of configurational changes in penicillin-binding protein structure; the strain was identified in 1967 and its rate of isolation now approaches 40%. *S. pneumoniae* has also evolved resistance to macrolides, clindamycin, and streptogramins.

Some patients with prior medical problems are more at risk for specific organisms. *H. influenzae* and *K. pneumoniae* are especially common isolates from pneumonias in alcoholic patients. Patients with chronic

Table 15-3 Point Scoring System Reflecting Risk in Community-Acquired Pneumonia (after Fine MJ et al, 1997)

Attribute	Points
AGE	
Male	Age (years)
Female	Age (years) − 10
ADMISSION FROM A NURSING FACILITY	10
COMORBID ILLNESSES	
Neoplastic disease	30
Liver disease	20
Congestive heart failure	10
Cerebral vascular disease	10
Renal disease	10
PHYSICAL EXAMINATION FINDINGS	
Altered mental status	20
Respiratory rate ≥ 30 bpm	20
Systolic blood pressure ≤ 90 mmHg	20
Temperature ≤ 35°C or ≥ 40°C	15
Pulse rate ≥ 125 bpm	10
LABORATORY AND RADIOLOGIC FINDINGS	
Arterial blood pH ≤ 7.35	30
Blood urea nitrogen ≥ 30 mg/dl	20
Sodium ≤ 130 mEq/l	20
Glucose ≥ 250 mg/dl	10
Hematocrit ≤ 30%	10
PaO_2 < 60 mmHg or oxygen saturation < 90%	10
Pleural effusion	10

Table 15-4 Fine Prediction Rule for Risk and Treatment Site in Community-Acquired Pneumonia (after Fine MJ et al, 1997)

Total Point Score	Risk Class	Mortality Rate (%)	Recommended Treatment Site
≤70	I	0.1	Outpatient
71–90	II	0.6	Outpatient
91–130	III	0.9–2.8	Probably outpatient
91–130	IV	8.2–9.3	Inpatient
>130	V	27–29.2	Inpatient

Atypical Community-Acquired Pneumonias

The term "atypical pneumonia" was originally used to describe a clinical syndrome of pneumonia which differed clinically and radiologically from typical pneumococcal pneumonia. Since atypical pathogens were more difficult to identify on Gram stain and cultures, and the term "atypical pneumonia" was coined. The atypical pneumonias can cause serious clinical syndromes with high morbidity and mortality and frequently require ICU care. Presently, the diagnostic tests for atypical pathogens include polymerase chain reaction, complement fixation, microimmunofluorescence, and enzyme immunoassay (for *C. pneumoniae* and *M. pneumoniae*); others include the serum IgM antibody ("cold agglutinin") for *Mycoplasma*, and direct fluorescent antibody (DFA) and indirect immunofluorescence antibody test (for *Legionella* spp.). The most established of these techniques is complement fixation which is relatively uncomplicated but has low sensitivity. The fluorescence techniques determine antibody titer in diluted serum samples but are subjective and costly. Enzyme-linked immunosorbent assays (ELISA) to not require dilution and because the results are measured in optical density (OD) units there is less subjectivity. Urinary antigen testing for *Legionella pneumophilia* serogroup 1 is a nonserologic test which becomes positive only after a few days of illness and may require a second test during the convalescent phase of illness to confirm the diagnosis, if such confirmation is necessary.

bronchitis are likely to present with *H. influenzae* or *M. catarrhalis*. Patients who have undergone splenectomy are at special risk for infection with encapsulated organisms such as pneumococcus.

Empiric initial antibiotic therapy for CAP must provide effect of coverage for *S. pneumoniae*; agents that also cover *Legionella* and *Mycoplasma* should be considered. Antibiotics of choice are ceftriaxone or cefotaxime with the addition of either a macrolide (e.g., azithromycin) or a fluoroquinolone.

Fine et al. have used both clinical investigation and meta-analysis to identify and quantify the effect of risk factors on mortality. The Fine criteria are described in Table 15-3. The Fine Prediction Rule is an algorithmic application of the Fine criteria to determine the optimal point of care (Table 15-4).

Blood cultures have low yield and are not recommended in the workup of uncomplicated CAP. On the other hand, in severe CAP, especially pneumococcal in origin, bacteremia is an important predictor of mortality.

The Infectious Disease Society of America (IDSA) and the American Thoracic Society (ATS) have promulgated guidelines for the treatment of CAP (Table 15-5).

CLINICAL CAVEAT

Presentation of Atypical Pneumonia
The hallmark presentation of atypical pneumonia is a nonproductive cough.

The type of environment may play an important role in the organisms to which the patient is exposed. Patients who are immunocompromised, who live in shelters, or who are incarcerated are at especially high risk for infection with *Mycobacterium tuberculosis*. Hunters and

Table 15-5   IDSA and ATS Guidelines for Empiric Treatment of Community-Acquired Pneumonia

Patient Class	IDSA	ATS
1. OUTPATIENTS (ORAL)		
a. Nonsevere pneumonia; *no* underlying cardiopulmonary disease	Macrolide *or* doxycycline *or* fluoroquinolone	Advanced macrolide
b. Nonsevere pneumonia; underlying cardiopulmonary disease *and/or* risk factors for DRSP		Beta-lactam *plus* macrolide *or* doxycycline; *or* fluoroquinolone alone
2. INPATIENTS (IV THERAPY)		
a. Nonsevere pneumonia; *no* underlying cardiopulmonary disease	Beta-lactam *plus* macrolide *or* doxycycline; *or* fluoroquinolone alone	Azithromycin *or* fluoroquinolone
b. Nonsevere pneumonia; underlying cardiopulmonary disease *and/or* risk factors for DRSP or enteric gram-negatives		Beta-lactam *plus* Azithromycin *or* doxycycline; *or* fluoroquinolone alone
3. ICU PATIENTS (IV THERAPY)		
a. Severe pneumonia; no risk of P. aeruginosa	Beta-lactam *plus* macrolide *or* fluoroquinolone	Beta-lactam *plus* azithromycin *or* fluoroquinolone
b. Severe pneumonia; risk of P. aeruginosa		Antipseudomonal beta-lactam *plus* fluoroquinolone

IDSA, Infectious Disease Society of America; ATS, American Thoracic Society.

people who work outdoors may be exposed to *Francisella tularensis* and develop tularemia, or *Yesinia pestis*, plague (see Chapter 33). Keepers of birds may contract psittacosis caused by *Chlamydia psittaci*. Inhalational anthrax occurs in wool sorters and tanners. However, *Bacillus anthracis*, a Gram-positive spore-forming bacillus, has also recently surfaced as a biological terror agent in the USA. Inhalational anthrax results in a hemorrhagic necrotic pneumonitis evolving 2–43 days following exposure. Lymphadenitis, pleuritis, and mediastinitis, however, are likely to predominate over pneumonitis. Fluoroquinolones are the drug of choice since tetracycline and penicillin-resistant strains have been isolated. Exposure to meat, especially from ungulates, is a risk for *Coxiella burnetii* pneumonia (Q fever) (see Chapter 33).

Viral Pneumonia

Viral pneumonias typically occur in the setting of an outbreak and occur predominantly in the winter and early spring. Patients at risk for viral pneumonias include those with underlying heart disease, chronic pulmonary disease, and pregnancy. Pulmonary infiltrates can occur in 20% of young adults with varicella but a frank pneumonia presentation is rare and is more suggestive of a bacterial superinfection (Figure 15-6). Herpetic pneumonias occur with high frequency in postoperative cardiac and transplant patients. The true incidence is probably under-recognized. The route of infection is probably the aspiration of saliva contaminated by the virus.

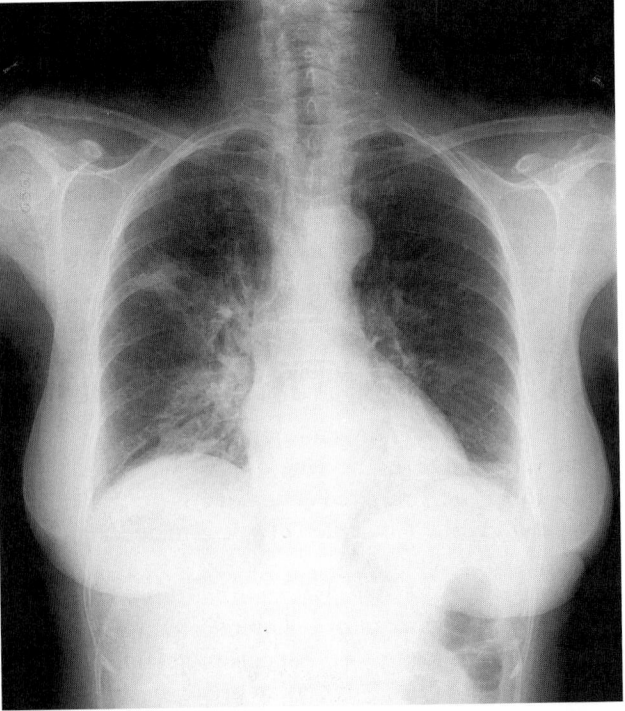

Figure 15-6   Influenzal viral pneumonia. There is evidence of consolidation in the right middle and lower lobes in the setting of pneumonia with positive viral titers.

The clinical picture is usually limited to hypoxia and dyspnea. The virus may be isolated in culture. Treatment is with antiviral agents such as acyclovir.

Pulmonary Hantavirus syndrome with the *Sin Nombre virus* was identified in 1993 in the American Southwest and is acquired through exposure to the deer mouse, its excrement, or contaminated dust; however, the disease has been reported throughout the USA. The syndrome is characterized by a nonspecific 3–6-day prodrome followed by hypoxemia and a sepsis syndrome. Although the clinical picture suggests a pneumonia, the microscopic picture is more consistent with pulmonary capillary leak syndrome such as occurs in ARDS. The case fatality rate for Hantavirus pulmonary syndrome is 50% or more.

Over the last two years there has been a growing concern over large-scale epidemics of viral pneumonias. The one with the greatest impact, severe acute respiratory syndrome (SARS), is a coronavirus infection that causes pneumonia and severe ARDS. It was first recognized in Southeast Asia in November 2002 from where it spread to other countries. Repeat epidemic episodes are likely. The SARS mortality rate worldwide is approximately 10.5%; the ICU admission rate ranged from 20% to 38%; over 60% of ICU patients require mechanical ventilatory support. The mortality rate of SARS patients admitted to the ICU ranges from 5% to 67%.

CLINICAL CAVEAT

SARS
- The most common clinical symptoms and signs of SARS are fever, cough, dyspnea, myalgias, and malaise.
- Common laboratory abnormalities include mild leukopenia, lymphopenia, and increased aspartate transaminase, alanine transaminase, lactic dehydrogenase, and creatine kinase.
- The chest radiograph pattern ranges from focal infiltrates to diffuse airspace disease. The risk of mortality increases with advanced age, comorbidities, a high lactic dehydrogenase, or a high neutrophil count at admission.

Emerging diseases are likely to become more of a global threat as viruses increasingly jump species and mutate rapidly.

Fungal Pneumonia

Fungal pneumonias represent a subset of CAPs caused by endemic fungi such as *Histoplasma capsulatum*, *Blastomyces dermatitidis*, and *Coccidioides immitis*. However, fungal pneumonias also represent opportunistic infections in immunocompromised populations and

are likely very important but largely under-diagnosed pathogens in nosocomial and especially ventilator-associated pneumonias. *Histoplasma* is found in soil contaminated with bird and bat excreta. Histoplasmosis is the most common systemic mycosis in the USA and is characteristically found in the Ohio and Mississippi river valleys. Although an estimated 500,000 people develop histoplasmosis in the USA annually, less than 1% develop a clinically symptomatic disease. In immunocompetent individuals with intact T-cell function, infection is usually subclinical and self-limited. In those patients who develop symptomatic histoplasmosis, the presentation is usually that of a flu-like syndrome with a nonproductive cough and pleuritic chest pain. Less than 5% of infected individuals develop rheumatologic syndromes such as pericarditis and arthralgias or inflammatory granulomatous mediastinitis. In patients with impaired immunologic function or patients who have received a high inoculum exposure, such as construction or agricultural workers, there may be an acute overwhelming pulmonary histoplasmosis characterized by profound hypoxemia and diffuse bilateral pulmonary infiltrates. Rare complications of histoplasmosis include chronic upper lobe cavitary pneumonic disease, fibrosing mediastinitis, and progressive disseminated histoplasmosis. Definitive diagnosis usually requires immunodiagnostic testing which is not definitive, or periodic acid Schiff staining. Treatment is either with itraconazole or amphotericin B; the concomitant systemic corticosteroid therapy should be considered (Figure 15-7).

Blastomyces is also found in moist soil rich with decaying organic material. Blastomycosis is endemic along the Mississippi and Ohio river basins as well as the Great Lakes. Approximately 75% of infected patients have isolated lung involvement and the remaining 25% develop a disseminated lymphohematogenous disease involving primarily the skin, bone, and genitourinary system. Pulmonary blastomycosis develops approximately six weeks after exposure and presents as a flu-like syndrome with a productive mucopurulent sputum. Chest radiographs reveal nonspecific diffuse reticulonodular infiltrates. Chronic common blastomycosis is similar to tuberculosis and is accompanied by night sweats, weight loss, and productive cough, and may progress to cavitary disease. Blastomycosis can be diagnosed by PAS or silver staining of sputum. Ketoconazole, itraconazole, or fluconazole are the mainstay therapies (Figure 15-8).

Coccidioides is found in semiarid desert soil. Coccidiomycosis is endemic in the southwestern USA and approximately 100,000 new cases occur annually in the Sonoran Desert and the Central (San Joaquin) Valley of California. Approximately 40% of infected individuals develop clinically evident disease in one to three weeks following exposure. The disease is typically a self-limited flu-like pneumonitis characterized by nonproductive

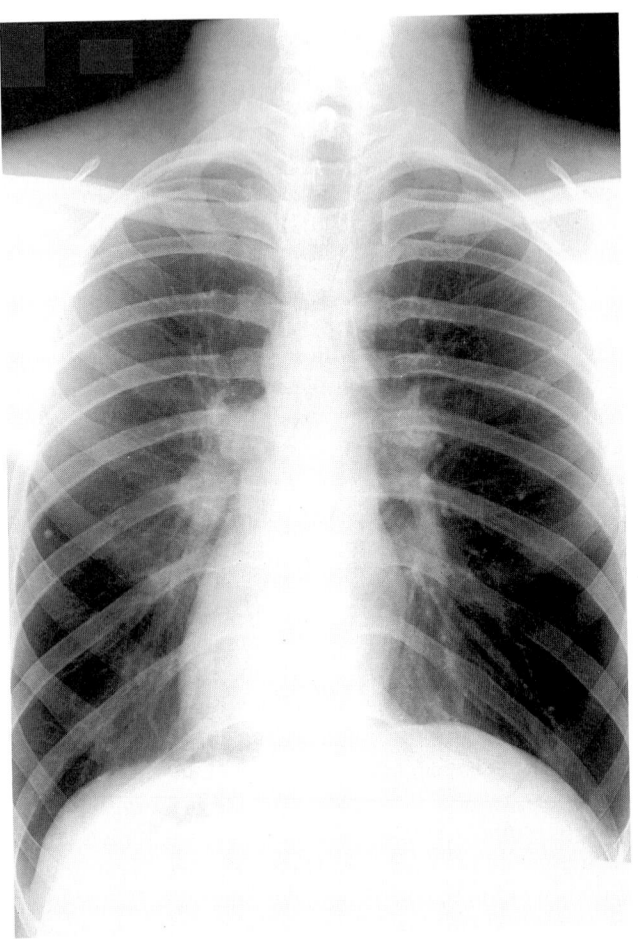

Figure 15-7 Histoplasmosis pneumonia. Characteristic large paratracheal and hilar adenopathy with calcifications. Old calcified foci are present in the peripheral lung fields. Infiltrates are patchy and poorly defined.

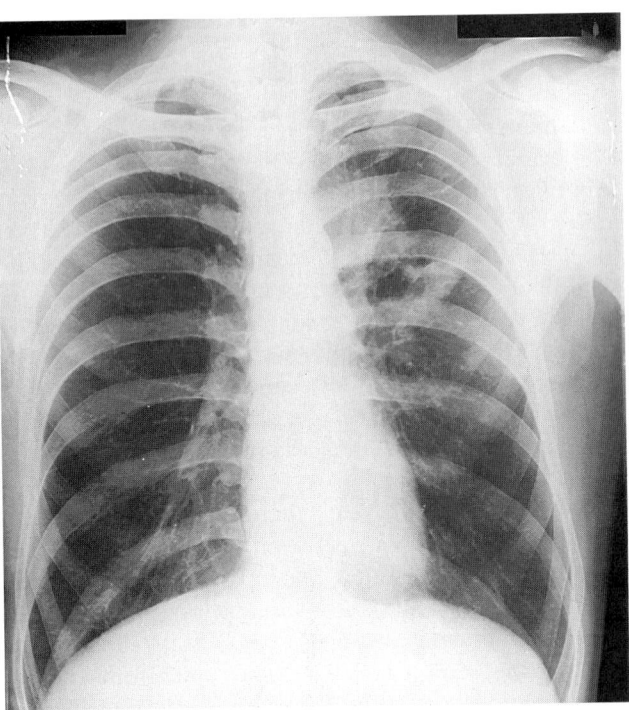

Figure 15-8 Blastomycosis pneumonia. Left mid-lung field density extending outwards from the left hilum demonstrates the focal alveolar infiltrates characteristic of approximately 75% of cases.

cough and pleuritic chest pain. Rheumatologic complications occur in about 20% of patients. Radiographic findings are typically patchy or nodular infiltrates which may coalesce to mimic those of other CAPs. Some 20% of patients develop pleural effusions and hilar adenopathy. About 5% of patients develop chronic pulmonary cavities or nodules which are considered a hallmark of coccidiomycosis. Immunocompromised patients are at especially high risk for disseminated disease which is manifested by plaques and papules, pustules, and chronic granulomatous meningitis. Serologic testing to IgM using precipitin or similar testing, complement fixation of IgG, or skin tests are commonly employed diagnostic modalities. Treatment is with ketoconazole, fluconazole, or amphotericin B (Figure 15-9).

Nosocomial Pneumonia

The definition of a nosocomial pneumonia is one that starts at least 48 hours after hospital admission. Nosocomial pneumonia or hospital-acquired pneumonia

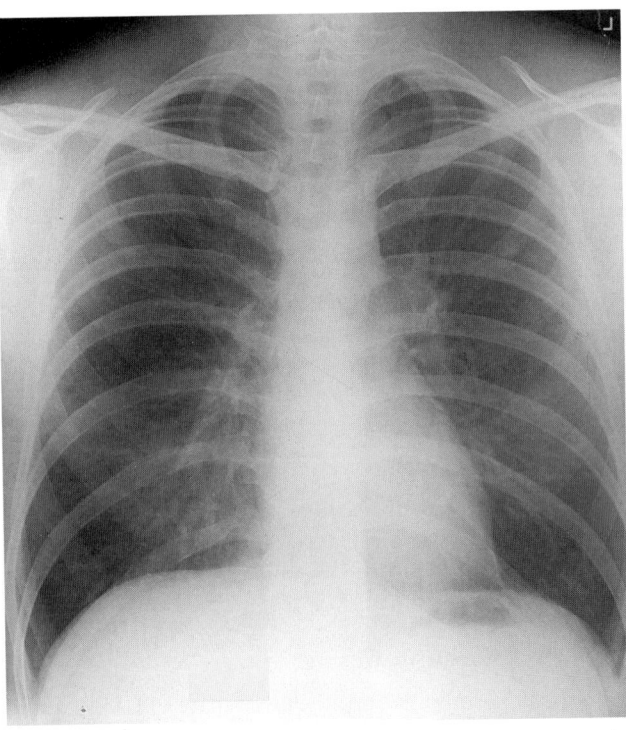

Figure 15-9 Coccidiomycosis. A patient from the San Joaquin Valley of California. Chest radiograph shows hilar prominence indicative of both adenopathy and a focal coin-lesion type of reaction in the mid-upper lung fields (coccidiomas).

is the main cause of nosocomial mortality; 60% of all nosocomial infections that result in death are due to nosocomial pneumonias.

In patients who are hospitalized for stroke, the development of pneumonia increases the 30-day risk of death threefold. The development of a nosocomial pneumonia increases the length of hospital stay by an average of 6–7 days; and the cost of treating a hospital-acquired pneumonia ranges from $5000 for patients treated on wards to $20,000–$40,000 per case of ventilator-associated pneumonia treated in ICUs.

CLINICAL CAVEAT

Nosocomial Pneumonia

- Clinical diagnosis is a relatively poor indicator of nosocomial pneumonia and chest radiography is also nonspecific.
- Empiric therapy for nosocomial pneumonia must provide adequate coverage against the core organisms responsible for the majority of nosocomial pneumonias in any given institution.
- Antibiograms that compile statistics regarding antibiotic efficacy profiles for pathogens in any given institution must also be consulted.
- Strategies to decrease the incidence of nosocomial pneumonia include the use of routine infection-control practices, vigorous handwashing and decontamination of equipment by hospital staff, nutritional assessment and support, and the isolation of patients with resistant respiratory pathogens.

Drug-resistant pathogens increasingly account for both community- and hospital-acquired pneumonia. The need for infectious disease (ID) services consultation is subjective and provider-specific. In institutions with restricted antibiotic formularies it may be necessary to obtain ID approval for the use of specific antibiotics; such approval is not synonymous with a formal ID consultation. An ID consultation might be considered in high-risk circumstances such as immunosuppressed patients, patients with complicated histories of frequent infections or the risk of pathogen resistance is high, and in situations where patients' conditions worsen despite aggressive antibiotic therapy.

Nosocomial pneumonias are often divided into hospital-acquired pneumonias (HAPs) which are nosocomial pneumonias that develop in patients who are not mechanically ventilated either on the wards or in the ICU; and ventilator-associated pneumonias (VAPs) which occur in those patients who are receiving mechanical ventilation. VAP usually refers to patients in the ICU; but VAPs may occur also in those patients who are receiving chronic mechanical ventilation outside the ICU.

Hospital-Acquired Pneumonia

HAP has an incidence of 0.5–1.0% of hospital admissions. Pneumonia is the second most common cause of, and accounts for up to 20% of, bacteremia and sepsis in hospitalized patients. Risk factors include advanced age, malnutrition, obesity, impaired immunity, depressed level of consciousness, and prior surgery. HAP due to anaerobes should be considered primarily in the setting of recent abdominal surgery, anaerobic infection, or suspected aspiration. Patients who are admitted with pneumonia from the community but come from an institutionalized setting or who have been recently hospitalized are treated as though they have HAP.

"*Severe HAP*" is defined based on admission to the ICU, respiratory failure based on the need for an $FIO_2 > 35\%$ to maintain $SpO_2 > 90\%$ or the need for mechanical ventilation, rapid radiologic progression of lung infiltrate, or evidence of severe sepsis with hypotension and/or end-organ dysfunction.

The core pathogens for HAP are *S. aureus*, *S. pneumoniae*, and the enteric Gram-negative bacilli (EGNB). The treatment of early-onset HAP must provide coverage against the core pathogens. The recommended regimens for the treatment of HAP include ceftriaxone, cefuroxime, or cefotaxime ± a macrolide. However, antimicrobial resistance is developing rapidly. Monotherapy with a fourth-generation cephalosporin may be cost-effective therapy for HAP. HAP *S. aureus* pneumonia due to methicillin-/oxacillin-resistant *S. aureus* (MRSA/ORSA) strains will likely require vancomycin or linezolid (Zyvox) for effective therapy.

Legionella or opportunistic *Aspergillus* should be suspected as a HAP in the setting of the administration of high-dose steroids or the new onset or worsening of pulmonary symptoms in hospitalized patients. Endemic *Aspergillus* infections have been recently related to hospital construction and renovation where immunocompromised or critically ill patients have been exposed to construction dust.

Ventilator-Associated Pneumonia

A nosocomial pneumonia that develops at least 48 hours after the initiation of mechanical ventilation is known as a VAP. Nosocomial pneumonia accrues an approximate 25% of adult ICU patients, at an incidence of 21 times greater than that of non-ICU patients. Approximately 17% of nosocomial pneumonias occur in the 1% of hospitalized patients who received mechanical ventilation. VAP has an incidence of 3–20% in patients receiving short-term mechanical ventilation. The cumulative incidence of VAP increases with the number of ventilator days. Statistically, the incremental risk of developing VAP during mechanical ventilation ranges from 1% to 3% per day.

Important risk factors for VAP include emergency surgery, intubation, recumbent positioning, oral pharyngeal secretions, pre-existing cardiopulmonary or neurologic disease, severity of illness, and tracheostomy. The duration of mechanical ventilation and the administration of systemic glucocorticoids independently predict risk of VAP. Patients who require emergency intubation, emergent re-intubation, or receive a tracheostomy are at higher risk of developing VAP. Occult VAP is a common cause of failure to wean from mechanical ventilation. Endotracheal tubes predispose to pneumonia formation because they bypass the normal filtering mechanisms in the upper airways and provide a direct conduit for the aspiration of pathogens into the lower respiratory tree, they have been shown to impair mucociliary clearance and epithelial ciliary function, they rapidly develop a contaminated biofilm which is then mechanically introduced distally routine suctioning, and the endotracheal tube cuff interferes with deglutition and also promotes the pooling of oral pharyngeal secretions above the endotracheal tube cuff. The high-volume low-pressure endotracheal tube cuffs used in clinical practice do not completely occlude the upper airway and therefore do not prevent either gross aspiration syndromes or microaspiration of oral pharyngeal secretions.

VAP, similar to any other nosocomial infection, must be managed especially aggressively in those patients who have implanted foreign bodies such as vascular graft material, arthroplasties, and pacemakers and defibrillators. The virulence of nosocomial pathogens and the potential for immunologic compromise in inpatients makes hematogenous seeding of foreign bodies especially likely and thereafter very difficult to treat.

VAP is also further characterized based on the time of onset of pneumonia. Early-onset VAP occurs within the first 96 hours of initiation of mechanical ventilation and is most commonly attributable to antibiotic-sensitive organisms such as *S. aureus*, *H. influenzae*, *S. pneumoniae*, and EGNB (Table 15-6). Late-onset VAP is pneumonia which is diagnosed 96 hours or more after the initiation of mechanical ventilation and is typically caused by MRSA, ORSA, *P. aeruginosa*, *Enterobacter* spp., or *Acinetobacter* spp. These organisms are more likely to be resistant and to contribute to morbidity and mortality. Therefore, the key core pathogens in VAP are generally *P. aeruginosa*, *S. pneumoniae*, *Acinetobacter* spp., *S. aureus*, and EGNB.

VAP is polymicrobial approximately 50% of the time. Empiric antibiotic therapy for VAP must account for both aggressive combination therapy based on an antibiogram specific to the ICU, as well as criteria for the duration of therapy. As microbiological data become available, usually within 48 hours, the empiric therapy should be tapered or modified accordingly. A key dilemma in the diagnosis of VAP is the differentiation

Table 15-6 Nosocomial Pathogens: Adapted from NNIS Data 1992–1999	
Pathogen	**Percentage**
Staphylococcus aureus	18.1
Pseudomonas aeruginosa	17.0
Enterobacter spp.	11.2
Klebsiella pneumoniae	7.2
Candida albicans	4.7
Escherichia coli	4.3
Haemophilus influenzae	4.3
Enterococcus spp.	1.7
All others	31.4

between endotracheal tube colonization, airway colonization, bronchitis, and true pneumonia. Colonization can be defined as the persistence of microorganisms at an anatomic site without evidence of host response or local invasion. The differentiation between pneumonia and colonization is especially difficult when the diagnosis is based on nonquantitative cultures obtained by simple endotracheal tube suctioning. A variety of microorganisms normally colonize the upper respiratory tract and these include *Viridans streptococci*, *Streptococcus pyogenes*, *Neisseria* spp., *Moraxella*, *Corynebacterium*, *Lactobacillus*, and *Candida* spp.

S. aureus is an extremely common cause of community- and hospital-acquired pneumonia. However, in hospitals its endemic rate of colonization is so high as to make it an almost ubiquitous hospital pathogen. MRSA and ORSA account for 70–80% of hospital isolates of *S. aureus*. Resistance is a function of both an altered penicillin and binding protein which confers beta-lactam resistance, as well as target modification which confers macrolides and possibly fluoroquinolone resistance. Vancomycin has become the mainstay therapy for *S. aureus*, but the emergence of vancomycin-resistant *S. aureus* (VRSA) and vancomycin (glycopeptide) intermediate-sensitive *S. aureus* (VISA or GISA) increasingly requires complex therapy with agents such as Quinupristin/dafopristin (Synercid) or Linezolid.

Gram-negative pathogens account for approximately 60% of clinical laboratory isolates in patients with nosocomial pneumonia. The enterobacteriaceae species that are most commonly seen include *K. pneumoniae*, *Proteus* spp., *Serratia* spp., *Citrobacter* spp., and *Escherichia* spp. These agents have been resistant to beta-lactams through the production of bata-lactamases; however, extended-spectrum beta-lactamases (ESBL) and beta-lactamases resistant to beta-lactamase inhibitors (inhibitor-resistant TEM-derived beta lactamases) have become significant. Vancomycin-resistant enterococcus (VRE or VREF) is increasingly prevalent. Both *Enterococcus faecium* and *E. faecalis* are becoming serious threats. However, the former is vastly more common than the latter at the present time. Linezolid and Synercid are important antibiotics against this class of organism. Vancomycin resistance in *Enterococcus* and *Staphylococcus* is a reflection of its overuse. It is estimated that 60–65% of vancomycin use is inappropriate.

Pseudomonas aeruginosa is an extremely common pathogen for HAP and VAP with a higher mortality rate than most other Gram-negative bacilli. Plasmid-mediated resistance is rapid. Pseudomonas pneumonia increases ICU mortality by a factor of 2.6–6.4. In patients who have *P. aeruginosa* or acinetobacter infections, crude ICU mortality exceeds 70%.

Fungal pneumonias are both under-diagnosed and under-treated in critically ill patients. Mycotic infection is known to occur in the presence of adjunctive antibiotic therapy, immunosuppression, and severe illness. Unfortunately, fungal infection is more likely be a post-mortem diagnosis than a clinical one. A key limitation is the inability to culture rapidly specimens containing fungal pathogens and perform sensitivity testing on isolates. The development of antifungal agents with decreased systemic toxicity has facilitated the treatment of mycoses in critically ill patients. Specific criteria for initiation and discontinuation of systemic fungal agents remain controversial.

CURRENT CONTROVERSY

Treatment of Ventilator-Associated Pneumonia
The risk of undertreatment is increased morbidity and mortality. The risk of overtreatment includes the development of resistant strains of bacteria, the significant cost of continued surveillance cultures, medications, consultations, drug level monitoring, and the increased potential for medication errors.

There is no gold standard method for the diagnosis of VAP. Studies have repeatedly been unable to demonstrate with statistical significance the clear value of any technique over any other. However, a number of diagnostic modalities are used in practice: endotracheal tube aspirates (ETA); bronchoscope-directed protected brushings (BDPB); protected brush specimen (PBS); bronchoscopic bronchoalveolar lavage (BBAL); and blind BAL or QTL which are quantitative tracheal lavage techniques. Endotracheal tube aspirates are the most commonly performed method of culturing respiratory secretions. Since endotracheal tube aspirates culture both contaminants and colonization as well as infectious pneumonia, the use of semiquantitative cultures and the determination of sputum neutrophil count can greatly increase their sensitivity. Bronchoscopy is an important adjunct to the

diagnosis of VAP, giving direct visualization of the airways which can reveal inflammation, mucus, and mucus plugging. A protected brush specimen can be obtained either blindly or with a bronchoscope. The protected brush is designed to reduce false positive cultures which are due to contamination from upper airway secretions and may represent only tracheobronchitis rather than true pneumonia. The protected brush is housed within a closed cannula. When the cannula is passed into the distal airways, the brush is advanced through the occluding plug of the cannula and is exposed directly to distal respiratory secretions. Structures are retracted into the cannula and removed for plating and culture. Quantitative cultures revealing colony growth $\geq 10^3$ colony forming units (cfu)/ml are considered positive and correspond to a bacterial density of 10^5–10^6 cfu/ml in undiluted respiratory secretions.

Bronchoalveolar lavage is performed through a bronchoscope by washing a specific lung segment with isotonic saline and collecting the effluent directly through the bronchoscope suction for culture. When the BAL is performed using a wedged catheter tip, which isolates the lung segment during lavage, the technique is known as a protected BAL. A minimum lavage volume of approximately 120 ml is recommended for adequate sampling; when smaller volumes of saline (10–50 ml) are used, the technique is called a mini-BAL. A threshold of 10^4 cfu/ml is considered positive for pneumonia when the BAL is used but this corresponds to the same bacterial titer in undiluted respiratory secretions as a protected brush. The sensitivity and specificity of BAL is considered to range from 70% to 100%. Open lung biopsy is the most definitive diagnostic procedure for histopathologic diagnosis of pneumonia in immunocompromised hosts.

KEY POINTS

Ventilator-Associated Pneumonia
- The single best predictor of mortality in patients with VAP is the resolution of pulmonary shunting as measured by the pAO_2/FIO_2 ratio.
- Successful prevention of VAP is a clearly more cost-effective strategy then surveillance and treatment.
- The avoidance of patient cross-contamination by vigorous handwashing is probably the most important precaution that health care workers can take to prevent spread of pneumonia and other infections in hospitals. Universal precautions should be considered universally.
- The use of endotracheal tubes designed to permit continuous removal of pooled subglottic secretions has been proven to decrease the incidence of VAP.

KEY POINTS—Cont'd

- Patient positioning in semi-recumbent rather than supine position decreases the incidence of VAP. The elevation of the head of the patient's bed can decrease the risk of aspiration.
- More controversial strategies include stress ulcer prophylaxis, selective digestive decontamination, aggressive oral and dental care, and frequent changes of ventilator circuits and filters.
- Potential future developments include the use of bioactive and drug-impregnated biomaterials for endotracheal tube construction.

Pleural or parapneumonic effusions are associated with up to 50% of bacterial pneumonias. These effusions can be free or loculated and may either resolve or develop into empyema. These effusions should be drained immediately if there is radiologic evidence of an air–fluid level. Parapneumonic effusions should be evaluated by paracentesis for Gram stain and culture, pH, LDH, protein, and glucose in order to differentiate between transudative and exudative fluid. Grossly purulent fluid should be drained.

The clinical pulmonary infections score (CPIS) has utility in both detecting the onset of VAP and also determining the sufficiency and adequacy of treatment. The CPIS also correlates with 28-day mortality. The diagnosis of pneumonia is generally based upon variations of the CPIS originally developed by Pugin et al. in 1990 (Table 15-7). The CPIS has a specificity (85–95%) similar to that of bronchoscopic diagnosis of pneumonia. The key parameters include temperature, quantity of secretions, leukocyte count, chest radiographic findings, hypoxemia, and BAL Gram stain and culture. A CPIS of >6 indicates infectious pneumonia with a sensitivity of 93% and specificity of 100%. Therefore, a CPIS of >6 almost excludes acute lung injury, pulmonary edema, or atelectasis as the etiology of a pulmonary infiltrate.

Pneumonia in Patients with Compromised Immune Status

The causes of pneumonia in the immunocompromised host include all pathogens listed above and extend to opportunistic pathogens. Other causes of pulmonary infection in immunocompromised patients include *Mycobacterium tuberculosis* and *M. avium-intracellulare*, *Cryptococcus*, *Toxoplasma*, and cytomegalovirus. Many of these infections also involve other organs such as the brain and the eye (Figures 15-10 and 15-11). Pneumonia in immunocompromised patients presents atypically. Dyspnea, hypoxemia, nonproductive cough, and a generalized radiographic infiltrate frequently constitute the presenting picture. Such patients may be hypothermic rather than febrile, and may have a leukopenia rather than leukocytosis. The responsible pathogen may be isolated in only 40% of immunocompromised patients. The early evolution of systemic sepsis in this population makes rapid diagnosis and intervention extremely important.

Pneumocystis carinii (PCP) is a protozoan pneumonia which is common in HIV-infected patients. The pneumonia

---

Table 15-7   Clinical Pulmonary Infection Score (CPIS) or Pugin Score

Variable	Range	Points
Temperature (°C)	≥36.5 and ≤38.4	0
	≥38.5 and ≤38.9	1
	≥39.0 and ≤36.0	2
Leukocytes/mm^3	≥4000 and ≤11,000	0
	≤4000 and ≥11,000	1
Secretions	<14 + volume of tracheal secretions	0
	≥14 + volume of tracheal secretions	1
	Purulent secretions	1
P$_A$O$_2$/FIO$_2$ (mmHg)	>240	0
	≤240	2
Chest radiograph	No infiltrate	0
	Diffuse/patchy infiltrate	1
	Localized infiltrate	2
Semiquantitative tracheal aspirate cultures	<1 pathogenic bacteria or no growth	0
	≥1 pathogenic bacteria	1
	Same organism as gram stain 1+ add	1

Modified from Pugin J, Auckenthaler R, Mili N et al: Diagnosis of ventilator-associated pneumonia by bacteriologic analysis of bronchoscopic and nonbronchoscopic "blind" bronchoalveolar lavage fluid. Am Rev Respir Dis 143:1121–1129, 1991.

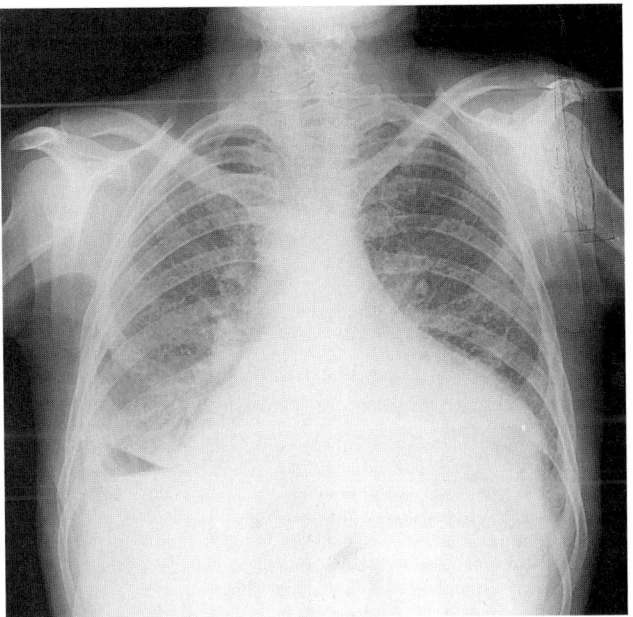

Figure 15-10 Miliary tuberculosis. Fine nodular lesions are apparent in bilateral lung fields.

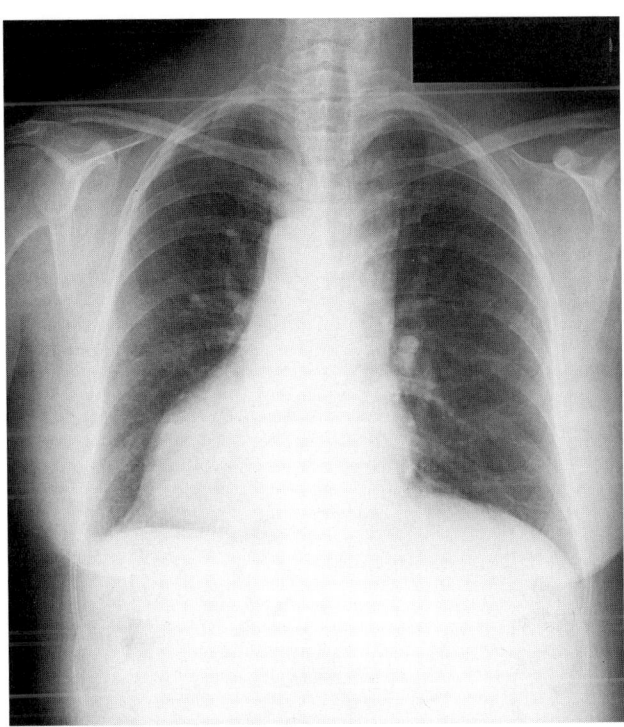

Figure 15-12 Early *Pneumocystis carinii* pneumonia. No radiographic pattern is pathognomonic and the early appearance is that of an "atypical" pneumonia.

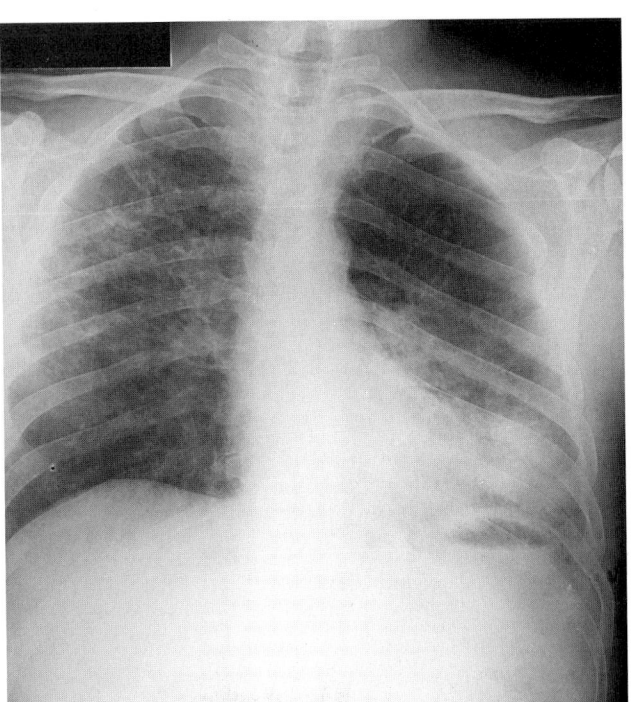

Figure 15-11 Cryptococcus pneumonia. Bilateral infiltrates with small thin-walled areas of cavitation. Radiographically, cryptococcus mimics nonspecific pneumonitis and presentation can vary from cavitations, miliary lesions, to larger infiltrates. Late-stage cryptococcus can be mistaken for pneumocystis, or lymphoreticular malignancy, and it also resembles ARDS.

can be rapidly progressive and lethal. The classic "ground glass" appearance on chest radiographs is nonspecific and may represent early ARDS. The initial antibiotic choice for PCP is trimethoprim-sulfamethoxazole (TMP-SMX) and co-administration of steroids must be considered. The initial response to therapy is frequently a clinical deterioration which may require intubation and mechanical ventilation. Treatment with TMP-SMX is considered to have failed if a favorable response is not apparent within three to five days. The second-line agent is intravenous pentamidine. Pentamidine is associated with significant side effects which include QTc prolongation, torsades de points, renal insufficiency and pancreatitis, neutropenia, as well as hyper- and hypoglycemia (Figures 15-12 and 15-13).

ADJUNCTIVE AND SUPPORTIVE THERAPEUTIC STRATEGIES

Fluid Resuscitation

In all patients with severe infective processes, supportive therapy is necessary to prevent secondary injury and the development of complications. Fluid resuscitation is a basic tenet of managing infection. Many patients are unable to "drink plenty of fluids" and therefore require intravenous hydration. Both systemic infection and

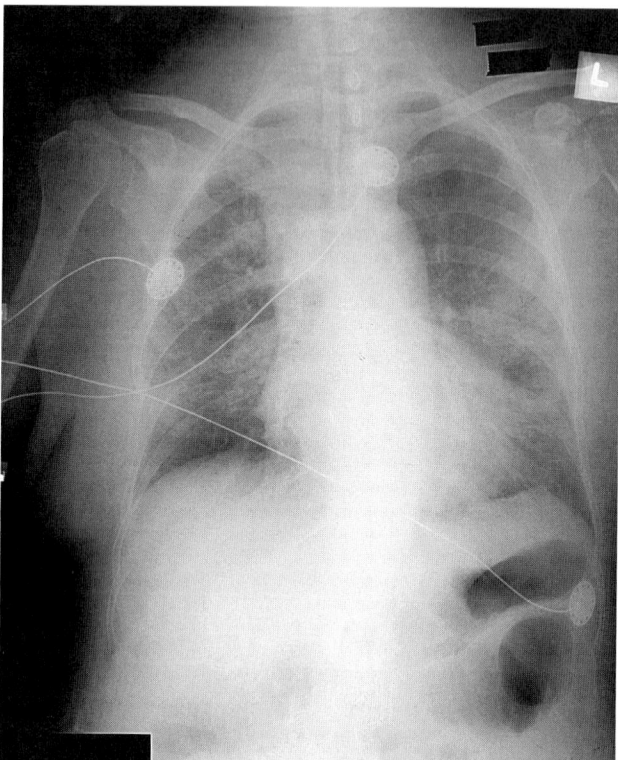

Figure 15-13 Late-stage *Pneumocystis carinii* pneumonia. Upright anteroposterior (AP) view. Widespread bilateral interstitial and alveolar infiltrates resembling ARDS. Interstitial markings result in a "honeycomb" appearance. An endotracheal tube is present.

systemic inflammatory response produce early peripheral vasodilatation and capillary leak which result in diminished intravascular fluid volume. Since increased stroke volume is usually not possible in such patients, the decreased intravascular volume is initially compensated for by tachycardia to maintain cardiac output and oxygen delivery to tissues. In patients who are unable to mount a compensatory tachycardia (diabetes, myocardial pump dysfunction, beta-blocker therapy, etc.) there are early signs of diminished peripheral perfusion and shock. In the setting of prolonged under-resuscitation, the inflammatory cascade is activated, regional hypoperfusion results, and acidosis and elevated serum lactate, acute renal failure due to acute tubular necrosis from regional underperfusion results, and the patient becomes progressively more difficult to resuscitate later.

Vasopressors should not be used as the mainstay of therapy for sepsis. Although vasopressors may be used to temporize while fluid resuscitation is ongoing, the substitution of vasopressors for fluid results in progressive tissue ischemia and organ failure. The development of progressive hypoxemia with intravascular volume therapy does not necessarily mean intravascular fluid overload – it is also consistent with a worsening of the pneumonia or the interval development of ARDS.

There are no data to support the use of colloid over crystalloid for intravascular volume resuscitation. However, emerging data may suggest that judicious use of colloids may help maintain intravascular oncotic pressure and decrease edema formation. Intravascular volume replacement therapy should be titrated to urine output, signs of improvement in organ perfusion (mental status, cyanosis resolution, etc.), serum lactate and acid–base balance, central venous filling or other preload measure correlated with cardiac output, or echocardiographic determination of end systolic volume and cardiac performance. A history of poor cardiac function, congestive heart failure, or pulmonary edema are not contraindications to intravascular volume replacement.

Nutritional Support

Patients with severe infection are highly catabolic and nutritional support should be instituted immediately, if possible. Many patients with pneumonia are already nutritionally depleted on initial presentation, and baseline nutritional status (pre-albumin, transferrin) should be documented. Daily calorie counts and serial nutritional indices may be required to ensure adequacy of nutritional support. Unless there is a definite contraindication to enteric feeding, it is the route of choice for nutritional support. Nutritional depletion has been shown to increase bacterial adherence to the airways, reduce alveolar macrophage function, impair neutrophil and macrophage recruitment, decrease levels of circulating complement factors, and reduce levels of airway IgA.

Pharmacologic Treatment

Antibiotic Principles

The ability of an antibiotic to exert its pharmacologic effect is related to penetration into infected tissue and achievement of adequate tissue concentrations. Inappropriate treatment of pneumonia is most often due to either nonsusceptibility or resistance of the pathogen to the chosen antibiotic regimen. Inappropriate initial antibiotic selection can range from 27% to 73% and has a dramatic impact on outcome measured by length of stay, multiple organ dysfunction syndrome, and mortality. Antibiotics that have good penetration into respiratory secretions that is not dependent on localized inflammation include the quinolones, azithromycin, clarithromycin, tetracycline, clindamycin, and TMP-SMX. Antibiotics that have impaired penetration into respiratory secretions and/or are dependent on inflammation for concentration within lung tissue include aminoglycosides and the beta-lactams (penicillins, cephalosporins, and carbapenems). Aminoglycosides have poor pulmonary penetration, and especially do not penetrate well into respiratory secretions. Therefore aminoglycosides should not be used as monotherapy for Gram-negative pneumonias. Azithromycin has replaced erythromycin in clinical practice because erythromycin has side effects of both QTc prolongation as well as enteric prokinesis which causes cramping discomfort. Fluoroquinolones are also associated with QTc prolongation, especially at higher doses.

Pathogen susceptibilities are often reported in terms of the minimum inhibitory concentration (MIC); the agent of choice will therefore depend on the MIC, guidelines and restrictions, and cost. Optimal pharmacologic action of antibiotics is that for which every concentration-dependent mechanism of action occurs when C_{max}/MIC is greater than 10.

In any patient who has failed to respond clinically after 48–72 hours of antimicrobial therapy, the therapeutic strategy must be reevaluated. Generally, this will require further workup including revaluation of culture and sensitivity data, consideration of superinfection, reconsideration of drug dosing or route of administration, and consideration of an alternative diagnosis. Evaluation of the patient's immunologic status may also be necessary.

Other routes of antibiotic therapy may be important in the care of ICU patients. Inhaled antibiotic therapy is probably underutilized. Inhaled antibiotics should be considered for severe HAP and in the treatment of refractory pneumonia in populations such as patients with cystic fibrosis.

Mechanisms of antimicrobial resistance include target-mediated resistance, enzymatic inactivation, cell membrane permeability alterations, and active expulsion of antibiotics from bacterial cells. Target-mediated resistance is a result of alterations in the number or affinity of antimicrobial binding sites within bacteria. Enzymatic inactivation results from the production of bacterial enzymes often carried by plasmids, which degrade antibiotic agents. Beta-lactamase production is the most common form of enzymatic resistance. Cell membrane permeability changes cause decreased antimicrobial uptake into bacterial cells. The promotion of active reflux of antibiotic out of bacterial cells is an energy-dependent mechanism which is carried on by plasmids and the creation of molecules known as transposons.

The rotation of first-line antibiotics of choice has been demonstrated to decrease the rate of evolution of pathogen resistance. Therefore, the choice of antibiotic should also be made in accordance with the preferred antibiotic in any particular cycle at any particular hospital.

Nonantibiotic Adjunctive Pharmacologic Therapy

In rare cases the use of immunomodulatory agents such as granulocyte colony-stimulating factor (GCSF) may need to be considered to enhance host polymorpho-nuclear leukocyte (PMN) response.

Bronchodilators are a very important adjunctive therapy in those patients with reactive airway disease who develop a superimposed respiratory tract infection. Since airway infection can predispose some patients to bronchospasm and thereby interfere with their ability to cough and clear secretions, bronchodilator therapy is beneficial in this population. Patients who use bronchodilator therapy regularly prior to admission may require an increase in the dose or frequency. Nonsteroidal bronchodilators can be either beta-2 agonists such as albuterol or anticholinergic such as Atrovent. The beta-2 sympathomimetics can still precipitate tachycardia. Lev-albuterol is a selective isomer with significantly less cardiac activity and possibly also a longer effective half-life.

Steroids are important bronchodilators in patients with underlying chronic obstructive pulmonary disease (COPD) or severe reactive airway disease. Methylprednisolone is the intravenous steroid bronchodilator of choice; prednisone is administered enterally. Patients for whom steroids have been chronically prescribed prior to admission require supplemental "stress doses" to avoid adrenal insufficiency in the setting of infectious stress. Mucolytic agents and expectorants may have a role when mucus clearance is difficult in the setting of dehydration or inspissated mucus is difficult for the patient to clear. N-acetylcysteine, recombinant DNase, and guaifenesin are prototypic mucolytic agents. N-acetylcysteine can precipitate bronchospasm and should be administered concomitantly with bronchodilators.

Humidification of inspired gases is important when the endotracheal tube bypasses the normal humidification and filtering systems of the upper airways. Humidification is important to avoid dry mucosal surfaces in patients with inflamed upper airways and humidification can improve expectoration of lower airway secretions. On the other hand, humidification systems must be carefully monitored for contamination with hypophilic organisms such as *Pseudomonas* and *Legionella*.

Stress ulcer prophylaxis must be considered in any hospitalized or critically ill patient exposed to metabolic stress; stress ulcer prophylaxis has been shown to decrease the incidence of gastrointestinal bleeding as a standard of care. The hypothesis that increasing gastric pH with stress ulcer prophylaxis increases incidence of nosocomial pneumonia due to aspiration of colonized gastric contents is no longer favored. Commonly used agents include proton pump inhibitors such as pantoprazole or others; H_2 blockers such as famotidine; or barrier agents such as sucralfate.

The use of oral care agents such as topical Mycostatin liquid may be beneficial because it focuses attention on oral care and the potential for bacterial and fungal overgrowth in the oral pharynx of integrated patients who have decreased salivary production and clearance. Also, oral care agents may have an antiseptic effect which decreases bacterial colonization. Patients who develop perioral or intraoral herpetic vesicles should have topical antiviral agents such as acyclovir applied.

Although pulmonary arteriolar vasodilators such as prostacyclin (PGI_2) and nitric oxide have been used in the management of severe cases of pneumonia, the use of these costly agents remains controversial and there is variability in their effectiveness. Hypoxic pulmonary vasoconstriction (HPV) is an adaptive response whereby a reflex vasoconstriction in the arteriolar supply to inflamed or diseased alveoli which have low alveolar oxygen concentrations results in minimization of pulmonary shunt fraction. Therefore, pulmonary arteriolar vasodilators which inhibit the HPV response are likely to increase blood supply to diseased hypoxic alveoli and actually increase shunt fraction and systemic hypoxemia.

GENERAL PRINCIPLES OF CHEST RADIOGRAPH INTERPRETATION

The portable anterior-posterior (AP) chest radiograph is the most commonly obtained radiologic study in the ICU. Although the critical care practitioner cannot be expected to render a complete final radiologic reading, it is incumbent on intensivists to be able reliably and independently to render preliminary interpretations which address specific questions regarding patients' clinical conditions. The chest radiograph is also key in the evaluation of a patient's response to therapy. The critical care notes should reflect independent readings as well as later confirmations or variations seen by radiologists.

KEY POINTS

Radiologic Interpretations

(a) Technique:
- (i) Anterior-posterior versus posterior-anterior versus lateral. Lateral decubitus films are sometimes obtained to determine fluid layering.
- (ii) Upright or supine. Upright films are necessary to better delineate pleural effusions and pneumothorax in and air under the diaphragm.
- (iii) Penetration: assessed objectively by comparison of lung fields and bony structures. Over penetration will emphasize the denser bony structures and obliterate subtle findings within the lung parenchyma.
- (iv) Rotation: relates to the patient's position on the radiographic plate. Rotation is best assessed by looking at clavicular symmetry.

(b) Hardware:
- (i) Endotracheal tube: should be midway between the clavicles and the carina within the trachea. It is important to note that the endotracheal tube will move approximately 2.5 cm in or out of the trachea with extension and flexion of the neck, respectively.
- (ii) Nasogastric and feeding tubes: must be followed within the esophagus into the stomach or small bowel. Tubes that enter the trachea will often pass through one mainstem bronchus.
- (iii) Tube thoracostomy: mention is usually made of the position of the tube, the intra- or extrathoracic placement of a last collecting hole of the chest tube, and resolution of the liquid or air collection which the tube was intended to treat.
- (iv) Other hardware: tracheostomy tubes, pacemakers, implantable cardiac defibrillation wires, intra-aortic balloon pump tips, prosthetic cardiac valves, evidence of vascular prostheses and stents, sternal wires, surgical clips, orthopedic prostheses, and airway stents. The mention of other foreign bodies, especially in trauma cases, is particularly important.

(c) Bony structures:
- (i) Fractures and dislocations of the clavicles, sternum, scapula, ribs, and vertebrae.
- (ii) Hyperostosis, osteopenia, or potential bony involvement of surrounding tumor or infection.

(d) Cardiovascular silhouette:
- (i) The AP portable radiograph is an unreliable indicator of cardiomegaly.
- (ii) The cardiac silhouette.
- (iii) The thoracic aorta. Special mention should be made of calcifications within the thoracic aorta and dilatation of the thoracic aorta.
- (iv) The pulmonary vasculature. Hilar accentuation. Pulmonary arterioles seen end-on are usually apparent and present as small opaque circles in the hilar regions and are normal findings. Evidence of vascular prominence, interstitial prominence, or alveolar flooding consistent with stages of congestive heart failure and pulmonary edema, respectively, must be noted.

KEY POINTS—Cont'd

    (v) The cardiovascular silhouette and trachea, taken together, are good indicators of mediastinal shift in the setting of consolidation (mediastinal shift toward the side of consolidation) and abnormal collections of air or fluid (mediastinal shift away from the side of the collection).

    (vi) The hilum: reflects both adenopathy as well as pulmonary vasculature and peribronchial tissue.

(e) Lung fields:

    (i) Expansion, hyperinflation, bullae, inspiratory effort, or atelectasis.

    (ii) Infiltrates, consolidation, cavitation, masses.

    (iii) Air bronchograms.

    (iv) Pleural collections.

(f) Diaphragm and surrounding abdominal tissue:

    (i) Air under the diaphragm is indicative of either a recent abdominal intervention such as recent surgery, paracentesis, or hysteroscopy; or it is a sign of a surgical emergency.

    (ii) A large gastric air bubble may require a nasogastric tube.

    (iii) Ileus may be apparent but is nonspecific and is an indirect incidental finding on a chest radiograph.

SELECTED READING

American Thoracic Society: Hospital-acquired pneumonia in adults: diagnosis, assessment of severity, initial antimicrobial therapy, and preventative strategies. A consensus statement. Am J Respir Crit Care Med 153:1711–1725, 1995.

Bartlett JG, Brieman RF, Mandell LA, File TM; Infectious Diseases Society of America: Community acquired pneumonia in adults: guidelines for management. CID 26:811–838, 1998.

Colice GL, Curtis A, Deslauriers J et al: Medical and surgical treatment of parapneumonic effusions: an evidence-based guideline. Chest 118:1158–1171, 2000.

Fine MJ, Stone RA, Lave JR et al: Implementation of an evidence-based guideline to reduce duration of intravenous antibiotic therapy and length of stay for patients hospitalized with community-acquired pneumonia: a randomized controlled trial. Am J Med 115:343–351, 2003.

Katzan IL, Cebul RD, Husak SH et al: The effect of pneumonia on mortality among patients hospitalized for acute stroke. Neurology 60:620–625, 2003.

Kirtland SH, Corley DE, Winterbauer RH et al: The diagnosis of ventilator-associated pneumonia. a comparison of histologic, microbiologic, and clinical criteria. Chest 112:445–457, 1997.

Luczycki S, Papadakos PJ, Szalados JE : Ventilator-associated pneumonia: pathophysiology, diagnosis, and treatment. Crit Care Shock 2:72–87, 2002.

Manocha S, Walley KR, Russell JA: Severe acute respiratory distress syndrome (SARS): a critical care perspective. Crit Care Med 31:2684–2692, 2003.

Masur H, Kaplan JE, Holmes KK; US Public Health Service; Infectious Diseases Society of America: Guidelines for preventing opportunistic infections among HIV-infected persons - 2002. Recommendations of the US Public Health Service and the Infectious Diseases Society of America. Ann Intern Med 137:435–478, 2002.

Niederman MS, Mandell LA, Anzueto A et al; American Thoracic Society: Guidelines for the management of adults with community-acquired pneumonia. Diagnosis, assessment of severity, antimicrobial therapy, and prevention. Am J Respir Crit Care Med 163:1730–1754, 2001.

Ost DE, Hall CS, Joseph G et al: Decision analysis and diagnostic strategies in ventilator-associated pneumonia. Am J Resp Crit Care Med 168:1060–1067, 2003.

Pugin J: Clinical signs and scores for the diagnosis of ventilator-associated pneumonia. Minerva Anesthesiol 68:261–265, 2002.

Pugin J, Auckenthaler R, Mili N et al: Diagnosis of ventilator-associated pneumonia by bacteriologic analysis of bronchoscopic and nonbronchoscopic "blind" bronchoalveolar lavage fluid. Am Rev Respir Dis 143:1121–1129, 1991.

Rex JH, Walsh TM, Sobel JD et al: Practice guidelines for the treatment of candidiasis. CID 30:662–78, 2000.

Wunderink RG, Waterer GW: Genetics of sepsis and pneumonia. Curr Opin Crit Care 9:384–389, 2003.

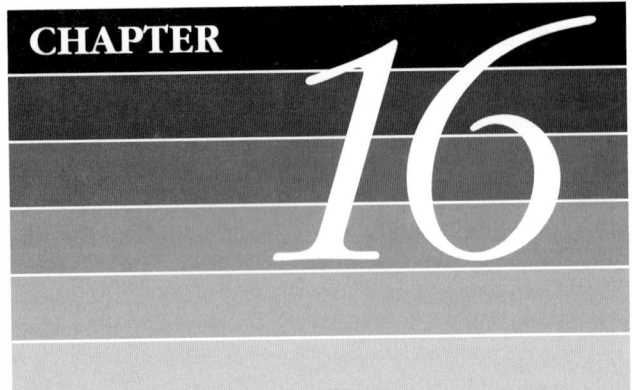

Acute Respiratory Distress Syndrome

PETER J. PAPADAKOS, M.D., F.C.C.P., F.C.C.M.

JACK J. HAITSMA, M.D., Ph.D.

Acute lung injury (ALI) and acute respiratory distress syndrome (ARDS) remain two of the most common conditions evaluated in the intensive care unit (ICU). ALI and ARDS are commonly encountered in the ICU and are associated with increased mortality, morbidity, and cost of care. ARDS is often seen in conjunction with multiple organ failure. The overall hospital mortality rate is between 20% and 50%. This wide range of mortality illustrates that there is a lack of understanding of the exact etiology and management of these conditions and further improvements and investigations into these conditions are needed. The exact incidence and prevalence of ALI and ARDS are unknown at present. Current reports put the number somewhere in the range of 150,000 cases in the USA or an estimated incidence of 75 cases per 100,000 population.

An American–European consensus conference has recently defined ALI and ARDS in an attempt to remove confusion related to terminology. This common language will allow investigators to evaluate and treat the same disorders and will greatly decrease confusion in the literature. Many investigators consider ALI and ARDS to represent a manifestation of a systemic disorder that arises from exaggerated proinflammatory pathways, culminating in the production of diffuse damage to the capillary endothelial cell and/or the alveolar epithelial barriers. In an attempt to improve outcomes in patients with ALI and ARDS, clinicians have used both local and systemic therapies to improve survival (Box 16-1).

RISK FACTORS

It has been recognized that ALI and ARDS may arise in association with a number of different clinical conditions. In reviewing the causes, sepsis continues to be the most commonly encountered factor: approximately 5–40% of septic patients develop ARDS. Shock, pneumonia, and the systemic inflammatory response syndrome (SIRS) are the most common risk factors. Other frequently encountered risk factors include multiple transfusions, aspiration injury, near drowning, pancreatitis, trauma, and many others. These clinical risk factors are synergistic, and when more than one of the clinical risk factors is present, the likelihood of ARDS is greater than the sum of the collective risk factors. Another major risk factor that has only recently come to light is the improper use of mechanical ventilation. Certain ventilator settings may lead to the development of ARDS. This so-called ventilator-induced lung injury (VILI) is highly important in that it may be preventable (Box 16-2).

CLINICAL MANIFESTATIONS

The initial clinical presentation may vary, primarily reflective of the underlying disease process and the overall condition of the patient. However, when ARDS becomes apparent the patient notes a significant distress associated with dyspnea and tachypnea and an increased work of breathing. Hypoxia is noted on the pulse oximeter or on the arterial blood gas (ABG).

The hallmark of ARDS is the presence of hypoxemia despite the administration of high concentrations of inspired oxygen, evidence of increasing shunt fraction,

Box 16-1 American–European Consensus Conference Definition of ALI and ARDS

Acute lung injury
- Acute onset of respiratory failure
- Bilateral chest infiltrates on chest x-ray
- Absence of elevated left heart pressure, no evidence of heart failure (pulmonary artery occlusion pressure (PAOP) < 18 mmHg)
- PaO_2/FIO_2 < 300 mmHg

Acute respiratory distress syndrome
- Acute onset of respiratory failure
- Bilateral chest infiltrates on chest x-ray
- Absence of elevated left heart pressure, no evidence of heart failure (PAOP < 18 mmHg)
- PaO_2/FIO_2 < 200 mmHg

Box 16-3 Common Pulmonary and Extrapulmonary Causes of ARDS

Direct pulmonary causes
- Pneumonia
- Acid aspiration
- Inhalation lung injury
- Chest trauma
- Near drowning

Extrapulmonary causes
- Sepsis, SIRS
- Shock, hypotension
- Pancreatitis
- Trauma
- Massive transfusion therapy
- Burns
- Postcardiopulmonary bypass

a decrease in compliance, and an increase in dead space ventilation. A chest radiograph in both ALI and ARDS shows the presence of diffuse bilateral pulmonary infiltrates. Chest computed tomography has been very helpful in elucidating that the injury is not homogeneous and has predominance in the dependent portions of the lung.

The precipitating injury need not directly involve the pulmonary system but can be triggered by other insults. For classification we separate the causes into pulmonary and extrapulmonary. There is some evidence that there is a difference in the mortality and morbidity based on whether the cause is pulmonary or extrapulmonary. The treatment may also be different (Box 16-3).

It is important to remember that ALI and ARDS is a clinical syndrome, and the diagnosis is made clinically using the consensus conference definition as a guide and not on a single radiograph, ABG measurement, or laboratory tests.

Box 16-2 Common Risk Factors for ARDS

- Sepsis and SIRS
- Pneumonia
- Prolonged hypotension and shock
- Trauma (long-bone fractures, lung contusion, fat embolism)
- Pancreatitis
- Near drowning
- Multiple emergency blood product transfusions
- Disseminated intravascular coagulation (DIC)
- Burn injury
- Postcardiopulmonary bypass

PATHOLOGIC MANIFESTATIONS

Alveolar type I cells compose the major gas exchange surface of the alveolus and are integral to the maintenance of the permeability barrier function of the alveolar membrane. Type II pneumocytes are the progenitors of type I cells and are responsible for surfactant production and homeostasis. During ALI and ARDS there is damage to the capillary endothelial and alveolar epithelial cells. This leads to cellular injury and alteration of the normal barrier function results in a permeable defect that gives way to flooding of the alveoli with protein-rich fluid and inflammatory cells. This results in the alteration of pulmonary mechanics, physiology, and gas exchange.

One of the most important changes is alteration of alveolar surfactant that results directly from the damage to the type II pneumocytes and from the inactivation and dilution of alveolar surfactant from the protein and fluid that may enter into the alveolar space. Surfactant dysfunction can lead to atelectasis and a further reduction in pulmonary compliance (resulting in bilateral chest infiltrates and disturbances in gas exchange).

Pathophysiology

The complex pathophysiologic process that culminates in the production of ALI and ARDS involves a delicate balance between the body's proinflammatory and anti-inflammatory responses to the inciting clinical event. This complex balance may also be genetically mediated in that some patients will release higher levels of cytokines when challenged by a stimulus. This cellular mediation is under active investigation and may be an avenue of therapy in the future (Box 16-4).

Box 16-4   Potential Mediators of ALI

- Polymorphonuclear leukocytes (PMLs)
- Leukotrienes
- Cytokines (interleukins 1, 2, 6, 8, 15; tumor necrosis factor (TNF); granulocyte colony-stimulating factor (GCSF))
- Platelet-activating factor (PAF)
- Toxic oxygen metabolites
- Endorphins
- CD-14
- Plasminogen activator inhibitor
- Vasoactive neuropeptides
- Histamine and serotonin
- Tissue macrophages and monocytes
- And many others currently under investigation

MANAGEMENT

The mainstay of management of patients with ALI and ARDS has been predominantly one of support. Although hypoxemia is the key feature of ARDS, mortality is predominantly due to multiple organ failure (MOF) and sepsis. The high mortality rates in patients with this condition have prompted active investigation into the physiologic processes involved in the production and propagation of the injury. Initial attention most be directed toward the underlying clinical condition. If there is an active infection then antimicrobial agents should be started and hemodynamic support provided. Hypotension and anemia should be corrected. The cornerstone still is the provision of good mechanical ventilatory support. Recent data from several clinical trials report significant survival benefit from a lung protective ventilatory support protocol.

CLINICAL CAVEAT

Ventilatory Management of ALI and ARDS

Start with a lung recruitment maneuver, use tidal volumes of 5–7 ml/kg, use a pressure control mode, and support the recruited alveoli with proper levels of PEEP.

Use of nonprotective ventilatory support strategies may have a role in a persistent proinflammatory response and the development of multiple organ dysfunction syndromes (MODS) and/or MOF. The cyclic opening and closing of alveoli in nonrecruited lung adds to the surfactant dysfunction. This may add to the loss of compartmentalization of the lung and transmigration of cytokines and infectious agents into and out of the lung. This in turn may lead to further complications and a poor outcome.

Ventilator-Induced Lung Injury

Over the last few years there has been a growing concern that the ventilatory support strategy in the management of patients with ALI and ARDS may augment the lung injury and impair the healing process. The Acute Respiratory Distress Syndrome Network (ARDS-NET) has been in the forefront of investigating aspects of mechanical ventilation. One very important finding was that in patients with ALI/ARDS mechanical ventilation with lower tidal volumes (5–7ml/kg) than those traditionally used (10–12 ml/kg) resulted in decreased mortality and increased the number of days without ventilator use.

Several other ongoing investigations have evaluated other aspects of mechanical ventilation and how they affect the lung. Investigators have found that cytokines and vasoactive substances are released with nonphysiologic-based modes of ventilation.

Open Lung Strategy

The repetitive recruitment/derecruitment of distal airways and alveoli has been shown to produce many physiologic affects. It cannot only produce shear forces secondary to large changes in pressure (ΔP) since the set tidal volume may be too high when given to a lung with atelectasis and decreased volume (functional residual capacity, FRC) but also can activate various mediators to be released that affect not only the lung but may trigger systemic effects and lead to MODS. These closed alveolar beds may also affect surfactant and produce more atelectasis and loss of barrier function. Therefore it is important for the clinician to recruit lung at the onset of mechanical ventilation and prevent it throughout mechanical ventilatory support.

Open Lung Concept

The law of Laplace links the pressure at the alveolar level to the surface tension and radius. In healthy individuals surfactant minimizes the surface forces and thus ensures alveolar stability at all alveolar sizes. During lung injury, all lungs present with some level of surfactant dysfunction, the degree of dysfunction determining the amount of pressure needed to expand the alveoli from a state of small radius (volume) to large radius (volume). It can further be derived from these laws that the pressure necessary to keep alveoli expanded is small at a high FRC, since FRC is directly correlated to the amount of open lung units and their size. If we apply a peak pressure (PIP) of 40–60 cmH$_2$O for ten breaths and then splint the lung open with either elevated positive

---

Box 16-5   Lung Opening Procedure (LOP)

- Set ventilator in pressure control mode
- Recruit with PIP of 40-60 cmH$_2$O (higher may be necessary with more injured lungs) for 10 breaths
- Splint the lung with PEEP set to the infection point (usually 10-15 cmH$_2$O)
- Adjust PIP down to lowest PIP to deliver 5-7 ml/kg tidal volume
- Titrate ventilator PIP and PEEP to give the smallest change in pressure (ΔP)

---

end-expiratory pressure (PEEP) or inverse ratio ventilation, we will stabilize the alveoli at a better position in the pressure/volume curve (Box 16-5). (See also Chapter 17.)

Experimental Therapies

In the 1990s a plethora of clinical trials were conducted to evaluate a host of "antimediators" that have targeted the potential proinflammatory compounds that can be identified in the blood or the lung in ARDS patients. However, to date there has not been major success for these compounds. However, many more compounds are under investigation.

Antioxidant therapy has also been under investigation. The agents vitamins C and E, procysteine, β-carotene, and N-acetylcysteine have been used in several ARDS trials. No survival benefit was found with any of these compounds.

As regards inhalation of nitric oxide (NO), several pilot studies showed a degree of success with this agent. Two large multicenter trials, however, did not show any benefit in survival with NO, but did show increases in oxygenation in the short term. Several centers still use this agent as a bridge therapy in critically ill patients.

Positioning is an important adjunct therapy; patients with ARDS may improve their oxygenation abnormality when they are placed in the prone position. This improvement is marked in patients with ARDS triggered from primary lung injury and may not be as marked in patients with ARDS triggered from a distal focus (non lung). Although placing the patient in the prone position results in improvement of oxygenation, it is important to remember that there are potential complications that result from this position. To date no randomized controlled trials have demonstrated an improvement in mortality associated with the prone position.

An old therapy that has resurfaced in the treatment of ARDS is the use of corticosteroids. Several reports have shown improvement in the repair phase of ARDS (fibroproliferative phase) with the use of steroids. This hypothesis is currently under evaluation by the NIH-sponsored ARDS-NET.

Since many of the problems associated with ALI/ARDS are triggered by injury to the surfactant system, there is now great interest in surfactant replacement therapy. The use of surfactant has been life saving in neonates so there may be a reason to use it in adults. Several ongoing studies are currently underway to evaluate several different surfactant preparations. This is a highly interesting avenue of investigation and may hold some promise in that this therapy is physiologically based.

CONCLUSIONS

ALI/ARDS continues to be a major problem in the ICU and generates a high level of mortality. It is important for the clinician to understand the underlying pathophysiology to develop treatment protocols in the management of these patients. Improvement in our understanding of mechanical ventilation may play an important role in decreasing mortality and time on mechanical ventilation. Lung recruitment and the prevention of VILI are at the forefront of treatment for this condition.

There are currently many investigations into the triggers of this condition and how they can be controlled. These investigations not only will generate new treatments but will also add to our understanding of the physiology of the lung.

CASE STUDY

ARDS in a Patient with Pneumonia

A 67-year-old presents to the ICU in respiratory distress, oxygen saturation of 85, and respiratory rate of 40. Due to the increased work of breathing the patient is electively intubated. A chest film shows bilateral infiltrates, ABG shows a PaO$_2$ of 67 on a FIO$_2$ of 100%. The patient had a five-day history of flu-like syndrome at home and developed a fever and chills prior to coming to the hospital. The patient's medical history is only positive for hypertension under good control with a β-blocker. The patient had traveled to Hong Kong the previous week. The patient was placed on pressure control mode and a LOP was done with a PIP of 60 cmH$_2$O for 10 breaths, and then the PIP was reduced to a pressure to generate tidal volumes of 6 ml/kg after the PEEP was set to 12 cmH$_2$O. The FIO$_2$ was rapidly titrated down. The patient grows out a staph species from the sputum and was started on Gram-positive antibiotic coverage, and was SARS negative. Over three days the patient stabilized and was weaned off the ventilator using a pressure support wean. The patient was extubated on day four but did require a BIPAP mask for 24 hours to decrease work of breathing. On day five the patient was transferred to a general ward and was discharged home on day eight in no distress.

SELECTED READING

Acute Respiratory Distress Syndrome Network: Ventilation with lower tidal volumes as compared with traditional tidal volumes for acute lung injury and with acute respiratory distress syndrome. N Engl J Med 342:1301-1308, 2000.

Amato MBP, Barbas CSV, Medeiros DM et al: Effect of a protective ventilation strategy on mortality in the acute respiratory distress syndrome. N Engl J Med 338:347-357, 1998.

Artigas A, Bernard GR, Carlet J et al: American-European consensus conference on ARDS, Part 2. Am J Respir Crit Care Med 157-163, 1998.

Dellinger RP, Zimmerman JL, Taylor RW et al: Effects of inhaled nitric oxide in patients with acute respiratory distress syndrome, results of phase 2 study. Crit Care Med 26:15-23, 1998.

Haitsma JJ, Papadakos PJ, Lachmann B: Surfactant therapy in ALI/ARDS. Curr Opin Crit Care 10:18-22, 2004.

Papadakos PJ, Lachmann B: Lung recruitment in ARDS. Mt Sinai J Med 6(1):73-77, 2000.

Pepe P: The clinical entity of adult respiratory distress syndrome. Crit Care Clin 2:377-385, 1986.

Slutsky AS, Tremblay LN: Multiple system organ failure: is mechanical ventilation a contributing factor? Am J Respir Crit Care Med 157:1721-1728, 1998.

Mechanical Ventilation

PETER J. PAPADAKOS, M.D., F.C.C.P., F.C.C.M.

BURKHARD LACHMANN, M.D., Ph.D.

Mechanical ventilation is the most common mode of life support in both the operating theatre and in the modern intensive care unit (ICU). It is present in all types of critical care units from postoperative units, surgical ICUs, trauma ICUs, medical ICUs, burn units, weaning centers, and neurologic/neurosurgical ICUs. Positive pressure mechanical ventilation became a standard technique for mechanical ventilation during the polio epidemic of the 1950s. As more and more complex patients survive resuscitation and are admitted to ICUs the level of ventilation required becomes more complex. Rapid and proper titration of mechanical ventilation plays an important role in many aspects of patient care. While the use of mechanical ventilation to treat acute or chronic respiratory failure has historically been important, interactive and noninvasive modes of ventilation are allowing more therapeutic options for many more types of patients and forms of respiratory failure. Advances in

ventilator technology with the introduction of computer control and feedback coupled with improved monitoring tools and a growing understanding of respiratory physiology have led to an explosion in our ability to care for patients. One of the most important advances is a growing knowledge of how the ventilator affects both normal and abnormal physiology. We have gained an understanding that mechanical ventilation plays an important role in the modulation of the inflammatory system and the release of cytokines and other vosoactive substances.

Anesthesiologists have added considerably to the literature of mechanical ventilation with their ability to see the effect of mechanical ventilation from the operating theatre to the postoperative unit especially during extensive surgical procedures.

This experience has allowed us to better understand the physiology of patients on ventilators and affect changes in their therapy.

Mechanical ventilation can also affect metabolism and with the delivery of oxygen both in healthy and unstable patients we can affect increases in oxygen delivery to organ systems and help in the regulation of the acid–base status. It can allow us to provide proper levels of pain control and sedation. Mechanical ventilation is therefore central in rational, effective, safe, and compassionate management.

INDICATIONS

Perhaps the most frequent application of mechanical ventilation is as a supportive therapy for respiratory failure. Respiratory failure is commonly classified into acute or chronic and these classes are then subdivided into inadequate oxygenation, inadequate ventilation, or both (Table 17-1).

The most important parameter to start mechanical ventilation is close observation of the patient and the

Table 17-1 Classification of Acute Respiratory Failure
Failure of oxygenation (hypoxemia)
Pneumonia
Hydrostatic pulmonary edema
Exacerbation of asthma
Pulmonary embolus
Failure of ventilation (hypercapnia)
Hypoventilation
Reduced respiratory drive
Drug intoxication
Head trauma, cerebral vascular accident
Impaired respiratory pump function
Respiratory muscle fatigue
Neuromuscular disease
Chest wall trauma/deformity
Increased dead space
Emphysema
Pulmonary embolus
Cystic fibrosis
Increased CO_2 production
Increased work of breathing (any cause)
Fever
Excessive carbohydrate intake

Table 17-2 Clinical Parameters Associated with Respiratory Failure

Respiratory Parameter	Usual Range	Respiratory Failure
Respiratory rate (breaths/minute)	12–25	>30
Vital capacity (ml/kg)	30–70	<15
Tidal volume (ml/kg)	5–8	<3-4
Oxygenation, PaO_2 (mmHg)	75–100	<60
Ventilation, $PaCO_2$ (mmHg)	35–45	>55 (see text)

Respiratory parameters that may act as a guide are respiratory rate above 30, tidal volume below 4 ml/kg, and a vital capacity below 15 ml/kg with subjective respiratory distress, which all suggest a need for respiratory support (Table 17-2).

MANIPULATION OF $PaCO_2$

In many situations mechanical ventilation is instituted in the absence of respiratory failure. The use of positive pressure ventilation to induce hypocarbia for the purpose of decreasing intercranial pressure (ICP) is a common therapy. This technique is useful both in neurologic and neurosurgical patients. Hyperventilation for the acute control of increased ICP is still the only emergent technique for patients at risk for herniation. It is however not useful after the acute phase.

PATIENTS REQUIRING SEDATION

In many surgical patients mechanical ventilation is required for postoperative care secondary to large fluid shifts, unstable vital signs, and a marked metabolic acidosis (lactate levels > 5). Patients in need of interaortic balloon pumping or the use of ventricular assist devices postcardiac surgery require sedation and mechanical ventilation. Massive trauma patients with unstable fractures, closed head injuries, or who require management of an open abdomen will need sedation titrated and ventilatory management secondary to these agents. Burn patients are another group who due to large amounts of narcotics and complex wound care may need several days of mechanical ventilation.

evaluation of the work of breathing. It does not require any equipment but does require a degree of clinical experience.

CLINICAL CAVEAT

Indication for Ventilator Support
Even with perfect blood gases, if a patient is working hard they will need a level of ventilatory support.

The range of acceptable blood gas values can vary widely, depending on the disease process causing respiratory failure and age. However, institution of mechanical ventilation is usually indicated before the development of laboratory values that demand immediate intubation and mechanical ventilation. The decision both to initiate and to discontinue mechanical ventilation is therefore a clinical judgment, made on the basis of careful evaluation of the patient and consideration of blood gas and metabolic abnormalities.

A general rule of thumb can be used to evaluate laboratory data, a PaO_2 < 60 mmHg (oxygen saturation <90%) on maximal oxygen supplementation, progressively increasing $PaCO_2$ values, and an acute respiratory acidosis with pH values below 7.25. Also other data such as worsening arrhythmias, hemodynamic instability, and decay in mental status all can suggest the need for mechanical ventilation and may stave off clinical deterioration.

CLINICAL CAVEAT

Heavy Sedation
If it is believed a patient will need heavy sedation or large dosages of narcotics it is best to electively intubate and mechanically ventilate them.

A large group of patients in all ICU environments needing a large amount of sedation that may cause respiratory depression are patients with complex histories of psychiatric disorders or patients that are withdrawing from drugs and alcohol. These patients may harm themselves and others if not acutely medicated.

BASIC MODES OF MECHANICAL VENTILATION

As ventilator technology has progressed, the ways of delivering positive pressure ventilation have proliferated. In daily practice, however, four basic modes of positive pressure ventilation are most commonly used. These modes can be classified on the basis of how they are triggered to deliver a breath, whether these breaths are targeted to a set volume or pressure, and how the ventilator cycles from inspiration to expiration (Table 17-3).

CONTROLLED MECHANICAL VENTILATION

Controlled mechanical ventilation (CMV) is the most common mode of ventilation in the patient under general anesthesia in the operating theater. It is an excellent starting block for the understanding of mechanical ventilatory parameters. CMV or volume control (VC) was the first volume-targeted mode. It is a pure "control" mode; that is, the minute ventilation (VE) is completely governed by the machine (VE = tidal volume (TV) × respiratory rate). The physician sets the respiratory rate, TV, inspiratory flow rate, ratio of inspiratory to expiratory time (I:E), positive end-expiratory pressure (PEEP), and the level of inspired oxygen (FIO_2). In VC, the patient is unable to trigger the ventilator to deliver additional breaths. This works well with patients under general anesthesia, unresponsive, or heavily sedated, but not for conscious patients, whose respiratory efforts are not sensed by the ventilator, which leads to patient discomfort and increased work of breathing. As a result, this mode has been largely abandoned outside of the operating theatre.

ASSIST-CONTROL VENTILATION

This mode is similar to VC mode except that the ventilator senses respiratory efforts by the patient. As in VC, the physician sets a respiratory rate, TV, flow rate, I:E ratio, FIO_2, and PEEP. Breaths are delivered automatically, regardless of the patient effort ("control"). In assist-control (AC), however, the ventilator detects the patient's effort and responds by delivering a breath identical to the controlled one ("assist"). The patient can therefore breathe faster than the back-up rate, but all breaths have the same tidal volume, flow rate, and inspiratory time. Hence AC mode allows better synchrony between patient and ventilator than VC mode, while still providing baseline minute ventilation. A better descriptive and accurate name for this mode is "volume-targeted assist-control ventilation."

Like all modes of mechanical ventilation, AC has several disadvantages. If the back-up respiratory rate is set too far below the patient's spontaneous rate, exhalation time progressively decreases, since the inspiratory time is fixed by the back-up rate and flow rate. In the extreme example, this may results in inadequate time for exhalation. As a result, lung volume remains above functional residual capacity (FRC), and a process called dynamic hyperventilation occurs. This increased lung volume is associated with elevation in the alveolar pressure at end-exhalation, or "auto-PEEP." Another problem occurs when patients with high minute ventilation requirements make persistent efforts while a breath is being delivered. If this effort is strong enough, the patient may trigger the ventilator again, a phenomenon known as "breath stacking." This can cause wide swings in airway pressure and

---

Table 17-3   Mechanical Functions in Positive Pressure Ventilators

Mode	Initiation	Limit	Cycle
VOLUME PRESET			
Controlled mechanical ventilation	Time	Volume	Volume/time
Assist-control ventilation	Pressure	Volume	Volume/time
Intermittent mandatory ventilation	Time	Volume	Volume/time
Synchronized intermittent mandatory ventilation	Time/pressure	Volume	Volume/time
PRESSURE PRESET			
Pressure-support ventilation	Pressure	Pressure	Flow
Pressure-control ventilation	Time	Pressure	Time

increase both the risk of barotrauma or biotrauma (ventilator-associated lung injury). Finally, in volume-targeted modes, the inspiratory rate is fixed. Many acutely ill patients strive for high inspiratory flow rates. If ventilator-delivered airflow is below patient demand, the work of breathing increases as the patient makes further futile efforts to augment inspiratory flow.

INTERMITTENT MANDATORY VENTILATION

In the early 1970s a new mode of partial ventilatory support, intermittent mandatory ventilation (IMV), was developed to facilitate weaning, the transition from mechanical support to normal spontaneous breathing. This mode has become very popular in the USA as a support mode.

The IMV mode delivers positive pressure mechanical breaths at a preset rate and allows spontaneous, unassisted breaths between mechanical breaths. It is time initiated, volume limited, and cycled by volume or time to provide mechanical breaths. To assist any spontaneous ventilation between mechanical breaths the ventilator has a secondary source of gas flow. This utilizes continuous gas flow within the circuit or has a demand valve that opens to allow gas to flow from a reservoir. Continuous gas flow at a rate greater than peak inspiratory flow rate imparts no additional work of breathing to the patient and requires a great volume of fresh gas flow to be used. The demand valve system, although more efficient in the conservation of fresh gas flow, imparts a significant work of breathing.

SYNCHRONIZED INTERMITTENT MANDATORY VENTILATION

Like AC mode, synchronized intermittent mandatory ventilation (SIMV) is also a volume-targeted mode and provides a guaranteed VE. For the mandatory breaths, tidal volume and respiratory rate are chosen, guaranteeing baseline minute ventilation. The practitioner also sets FIO_2, PEEP, and flow rate as with other modes. SIMV is similar to IMV with the addition of computer control to synchronize mechanical breaths with spontaneous efforts to reduce the likelihood of breath stacking. If a sufficient effort occurs shortly before the mandatory breath is delivered (a time interval known as the "synchronization period") a breath identical to the mandatory breath is delivered. If a patient effort occurs outside this synchronization period, the airway pressure, flow rate, and tidal volume are purely patient-generated, and the ventilator provides no assistance. While this reduces

---

Box 17-1 Synchronized Intermittent Mandatory Ventilation

- Volume-controlled mode in which operator sets TV, flow rate, and respiratory rate.
- Mandatory breaths are positive pressure breaths that provide full ventilatory assistance and deliver the set TV; the patient does not control TV during mandatory breaths.
- Mandatory breaths are either time-triggered or synchronized to patient triggering.
- Spontaneous breaths are allowable between mandatory breaths, but patients receive no positive pressure assistance during spontaneous breaths.
- Provides preset ventilatory backup to guarantee minimum VE.

---

the likelihood of air trapping and breath stacking, it can increase the work of breathing. An interesting factor is if the mandatory respiratory rate is less than approximately 80% of the patient's actual rate, the high level of work expended during the spontaneous breaths will also be expended during the mandatory breaths. This is based due to the physiology of the respiratory center in the brain, which has a lag time and is unable to alter its output on a breath-to-breath basis. So if high neurologic output is required for a significant percentage of breaths, that same output will be given for all breaths including the artificial breaths delivered by the ventilator. Therefore, attempting to "exercise" the respiratory muscles by setting the SIMV rate at half of the patient's spontaneous rate is counterproductive, because it simply increases the work of breathing and results in respiratory muscle fatigue and may result in weaning failure (Box 17-1).

CLINICAL CAVEAT

The Work of Breathing

The most important factor that leads to proper patient–ventilator synchronization is properly supporting the patient's spontaneous breathing. Proper support leads to decreased work of breathing.

SIMV is the most commonly used mode of mechanical ventilation for uncomplicated patients who require only short periods of support. The pure use of volume-cycled ventilation may not be ideal for long-term support and in patients with complex problems such as acute respiratory distress syndrome (ARDS). In weaning this mode should be married to pressure-support ventilation, which is discussed later.

PRESSURE-CONTROL VENTILATION

A more accurate name for pressure-control ventilation (PCV) mode is "pressure-targeted assist-control ventilation." The mode is similar to AC mode described above, except that a defined inspiratory pressure (IP) is set, instead of a tidal volume. This allows absolute control over peak pressure source. Pressure control is a more natural form of artificial ventilation in that it mimics the natural way we breathe. The basic setting are similar to AC: respiratory rate, I:E ratio, FIO_2, PEEP, and trigger sensitivity.

Inspiratory flow rate is not fixed in PCV. It varies with IP, inspiratory time, respiratory mechanics, and patient effort. This can be advantageous, because flow rate increases with patient effort, unlike the volume-targeted modes, in which flow rate is fixed. Therefore patients with high-ventilation requirements may feel more comfortable on PCV, because they can regulate and increase flow as needed. This variable flow rate has another potential advantage: the flow pattern changes as respiratory system compliance decreases as inflation proceeds and compliance decreases. The major down side of this mode is that if compliance changes the TV delivered are variable. Therefore TV changes and can be either too high or too low to meet patient demands. To combat this newer more complex ventilators have created an ability to maintain set TV in pressure-control mode.

PRESSURE SUPPORT

Pressure support ventilation (PSV) is a pressure-triggered mode in which the patient's inspiratory effort is supported by a preset inspiratory pressure (in the usual range 5–15 cmH_2O). Inspiration is initiated by the patient and is terminated when the flow falls below a specific level. In this mode the patient determines the respiratory rate, inspiratory time, and TV. Unlike the previous modes PSV assists only breaths initiated by the patient. Therefore, patients with unstable respiratory function or respiratory drive may not be adequately ventilated with pressure support alone. Patients who are heavily medicated with narcotics and sedatives may not benefit from this mode alone.

In theory since the patient controls the rate, length, depth, and flow profile of each breath, it has been claimed that PSV is more comfortable than other modes of ventilation. Even at low levels, PSV improves the efficiency of spontaneous respiratory rate, more efficient muscle activity, and less oxygen consumption.

PSV may be used solely to overcome the work of breathing imposed by the endotracheal tube and ventilator circuit (specific values vary from machine to machine but a range is 8–10 cmH_2O). If a patient is doing well at a low level of PSV it may be predictive that the patient will do well with extubation. PSV is used in combination with other modes to provide patient comfort, decrease work of breathing, and affect weaning outcome.

CLINICAL CAVEAT

Pressure Support

Most patients on artificial mechanical ventilation will need the addition of pressure support to provide patient comfort and aid in weaning. Pressure support is also used to counteract the resistance of endotracheal tubes and decrease the work of breathing in spontaneous breaths.

NEW MODES OF VENTILATION

In recent years more complex ventilators have been introduced to better support a growing number of patients with complex lung mechanics. With the addition of microcomputers and feedback loops in ICU ventilators they are better able to control and support respiratory parameters that were manually adjusted only a few short years ago. It is hoped that this technology will aid in the management of patients and also reduce ventilator-induced lung injury (VILI). Some of these modes build on the basic modes of pressure control and assist control by providing technologic advances that correct the limitations that they have historically had.

Pressure-Regulated Volume Control

Pressure-regulated volume control (PRVC) is a mode that is a combination of decelerating flow of pressure control with volume guarantee. This mode allows for nearly continuous monitoring of lung mechanics. Inspiratory pressure is regulated to a value based on the volume–pressure calculation of the previous breath compared with the preset target volume. As compliance changes, the pressure is regulated to the lowest possible limit as long as the target pressure is reached.

Pressure-Controlled Inverse Ratio Ventilation

To prevent gas trapping, at least as much time is allowed for exhalation as for inhalation; however, for certain patients, gas exchange may improve markedly when the ratio is extended to values greater than 1:1. This mode is usually only used in patients with severe respiratory failure, hypoxemia, and ARDS. Pressure-controlled inverse ratio ventilation (PCIRV) is currently used as a technique of last resort but may have a role in the earliest phase of lung failure when lungs are most recruitable. It may be important to decrease cyclic opening and closing of alveolar units and play a role in lung protection by keeping recruited alveoli open, thereby decreasing shear forces.

Airway Pressure-Release Ventilation and Biphasic Airway Pressure

Airway pressure-release ventilation (APRV) and biphasic airway pressure (BiPAP) can be thought of as variants of IRV intended for use with spontaneously breathing patients. BiPAP is widely used to support patients with sleep apnea and also used with success in patients prone to atelectasis. It has been found useful in trauma patients with multiple broken ribs from developing pneumonia. This mechanism is used to provide added ventilatory support for patients who need continuous positive airway pressure (CPAP) for oxygenation but cannot provide adequate ventilatory drive without machine assistance. Both APRV and BiPAP allow ventilatory efforts around CPAP. It allows for depressurization of the system, either partially or completely, for short periods at a set frequency. After this release, fresh gas enters until pressure equals the set upper limit. BiPAP differs from APRV in that it allows for an option to have the patient breathe for extended periods of time spontaneously at either level of pressure.

As with IRV, these modes may generate sustained higher mean airway pressure, which may exert traction. The efficacy of pressure-release cycles depends on the duration of the release, the mechanical properties of the chest, the level to which airway pressure is allowed to fall, and the cycling frequency between the two pressure baselines.

A problem with these systems is that as ventilatory support increases; mean airway pressure falls decreasing some of the oxygen-exchange advantages of the higher CPAP levels. This mode may not be useful for patients with significant airflow obstruction or greatly reduced lung compliance.

Jet Ventilation, High Frequency

The goal of high-frequency ventilation (HFV) is to effect oxygenation and ventilation at relatively low peak pressure, thereby minimizing trauma due to higher inspiratory pressure and volume. Tidal volumes that approximate to or are less than anatomic dead space may be used. Distinct types of HFV include high-frequency jet ventilation (HFJV) and high-frequency oscillation (HFO). In general, sedation analgesia and neuromuscular blockade are maintained during the use of these modes to prevent spontaneous breathing and maximize the efficiency of these techniques.

> **Box 17-2 Mode of Ventilation**
>
> The mode of ventilation used should be individualized to specific patient's needs. The primary goal should be to recruit lung affected by atelectasis and prevent further collapse.

HFO is currently the most used in the ICU. HFO can recruit lung units by employing mean airway pressures equal to or greater than conventional ventilation without exposing the lung to comparably high peak pressures. HFO has been associated with decreased incidence of barotrauma in patients requiring high levels of support. Despite enormous interest these modes have not replaced more conventional modes of ventilation (Box 17-2).

HOW TO SET THE VENTILATOR

The way one initially sets the ventilator will play an important role in patient care and will affect patient physiology. There is much evidence that the mode and style of artificial ventilation will affect not only patient comfort but also time of support. The settings may produce volume and pressure trauma if improper levels of tidal volume and pressure are set. There is growing evidence that the initial tidal volume can affect morbidity and mortality. Atelectasis and alveolar collapse can affect levels of surfactant in the lung and also be important in the release of cytokines and the transmigration of bacteria both into and out of the lung. So a rational approach must be taken when treating patients with respiratory failure who are admitted to the ICU (Box 17-3).

The use of ventilator graphic displays has greatly improved monitoring of lung function. These flow volume loops give us the ability to evaluate lung compliance, set levels of PEEP, evaluate I:E ratios, and titrate ventilator support with clear end points.

> **Box 17-3 Basic Ventilator Settings**
>
> - Set the FIO$_2$ to 100%
> - Set a tidal volume of 5–7 ml/kg
> - Set a rate of 14
> - Use a pressure-control mode
> - Set the PEEP to 10 cmH$_2$O or best PEEP if one has pressure/volume graphics
> - Get an arterial blood gas on these settings after 15 minutes and adjust oxygen and rate as needed.

Traditional approaches to mechanical ventilation used tidal volumes of 10–15 ml/kg body weight. Since 2000 a large multicenter trial, the Acute Respiratory Syndrome Network, has challenged this common practice. The findings showed that patients fared better when placed on normal physiologic tidal volumes of 5–7 ml/kg body weight. This so-called low tidal volume ventilation again points out that even the basic concepts of mechanical ventilation need to be studied.

CLINICAL CAVEAT

Tidal Volume
The ventilator should be set with normal physiologic tidal volumes of 5–7 ml/kg versus the traditional 10–15 ml/kg.

It is best to start to place the patient on a FIO_2 of 100% on arrival to the ICU as a baseline to evaluate the patient's lung physiology. The level of hypoxia can also be evaluated at this time. The level of shunt can also be rapidly evaluated at this level of oxygen. This data will also allow the practitioner to decide if lung recruitment is necessary. The use of PEEP to allow recruited alveolar beds to remain open can also be elucidated from the baseline arterial blood gas that is used on this concentration of oxygen.

TITRATION OF POSITIVE END-EXPIRATORY PRESSURE

PEEP refers to pressure in the airway at the end of expiration that exceeds atmospheric pressure. The term is applicable to patients receiving mechanical ventilation. For spontaneously breathing subjects, the term CPAP is used when inspiratory and expiratory portions of the circuit are pressurized above atmospheric pressure. PEEP is used mainly to stabilize lung units and improve oxygenation in patients with hypoxia and replicate normal lung physiology (Box 17-4).

PEEP can be titrated best through the use of the pressure–volume curve using inflection points. The ideal point is between the lower and upper inflection where lung compliance is maximal. Airway pressures below the lower inflection point are associated with low compliance, alveolar collapse, and atelectasis. At airway pressures above the upper inflection point, compliance also decreases, the limit of lung distention is approached, and the risk of barotrauma is high but oxygenation is best. A good strategy for optimized mechanical ventilation and PEEP is to select a PEEP level just above the lower inflection point, and maintain plateau airway pressures below the upper inflection point (Figure 17-1).

There is no evidence that PEEP levels below or equal to 10 cmH_2O will affect ICP in patients with head injury.

Box 17-4   Key Effects of Positive End-Expiratory Pressure

BENEFICIAL:
- Usually improves oxygenation
- Stabilizes lung units
- Minimizes potential for ventilator-induced lung injury

ADVERSE:
- May worsen gas exchange
- Decreases preload thereby decreasing cardiac output in patients with low intervascular volume
- Interferes with assessment of hemodynamic pressures

In patients with both acute lung injury and closed head injury PEEP is titrated to maximize both oxygenation and ICP pressure (Box 17-5).

One should monitor for auto-PEEP, or intrinsic PEEP, which is due to inadequate time for lung emptying in the setting of increased airway resistance and expiratory flow limitation.

Adverse effects, especially in volume-targeted modes, include increased work of breathing, risk of barotrauma or volutrauma, and hemodynamic compromise. Auto-PEEP should be monitored closely; the newer generation of ventilators can provide automated assessment of auto-PEEP (Box 17-6).

LUNG RECRUITMENT

Every effort should be made to ensure that there is no atelectasis present in patients on artificial ventilation.

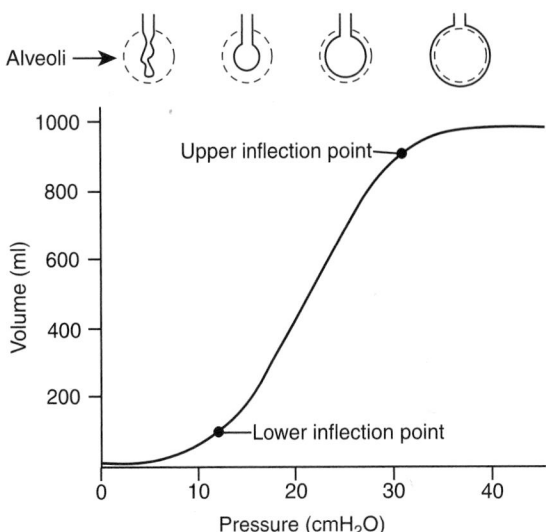

Figure 17-1   Calculation of inflection point.

Box 17-5 Key Indications for Positive End-Expiratory Pressure

- Acute lung injury and acute respiratory distress syndrome.
- Cardiogenic pulmonary edema.
- Atelectasis associated with severe hypoxemia.
- Other forms of severe hypoxemic respiratory failure.

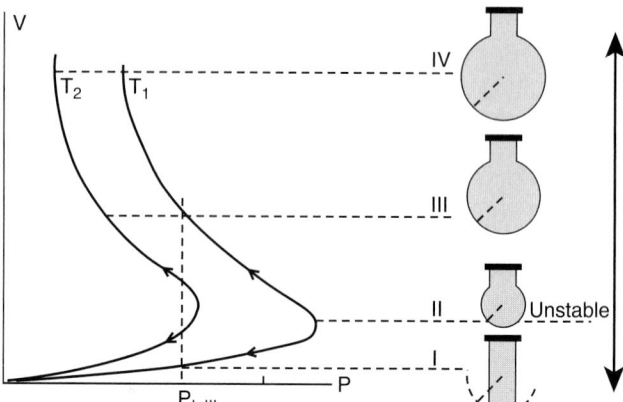

Figure 17-2 Physiologic behavior of the alveolus. The pressure (P)–volume (V) relation is displayed on X–Y axes. The status of the bronchoalveolar unit is shown on the right-hand side. The arrows show the direction from closed (bottom) to open (top). The ideal alveolar status is IV or III.

The use of an open-lung strategy will not only improve oxygenation but also may also decrease the levels of cytokines and prevent the loss of surfactant. There is evidence that this strategy also prevents the transmigration of both cytokines and infectious agents across the lung. This lung recruitment should be applied to all patients no matter what mode of ventilation is applied (Figure 17-2).

CONCLUSIONS

The management of mechanical ventilation is no longer a hit-or-miss procedure but a therapy, which has physiological end points along with the basic goals of oxygenation and removal of carbon dioxide. Which ventilator settings are chosen from the outset will have a great impact on patient management. Proper settings will allow for improved oxygenation on the lowest FIO_2 with the least atelectasis. Proper titration will decrease biotrauma and may affect cytokine levels thereby affecting other organs. The proper settings will allow for the patient to be rapidly weaned from the ventilator. The physician should work with the respiratory therapists in the ICU to manage the patient in an ongoing manner. This is because a patient's condition is ever changing and may need adjustments throughout the day. The therapist is also specially trained to manage the ever-advancing technology of modern ICU ventilators.

Box 17-6 Treatment Strategies for Minimizing Auto-Positive End-Expiratory Pressure in Volume-Targeted Ventilation

- Aggressive bronchodilator therapy.
- Pain control, sedation; consider selective use of neuromuscular blockade.
- Minimize I:E; e.g., increase expiratory time and inspiratory flow rate, reduce tidal volume, reduce respiratory rate.
- In selected cases, judicious application of (extrinsic) PEEP will counter intrinsic PEEP and decrease the work of breathing (asthma, chronic obstructive pulmonary disease).
- In some selected patients with severe lung injury auto-PEEP can be used to advantage especially patients where the strategy of PCIRV is used.

CASE STUDY

Management of a Patient with Multiple Trauma

A 25-year-old man involved in a high-speed head-on collision presents to the emergency room with acute respiratory distress and abdominal pain. The patient was intubated with in-line traction. Trauma evaluation showed a right femur deformity, chest deformity, and abdominal rebound. An emergent x-ray showed multiple rib fractures bilaterally, a right femur fracture, and no evidence of a spinal injury. A CT scan showed atelectasis and a pulmonary contusion, and a grade II liver injury. The initial blood gas on a FIO_2 of 100% was a PaO_2 of 64 and $PaCO_2$ of 38. The patient was placed on pressure control after a lung-opening procedure (LOP) with an opening pressure of 60 cmH_2O for ten breaths. The pressure control was titrated to generate a tidal volume of 6 ml/kg, a ventilatory rate of 14, and the initial PEEP was set at 10 cmH_2O. The repeat arterial blood gas was now a PaO_2 of 475 and a $PaCO_2$ of 34. The FIO_2 was lowered to 50% and the rate decreased to 12. An epidural catheter was placed for pain management and the patient tolerated operative management of the fracture on hospital day two without a problem. The patient was weaned using pressure support over the course of five days and was extubated without a problem. He was transferred to general surgical ward on day six.

SELECTED READING

Acute Respiratory Distress Syndrome Network: Ventilation with lower tidal volumes as compared with traditional tidal volumes for acute lung injury and the acute respiratory distress syndrome. New Engl J Med 242:1301–1308, 2000.

Apostolakos MJ, Levy PC, Papadakos PJ: New Modes of mechanical ventilation. Clin Pulmon Med 2(2):121–128, 1995.

Botz GH, Sladen RN: Conventional modes of mechanical ventilation. Int Anesthesiol Clinics 38(1):19–27, 1997.

Dreyfuss D, Saumon G: Ventilator-induced lung injury: lessons from experimental studies. Am J Resp Crit Care Med 157:294–323, 1998.

Lachmann B: Open up the lung and keep the lung open. Intens Care Med 18:319–321, 1992.

Papadakos PJ, Lachmann B, Bohm S: Pressure control ventilation: consensus and new horizons. Clin Pulmon Med 5(2):59–65, 1998.

Richard JC, Maggiore SM, Jonson B et al: Influence of tidal volume on alveolar recruitment. Respective role of PEEP and a recruitment maneuver. Am J Respir Crit Care Med 158:1571–1577, 1998.

CHAPTER 18

Weaning from Mechanical Ventilation

MICHAEL J. APOSTOLAKOS, M.D.

Pathophysiology of Weaning Failure
Approach to Weaning from Mechanical Ventilation
Predictive Criteria of Weaning Outcome
Withdrawal of Mechanical Ventilation
Modes of Mechanical Ventilation During Weaning
Summary

A significant proportion of patients admitted to intensive care units (ICUs) undergo intubation with mechanical ventilation. The majority of such patients are extubated quite readily. However, as many as 20% of mechanically ventilated patients will fail their first attempt at weaning. More than 40% of the time on mechanical ventilation is spent trying to wean the patient from the ventilator. The causes of prolonged ventilator dependency are listed in Table 18-1. As mechanical ventilation is associated with a host of complications, every effort should be made to discontinue mechanical ventilation as soon as the patient can resume and sustain spontaneous ventilation. However, choosing the appropriate time for discontinuation of mechanical ventilation may prove difficult. If chosen too early, severe cardiopulmonary decompensation may further delay extubation. If chosen too late, the patient remains at risk for ventilator-associated complications such as pneumonia. Various clinical and laboratory factors used to evaluate respiratory capacity have been used as predictive factors in weaning. These are utilized in an attempt to optimize weaning. This chapter reviews the causes of weaning failure and an approach to liberating patients from mechanical ventilation.

PATHOPHYSIOLOGY OF WEANING FAILURE

Weaning from mechanical ventilation depends on the strength of the respiratory muscles, the load applied to the muscles, and the central drive to breathe.

Respiratory failure may occur from any of these. For example, Guillain-Barré syndrome can lead to muscle weakness, acute bronchospasm to increased respiratory load, and a narcotic overdose to a decreased central drive. All of these may lead to respiratory failure. The factors of strength, load, and drive constantly interact. Disorders may occur in isolation or in concert.

The relationship between respiratory load and muscle strength can be viewed as a balance. If muscle strength is too weak or load is too heavy, muscular contraction cannot be maintained and the muscles acutely fail. This is termed fatigue. The dominant feature of the pathophysiology of weaning failure is high levels of load relative to the strength of the respiratory muscles. For those who fail, as the weaning progresses, load increases as compared to those who succeed with the weaning trial. Almost always the drive to breathe is high in such cases.

APPROACH TO WEANING FROM MECHANICAL VENTILATION

The first step in weaning a patient from mechanical ventilation is identifying and treating the process that caused the patient to go on the ventilator in the first place (Table 18-2). Common causes of respiratory failure leading to mechanical ventilation include pneumonia, sepsis, congestive heart failure, status epilepticus, and major surgery. Major effort should be directed to reverse this underlying process while ventilating the patient in a nontoxic manner. It should be remembered that mechanical ventilation is a supportive but not a therapeutic endeavor.

Common problems found in weaning patients include fluid overload, altered mental status, acid–base changes, and electrolyte disturbances. These need to be corrected if weaning is to be successful.

Table 18-1 Causes of Ventilatory Dependency

Hypoxemic respiratory failure
    Impaired pulmonary gas exchange
    Nonpulmonary shunt
    Decreased oxygen content of venous blood
    Hypoventilation
Respiratory muscle pump failure
    Decreased neuromuscular capacity
    Increased respiratory pump load
Psychological factors
    Anxiety
    Depression
    Motivation

Modified from Tobin MJ: Weaning patients from mechanical ventilation.
How to avoid difficulty. Postgrad Med 89:171-178, 1991.

Volume overload is common following treatment for systemic inflammation in patients with severe infection and major surgery. This extra volume leads to chest wall edema and pulmonary edema with resultant reduction in functional residual capacity and alveolar collapse. This leads to ventilation/perfusion mismatch and shunting with resultant hypoxemia and a need for increased positive end-expiratory pressure (PEEP) to keep alveoli open. Generally, fluid is mobilized quite readily once the systemic inflammation has been controlled; however, at times diuretics are required to mobilize this extra fluid.

The etiology of altered mental status in mechanically ventilated patients is often multifactorial. Causes of altered mental status include pain, anxiety, and delirium,

Table 18-2 Steps in Managing Patients Who Have Difficulty Weaning from Mechanical Ventilation

Determine cause of ventilatory dependency
Rectify correctable problems
    Pulmonary gas exchange
    Fluid balance
    Mental status
    Acid–base status
    Electrolyte disturbance
Use team approach
Utilize weaning protocol
Utilize daily trials of spontaneous breathing
Consider psychological factors
Optimize posture
Optimize pulmonary care
Ensure adequate nutritional support
Optimize general patient care
Provide ambulation

Modified from Tobin MJ: Weaning patients from mechanical ventilation.
How to avoid difficulty. Postgrad Med 89:171-178, 1991.

as well as toxic/metabolic processes. Oversedation with longer-acting sedatives has been associated with longer time on mechanical ventilation. Many institutions have developed guidelines to assist with sedative administration in mechanically ventilated patients in an attempt to limit this possibility. Successful guidelines utilize a sedation score (e.g., Ramsay scale) to direct bedside caregivers to the goal of sedation and have automatic reductions in sedation dosage (or hold orders) to limit oversedation.

For otherwise stable weaning patients, their pH should be normal (7.35–7.45). Acute illness and the therapy of such can lead to alteration of pH, but this should correct with the treatment of the underlying condition. However, patients with chronic hypercapnia require special mention. Minute ventilation delivered by the ventilator should be adjusted to maintain the patient's usual arterial carbon dioxide level. If a patient with chronic hypercapnia is lowered to the normal range during mechanical ventilation, renal compensation by excretion of bicarbonate occurs and pH normalizes. Subsequently, when the patient resumes spontaneous breathing arterial carbon dioxide tension increases and acute respiratory acidosis may occur because the reduced bicarbonate stores are inadequate for buffering.

Electrolyte disturbances can also adversely affect weaning. Most notably hypocalcemia, hypophosphatemia, and hypomagnesemia have been associated with weakness, which can limit weaning. These disturbances must be corrected prior to weaning attempts.

Malnutrition is particularly common in ventilator-dependent patients. This has a variety of detrimental effects on the respiratory system. On the other hand, nutritional repletion has been shown to increase muscle mass and decrease fatigability of nonrespiratory muscles. Malnutrition produces a decrease in the ventilatory response to hypoxia, a reduction in muscle mass, and a loss of muscle strength and endurance. Host defense compromise related to nutritional depletion may contribute to pneumonia. For malnourished, critically ill patients, nutritional supplementation has been shown to increase patient inspiratory force. Several retrospective studies suggest that appropriate nutritional support may facilitate weaning. Controlled study is required to address fully the role of nutritional support in facilitation of weaning from mechanical ventilation.

Before weaning trials, airway secretions should be suctioned and bronchodilators administered. Beneficial effects of bronchodilators delivered via a spacer device have been noted in patients being weaned from mechanical ventilation regardless of whether the patient had preexisting chronic airway obstruction.

Psychological considerations are also extremely important in achieving a successful weaning outcome. Informing the patient of the weaning plan may decrease patient stress. The presence of a team member providing assurance and explanation during a trial of spontaneous breathing or a decrease in the level of mechanical ventilator support may be valuable. If patients are alert, they should be informed of progress. Environmental stimulation such as the use of a television, radio, or books should be provided. Sleep should be ensured because deprivation causes impairment of the respiratory control system in addition to general discomfort.

Optimal patient posture during weaning from mechanical ventilation varies according to the underlying pathophysiology. Patients with intercostal muscle weakness resulting from low cervical spinal cord lesions show an increase in lung volumes on changing from the upright to the supine posture. Supine posture forces abdominal contents upward displacing the diaphragm cephalad. The diaphragm can then contract downward across a longer distance increasing the volume of gas moved. Conversely, patients with diaphragmatic paralysis do better in the upright position. Vital capacity falls by 50% when these patients are supine. The displacement of the paralyzed diaphragm cephalad leads to a decreased functional residual capacity (FRC) and places the ancillary muscles of respiration at a mechanical disadvantage.

Ventilator settings during periods of mechanical ventilation may affect progress with subsequent weaning trials. A major purpose of mechanical ventilation between weaning trials is to provide rest for the respiratory muscles. With most modes of ventilation (assist-control, synchronized intermittent mandatory ventilation (SIMV), and pressure support ventilation (PSV)) inspiratory muscles do not stop contracting once the ventilator has been triggered. Thus, the inspiratory muscles are not simply "resting." Adjustment of the ventilator settings is necessary to minimize respiratory work. Even when optimally adjusted, patients may still perform a considerable portion of the work of inflation during assisted ventilation.

PREDICTIVE CRITERIA OF WEANING OUTCOME

CURRENT CONTROVERSY

Criteria for Readiness to Wean
The best criterion for readiness to wean from mechanical ventilation remains controversial.

Conventional criteria for readiness to wean are relatively easy to measure but their specificity and sensitivity are relatively poor. These include vital capacity (VC),

tidal volume (TV), minute ventilation (MV), maximum voluntary ventilation, respiratory frequency, and maximal inspiratory pressure.

VC is the greatest volume of gas that a patient is able to exhale in taking a maximum inspiration from residual volume. TV is that volume of gas moved during a normal respiratory cycle. The threshold values for these two parameters predictive of weaning remain controversial but are of the order of 5–8 ml/kg for TV and 10–15 ml/kg for VC. Measurement of VC is relatively difficult because it depends on considerable cooperation from the patient. Given the large degree variability in VC, it is not surprising that some studies have shown that VC often failed to predict weaning outcome with a high degree of accuracy. Although slightly better, using a TV cutoff of 4 ml/kg, the positive predictive value was 0.67 and negative predictive value was 0.85, left significant room for improvement.

In a resting, healthy adult MV is about 6 l/minute. Maximum voluntary ventilation (MVV) is the volume of air that can be inhaled and exhaled with maximum effort over one minute. Normal values for MVV range from 50 to 250 l/minute. The relationship between resting MV and MVV indicates the proportion of the patient's ventilatory capacity required to maintain a certain level of $PaCO_2$ and also indicates the reserve available for further respiratory demands. The combination of a MV of <10 l/minute and the ability to double this value during an MVV maneuver was associated with the ability to wean successfully. However, both of these tests are associated with significant false positive and false negative rates. Furthermore, the MVV can be difficult to obtain in the critically ill patient, as they may be unable to cooperate.

One simple assessment of respiratory muscle function can be made by measuring muscle strength. Respiratory muscle strength can be measured at the patient's bedside by recording the maximal inspiratory pressure (MIP) by means of an aneroid manometer. Maximum static inspiratory pressures for healthy young men and women are approximately −120 cmH$_2$O and −90 cmH$_2$O, respectively. Maximal inspiratory efforts may be performed easily in uncooperative intubated patients by using a one-way valve connected to the manometer, which allows the patient to exhale freely but forces the patient to inhale against the manometer. A MIP < −30 cmH$_2$O is associated with successful extubation but a MIP > −20 cmH$_2$O is associated with the inability to maintain spontaneous breathing. Studies have shown these values to have a better negative predictive value than positive predictive value.

Several more recent predictive criteria of weaning outcome have been described. These include measurements of transdiaphragmatic pressure, airway occlusion pressure, gastric intramural pH (pHi), and several integrative indices. However, these techniques all share in common the requirement for specialized equipment, difficulty of measurement, or complicated equations, which make bedside utility poor.

One exception to the above is the rapid shallow breathing index described by Tobin and Yang. They had found that MV is well maintained in patients who fail a weaning trial, but its components TV and respiratory frequency are combined in a manner that results in inefficient gas exchange. In general, patients who fail weaning trials drop their TVs and increase their respiratory rates. Yang and Tobin have shown that the rapid shallow breathing index as reflected by frequency (breaths/minute)/tidal volume (liters) is the most accurate predictor of weaning outcome. Using a threshold of <105, the frequency (f)/tidal volume (V_T) ratio had a positive predictive value of 0.78 and a negative predictive value of 0.95.

The advantages of the f/V_T ratio as a weaning predictor are that it is easy to measure and not dependent on patient cooperation or effort. The f/V_T ratio was evaluated while patients were spontaneously breathing through the endotracheal tube. A bedside spirometer was used to measure V_T. The predictive value of this index may be lower if measured while patients are on the ventilator with either continuous positive airway pressure (CPAP) or pressure support.

WITHDRAWAL OF MECHANICAL VENTILATION

Withdrawal of mechanical ventilation is considered when the underlying process responsible for the acute respiratory failure is improving or resolved, the patient is in good clinical condition, and gas exchange is adequate (e.g., $PaO_2 \geq 60$ mmHg with $FIO_2 \leq 0.50$ and PEEP ≤ 7.5 cmH$_2$O).

Several clinical parameters discussed above have been used to predict weaning outcome so that the presence of favorable weaning parameters supports the decision to undertake a weaning attempt. This is a trial of spontaneous ventilation prior to extubation. Usually, such a trial is conducted by disconnecting the patient from the ventilator and observing respiratory rate, presence or absence of abdominal paradox, activity of accessory inspiratory muscles, level of consciousness, and monitoring oxygen saturation by pulse oximetry while the patient breathes spontaneously.

Spontaneous breathing trials have been described using a simple T-tube or low-level pressure support (PS) or CPAP at levels ≤7 cmH$_2$O. The T-tube is simply the endotracheal tube connected to flow by oxygen. PS or CPAP are used to reduce the workload imposed on the respiratory muscles and compensates for the extra work of breathing imposed by the endotracheal tube and the ventilator inspiratory valve and circuit. Trial length varies from 30 minutes to 2 hours. Intolerance is judged by tachycardia or bradycardia (>20% increase or decrease from baseline), tachypnea (>35 breaths/minute), hypoxemia (<90% saturated), hypertension (>180 mmHg systolic), hypotension (<90 mmHg systolic), and/or subjective shortness of breath (anxiety, diaphoresis, agitation).

Despite selecting the patients able to undergo a trial of spontaneous breathing according to weaning criteria and monitoring them during the trial looking for intolerance, it is common for marginal patients to require reintubation within 48 hours of extubation. The frequency of extubation failure as defined by reintubation within 48 hours of extubation varies from 4% to 19%. The spontaneous breathing trial evaluates respiratory mechanical function in the presence of an artificial airway. Patients with altered mental status, recurrent aspiration, or copious secretions may achieve ventilator independence but require continued airway protection. Thus, the decision to extubate a patient requires, in addition to a successful spontaneous breathing trial, sufficient level of consciousness and adequate clearance of secretions.

MODES OF MECHANICAL VENTILATION DURING WEANING

CURRENT CONTROVERSY

Weaning Mode
  The optimal mode of mechanical ventilation used during weaning is controversial but IMV weaning appears to slow the process.

Much has been written regarding the mode of mechanical ventilation to be used during weaning. There remain three methods in widespread use: progressive T-piece trials, intermittent mandatory ventilation (IMV), and PSV. At this point no standardized approach to wean patients from mechanical ventilation has been developed, and the choice of technique varies with the physician.

Recent studies suggest that IMV weaning prolongs time on the ventilator. This is likely due to the fact that the physician slowly decreases the IMV rate over time. By the time the IMV rate is slowed to the point where a spontaneous breathing trial is performed, valuable time is lost.

Results with the use of PS trials have been variable. Those studies with well-defined protocols and rapid reduction of PS to lead to spontaneous breathing trials show equivalence to daily T-piece trials.

Daily T-piece trials have consistently been superior to IMV weaning and at least equivalent to PS weaning in several large studies. Twice or more times daily T-piece trials have not been shown to be more advantageous than daily trials. They may actually be harmful in that they may lead to fatigue.

Several recent studies have shown that protocol-directed weaning by nurses or respiratory care practitioners is superior to independent physician-directed weaning. This is likely due to the fact that providers are easily distracted by more acute patients and "stable" weaning patients may not undergo their daily trial of spontaneous breathing unless it is under protocol direction.

CLINICAL CAVEAT

Weaning from Mechanical Ventilation
- Use team approach
- Utilize weaning protocol
- Perform daily trials of spontaneous breathing once patients have reached oxygenation criteria to extubate ($FIO_2 \leq 50\%$ and $PEEP \leq 7.5$ cmH_2O).

CASE STUDY

A 65-year-old male was admitted to the MICU 5 days ago with streptococcal pneumonia, septic shock, and respiratory failure. He was aggressively treated with antibiotics, intravenous fluids (>15 liters crystalloid), levophed, activated protein-C, and mechanical ventilation. Initially he required $FIO_2 > 80\%$ and $PEEP > 12$ cmH_2O due to acute lung injury from the pneumonia and sepsis. Over the next 48 hours his blood pressure stabilized allowing levophed and intravenous fluids to be discontinued. By day 3 the patient began auto-diuresing and FIO_2 and PEEP were reduced. The patient had a history of mild chronic obstructive pulmonary disease but no cardiac disease. On day 5 the patient remains 5 liters over his admission weight. His current vent settings are:

IMV rate, 8; tidal volume, 500 ml: pressure support, 10 cmH_2O (resulting in spontaneous tidal volumes of 450 ml); PEEP, 7 cmH_2O; and FIO_2, 40%. His arterial blood gas is pH = 7.37, PCO_2 = 41, and PO_2 = 110. He is comfortable and breathing at a total respiratory rate of 14.

QUESTIONS

1. Is this patient ready to wean?
2. If yes, how would you proceed?
3. If the patient fails a trial of spontaneous breathing, what factor(s) would need to be reassessed and/or treated to optimize the patient for the next trial of spontaneous breathing?

SUMMARY

A preferred approach to weaning patients from mechanical ventilation involves a team approach of all caregivers (nurses, respiratory therapists, physical therapists, nutritionists, and physicians) in a protocol-driven fashion giving authority to the front-line staff to wean the patient as tolerated by the protocol. The protocol generally leads rapidly to a daily trial of spontaneous breathing (T-piece or PS) in any ventilated patient who meets the criteria. If the patient passes the spontaneous breathing trial, the patient is extubated. Failures of extubation are reassessed and reversible factors are addressed and a subsequent spontaneous breathing trial is undertaken when the patient is ready (usually daily).

SELECTED READING

Dries DJ: Weaning from mechanical ventilation. Trauma 43:372–384, 1997.

Esteban A, Frutos F, Tobin MJ et al: A comparison of four methods of weaning patients from mechanical ventilation. N Engl J Med 332:345–350, 1995.

Esteban A, Alia I, Gordo F: Weaning: what the recent studies have shown us. Clin Pulm Med 3:91–100, 1996.

Goldstone J: The pulmonary physician in critical care: 10. Difficult weaning. Thorax 57:986–991, 2002.

Jaeschke RZ, Meade MO, Guyatt GH et al: How to use diagnostic test articles in the intensive care unit: diagnosing weanability using f/Vt. CCM 25:1514–1521, 1997.

Tobin MJ: Weaning patients from mechanical ventilation. How to avoid difficulty. Postgrad Med 89:171–178, 1991.

CHAPTER 19

Nontraumatic Brain Injury

A. RAFFAELE DE GAUDIO, M.D.

GUGLIELMO CONSALES, M.D.

The term "stroke" includes every clinical condition characterized by alterations in the cerebral circulation. According to these alterations stroke may be classified as ischemic or hemorrhagic. Ischemic stroke accounts for about 85% of strokes and is most commonly caused by atherothrombotic brain infarction (61%) or cerebral embolism (24%). The mortality from ischemic stroke is 7.6% within 30 days. Hemorrhagic stroke represents about 15% of strokes and includes intraparenchymal and subarachnoid hemorrhages. The mortality from hemorrhagic stroke is 37.5% within 30 days (Box 19-1).

Every year in the USA about 600,000 people suffer a stroke; among these about 500,000 are first attacks and 100,000 are recurrent attacks. In 1998 stroke was the cause of 158,448 deaths in the USA, accounting for about 1 of every 14.8 deaths. Among these deaths, 47% occur out of hospital. According to these data and when considered separately from other cardiovascular diseases, stroke ranks as the third leading cause of death, behind heart diseases and cancer. At all ages more women than men die of stroke. In 1998 among the deaths from stroke, 38.6% were men and 61.4% were women. About 4,500,000 stroke survivors are alive today in USA and

---

Box 19-1   Classification of Stroke

- Ischemic stroke
- Hemorrhagic stroke
  - Intraparenchymal hemorrhage
  - Subarachnoid hemorrhage

Box 19-3   Classification of Ischemic Stroke

- Atherosclerosis of large-calibre vessels (caused by embolism or thrombosis)
- Cardiac embolism
- Small vessel occlusion (lacunae)
- Stroke deriving from other causes (arterial dissection, coagulopathy, arterial–arterial embolism, venous occlusion, etc.)
- Stroke deriving from unknown cause

---

many of these survivors have serious, long-term disability; in fact while 50–70% of stroke survivors regain functional independence, 15–30% are permanently disabled with high social costs. Risk factors for stroke include age above 65 years old and black race. A multidisciplinary approach to stroke involving neurologists, neurosurgeons, internists, and intensivists gives the best results.

This chapter reviews the pathophysiology and the intensive management of stroke.

ISCHEMIC STROKE

Definition and Pathophysiology

Ischemic stroke is defined as a clinical condition characterized by ischemic alterations in the cerebral circulation. According to the clinical pattern ischemic cerebrovascular disease may be classified as transient ischemic attack (TIA), progressing stroke, or stabilized stroke (Box 19-2).

Different clinical presentations and localizations of cerebral lesions may identify several subtypes of ischemic stroke with different outcome and recurrence probability. Classification based on clinical, radiological, and Doppler scanning findings has been recently proposed (Box 19-3).

Ischemic strokes deriving from the occlusion of large arteries are caused by atherosclerosis of the carotid artery

or the vertebrobasilar artery. The atherosclerotic occlusion of small perforating branches results in small ischemic areas termed "lacunae": if they involve functional areas, clinical signs will occur. A global reduction in cerebral blood flow deriving from severe hypotension or cardiac arrest may cause watershed infarctions involving the most distal areas of the parenchyma perfused by cerebral arteries.

Anterior Circulation Ischemia

The vessel most involved in the anterior circulation ischemia of the brain is the middle cerebral artery or its branches; however, also the occlusion of the anterior cerebral artery may result in symptoms of anterior circulation ischemia. The clinical pattern of anterior circulation ischemia depends on the size and the site of the ischemic area. This area may be represented by the whole territory perfused by a cerebral artery, or by smaller areas (lacunar infarctions), or by the more distal areas (watershed infarctions) (Box 19-4).

When the occlusion involves just the superior branches of the middle cerebral artery, hemiparesis and hemisensory loss involving only the inferior limb are associated with motor aphasia or neglect syndrome. The occlusion of the inferior branches of the middle cerebral

---

Box 19-2   Classification of Cerebrovascular Disease

- Transient ischemic attack (TIA) includes neurological dysfunctions secondary to cerebrovascular disease lasting less than 24 hours
- Progressing stroke includes neurological dysfunctions secondary to cerebrovascular disease that worsen in a period of hours (anterior circulation impairment) or days (posterior circulation impairment)
- Stabilized stroke includes a clinical state that remains stable for at least 24 hours (anterior circulation impairment) or 72 hours (posterior circulation impairment)

Box 19-4   Results of Ischemia

Ischemia of the whole territory perfused by the middle cerebral artery results in:
- Contralateral hemiplegia
- Contralateral hemisensory loss
- Conjugated deviation of the eyes toward the injured side
- Homonymous hemianopia
- Global aphasia if the stroke involves the dominant hemisphere
- Neglect syndrome if it involves the nondominant hemisphere

artery results in mild and transient motor and sensitive symptoms while hemianopia may be associated with sensorial aphasia (dominant hemisphere involvement) or confusion (nondominant hemisphere involvement). The occlusion of small branches may result in small ischemic areas and minimal clinical signs.

Anterior circulation ischemia may rarely derive from the occlusion of the anterior cerebral artery. If this is the case, paresis and sensory loss will involve the contralateral inferior limb with a minimal involvement of the eyes.

Lacunar infarctions of lenticulostriate arteries results in the ischemia of the internal capsule with a pure motor stroke or hemiparesis associated with ataxia or dysarthria. These clinical signs often derive also from ischemic lesions in the brain stem.

Watershed infarctions occurring in the areas between the territory of the middle cerebral artery and the territory of the anterior cerebral artery cause hyposthenia in the contralateral inferior limb associated with a milder hyposthenia of the superior limb and no involvement of the eyes. Motor aphasia in the case of dominant hemisphere involvement or mood alterations in the case of nondominant hemisphere involvement may occur. Watershed infarctions involving the territories between the areas dependent on the middle cerebral artery and posterior cerebral artery result in the homolateral loss of the visual field associated with sensorial aphasia (dominant hemisphere) or unilateral neglect syndrome and agnosia (nondominant hemisphere). Subcortical watershed infarctions involve the cerebral white matter between the deep and superficial perforating branches of the middle cerebral artery and cause paresis and sensory loss of the face and the superior limb.

Vertebrobasilar Ischemia

The clinical pattern deriving from vertebrobasilar ischemia is characterized by the slow and progressive development of symptoms often related to the involvement of the cranial nerves. Headache and dizziness are common. If ischemia involves the reticular activating system sudden alterations of consciousness and coma may occur.

The occlusion of the posterior-inferior cerebellar artery results in the Wallenberg syndrome (Box 19-5).

Embolic events may cause cerebellar infarctions resulting in cerebellar edema that may progress to the compression of the fourth ventricle with obstructive hydrocephalus and herniation of the posterior fossa content which is a neurosurgical emergency that needs the placement of a ventricular drain tube or the performance of decompressive craniotomy.

Lacunar strokes may result in a pure sensitive stroke (thalamic involvement) or a pure motor stroke (pontin involvement). Pontin lesions may also result in ataxic hemiparesis. A peculiar clinical pattern is the locked in

---

> ### Box 19-5 Wallenberg Syndrome
>
> This syndrome includes:
> - Homolateral Horner's syndrome (enophthalmus, miosis, ptosis)
> - Homolateral loss of face sensibility to pain and heat
> - Contralateral hemisensory loss
> - Dizziness
> - Nystagmus
> - Eye deviation
> - Dysphagia
> - Dysphonia

---

syndrome caused by the occlusion of the major branch of the basilar artery resulting in pontin ischemia without mesencephalic involvement. Locked in syndrome is characterized by the at least partial persistence of consciousness associated with the impairment of every motor activity except eye movement. Vertebral artery dissection and subclavian artery steal syndrome may precipitate symptoms of vertebrobasilar ischemia. The dissection of the vertebral artery usually is traumatic and has good outcome with anticoagulant therapy. The subclavian artery steal syndrome is caused by a stenosis in the subclavian artery, proximal to the vertebral artery. Symptoms related to vertebrobasilar ischemia may develop during physical activity involving the superior limbs. These symptoms are usually transient, but surgical or endovascular treatment of the stenosis may be necessary.

Prehospital and Emergency Room Care

The early phase of nontraumatic brain injury may be associated with the impairment of vital functions that makes patients with stroke critical. Large infarctions in the territory of the middle cerebral artery and vertebrobasilar circulation as well as stroke-related seizures may compromise airway patency and ventilation. These situations are often associated with loss of protective reflexes and pulmonary inhalation. In small infarctions ventilation impairment is usually less severe. In any case, prehospital and emergency room care should always begin with an assessment of airway patency and ventilation. Severe heart failure is rarely precipitated by ischemic stroke, while heart diseases may be the cause of stroke because of arrhythmias or acute myocardial infarction. Systemic arterial pressure usually increases in the first hours after ischemic stroke, but usually this increase is transient. Large strokes are associated with cerebral edema that causes intracranial hypertension and mass effect resulting in brain shift and brain herniation. Patients with stroke are at high risk of seizures that may be difficult to treat. Hyperglycemia is a usual finding in

Box 19-6 Prehospital and Emergency Room Care After Ischemic Stroke

- Airway management
- Systemic blood pressure control
- Intracranial pressure management
- Diagnostic workup

nontraumatic brain injury and is associated with poor outcome, and therefore it should be avoided (Box 19-6).

Airway Management

Orotracheal intubation and ventilation support should be considered when airway patency or ventilation are in doubt. There are several indications for tracheal intubation in patients with stroke.

CLINICAL CAVEAT

Indications for tracheal intubation after stroke:
- $PaO_2 < 50\text{–}60$ mmHg
- $PacO_2 > 50\text{–}60$ mmHg
- Vital capacity < 500–800 ml
- Signs of respiratory fatigue (respiratory rate > 30 breaths/minute, dyspnoea, respiratory acidosis, use of the accessory respiratory muscles)
- Significant alterations of consciousness
- Inhalation risk
- Impairment of airway patency

Patients who do not need tracheal intubation often have a decreased PaO_2 and therefore supplemental oxygen should be given also in spontaneous breathing patients. A nasogastric tube should be placed to decrease the risk of inhalation. Many patients with nontraumatic brain injury are confused and show psychomotor agitation that may require sedative drugs. Imaging examination sometimes requires deep sedation. Any time a sedative drug is used in a brain-injured patient its respiratory effects should be carefully monitored using clinical examination and arterial oxygen saturation monitoring. The use of these drugs may make tracheal intubation necessary to achieve the complete control of airways and ventilation. An appropriate control of volemia is mandatory even if a severe cardiovascular failure associated with ischemic stroke is usually confined to cases of cardiogenic stroke, arrhythmias, and concomitant myocardial infarction. A central venous catheter and a urinary catheter are necessary to address fluid management.

Systemic Blood Pressure Control

The incidence of systemic hypertension in patients with stroke is 70%. Antihypertensive therapy should be used only if the systolic blood pressure is above 220 mmHg or the diastolic blood pressure is above 120 mmHg. If stroke is associated with acute myocardial infarction, aortic dissection, or aortic aneurysms, antihypertensive treatment should be initiated even at lower pressure values. Strict blood pressure control is also mandatory if thrombolytic treatment is used. It is commonly accepted that an acute reduction in systemic blood pressure results in a sudden reduction in cerebral blood flow that may worsen the damage to ischemic penumbra that is the area closed to the necrotic tissue. This reduction in cerebral blood flow may occur also at high values of systemic pressure especially in patients with chronic hypertension that is associated with a shift of the autoregulation of cerebral blood flow to higher values of perfusion pressure. Autoregulation is also abnormal with a pressure-dependent cerebral flow in the injured and perilesional areas. An optimal systemic blood pressure that would ensure an appropriate cerebral perfusion pressure and cerebral blood flow is far from being set. According to general agreement systolic arterial blood pressure should always be above 150–160 mmHg.

CLINICAL CAVEAT

Antihypertensive drugs in patients with stroke:
- Beta-blockers
- Alpha-2 agonists
- Nitrates
- Calcium antagonists
- Alpha-1 inhibitors

Beta-blockers

Labetalol is a blocker of both beta receptors and apha-1 receptors. The action on the latter receptors causes vasodilatation that is not associated with tachycardia because of the block of beta receptors. Boluses of 0.05–0.5 mg/kg cause a reduction in arterial blood pressure lasting a few minutes within 5–10 minutes. A continuous intravenous infusion at a dose of 0.5–2 mg/kg/hour can also be used. Asthma, acute heart failure, bradycardia, and conduction abnormalities contraindicate the use of beta-blockers.

Alpha-2 Agonists

Clonidine is an alpha-2 agonist drug that acts centrally inhibiting the neurons of the bulbar vasomotor center. This causes diffuse vasodilatation of resistance and capacitance vessels and a reduction in heart rate and cardiac output. Clonidine is a short-acting drug if used in a single dose of 0.075 mg. Sedation and xerostomia are collateral effects of clonidine.

Nitrates

Nitroglycerine induces vasodilatation mediated by nitric oxide pathways. The short effect of this drug allows an intravenous continuous infusion at a dose of 5–10 μg/minute. Nitroprussate is a venous and arterial vasodilator used intravenously at a dose of 0.5–10 μg/kg/minute. It is usually not used in brain-injured patients because it causes cerebral vasodilatation associated with a depressed response to CO_2.

Calcium Antagonists

Nifedipine is a calcium antagonist that may be used sublingually at a dose of 10 mg.

Alpha-1 Inhibitors

Urapidil is an alpha-blocker that produces prevalently arterial vasodilatation associated with a minor venous vasodilatation without significant changes in heart rate and cardiac output. Urapidil can be used in boluses of 12.5 mg or by continuous intravenous infusion.

Even if hypotension decreases cerebral perfusion pressure and cerebral blood flow and may worsen ischemic injuries, severe hypertension when uncontrolled increases perilesional cerebral edema and poses at high risk for the hemorrhagic progression of stroke especially in patients treated with anticoagulants that are contraindicated if hypertension is uncontrolled.

Intracranial Pressure Management

Intracranial hypertension should be promptly identified and treated because it may result in dramatic consequences such as brain herniations. The treatment of intracranial hypertension includes invasive monitoring of arterial blood pressure and intracranial pressure and should be performed in an intensive care unit (ICU) (Box 19-7).

Box 19-7   Methods for the Control of Intracranial Hypertension

- Sedation
- Analgesia
- Appropriate head position
- Osmotic diuretics
- Tris-hydroxymetil aminomethane (THAM)
- Hyperventilation
- Muscle relaxation
- Barbiturates
- Hypothermia
- Decompressive craniotomy

Sedation and analgesia are useful to prevent sudden increases in intracranial pressure because they reduce the adrenergic discharge associated with pain and they control the psychomotor agitation.

Appropriate *head position* with a head-up tilt of 20–30° without lateral deviations of the head improves venous return through jugular veins and it is considered a basic step in intracranial hypertension treatment. Indeed an increase in venous return from the brain is associated with a reduction in cerebral perfusion pressure when head tilt is applied. The reduction in cerebral perfusion pressure may induce the vasodilatation of cerebral vessels resulting in further intracranial hypertension. A head-up tilt of 30° has become a good practice of general intensive care also for the prevention of nosocomial pneumonia. It should be associated with a careful management of systemic arterial blood pressure to prevent cerebral hypoperfusion.

The most popular osmotic diuretic is *mannitol*, which inhibits water and sodium absorption in the kidney resulting in osmotic diuresis. Mannitol induces an osmotic gap between the intravascular compartment and the brain parenchyma resulting in a movement of water from the extravascular compartment into cerebral capillaries with a reduction in intracranial hypertension. The blood–brain barrier must be intact for these effects to occur. Mannitol acts also as plasma expander reducing hematocrit and viscosity. These effects improve cerebral blood flow and cerebral oxygen delivery. Moreover, mannitol has also antioxidant properties that may result in a neuroprotective effect. When used in continuous intravenous infusion it may alter the blood–brain barrier. This alteration may allow mannitol to exit into the extravascular compartment worsening cerebral edema. Plasmatic osmolarity should be below 320 mosm/l when mannitol is used because of the risk of tubular necrosis. Therefore mannitol can be used for the treatment of an unequivocal intracranial hypertension at a dose of 0.25–1 g/kg. This regimen produces effects lasting 6–8 hours within 2 minutes. Euvolemia, serum osmolarity below 320 mosm/l, diuresis, and renal function monitoring should always be ensured when mannitol is used. Furosemide may exaggerate the collateral effects of mannitol and should not be used in intracranial hypertension. Tris-hydroxymetil aminomethane (THAM) increases pH resulting in a decrease in intracranial hypertension. A dose of 60 mmol administered in 45 minutes decreases intracranial pressure within 15 minutes. Provided there is a careful monitoring of blood pH, THAM can be used with a continuous intravenous infusion of 3 mmol/hour.

Hyperventilation increases pH, reducing $PaCO_2$. A decreased $PaCO_2$ causes cerebral vasoconstriction with a reduction of both intracranial hypertension and cerebral blood flow. Hyperventilation produces transient effects because a readjustment in brain pH occurs after 24 hours. Moreover, the effects of hyperventilation depend on the cerebral vessel response to CO_2 that may be altered in patients with stroke resulting in cerebral hypoperfusion of perilesional areas. Because the transient effect of hyperventilation on intracranial hypertension sacrifices cerebral blood flow, the benefits resulting from hyperventilation may be limited. In any case, $PaCO_2$ should be maintained between 35 and 40 mmHg because higher values exacerbate intracranial hypertension.

Barbiturates and propofol can induce a pharmacologic coma with the electroencephalographic features of burst suppression. This produces a profound reduction in cerebral metabolism and in cerebral blood flow because of cerebral autoregulation resulting in a decreased intracranial pressure. Careful hemodynamic monitoring should be used when barbiturates or propofol are used at high doses because of the cardiovascular effect of these drugs.

Hypothermia shows neuroprotective effects because it decreases cerebral metabolism. Hypothermia reduces also the alterations of the blood–brain barrier after cerebral ischemia decreasing cerebral edema and intracranial hypertension. Unequivocal outcome benefits from the use of hypothermia in patients with stroke are still lacking.

Decompressive craniotomy has shown experimental effectiveness in large cerebral infarctions. It should be considered when every other treatment has failed but neurologic impairment is not already irreversible.

Diagnostic Workup

The role of diagnostic workup in the management of nontraumatic brain injury is very important to choose the appropriate treatment. The use of specific therapy such as thrombolytic therapy increases further the importance of early diagnostic workup. Among neuroimaging techniques, computed tomography (CT) scanning is the first choice in patients with stroke and it should be performed as soon as possible. Initially CT scanning should identify or exclude the presence of intracranial hemorrhages or nonvascular lesions (neoplastic tissue). CT scanning is then important to identify the location and extension of the neurologic lesion. Ischemic lesions will not show direct signs on CT scanning until 12–24 hours after stroke; sometimes the occluded artery may result in a hyperdense image even if calcified vessels may cause false positive findings. Even large ischemic strokes are not evident on CT scanning in the first hours; 60% of cerebral infarctions will be evident on CT scanning 24 hours after symptom presentation, while 100% of cerebral infarctions are evident 7 days after presentation.

The mass effect associated with large ischemic lesions is promptly evident on CT scanning even when the direct signs of ischemia are not present. If the initial CT scanning is negative and in the case of neurologic deterioration CT scanning should be repeated after 24 hours until 7 days after clinical presentation. The early finding of either hypodensity or mass effect has a negative prognostic value. The diagnostic benefit resulting from contrast enhancement in the early phase of stroke is controversial, while it is widely accepted for the later assessment of stabilized strokes. CT scanning is the first choice among neuroimaging techniques for the early diagnostic workup of patients with stroke because it is widely diffused, easy to read, and not very expensive. NMR could give good diagnostic information especially in anterior lesions but it may be difficult to perform in the early phase of stroke because of the instability of the patient's condition.

Besides neuroimaging, the early diagnostic workup for patients with stroke should include electrocardiogram and eventually echocardiogram in order to identify an eventual cardiogenic cause of stroke. Laboratory examinations should include complete blood count, glycemia, coagulation tests, electrolytes, blood gases, and indexes of renal and hepatic function. Doppler examination of the anterior and vertebrobasilar circulations may be useful as well as transcranial Doppler. Electroencephalogram may be useful to demonstrate seizure activity. Lumbar puncture should be performed if subarachnoid hemorrhage is suspected with a negative CT scanning. Radiographic examination of the chest should also be performed, while X-rays of the cervical spine should be reserved for patients who are unconscious or with cervical pain or lesions (Box 19-8).

Box 19-8 Diagnostic Workup for Ischemic Stroke

- CT scan of the head
- Electrocardiogram
- Chest x-rays
- X-rays of the cervical spine (in case of loss of consciousness or neck pain)
- Complete blood count
- Coagulation tests
- Electrolytes
- Glycemia
- Blood gas analysis
- Liver and kidney function tests
- Lumbar puncture (in case of suspected subarachnoid hemorrhage with negative CT scan)
- Electroencephalography

INTENSIVE CARE UNIT CARE

The target of the treatment of stroke is to limit neuronal damage in order to allow the best neurologic recovery that is possible for each patient. Clear experimental evidence has focused on the time elapsing from symptom presentation and treatment initiation. If this time is short, therapy is more likely to succeed. A "brain attack" approach that considers stroke as an emergency has been developed because the time window that allows a successful treatment is limited to 3–6 hours for anterior circulation ischemia and 6–12 hours for posterior circulation ischemia. When time becomes the key of a successful treatment, organizational and educational aspects of the health system become important. The diagnostic suspicion of stroke should be met by an emergency department able to face stroke with the same effectiveness as myocardial infarction. Diagnostic and therapeutic protocols are useful tools in this intent (Box 19-9).

ICUs dedicated to stroke termed "stroke units" are growing everywhere and are demonstrated to reduce mortality and neurologic outcome after stroke. ICU care for patients with stroke includes specific therapies like thrombolytic, anticoagulant, and triple H therapy, and a careful general care (Box 19-10).

Box 19-9 Indications for Intensive Care Unit Admission After Ischemic Stroke

- Progressing symptoms
- Unstable hemodynamic parameters
- Embolic occlusion of intracranial carotid or of the middle cerebral artery
- Multiple embolisms
- Unstable endocarditis
- Intracranial hypertension
- Arterial dissection
- Thrombolytic or hypervolemic therapy
- Comorbidities
- Severe arrhythmias
- Concomitant myocardial infarction
- Hypertensive bursts
- Severe hypotension
- Sepsis
- Severe dehydration
- Renal failure
- Electrolytic abnormalities
- Endocrine abnormalities

Box 19-10 Specific Intensive Care Unit Therapy

This includes:
- Thrombolytic
- Anticoagulant
- "Triple H"

SPECIFIC THERAPY

Thrombolytic Therapy

The dissolution of the thrombus occluding the cerebral vessel would restore the patency of the vessel occluded and cerebral perfusion to the ischemic areas. Several thrombolytic agents like streptokinase, urokinase, and recombinant tissue plasminogen activator (rt-PA) have been used with success in the treatment of myocardial infarction. Myocardial vessels have a thicker wall containing a larger number of smooth muscle cells while cerebral vessels have a thin wall with few smooth muscle cells that make them susceptible to break under reperfusion. Thrombolytic agents activate plasminogen resulting in fibrine dissolution. They can be used systemically with an intravenous infusion or locally with intra-arterial instillation. Thrombolytic therapy can be used if the time elapsed from symptom presentation is less than 3–6 hours for anterior circulation ischemia or 12 hours for posterior circulation ischemia.

CLINICAL CAVEAT

Thrombolytic therapy is indicated if the time elapsed from clinical onset is:
- Less than 3–6 hours for anterior circulation ischemia
- Less than 12 hours for posterior circulation ischemia

Absolute and relative contraindications must also be excluded before thrombolytic therapy. Acute bleeding and cerebrovascular disease or surgery in the last two months are absolute contraindications. Other contraindications include severe recent trauma, uncontrolled arterial hypertension, mild or severe neurologic impairments, major infarction on CT scan, coagulation defects, postpartum period, and cardiopulmonary resuscitation complicated by rib fractures.

Several controlled trials evaluated the effectiveness of thrombolytic therapy in stroke. While streptokinase has shown increased mortality resulting from hemorrhagic complications, intravenous rt-PA has shown improvements in functional outcome without any significant

CLINICAL CAVEAT

Contraindications for rt-PA after ischemic stroke:
- Therapy with oral anticoagulants or INR > 1.7
- Therapy with heparin in the past 48 hours or prolonged aPTT
- Platelets count < 100,000/mm^3
- Stroke or head trauma in the past 3 months
- Surgery in the past 14 days
- Systolic pressure > 185 mmHg or diastolic pressure > 110 mmHg
- Rapid improvement of clinical examination
- Mild neurologic deficits
- Previous intracranial hemorrhage
- Glycemia > 400 mg/dl or <50 mg/dl
- Seizures
- Gastrointestinal or urinary tract bleeding in the past 21 days
- Recent myocardial infarction

increase in mortality in European and North American trials, although with an increase in hemorrhagic complications. The dose of rt-PA is usually 0.9 mg/kg (maximum 90 mg) given over 1 hour. The American Heart Association, the American Academy of Neurology, and the Canadian Stroke Consortium recommend rt-PA in patients with stroke within 3 hours of symptom presentation. Any suspicion of intracranial hemorrhage as well as any precipitating condition contraindicates thrombolytic therapy. rt-Pa can be used in patients treated with aspirin. Even if heparin, antithrombotic, and antiaggregant drugs are not recommended when thrombolytic therapy is used, good results in patients with posterior circulation ischemia treated with rt-PA followed by the infusion of heparin have been obtained. Intra-arterial thrombolytic therapy is an attractive alternative to systemic thrombolysis even if it requires cerebral angiography. Technical difficulties could therefore limit its use. Intra-arterial thrombolysis can probably be safely used within 6 hours regarding anterior circulation strokes and within 12 hours regarding posterior circulation strokes. Basilar artery occlusion carries a mortality of 90% if untreated. Nonrandomized studies have shown reduced mortality and morbidity with intra-arterial basilar thrombolysis. Organizational limits remain a major barrier to the wide use of thrombolysis in patients with stroke because of its short therapeutic time window.

Anticoagulant Therapy

Theoretically heparin would be useful when large arterial vessels are occluded to prevent distal embolism and in patients with embolic strokes provided that hemorrhagic lesions have been excluded. However, heparin either unfractionated or of low molecular weight resulted in no significant reductions in death or disability after stroke when it was used within 24–48 hours after stroke onset, even in subgroups of patients with atrial fibrillation. While heparin reduces the incidence of recurrent ischemic stroke and venous thromboembolism, it increases the incidence of intracranial bleeding. Probably the safety of heparin may be improved by carefully monitoring coagulation indices. Deferred use of heparin for thromboembolism prevention is widely practiced in immobile patients.

Antiplatelet Drugs

Several clinical trials advocate the use of aspirin 150–300 mg within 48 hours after stroke onset. Aspirin prevents early recurrent ischemic stroke, reduces death and disability at 3–6 months, and increases the probability of full functional recovery. Aspirin causes an increase of as small as 0.2% in the risk of intracranial hemorrhage. The beneficial effects of aspirin have no significant heterogeneity across any subgroup including patients with intracranial hemorrhage. The modest benefit associated with aspirin shows no time dependency within 48 hours and it reflects early secondary prevention rather than any influence over the acute pathophysiology of stroke.

Triple H Therapy

A therapeutic strategy based on hypervolemia, hypertension, and hemodilution has been advocated for subarachnoid hemorrhage but may be useful also in the treatment of ischemic stroke. This therapy is based on the fact that cerebral blood flow is dependent on systemic arterial pressure and blood viscosity when autoregulation is impaired. Large amount of colloids and crystalloids are used to achieve hypervolemia and hemodilution that reduce blood viscosity improving cerebral blood flow. Inotropes such as dopamine are used to maintain a supranormal systemic arterial pressure resulting in a high cerebral perfusion pressure. Triple H therapy requires a careful monitoring of cardiovascular performance especially in patients with heart disease (Box 19-11).

Box 19-11   Triple H Therapy

This usually requires:
- Colloids (50–1500 ml)
- Crystalloids (5000–10,000 ml)
- Blood transfusions (if necessary)
- Dopamine or dobutamine (10–30 μg/kg/minute)

Box 19-12   General Intensive Care Unit Care in Ischemic Stroke

Important aspects of general ICU care in ischemic stroke include:
- Electrolytes and fluid management
- Nutritional support
- Glycemic control
- Temperature control
- Prevention and management of seizures
- Prevention and management of infectious complications
- Prevention and management of thromboembolism

GENERAL CARE

The aspects of general ICU care as regards ischemic stroke are summarized in Box 19-12.

Electrolytes and Fluid Management

An appropriate fluid management is very important for patients with stroke because the quality and the quantity of administered fluids may influence cerebral metabolism and perfusion and intracranial volumes. Physiologically cerebral perfusion is coupled to cerebral metabolism and it is not dependent on systemic hemodynamic changes because of cerebral autoregulation. When the brain is injured cerebral autoregulation is altered and systemic arterial pressure becomes a fundamental factor in determining cerebral blood flow. Therefore, regarding quantity, fluid management should be addressed to euvolemia in order to avoid hemodynamic instability that may decrease cerebral blood flow. Physiologically endothelium of cerebral vessels has peculiar permeability features that characterize the blood–brain barrier. In particular, cerebral endothelium is selectively permeable to small molecules. During brain injury a disruption of the blood–brain barrier causes an increase in extravascular fluid. Fluid osmolarity is the major determinant of water flux across the blood–brain barrier. Therefore, regarding quality, fluid management in patients with stroke should be based on isohypertonic fluids such as normal saline. The use of hypotonic fluids such as glucose 5% in water should be avoided and restricted to hyperosmolar states. No definite results support the use of either colloids or crystalloids. HyperHaes is a mixture of a 7% NaCl solution with colloidal fluids that mobilizes quickly free water into the vascular compartment and could be useful in reducing cerebral edema and intracranial hypertension.

CLINICAL CAVEAT

Strategies for fluid management in ischemic stroke:
- Quantity of fluids: the goal is euvolemia
- Quality of fluids: isohyperosmolar fluids
- No definite results support the use of either colloids or crystalloids
- A mixture of hyperosmolar crystalloids and colloids may reduce cerebral edema and intracranial hypertension

---

Nutritional Support

Patients with stroke have a hypercatabolic state that requires a careful nutritional support. Even if the patient is conscious, spontaneous nutrition is not recommended because the risk of inhalation is high in patients with stroke. Early enteral nutrition should be initiated as soon as possible. Enteral nutrition should provide 25–30 kcal/kg and 1.5 g/kg of proteins every day. A nasogastric tube, even in tracheal intubated patients, does not exclude inhalation and percutaneous gastrostomy or jejunostomy should be considered.

Glycemic Control

Either hyper- or hypoglycemia may be deleterious for the central nervous system, and a strict glycemic control is therefore necessary. Hyperglycemia may increase lactate production that worsens neuronal acidosis and brain damage. Therefore insulin should be used to keep glycemia in the normal range when hyperglycemia occurs.

Temperature Control

Hyperthermia increases the extension of ischemic lesions and worsens outcome. Hyperthermia-related damage may depend on the increased production of oxygen free radicals and neuromediators. Hyperthermia alters the blood–brain barrier and exacerbates excitotoxicity in perilesional areas. Therefore hyperthermia should be promptly controlled using physical and pharmacologic methods. Deliberate therapeutic hypothermia is still controversial.

Prevention and Management of Complications

Ischemic stroke may be associated with seizures, infectious complications, deep venous thrombosis, and pulmonary embolism (Box 19-13).

Seizures. Stroke is a frequent cause of seizures and the most common cause of status epilepticus in adults.

Box 19-13   Common Complications of Ischemic Stroke

- Neurological:
  - Cerebral edema
  - Hydrocephalus
  - Hemorrhagic transformation
  - Seizures
- Medical:
  - Pulmonary inhalation
  - Hypoventilation
  - Pneumonia
  - Myocardial ischemia
  - Arrhythmias
  - Thromboembolism
  - Urinary tract infections
  - Malnutrition
  - Anchylosis

Early seizures occur in the first week after the onset of stroke; late seizures occur later. Seizures are the expression of ischemic damage. They can aggravate brain injury. Therefore seizures should be aggressively treated using benzodiazepines and phenitoine.

Infectious complications are frequent and directly related to outcome. The cause of death in 15–25% of patients with stroke is bacterial pneumonia resulting from inhalation. Urinary tract infections are very frequent as well because of bladder catheterization. Head-up tilt is useful for the prevention of pneumonia in patients with stroke. Inhalation should be promptly identified. Antibiotic administration may start on an empirical base and then be turned to a specific strategy when the cultural results are available.

Deep venous thrombosis and pulmonary embolism. Pulmonary embolism is the cause of death in 25% of patients with stroke. Deep venous thrombosis is the main cause of pulmonary embolism and therefore should be appropriately prevented in immobilized patients. Unfractionated or low-molecular-weight heparin is effective in the prevention of deep venous thrombosis and pulmonary embolism and should always be considered in immobilized patients. Mechanical methods to improve venous return from the inferior limbs, such as elastic stockings, may be also useful.

SURGICAL THERAPY

Acute carotid endarterectomy. Carotid endarterectomy is the treatment of choice for stenotic atherosclerotic lesion of the carotid artery. Its use in ischemic stroke is controversial because of the risk of hemorrhagic progression of stroke. Acute ischemic stroke caused by carotid occlusion occurring inside the hospital either spontaneously or following angiography or elective carotid surgery may be an indication for surgical revascularization. Acute carotid endarterectomy may be used also in severe stenosis of the carotid artery with a floating thrombus if the patient has progressing neurologic symptoms.

NEURORADIOLOGIC PROCEDURES

Angioplasty and stenting. Intravascular treatment of symptomatic lesions of the cerebral circulation is an attractive alternative to surgery. These procedures are reserved to patients with high perioperative risk or with inoperable lesions. Stenting may be a useful complement to angioplasty in order to keep the vessel patent. Angioplasty and stenting are invasive techniques with several possible complications including microembolism, artery dissection, thrombosis, intracranial hemorrhage, and hemorrhagic progression of the ischemic stroke.

SPONTANEOUS INTRAPARENCHYMAL HEMORRHAGE

Definition, Etiology, and Pathophysiology

Intraparenchymal hemorrhage accounts for 8–13% of strokes. Its incidence is decreasing probably because of the earlier and stricter control of hypertension; in any case it is still associated with high mortality rates.

The causes of spontaneous intraparenchymal hemorrhage include arterial hypertension, vascular abnormalities, coagulopathies, neoplasia, vasculopathies, drugs, hemorrhagic progression of ischemic stroke, postoperative and post-traumatic hemorrhages, pregnancy, neonatal intraventricular hemorrhage, and other causes (Box 19-14).

Box 19-14   Causes of Intraparenchymal Hemorrhage

- Chronic arterial hypertension
- Vascular abnormalities
- Coagulopathies
- Neoplasia
- Vasculopathies (amyloid angiopathy, vasculitis, moya-moya disease)
- Drugs (sympathomimetics, anticoagulants, fibrinolytics)
- Postoperative hemorrhages
- Hemorrhagic transformation of ischemic stroke
- Post-traumatic hemorrhage
- Pregnancy
- Other causes

Chronic arterial hypertension is the most common cause of spontaneous intraparenchymal hemorrhage, although this etiologic role has decreased during recent decades because of antihypertensive therapy. Arterial hypertension results in alterations of cerebral vessels especially perforating arteries and small subcortical arteries. Lipids accumulate in the subintimal layer also damaging the muscularis layer of the media. These abnormalities weaken the vessel wall resulting in the small aneurysms of Charcot Bouchard. Perforating arteries are terminal branches departing perpendicularly from cerebral vessels. Therefore they are exposed to high hemodynamic stress especially at high arterial pressures that may precipitate the rupture of these weak vessels. Given the distribution of perforating and subcortical arteries, intraparenchymal hemorrhages caused by hypertension occurs usually in basal nuclei, thalamus, cerebellum, and pons, while they are less common in the hemispheres.

Vascular abnormalities resulting in intraparenchymal hemorrhage include intracranial aneurysms and vascular malformations. Although the rupture of an intracranial aneurysm usually results in subarachnoid hemorrhage, it can also cause intraparenchymal hemorrhage especially in case of rebleeding. Intraparenchymal and subarachnoid hemorrhage can be associated. Intracranial aneurysms are more common at the bifurcation of the mean cerebral artery, in the posterior communicant artery, at the bifurcation of the internal carotid artery, and in the anterior cerebral artery. Therefore in these cases intraparenchymal hemorrhage occurs in frontal and temporal lobes. Aneurysms are generally congenital but they may be also post-traumatic. In the latter case they can bleed for weeks, months, and even years after the initial trauma. It is also possible that septic embolism from the heart results in micotic aneurysms.

Vascular malformations include arterial-venous malformations, capillary telangiectasis, cavernous angiomas, and venous angiomas. Arterial-venous malformations are characterized by a direct communication between the arterial and venous systems without interposed capillaries: this results in increased pressures in the venous portion with dilation and high risk of rupture. They usually occur in the cerebral hemispheres involving branches of the cerebral mean artery. The rupture of arterial-venous malformations is more common in patients aged between the second and the fourth decade. Capillary teleangiectases are capillaries abnormally dilated. They are usually localized in the pons or in the floor of the fourth ventricle and may result in spontaneous bleedings. Cavernous angiomas are vascular dilations localized especially over the cerebral hemispheres. They rarely cause massive bleedings; usually they determine headache, seizures, and neurologic focal signs. Venous angiomas are abnormal radial veins confluent toward a central vein. They occur in the frontal and parietal lobes and rarely bleed (Box 19-15).

> **Box 19-15 Vascular Abnormalities Resulting in Intraparenchymal Hemorrhage**
>
> - Intracranial aneurysms
> - Vascular malformations
>   - Arterial-venous malformations
>   - Capillary telangiectasis
>   - Cavernous angiomas
>   - Venous angiomas

Intracranial tumors are a frequent cause of intraparenchymal hemorrhages because they have a large and fragile vascular tissue and large areas of necrosis. They may be metastatic lesions or malignant glyomas; benign tumors rarely bleed. Intracranial neoplasia should be suspected if subcortical clotting, abnormal tissue surrounding the hematoma, edema with mass effect, and multiple lesions appear on CT scanning. Either congenital or acquired coagulopathies may result in intraparenchymal hemorrhage especially if the platelet count is below $10,000/\mu l$ or the activity of a coagulation factor is decreased below 1%. Intraparenchymal hemorrhage may be a dramatic complication of anticoagulant and thrombolytic treatments. Anticoagulants increase 8–12 times the risk of intracranial hemorrhage that in these cases is localized in the hemispheric white matter and in the cerebellum. Thrombolytic drugs may cause multiple hemispheric hemorrhages.

Vasculitis is another important cause of intraparenchymal hemorrhages. Sympathomimetic drugs may cause hypertension resulting in intraparenchymal hemorrhages.

Moya Moya disease is a progressive vascular disease involving the internal carotid artery and sometimes the vertebral arteries. It results in the occlusion of the vessels involved with ischemic or hemorrhagic symptoms.

Clinical Symptoms and Signs

The clinical pattern of spontaneous intraparenchymal hemorrhage is characterized by an acute onset without warning signs and by a rapid evolution in minutes or hours, rarely in days. The incidence of alterations of consciousness in intraparenchymal hemorrhage is 60% and coma occurs in two-thirds of these patients. Systemic hypertension is common also in nonhypertensive patients and represents a reflex response to the intracranial hypertension caused by the mass effect of the hematoma (Cushing reflex). The goal of this hypertensive response is to maintain cerebral perfusion pressure, but persistent systemic hypertension may result in vasogenic edema and rebleeding. On the other hand, hypotension must be avoided because it precipitates ischemic lesions in perilesional areas, given the alterations of cerebral autoregulation. Therefore systemic arterial pressure should be maintained in the normal range. Headache occurs at the onset in 30% of patients and later in 60% of cases. Vomiting is more common in hemorrhagic strokes than in ischemic ones. Seizures are common especially in hemispheric hemorrhages. They are usually present at the onset or occur early; late seizures are rare. The clinical pattern is dependent on the site and the size of the hemorrhage.

CLINICAL CAVEAT

Clinical symptoms and signs of intraparenchymal hemorrhage:
- Alterations of consciousness
- Coma
- Systemic hypertension
- Headache
- Vomiting
- Seizures

Supratentorial Hemorrhage

Intraparenchymal hemorrhages occurring in the supratentorial area may involve the cerebral cortex, the cerebral hemispheres, and basal nuclei. Cortical hemorrhages are usually multiple and produce neurologic signs dependent on the site of injury (alterations of mobility or sensitivity); seizures are common. Hemispheric hemorrhages are caused by hypertension in 31% of cases. Changes of consciousness are rare, although coma may occur if the hemorrhage is large. If the frontal lobe is involved, contralateral motility is altered (the superior limb is more frequently involved than the inferior limb or the face) and headache, abulia, and disorientation in time and space may occur. Patients with hemorrhage of the parietal lobe present headache and deficit in the contralateral sensitivity. If the dominant hemisphere is involved the patient may have difficulty in naming, writing, reading, and calculating, while if the nondominant hemisphere is involved neglect syndrome occurs. Hemorrhages in the dominant temporal lobe cause sensitive dysphasia with difficulties in the comprehension but not in the repetition of words. Ear pain may occur. Hemorrhage in the occipital lobe produces hemianopia and pain in the homolateral eye, and sometimes hallucinations with bright colors may occur.

Intraparenchymal hemorrhage involving putamen headache is rare, while alterations in motility are common. Large hemorrhages in this area cause contralateral flaccid hemiplegia and hemianesthesia, deviation of the eyes toward the injured side, and hemianopia. Dysphasia or motor aphasia occur if the dominant hemisphere is involved, neglect syndrome if the nondominant hemisphere is involved. Very large hemorrhages disconnect diencephalons from the reticular system and cause stupor or coma associated with mydriasis and positive Babinski's reflex.

Hemorrhages involving the caudate are rare. Confusion, vomiting, and headache are common in these cases. If the intraparenchymal hemorrhage involves the thalamus, there is a contralateral alteration of the sensitivity of the head, the face, the superior limb, and the chest. If the injury extends to subthalamic areas, ocular signs (deviation of the eyes, nystagmus) are common, while the involvement of the internal capsule results in alterations in motility. Thalamic lesions of the dominant hemisphere cause aphasia, while those of the nondominant hemisphere produce unilateral neglect syndrome.

Infratentorial Hemorrhage

Intraparenchymal hemorrhages of the mesencephalon are rare. Sometimes they may cause an important mass effect, but usually they are benign. The third and fourth cranial nerves are typically involved. If intraparenchymal hemorrhage involves the highest portion of the mesencephalon, Parinaud syndrome may occur with paralysis in looking up, mydriasis, intact convergence movements, and eyelid movements.

Intraparenchymal hemorrhages involving the pons may have devastating consequences. Even small hemorrhages result in loss of consciousness and tetraplegia with positive plantar reflex, miosis, and absence of horizontal eye movements after oculocephalic and oculovestibular reflex elicitation. Ocular bobbing, a sudden down-deviation of the eyes followed by a slow return to the resting position, is pathognomonic. Severe alterations in the respiratory pattern are always present while an abnormal deglutition facilitates inhalation. Thermoregulation is often impaired with severe hyperthermia and shivers so intense that they may be confused with seizures. Survival is often limited to the first 24 hours, but some patients progress to a vegetative state or, if injury is limited, to locked in syndrome.

Bulbar hemorrhages are rare. They cause dizziness and headache followed by hemiparesis. They may be associated with nystagmus, abnormal deglutition, weakness of the limbs, and cerebellar ataxia.

Cerebellar Hemorrhage

The clinical pattern associated with intraparenchymal hemorrhages involving the cerebellum is variable: small hemorrhages may give mild neurologic signs, but if compression of the brain stem occurs consciousness and vegetative functions become impaired and obstructive hydrocephalus may develop resulting from the compression of the ventricular system. When compressive complications occur, immediate surgical evacuation of the hematoma is necessary. The onset of cerebellar hemorrhage in conscious patients is usually associated with headache, dizziness, dysarthria, and difficulties in walking and standing upright. Less common findings are ataxia, positive plantar reflex, paralysis of the facial nerve, paralysis of eye movement, and nystagmus. When nausea and vomiting are severe, the most useful sign of cerebellar involvement is the difficulty in walking and standing upright. When the brain stem is involved, consciousness is invariably altered.

Diagnostic Workup

CT scanning is fundamental for the diagnosis of spontaneous intraparenchymal hemorrhage. It allows the identifications of even small hemorrhages because of the spontaneous enhancement of the proteic components of hemoglobin. With CT scanning it is possible to identify the site of the intraparenchymal hemorrhage and the eventual presence of mass effect and brain shift. Ventricular or subarachnoid extension and secondary hydrocephalus associated with intraparenchymal hemorrhage are also evident on the CT scan (Box 19-16).

Brain shift is very important because it correlates with the level of consciousness and with the development of cerebral herniations. CT scanning also allows a rapid calculation of the size of the hematoma using simple formulas such as the ABC/2 formula of Kothary (Box 19-17).

NMR is particularly useful in the diagnosis of vascular malformations and cerebral tumors, although CT scanning is more sensitive for the identification of hemorrhages occurring in the last 12 hours because the blood is isointense on NMR in the early phase of hemorrhages.

Acute and Intensive Care Unit Management

Acute treatment of patients with intraparenchymal hemorrhage has the goal of obtaining stable vital parameters. Ventilation is abnormal in many patients with head injury and the reflexes for airway protection are often ineffective. Therefore tracheal intubation and mechanical ventilation are often necessary. In patients with an effective spontaneous ventilation supplemental oxygen is recommended to reduce the risk of cerebral hypoxia (Box 19-18).

Usually patients with intraparenchymal hemorrhage have systemic arterial hypertension in the early phase after hemorrhage. This is probably a reflex response to maintain cerebral perfusion pressure. Although persistent systemic hypertension may result in vasogenic edema and rebleeding, hypotension must be avoided because it precipitates ischemic lesions in perilesional areas. Therefore sudden decreases in systemic arterial pressure should be avoided. A systolic arterial pressure of around 160 mmHg has been advocated in conscious patients and around 180 mmHg in comatose patients; these values should be even higher, although below 210 mmHg, in patients with chronic arterial hypertension. Another important target is to obtain stable values of arterial pressure; treatment with labetalol, nitrates, esmolol, and angiotensin converting enzyme (ACE) inhibitors is useful for the prevention of paroxysmal hypertension that may contribute to rebleeding. Precipitating causes of hypertension should be avoided also providing appropriate sedation and analgesia. Coagulation deficits increase the risk of intraparenchymal hemorrhage and should be treated immediately

---

Box 19-16   CT Scanning in Intra-parenchymal Hemorrhage

This shows:
- The site of the hemorrhage
- The extent of brain shift
- The subarachnoid extension (if present)
- Secondary hydrocephalus (if present)

Box 19-17   ABC/2 Formula of Kothary

Volume of hematoma = $(A \times B \times C)/2$
- A = the maximum diameter of the hematoma in a single scan
- B = the maximum diameter perpendicular to A
- C = the number of scans that show the hematoma times the thickness of each scan

---

Box 19-18   Goals of Acute and Intensive Care Unit Management of Intraparenchymal Hemorrhage

- Restoration of an appropriate ventilation
- Arterial pressure control
- Treatment of coagulation deficits
- Intracranial pressure monitoring
- Prevention and treatment of seizures
- Surgical treatment if the medical treatment fails to control intracranial hypertension and to prevent neurological deterioration

discontinuing anticoagulant or thrombolytic drugs, administering plasma, coagulation factors, or protamine. Intracranial pressure monitoring is useful to guide medical treatment of patients with intraparenchymal hemorrhage and to identify early the cases requiring surgical treatment. When there is intracranial hypertension a head-up tilt of 20–30° improves venous return and mannitol administrations at a bolus dose of 1–1.5 g/kg followed by doses of 0.5 g/kg every 4–6 hours should be considered. Mechanically ventilated patients may be treated with temporary hyperventilation. Intraventricular catheters may be used to drain cerebrospinal fluid in the attempt to reduce intracranial hypertension.

Antiepileptic drugs are administered to all patients with intraparenchymal hemorrhage even if conclusive data for the doses and the duration of the antiepileptic therapy are lacking.

Corticosteroids are not recommended because they cause many complications and no demonstrable beneficial effect.

When medical treatment fails to control intracranial hypertension and to prevent neurologic deterioration, surgical treatment is indicated. Surgery is usually not necessary in conscious patients, while it is advisable when massive intraparenchymal hemorrhages are associated with severe neurologic impairments involving the function of the brainstem. Stereotaxic drainage is an alternative to open ceiling drainage. Recently, surgical evacuation of the hematoma has been associated with fibrinolytic drugs that have been used to obtain dissolution of the clotting.

Outcome

The clinical pattern that characterizes the onset and the early phase of the intraparenchymal hemorrhage is the most important prognostic factor. Outcome is significantly worse in comatose patients. Other negative prognostic factors include a volume of hemorrhage above 60 ml, the localization in deep structures, brain shift, and the age of the patient.

SUBARACHNOID HEMORRHAGE

Definition, Etiology, and Pathophysiology

Subarachnoid hemorrhage accounts for 6–8% of cerebral strokes. It is defined as a collection of blood in the subarachnoid space between pia mater and arachnoid involving the base cisterns and the hemispheric and interhemispheric fissures. In the most severe cases blood may reach cerebral ventricles, and in 30% of cases subarachnoid hemorrhage is associated with intraparenchymal hemorrhage.

The annual incidence of subarachnoid hemorrhage is 15–20 per 100,000 population, and it is higher in women than in men (1.7:1). The incidence of subarachnoid hemorrhage shows a peak in the sixth decade. The mortality from subarachnoid hemorrhage is high, even if during recent years it has decreased. Mortalities after 30 days and after one year are equivalent, so subarachnoid hemorrhage causes death mostly within the first month. One-half of patients with subarachnoid hemorrhage either die or have severe inability, while one-third survive with a good functional recovery. Among strokes, subarachnoid hemorrhage shows the best response to surgical and medical intensive care.

The cause of subarachnoid hemorrhage may be the rupture of intracranial aneurysms (75–80%), the rupture of vascular malformations (4–5%), arteriopathies, infections (meningitides and meningoencephalitis), intoxications (alcohol, carbon monoxide, cocaine, epinephrine, amphetamines, monoamine oxidative inhibitors, opioids), traumas (head trauma, electrocution, seizures, burns, strangulations), cancer (ependimoma, glyoma, melanoma, metastasis), venous thrombosis and blood disorders (sickle cell anemia, leukemia, lymphoma, anticoagulants, aspirin, disseminated intravascular coagulation) (Box 19-19).

Intracranial aneurysms have an incidence of 2–5% and, according to Carmichael's hypothesis, degenerative factors acting on a congenitally abnormal vessel contribute to their formation. Risk factors for intracranial aneurysms are smoking, hypertension, alcohol, contraceptives, and hormonal changes associated with the menopause. Intracranial aneurysms may be saccular (berry), fusiform, or dissecting (Box 19-20).

Saccular (berry) aneurysms are the most frequent and represent the most common cause of subarachnoid hemorrhage. They are often associated with type III collagen deficiency related to congenital diseases including aortic

---

Box 19-19   Causes of Subarachnoid Hemorrhage

- Rupture of intracranial aneurysms
- Rupture of vascular malformations
- Arteriopathies
- Infections (meningitides and meningoencephalitis)
- Intoxications (alcohol, carbon monoxide, cocaine, epinephrine, amphetamines, monoamine oxidative inhibitors, opioids)
- Traumas (head trauma, electrocution, seizures, burns, strangulations)
- Neoplasias (ependimoma, glyoma, melanoma, metastasis)
- Venous thrombosis
- Blood disorders (sickle cell anemia, leukemia, lymphoma, anticoagulants, aspirin, disseminated intravascular coagulation)

Box 19-20 Intracranial Aneurysms

These may be:
- Saccular (berry)
- Fusiform
- Dissecting

coarctation, polycystic kidney disease, Marfan's syndrome, Ehlers–Danlos syndrome, and fibromuscular dysplasia of the renal arteries. Saccular aneurysms occur at the bifurcation of cerebral arteries, more frequently in the anterior circulation (anterior communicant artery, posterior communicant artery, middle cerebral artery, carotid artery). These aneurysms may rarely compress closed structures causing symptoms before their rupture. Thrombosis may occur inside the aneurysm causing acute headache, stiff neck, and inflammatory cells in the cerebrospinal fluid. The annual rupture risk for saccular aneurysms is 1.4–3% and it is not related to the aneurysm size or site.

Fusiform aneurysms are associated with atherosclerotic alterations involving the media and elastica of the arterial wall. The preferred sites are the basilar artery and the intracranial segment of the carotid artery. The rupture of fusiform aneurysms is rare, while thrombosis may occur inside the aneurysm causing embolism. Fusiform aneurysms may compress the brainstem and structures inside the sinus carvenosum such as the second, third, fourth, fifth, and sixth cranial nerves.

Dissecting aneurysms are an infrequent cause of subarachnoid hemorrhage. They can cause ischemic symptoms derived from thromboembolism.

Clinical Symptoms and Signs

The typical clinical presentation of subarachnoid hemorrhage includes acute and severe headache with stiff neck often associated with photophobia, nausea, and vomiting. An initial loss of consciousness is very frequent; sometimes it recedes, other times it persists. Patients with perimesencephalic subarachnoid hemorrhage usually present a subacute headache (progressing over minutes) not associated with alterations of consciousness. Before the rupture of the aneurysm, clinical symptoms like headache, nausea, neck ache, chest, back and leg pain, photophobia, and lethargy may be the consequence of minor bleedings or warning leaks. Ischemic symptoms like dizziness, focal sensory or motor changes, and speech and cognitive abnormalities may derive from thromboembolism. Aneurysmal enlargement may result in the compression of surrounding structures such as cranial nerves or brain parenchyma. In these cases symptoms

like visual field deficits, eye movement alterations, eye, ear, or face pain, and seizures may occur. Between 30% and 60% of patients with intracranial aneurysm will have warning signs prior to the rupture of the aneurysm; however, they will be often misinterpreted as hemicranias, hypertensive encephalopathy, cerebral cancer, meningitides, sinusitis, and cervical spine pathology.

CLINICAL CAVEAT

Clinical symptoms and signs of subarachnoid hemorrhage:
- Acute and severe headache
- Stiff neck
- Photophobia
- Nausea
- Vomiting
- Loss of consciousness

Before the rupture of the aneurysm minor bleedings may cause:
- Headache
- Neck ache
- Chest pain
- Back pain
- Leg pain
- Photophobia
- Lethargy

Classification

Several clinical classifications of subarachnoid hemorrhage have been proposed to assess objectively the clinical progression of each patient and to achieve an early outcome determination. The most common classifications are the Hunt and Hess grading system (Box 19-21) and the World Federation of Neurologic Surgeons grading system (Box 19-22). The latter uses the Glasgow Coma Scale and is more objective, while the Hunt and Hess grading system uses a more subjective evaluation of

Box 19-21 Hunt and Hess Grading System

- Grade I – normal neurologic examination, mild head ache, and slightly stiff neck
- Grade II – moderate to severe headache and stiff neck; no confusion or neurologic deficit except for cranial nerve palsy
- Grade III – persistent confusion and/or focal neurologic deficit
- Grade IV – persistent stupor; moderate to severe neurological deficit
- Grade V – coma with moribund appearance

Box 19-22 World Federation of Neurologic Surgeons Grading System

- Grade I – GCS 15 without motor deficit
- Grade II – GCS 13–14 without motor deficit
- Grade III – GCS 13–14 with motor deficit
- Grade IV – GCS 7–12 with or without motor deficit
- Grade V – GCS 3–6 with or without motor deficit

Box 19-24 Diagnostic Workup for Subarachnoid Hemorrhage

- CT scanning in the first hours after clinical onset
- Lumbar puncture if CT scanning is negative and the clinical suspicion of subarachnoid hemorrhage still exists
- Angiography of the cerebral vessels if CT scanning or lumbar puncture are positive for subarachnoid hemorrhage

---

the clinical state. Another classification based on the Glasgow Coma Scale has been proposed from John Hopkins University (Box 19-23).

Diagnostic Workup

The suspicion of subarachnoid hemorrhage must be confirmed by an appropriate diagnostic workup including CT scanning. NMR has a limited utility in the acute phase. When CT scanning is performed in the first hours following the onset of subarachnoid hemorrhage it has a sensitivity of 95%. False negatives rise to 10% after 3 days, and to 50% after 7 days. The blood may be drained from the subarachnoid space within 24 hours in 2–5% of cases while the blood in the cerebral parenchyma or in the cerebral ventricles persists longer. The identification of the aneurysm location is easier if intraparenchymal blood is present. Intraventricular blood is a sign of severe hemorrhage.

When CT scanning is negative, lumbar puncture is necessary. After aneurysmal rupture the blood appears in the cerebrospinal fluid within a few minutes and disappears within 7–10 days. Oxyhemoglobin is present in the supernatant of the cerebrospinal fluid 2–4 hours after the aneurysmal rupture and persists for 4 weeks. Xanthochromia makes the difference between a positive lumbar puncture and traumatic bleeding during lumbar puncture.

If CT scanning or lumbar puncture are positive for subarachnoid hemorrhage the angiography of the cerebral vessels should be performed to identify the site of bleeding, while it is not indicated if both CT scanning and lumbar puncture are negative and less than 2 weeks have elapsed from the clinical onset. Early angiography should be performed also in patients with severe clinical symptoms eligible for endovascular treatment; late angiography is less reliable because of vasospasm. If angiography fails to identify the site of bleeding it should be repeated after a few days: a previously unidentified aneurysm will be diagnosed in 10% of these cases. Cerebral angiography poses the risk of nephro- and neurotoxicity. Intravenous fluids reduce nephrotoxicity that is most common in patients treated with ACE inhibitors and nonsteroidal anti-inflammatory drugs (NSAIDs). Neurotoxicity may cause confusion, abnormal speech, and changes of consciousness. Whenever angiography is not possible, NMR or CT scanning with contrast enhancement should be performed (Box 19-24).

Management of Neurologic Complications

Neurological complications following subarachnoid hemorrhage include vasospasm, rebleeding, intracranial hematoma, hydrocephalus, persistent intracranial hypertension, and seizures (Box 19-25).

Vasospasm

In around 60% of patients with subarachnoid hemorrhage vasospasm of the major cerebral arteries is evident

---

Box 19-23 Johns Hopkins University Scale

- Grade I – GCS 15
- Grade II – GCS 14–12
- Grade III – GCS 11–9
- Grade IV – GCS 8–6
- Grade V – GCS 5–3

Box 19-25 Neurological Complications of Subarachnoid Hemorrhage

- Vasospasm
- Rebleeding
- Intracranial hematoma
- Hydrocephalus
- Persistent intracranial hypertension
- Seizures

angiographically, and half of patients with vasospasm will present delayed ischemic deficits that may progress to cause death. Acute vasospasm occurs a few hours after hemorrhage, while chronic vasospasm occurs 3-4 days after hemorrhage and recedes after 14 days. The term vasospasm is misleading because it is not a spasm of the muscularis layer of the vessels but a proliferative arteriopathy resulting in the obstruction of the vessels and in the alteration of the cerebral autoregulation. This arteriopathy seems to be induced by the presence of hemoglobin in the subarachnoid space which results in a peroxidative damage involving free radicals. The quantity of blood in the subarachnoid space seen on CT scanning is predictive of vasospasm. Delayed ischemic deficit causes an alteration in consciousness progressing over minutes or hours; focal deficits are less frequent. Serial transcranial Doppler is an effective monitor of cerebral blood flow in these instances and should be associated with clinical assessment. Vasospasm may be treated with calcium antagonists, triple H therapy, or angioplasty.

CLINICAL CAVEAT

Treatments of vasospasm associated with subarachnoid hemorrhage:
- Calcium antagonists
- Triple H therapy
- Angioplasty

While other calcium antagonists are less useful, nimodipine is effective in the prevention of delayed ischemic deficits. Nimodipine prevents cytotoxicity blocking calcium channels over neuronal membranes, and, although it does not reduce the incidence of symptomatic vasospasm, nimodipine improves cerebral blood flow through collateral branches resulting in a better functional outcome. Nimodipine may be used at a dose of 60 mg through a nasogastric tube every 4 hours for 21 days or by a continuous intravenous infusion of 2 mg per hour for 14 days. Collateral effects are usually mild, including: hypotension, flushing, edema, headache, increases in pulmonary shunting, and decreases in gastrointestinal motility. Hypotension should be treated to prevent negative effects on cerebral perfusion. Several authors advocated triple H therapy to decrease ischemic lesions from vasospasm. Triple H therapy is based on deliberate hypertension, hypervolemia, and hemodilution. The rationale for this therapy is that vasospasm impairs cerebral autoregulation and makes cerebral blood flow dependent on systemic arterial pressure and hematic viscosity. It is still a matter of controversy as to which is the most important among the three targets;

however, triple H therapy is largely accepted. An appropriate fluid management is fundamental in order to obtain hypertension and hypervolemia. Conclusive data about the kind of fluid to be used are lacking. The long-lasting controversy between colloids and crystalloids has still not produced an evidence-based endpoint. Usually colloids and crystalloids are used together in a dose ratio of 1:3. Isotonic fluids with an adequate amount of sodium are necessary given the dangers of hyponatremia in these patients. Once provided a hypervolemic state, hypertension may require inotrope or vasopressor drugs. Hypertension is associated with an important cardiovascular risk and careful hemodynamic monitoring should be used to obtain a pulmonary capillary wedge pressure (PCWP) equal to 15-18 mmHg. Transcranial Doppler may be useful in patients with subarachnoid hemorrhage to identify when deliberate hypertension is necessary to ensure an appropriate cerebral blood flow. The use of transcranial Doppler to guide deliberate hypertension may be especially beneficial in patients with cardiovascular disease in whom long-lasting hypertension is detrimental. Transluminal angioplasty is able to limit ischemic damage associated with vasospasm. When it is used within 6-12 hours after the onset of ischemic deficit, angioplasty is especially useful in patients not responsive to triple H therapy. Timing is important because when the vasospasm-related morphological changes of the cerebral vessels have occurred, angioplasty is less effective (Box 19-26).

During neuroradiologic procedures it is possible to administer intra-arterially papaverine, which in several cases seems to be useful.

Tirilazilad is a free radical scavenger that has been used in the treatment of the vasospasm from subarachnoid hemorrhage. Results seem to be better in males than females, probably because of a shorter half-life in women. Phenitoine may also reduce the half-life of tirilazilad.

Rebleeding
Rebleeding occurs in 20% of cases of subarachnoid hemorrhage and is associated with high mortality (70%).

Box 19-26 Angioplasty

This is indicated if:
- The neurologic deficit has no other possible cause than vasospasm
- The ischemic deficit is not responsive to triple H therapy
- The vasospasm is angiographically evident in an accessible area
- A recent infarction is absent

The risk for rebleeding is higher during the 24–48 hours after the first hemorrhage. Clinically the level of consciousness declines acutely and headache suddenly worsens associating with confusion. If the patient is already comatose, mydriasis and seizures occur, respiratory pattern changes, and apnoea may result. The control of hypertension has an important role in the prevention of rebleeding after subarachnoid hemorrhage, although the treatment of systemic hypertension is complex and controversial. Cerebral ischemia is more likely if patients receive antihypertensive treatment, but the incidence of rebleeding is higher if systolic arterial pressure is higher than 160 mmHg. Patients with a stable mean arterial pressure higher than 130 mmHg that is not related to pain, anxiety, or discomfort from mechanical ventilation should receive an antihypertensive treatment based on labetalol or esmolol. Surgical repair of the aneurysm is the best way to prevent rebleeding.

Intracranial Hematoma

Among patients with subarachnoid hemorrhage, around 15–20% also present with intracranial hematoma. Immediate surgical drainage is necessary if signs of brain compression occur, otherwise intracranial hematoma is drained when aneurysm is repaired.

Hydrocephalus

The incidence of hydrocephalus in patients with subarachnoid hemorrhage is 20%. It may be acute, subacute, or late. Acute hydrocephalus is evident on the first CT scanning and is usually associated with intraventricular hemorrhage. The treatment of acute hydrocephalus is based on immediate ventricular drainage avoiding a sudden decrease in cerebrospinal fluid that may precipitate rebleeding, while lumbar puncture should be avoided. Subacute hydrocephalus occurs during the first week after the onset of subarachnoid hemorrhage. Usually subacute hydrocephalus is communicant and is not associated with neurologic impairment. While subacute hydrocephalus should be monitored with serial examinations, its treatment is reserved for the cases associated with neurologic signs because it usually resolves spontaneously. Late hydrocephalus occurs weeks to months after the first bleeding and it is usually associated with a typical clinical triad: ataxia, dementia, and incontinence. A permanent ventricular shunting should be considered.

Persistent Intracranial Hypertension

Subarachnoid hemorrhage is usually associated with a sudden increase in intracranial pressure that may become higher than arterial pressure resulting in the transient loss of consciousness usually present in the acute phase. This may be a defensive mechanism that would limit bleeding. If the amount of blood in the subarachnoid space is high enough it may cause persistent intracranial hypertension resulting in cerebral death.

Seizures

The incidence of seizures in the acute phase of subarachnoid hemorrhage is 10–15%. If seizures occur after the acute phase, rebleeding should be excluded with appropriate examinations because seizures may be the sign of rebleeding. Seizures are usually associated with severe acute hypertension that may be the cause of rebleeding and should be prevented.

Medical Complications

Arrhythmias (QT tract alterations, atrial flutter and fibrillation, supraventricular tachycardia, and ectopic beats) and electrocardiographic alterations like T wave inversion and ST-T tract changes are associated with 50% of the cases of subarachnoid hemorrhage. Ischemic myocardial lesions including necrosis have been observed with an incidence around 1%. Acute pulmonary edema occurs in 2% of cases. Probably cardiovascular complications result from the high plasmatic levels of catecholamines observed in patients with subarachnoid hemorrhage. Cardiac and pulmonary complications may be precipitated by triple H therapy. Another common medical complication associated with 4–30% of cases is hyponatremia. This has been considered the result of inappropriate secretion of ADH, but it is usually caused by a cerebral salt wasting syndrome often associated with subarachnoid hemorrhage. Alterations in the production of vasopressin, atrial, and cerebral natriuretic hormone contribute to this salt wasting syndrome. Hyponatremia and hypovolemia are associated with delayed ischemic deficit while hyponatremia and hypervolemia are associated with cerebral edema and intracranial hypertension. Other medical complications often associated with subarachnoid hemorrhage are stress ulcers and deep venous thrombosis (Box 19-27).

Box 19-27 Medical Complications of Subarachnoid Hemorrhage

- Arrhythmias
- Electrocardiographic alterations
- Ischemic myocardial lesions
- Acute pulmonary edema
- Hyponatremia
- Hypovolemia
- Hypervolemia
- Stress ulcers
- Thromboembolism

SELECTED READING

Adams HP: Treating ischemic stroke as an emergency. Arch Neurol 55:457-461, 1998.

Adams HP, Brott TG, Crowell RM et al: Guidelines for the management of patients with acute ischemic stroke. Stroke 25(9):1901-1914, 1994.

Archer DP, Shaw DA, Leblanc RL et al: Haemodynamic considerations in the management of patients with subarachnoid hemorrhage. Can J Anaesth 38(4): 454-470, 1991.

Berger C, Schwab S: Stroke - a medical emergency. Eur J Emergency Med 6:61-69, 1999.

Bleck TP: Medical management of subarachnoid hemorrhage. New Horizons 5(4):387-396, 1997.

Brisman MH, Bederson JB: Surgical management of subarachnoid hemorrhage. New Horizons 5(4):376-386, 1997.

Castillo V, Bogousslavsky J: Early classification of stroke. Cerebrovasc Dis Suppl 3:5-11, 1997.

Chaves CJ, Pessin MS, Caplan LR et al: Cerebellar hemorrhagic infarction. Neurology 46:346-349, 1996.

Davenport RJ, Dennis MS, Wellwood I et al: Complications after acute stroke. Stroke 27:415-420, 1996.

Gebel JM, Broderick JP: Intracerebral hemorrhage. Neurologic Clin 18(2):419-438, 2000.

Guy J, McGrath BJ, Borel CO et al: Perioperative management of aneurysmal subarachnoid hemorrhage: 1. Operative management. Anesth Analg 81:1060-1072, 1995.

Higashida RT, Furlan AJ; Assessment Committees of the American Society of Interventional and Therapeutic Neuroradiology and the Society of Interventional Radiology: Trial design and reporting standards for intra-arterial cerebral thrombolysis for acute ischemic stroke. Stroke 34:e109-e137, 2003.

Mayberg MR, Batjer HH, Dacey R et al: Guidelines for the management of aneurysmal subarachnoid hemorrhage. Stroke 25:2315-2328, 1994.

McGrath BJ, Guy J, Borel CO et al: Perioperative management of aneurysmal subarachnoid hemorrhage: 2. Postoperative management. Anesth Analg 81:1295-1302, 1995.

Muir KW: Medical management of stroke. J Neurol Neurosurg Psychiatry 70:i12-i16, 2001.

Obana WG, Andrews BT: The intensive care management of non traumatic intracerebral hemorrhage. In Andrews BT, editor: *Neurosurgical Intensive Care*, New York: McGraw Hill, 1993, pp 311-327.

Practice advisory: Thrombolytic therapy for acute ischemic stroke - summary statement. Neurology 47:835-839, 1996.

Ropper AR, Shutz H: Spontaneous intracerebral hemorrhage. In Hacke W, editor: *Neuro Critical Care*, Berlin: Springer-Verlag, 1994, pp 621-631.

Voelker JL, Kaufman HH: Intraparenchymal hemorrhage. New Horizons 5(4):342-451, 1997.

Wahlgren NG: Pharmacological treatment of acute stroke. Cerebrovasc Dis 7(Suppl 3):24-30, 1997.

Weaver JP, Hanley D, Danchev D et al: Subarachnoid hemorrhage. In Ripple JM, Irwin RS, Fink MP et al, editors: *Intensive Care Medicine*, Boston: Little Brown, 1996, pp 2051-2058.

Yamaguchi T, Minematsu K, Hasegawa Y: General care in acute stroke. Cerebrovasc Dis 7(Suppl 3):12-17, 1997.

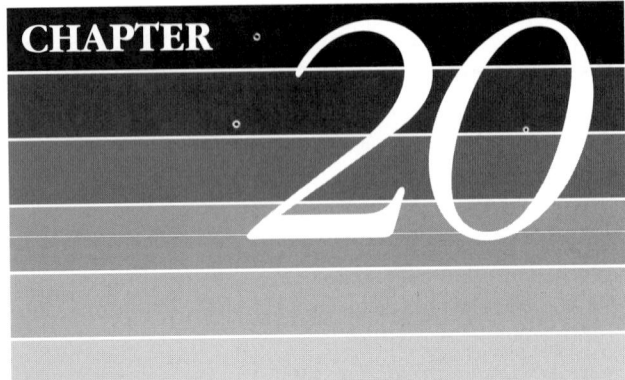

CHAPTER 20

Traumatic Brain Injury

A. RAFFAELE DE GAUDIO, M.D.

SIMONE RINALDI, M.D.

EPIDEMIOLOGY

Traumatic brain injury (TBI) is considered a "silent global epidemic" because the incidence of TBI is between 180 and 250 per 100,000 population per year (in the USA) and it may be even higher in Europe. Each year TBI causes more than 50,000 deaths for a rate of 20.6 per 100,000 population, more than 33% of all injury-related deaths. Moreover, neuropsychologic impairments and other disabilities requiring extensive rehabilitation services and long-term care are common among survivors. Groups at high risk for TBI include males, especially adolescents and young adults, and individuals living in regions with socioeconomic deprivation. The age-specific TBI incidence curve shows a biphasic pattern with a peak in the second and third decades and another one over the seventh decade. Mortality rate from TBI is higher among persons aged over 75 years and among males. Causes of TBI may be motor vehicle-related, fall-related, or firearm-related. Industrial accidents, non-motor vehicle-related trauma, and assaults are other possible causes. The pattern of TBI shows marked variations across the world. For example, in western Europe vehicular-related TBIs are decreasing because of preventive strategies (mandatory helmets, speed control, etc.). The highest motor vehicle-related TBI death rates are among persons aged 15–19 and 20–24 years. Among persons aged over 75 years, falls are the leading cause of fatal TBIs. Death rates among persons with these injuries are considerably higher among males than females.

CLASSIFICATION

TBI is a clinical entity caused by a direct and/or indirect mechanical insult, characterized by signs of diffuse or localized brain dysfunction which may occur early or late after the mechanical insult. From an anatomic/pathologic perspective TBI may be classified according to the associated lesions of the skull and the brain parenchyma (Box 20-1).

From a clinical point of view TBI may be classified according to the Glasgow Coma Scale (GCS) (Box 20-2).

Recently, the modified Head Injury Severity Score (HISS) has been proposed. This system classifies TBI as:

- minimal if GCS is equal to 15 and TBI has not been associated with loss of consciousness;

Box 20-1 Anatomic/Pathologic Classification of Traumatic Brain Injury

- Skull vault fracture
- Skull base fracture
- Other skull fractures
- Multiple fractures involving skull or face with other bones
- Concussion
- Cerebral laceration and contusion
- Subdural, subarachnoid, and extradural hemorrhage after injury
- Other unspecified intracranial hemorrhage after injury
- Intracranial injury, not otherwise specified
- Late effects of fracture of the skull and face
- Late effects of intracranial injury without skull fracture
- Other open wound to the head

Box 20-2 Glasgow Coma Scale

BEST EYES OPEN SCORE

Spontaneously, 4
On command, 3
To pain, 2
No response, 1

BEST VERBAL RESPONSE

Orientated, 5
Confused, 4
Inappropriate words, 3
Incomprehensible, 2
No response, 1

BEST MOTOR RESPONSE

Obeys to command, 6
Localized pain, 5
Flexion withdrawal, 4
Abnormal flexion, 3
Extension, 2
No response, 1

- mild if GCS is equal to 14 or 15 and if TBI has been associated with brief (<5 minutes) loss of consciousness or amnesia;
- moderate if GCS is between 9 and 13 and loss of consciousness has lasted more then 5 minutes or a focal neurologic deficit is present; and
- severe if GCS is below 8.

PATHOPHYSIOLOGY

The pathophysiology of TBI depends on three different pathologic instances: the brain damage at the time of injury (primary damage), the insults the brain receives during the postinjury phase (secondary damage), and the extracranial lesions. All these move together to cerebral tissue hypoxia and ischemia which are the leading causes of brain death.

Primary Damage

Primary damage is the brain injury that occurs at the time of the initial mechanical insult. This is a major determinant of outcome from TBI, but, unless it consists of a surgically evacuable mass lesion, it is usually irreversible. Primary damage includes scalp lacerations and skull fractures, brain contusion and lacerations, intracranial traumatic hemorrhage (extradural, subdural, and intracerebral hematoma), and diffuse axonal injury (Box 20-3).

Box 20-3 Primary Damage

Primary damage includes:
- Scalp lacerations
- Skull fractures
- Brain contusion and lacerations
- Intracranial traumatic hemorrhages (extradural, subdural, and intracerebral)
- Diffuse axonal injury

Box 20-4 Skull Base Fractures

Skull base fractures may involve:
- Anterior cranial fossa with lesions of the first, second, third, and fourth cranial nerves and ecchymosis over the orbitary region
- Medial cranial fossa with lesions of the fifth, seventh, and eighth cranial nerves, otorrhagia and otorrhoea
- Posterior cranial fossa with lesions of the ninth, tenth, eleventh, and twelfth cranial nerves

---

Scalp Lacerations and Skull Fractures

Because of the scalp's rich vascularization, scalp lacerations may be associated with underestimated blood loss. The site and the size of skull fractures depend on the impact site and the speed and the shape of the damaging agent. Skull fractures may be categorized as blunt (if the skin is intact) or penetrating (if the skull vault appears through the scalp laceration) or, according to their site, as skull vault fractures and skull base fractures. Skull vault fractures may radiate to the base and may be linear or depressed.

Skull base fractures may involve the anterior, medial, or posterior cranial fossa. If the skull base fracture is associated with a dural lesion cerebrospinal fluid may drain to the nose or ear producing oto- or rhinoliquorrhea that may be complicated by meningitides requiring sometimes a surgical treatment. If the anterior cranial fossa is fractured, lesions of the first, second, third, and fifth cranial nerves may occur (sphenoidal fissura syndrome); an ecchymosis over the eyelid, the orbitary, and the subconjunctival region appears usually 2–3 days after the trauma. When the medial cranial fossa is fractured, the internal auditory meatus and the middle ear are often involved with otorrhagia and otorrhoea if the tympanic membrane is injured. Lesions to the fifth, seventh (peripheral paralysis of the facial nerve), and eighth cranial nerves may occur. Sinum cavernosum may be involved resulting in carotid injuries and fistula between carotid artery and sinum cavernosum. When there is a posterior cranial fossa fracture, lesions to the ninth, tenth, eleventh, and twelfth cranial nerves may occur with phonation and deglutition problems. Growing fractures are skull fractures associated with dural and arachnoid lesions; a pulsatile tender mass usually develops in a few weeks (Box 20-4).

Brain Contusions and Lacerations

Brain contusions and lacerations are traumatic lesions to the brain parenchyma, usually in the frontal and temporal lobes. Brain contusion is characterized by the breakage of cortical capillaries and pia mater resulting in a little hemorrhage and ecchymosis over the brain. Brain laceration instead is characterized by a macroscopic lesion to the brain parenchyma that appears necrotic and mixed to blood clots. Brain laceration may be either limited to a subcortical area or extended to a cerebral lobe and cerebral ventricles. Intra- or extraparenchymal hemorrhages, cerebral edema, and necrosis are often associated with these lesions.

Extradural Hematoma

Extradural hematoma is a mass of blood between dura mater and the skull bone. Extradural hematomas are localized mostly in the temporal and parietal areas because they are very exposed to traumatic injuries and because meningeal artery branches run through this region. More than 50% of extradural hematomas are arterial in origin, deriving usually from the medial meningeal artery. They also may be venous either from bone or dura mater vessels. Usually they are associated with skull fractures and, in around 40% of cases, with brain contusions and lacerations or intraparenchymal hematomas. Clinically extradural hematoma results in consciousness alterations often stable or progressing to coma. The classic pattern of loss of consciousness, symptom-free interval (minutes to days), and coma is not the most frequent clinical pattern. Usually extradural hematomas also present site-related signs like contralateral hemiparesis, hemiplegy, Babinski, and homolateral mydriasis with anisocoria (in 60% of cases). Signs related to cerebral herniation may present sooner or later after trauma. Urgent surgical treatment is the primary therapy for extradural hematoma because outcome is determined by the size of the blood mass, and also by the extent to which the secondary distortion of the brain stem has progressed before surgery has been undertaken (Box 20-5).

Box 20-5 Clinical Signs of Extradural Hematoma

Clinical signs of extradural hematoma include:
- Alterations of consciousness
- Contralateral hemiparesis
- Contralateral Babinski
- Homolateral mydriasis with anisocoria
- Signs of cerebral herniation

Subdural Hematoma

Subdural hematoma is a blood mass between dura mater and arachnoides. Usually it is associated with a hemorrhagic brain laceration; extradural or intraparenchymal hematomas may coexist. It is more frequent in the elderly. It is localized usually in the interhemispheric scissure, expanding to the frontal, parietal, and temporal lobes. Brain atrophy may allow the brain to move according to the trauma-related accelerations and decelerations; this movement would stretch the "bridge veins" between dura mater and cerebral parenchyma making them bleed. The blood may also originate from cerebral cortex arteries and veins. Subdural hematoma is rarely alone and acute; usually it is associated with brain contusions and lacerations that may take part in the hematoma development. Disorders of consciousness are often early and severe. A minor disorder of mentation is not unusual, although it often progresses to coma. Homolateral mydriasis and contralateral hemiparesis may often be present in association with signs of brainstem lesions like decerebration. Neurovegetative signs including hyperthermia, hypertension, and electrocardiographic abnormalities are also common. Surgical treatment is the therapy of choice for subdural hematoma.

Intracerebral Hematoma

Intracerebral hematoma is a blood mass totally inside the brain parenchyma, without extension to the brain surface. At the moment of traumatic impact a breakage of intracerebral vessels results in intracerebral hemorrhages. Intracerebral hematoma derives from these multiple intracerebral traumatic hemorrhages. Frontal and temporal lobes are the most frequent locations although even deeper areas such as basal nuclei may be involved. Usually intracerebral hematomas are associated with brain lacerations and contusions as well as diffuse axonal injury. The clinical picture usually includes disorders of consciousness, hemiplegy, anisocoria, and brainstem involvement. A surgical approach to intracerebral hematoma is not always possible and outcome is usually poor.

Diffuse Axonal Injury

Diffuse axonal injury is a diffuse injury to the white cerebral matter. Damaged axons display injuries progressing to axonal disconnection. Time allows a glial reaction with myelin degeneration. Probably stretching stress during the acceleration–deceleration phases of traumatic impact causes axonal breakage and a focal influx of Ca^{2+} promoting proteolytic processes involving cysteine proteases, calpain, and caspase that modify the axonal cytoskeleton, causing irreversible damage. The clinical picture of diffuse axonal injury is a severe neurologic failure with post-traumatic coma evolving into a persistent vegetative state without macroscopic

---

Box 20-6   Secondary Damage

Secondary damage includes:
- Cerebral edema
- Ischemic brain damage
- Brain shift and herniation
- Hydrocephalus

---

encephalic lesions. Surgical treatment is impossible, and medical treatment gives frustrating results and outcome is poor. Inhibition of proteolytic processes may be a therapeutic strategy in the future.

Secondary Damage

Secondary damage includes the insults that the brain receives in the postinjury phase of trauma. Every clinical complication that reduces cerebral nutrients and oxygen delivery (hypotension, hypoxia, anemia, hypoglycemia, hypocapnia, etc.) or increases cerebral oxygen consumption (hyperthermia, seizures) contributes to secondary damage. Secondary brain damage includes cerebral edema, ischemic brain damage, brain shift and herniation, and hydrocephalus (Box 20-6).

Cerebral Edema

Brain swelling is a very dangerous secondary damage because it may progress to brain ischemia and herniation given that the nervous parenchyma is embedded in the noncompliant box of the skull. The brain is particularly susceptible to edema because it is not supplied with a lymphatic system to drain extraneous fluid in the interstitial compartment. Ion and water movement between the vessels and the brain occurs across the blood–brain barrier which depends on the capillaries of the brain. Here endothelium has tight junctions and few endocytotic vesicles. This kind of endothelial differentiation derives from the cross-talk with astrocytes. Cerebral edema may be vasogenic, cytotoxic, and interstitial (Box 20-7).

Box 20-7   Cerebral Edemas

Cerebral edemas include:
- Vasogenic edema resulting from fluid spilling across the vessels to the extracellular compartment
- Cytotoxic edema resulting from an increase in the intracellular water caused by ischemia
- Interstitial edema occurring in some kinds of hydrocephalus because of fluid accumulation in periventricular areas

- Vasogenic edema is the result of fluid spilling across the vessels to the extracellular compartment. Usually the vessels producing vasogenic edema show an abnormal barrier function. Brain contusions and lacerations usually are surrounded by injured vessels with poor barrier function. Moreover ischemia may alter endothelial barrier function resulting in vasogenic edema that increases intracranial pressure and ischemia with a negative closed loop mechanism. Vasogenic edema affects preferentially white cerebral matter that appears swollen.
- Cytotoxic edema results from an increase in the intracellular water. Cerebral gray matter is usually more susceptible to cytotoxic edema as consequence of either ischemia or hypo-osmolarity. Ischemia impairs neuronal metabolism and membrane ionic pump function. Hypo-osmolarity shifts water into neuronal cells that appear swollen.
- Interstitial edema occurs in some kinds of hydrocephalus when fluids cross ependimal cells and accumulate in the periventricular areas.

Ischemic Brain Damage

Ischemic brain damage is one of the most important factors precipitating TBI. Most ischemic brain damage is secondary to brain swelling, brain shift, and brain herniation, rather than the direct effect of the primary damage upon the brain.

TBI is strongly linked to ischemic brain damage. Ischemic brain damage results from pathogenetic mechanisms associated also with TBI, including excitotoxicity, inflammation, free radicals, and apoptosis. Production of heat shock proteins and endogenous antioxidants are defensive mechanisms triggered by cerebral ischemia and TBI (Box 20-8).

Phospholipase stimulation may cause alterations in membrane phospholipids compromising the ability to accumulate excitotoxic amino acids. Inhibitors of both cyclooxygenase and lipoxygenase pathways have been shown to reduce cerebral deficits following ischemia and trauma. Excitotoxicity is considered to be caused mainly by the inappropriate release of glutamate. Multiple human clinical trials focused on glutamate antagonists for the treatment of TBI and ischemia. Even nonneuronal cells (brain glia and lymphocytes) can release substances that bind to glutamate receptors. Excitotoxicity may be ongoing for several days, rather than just in the initial phase of TBI. Hence arresting excitotoxic processes may modulate progressive brain injury in the initial days after TBI. Ischemic brain injury associated with TBI causes neuronal apoptotic death. A calcium-binding peptide produced by astrocytes may be implicated in neuronal apoptosis. Ischemic brain damage adversely affects outcome morbidity, and the difficulty in preventing ischemic damage in cases with marked brain shift leads to poor outcome in patients with TBI.

Brain Shift and Herniation

Intracranial hypertension is often associated with TBI because blood masses may evolve in brain shift and herniation. Cerebral masses move areas of cerebral parenchyma across dural folds resulting in brain shift and herniation. If one hemisphere expands the cingulate gyrus may herniate below the falx cerebri or the temporal lobe may herniate between the tentorium cerebelli and the brainstem. The latter herniation may injure the third cranial nerve with anisocoria and homolateral mydriasis. Moreover the contralateral cerebral pedicle may be compressed against tentorium cerebelli determining paralysis homolateral to the cerebral lesion (Kernoan Woltman syndrome). Even if initially the respiratory pattern is not affected by this kind of herniation, later pathologic respiratory patterns like Cheine–Stokes breath may occur. Cerebellum may herniate into the foramen magnum with a coning mechanism impairing respiration and other brainstem functions. Brainstem compression resulting from cerebellum herniation may be fatal. Cerebral parenchyma may also herniate across skull defects. Brain shift compresses superficial cerebral arteries against dural folds determining occlusion and cerebral ischemia (Box 20-9).

Hydrocephalus

Hydrocephalus is a dilatation of the cerebral ventricles with increased cerebrospinal fluid. TBI may obstruct cerebrospinal fluid flow. When this obstruction occurs

---

Box 20-8 Ischemic Brain Damage

Ischemic brain damage results from:
- Excitotoxicity
- Inflammation
- Free radicals
- Apoptosis
  Heat shock proteins and endogenous antioxidants are defensive mechanisms.

Box 20-9 Brain Herniation

Brain herniation includes:
- Herniation of the cingulate gyrus below falx cerebri
- Herniation of the temporal lobe between tentorium cerebelli and the brainstem
- Herniation of the cerebellum into the foramen magnum
- Herniation of the cerebral parenchyma through skull defects

Box 20-10   Extracranial Lesions

Extracranial lesions that may complicate traumatic brain injury:
- Thoracic lesions
- Abdominal traumas
- Extremity fractures

in the intraencephalic liquoral spaces, hydrocephalus is noncommunicant. If obstruction occurs in the subarachnoid space, hydrocephalus is communicant. Ventricular dilatation secondary to severe hydrocephalus may produce cerebrospinal fluid spillage in periventricular brain parenchyma resulting in interstitial cerebral edema.

Extracranial Lesions

TBI is often associated with extracranial lesions that may contribute to outcome. Thoracic lesions should always be considered and are particularly dangerous in association with TBI because they cause by themselves hypoxia and hypercapnia. Moreover hypertensive pneumothorax determines a decrease in cardiac output and an increase in intracranial pressure resulting in severe brain hypoperfusion. Abdominal traumas may be associated with significant blood loss that causes anemia and hypotension, factors contributing to secondary damage after TBI. Extremity fractures are also associated with underestimated hypovolemia that may impair brain perfusion after TBI (Box 20-10).

PATHOPHYSIOLOGY OF CEREBRAL BLOOD FLOW

TBI is always associated with alterations in cerebral blood flow because the physical injury and the consequent inflammatory response impair the normal functions of cerebral vessels and neurons. In particular, a **hypoperfusion phase** is usually followed by a **hyperemic** or **vasospastic phase**. The first 72 hours following TBI are usually characterized by a reduction in cerebral blood flow resulting from intracranial and extracranial mechanisms. This hypoperfusion phase produces ischemic brain damage with cytotoxic cerebral edema and increased intracranial pressure. Following this hypoperfusion phase 25–30% of patients experience a hyperemic phase with an increased cerebral blood flow that persists during 7–10 days after TBI. Probably it is associated with a recovery of autoregulatory mechanisms. Intracranial inflammation and the consequent impairment of the blood–brain barrier lead to patients being at risk for vasogenic cerebral edema in this hyperemic phase. The hypoperfusion phase may be followed in

Box 20-11   Pathophysiology of Cerebral Blood Flow in Traumatic Brain Injuries

The pathophysiology of cerebral blood flow in traumatic brain injuries includes:
- Hypoperfusion phase, usually characterizes the first 72 hours after trauma
- Hyperaemic phase, occurs in 25–30% of patients after the hypoperfusion phase, persists for 7–10 days after trauma
- Vasospastic phase, occurs in 10–15% of patients following the hypoperfusion phase

10–15% of patients by a persistent vasospastic phase with cerebral hypoperfusion due to arterial vasospasm (Box 20-11).

Autoregulation of Cerebral Blood Flow

If the cerebral perfusion pressure ranges between 50 and 150 mmHg, the cerebral vessels maintain a constant cerebral blood flow according to the actual cerebral metabolism. This property of cerebral blood flow is known as cerebral blood flow autoregulation. In hypertensive patients the pressure range of autoregulation is higher for morphologic and functional changes in the arterial walls. In TBI autoregulation is altered particularly during the early hypoperfusion phase when cerebral perfusion pressure is directly dependent on systemic blood pressure and probably should be higher than 60–70 mmHg to guarantee an appropriate cerebral blood flow. During the later hyperemic phase, autoregulation starts to recover but high cerebral perfusion pressure may result in vasogenic edema and increased intracranial pressure so a lower range of cerebral perfusion pressure between 50 and 70 mmHg is safe. Mechanical, metabolic, and neurogenic factors influence normal autoregulation. The mechanical factor is the automatic and myogenic adaptation of arteriolar resistances to transmural pressure changes. Transmural pressure is the difference between pressures inside and outside the vessel; the pressure inside the vessels is considered the medium arterial pressure and the pressure outside the vessels is considered the intracranial pressure. If transmural pressure increases, vessels constrict; if it decreases, vessels vasodilate. When vessels change their caliber intracranial blood volume also changes. If intracranial arterial blood volume increases, cerebrospinal fluid shifts compressing intracranial veins and reducing intracranial venous blood volume. The metabolic factor is the coupling between cerebral blood flow and cerebral metabolism that guarantees appropriate substrate delivery for cerebral metabolism (Box 20-12).

Box 20-12   Autoregulation of Cerebral Blood Flow

Autoregulation of cerebral blood flow is influenced by:
- Mechanical factor - the automatic and myogenic adaptation of arteriolar resistances to transmural pressure changes
- Metabolic factor - the coupling between cerebral blood flow and cerebral metabolism
- Neurogenic factor

Box 20-13   Intracranial Pressure and Cerebral Perfusion Pressure: The Relationship

- According to the Monroe-Kelly law, the sum of cerebral parenchyma volume, cerebrospinal fluid volume, and blood vessel volume is constant.
- If one of these three contents of the skull increases in volume, intracranial pressure also increases.
- The cerebral perfusion pressure (CPP) is considered the difference between the systemic mean arterial pressure (MAP) and the intracranial pressure (ICP): $CPP = MAP - ICP$

Carbon dioxide is the most important substance acting on the metabolic factor of autoregulation because it crosses the blood–brain barrier rapidly influencing extracellular pH that influences vessel caliber. If $PaCO_2$ increases by 1 mmHg, cerebral blood flow increases 4% and intracranial vascular volume increases 0.04 ml/100 g. TBI is often characterized by an uncoupling between cerebral metabolism and cerebral blood flow. In acute traumatic injury often there is a reduction in cerebral metabolism sometimes associated with an increase in cerebral blood flow because of an abnormal autoregulation. TBI is associated also with an impaired hypocapnic vasoconstriction localized more in injured areas than all over the brain. Hypercapnia will determine an "intracranial steal phenomenon" because the vasodilatation of healthy areas steals blood from the injured areas. Instead, hypocapnia may cause an "inverse steal phenomenon" causing a redistribution of blood flow to the injured areas. This is the rationale for therapeutic hypocapnia in TBI. In any case hypocapnia may cause ischemia in previously healthy areas especially during the early hypoperfusion phase, so appropriate neuromonitoring is necessary when hyperventilation is used.

Intracranial Pressure and Cerebral Perfusion Pressure

The skull is a rigid box with an incompressible content including cerebral parenchyma (80%), cerebrospinal fluid (10%), and blood vessels (10%). The incompressibility of the content and the rigidity of the container is the basis of the Monro–Kelly law stating that the sum of cerebral parenchyma volume, cerebrospinal fluid volume, and blood vessel volume is constant. If one of the three contents increases in volume, initially the others decrease, then, when the total content volume increases, intracranial pressure also increases. Cerebral perfusion pressure, a major determinant of cerebral blood flow, is highly influenced by intracranial pressure. Cerebral perfusion pressure, in fact, is the difference between the arterial pressure in the feeding arteries as they enter the subarachnoid space and the pressure in the draining veins before they enter dural sinuses. These pressures are difficult to measure, so cerebral perfusion pressure (CPP) is considered the difference between the systemic mean arterial pressure (MAP) and the intracranial pressure (ICP), taken as an estimate of tissue pressure: $CPP = MAP - ICP$ (Box 20-13).

Simultaneous measurement of both invasive arterial pressure and intracranial pressure has therefore become a useful monitoring technique in patients with TBI to determine the cerebral perfusion pressure.

Given that an estimation of the cerebral perfusion pressure based on intracranial pressure is misleading if the intracranial pressure is low, recently it has been proposed to measure the critical closing pressure. The cerebral critical closing pressure may be determined in a minimally invasive way using transcranial Doppler flow tracings and invasive arterial pressure. In up to 50% of patients with TBI intracranial pressure may lead to an overestimation of the cerebral perfusion pressure when compared to critical closing pressure.

Vasodilatation and Vasoconstriction Cascades

The physiologic concept of vasodilatation and vasoconstriction cascades is the base for a recent therapeutic strategy for TBI. The vasodilatation cascade depends on a reduction in cerebral perfusion pressure that has an autoperpetuating trend. In fact, if the cerebral perfusion pressure decreases, cerebral vessels dilate in an attempt to maintain cerebral blood flow as a result of normal autoregulation. This vasodilation results in an increased cerebral blood volume that increases intracranial pressure and finally reduces the cerebral perfusion pressure. This vasodilatation vicious circle may be interrupted triggering the vasoconstriction cascade by increasing arterial blood pressure. The increase in arterial blood pressure leads to an increase in cerebral perfusion pressure resulting, according to normal autoregulation,

Box 20-14   Vasodilatation Cascade

The vasodilatation cascade:
- Reduction in cerebral perfusion pressure
- Vasodilatation of cerebral vessels
- Increased cerebral blood volume
- Increased intracranial pressure
- Reduction in cerebral perfusion pressure

The vasoconstriction cascade:
- Increased arterial blood pressure
- Increased cerebral perfusion pressure
- Vasoconstriction of cerebral vessels
- Decreased cerebral blood volume
- Decreased intracranial pressare
- Increased cerebral perfusion pressure

in vasoconstriction of cerebral vessels. This vasoconstriction reduces cerebral blood volume and then intracranial pressure resulting finally in an increase in cerebral perfusion pressure (Box 20-14).

MANAGEMENT OF TRAUMATIC BRAIN INJURY

Prehospital and Emergency Room Care

Prehospital and emergency room care of TBI should be directed by the Advanced Trauma Life Support (ATLS) guidelines for the early management of trauma. Prehospital care of TBI includes airway management and treatment of hypoxia, hypotension, and fluid resuscitation and neurologic assessment only after cardiorespiratory stability has been guaranteed. Emergency room care includes cardiorespiratory stability optimization, considerations related to the multiple trauma patient, neurologic assessment followed by brain-specific therapies, and early diagnostic workup with indications for surgery (Box 20-15).

Box 20-15   Prehospital Care of Traumatic Brain Injury

Prehospital care of traumatic brain injury includes:
- Airway management
- Treatment of hypoxia
- Treatment of hypotension
- Neurologic assessment after cardiorespiratory stability

Emergency room care includes:
- Cardiorespiratory stability optimization
- Neurologic assessment
- Eventual brain-specific therapies
- Early diagnostic workup

Hypoxia and Airway Management

Orotracheal intubation is the gold standard for airway management and hypoxia treatment of patients with severe traumatic brain injury (GCS < 9), marked agitation, or severe extracranial trauma. Nasotracheal intubation is contraindicated in suspected fractures of the skull base because the lesion of the cribriform plate could create a communication with intracranial structures. Orotracheal intubation should be performed using a rapid sequence induction with cricoid pressure (Sellick maneuver) and in-line immobilization of the cervical spine. All patients with TBI are assumed to have a potential cervical spine injury and should be immobilized in a rigid collar until a cervical spine fracture is definitely excluded by appropriate radiologic imaging examination. After appropriate orotracheal intubation TBI patients should be ventilated in 100% oxygen to maintain PaO_2 above 100 mmHg; ventilation should be adjusted to maintain a normal $PaCO_2$ of 35–40 mmHg. Hyperventilation in early resuscitation is not indicated, the priorities being appropriate oxygenation and hemodynamic stability.

Hypotension and Fluid Resuscitation

In TBI hypotension may be a dangerous trigger of secondary damage. Concomitant multiple system trauma is often associated with TBI resulting in significant blood loss, hemodynamic instability, and shock. Prompt restoration of circulating blood volume to prevent secondary damage deriving from cerebral hypoperfusion is a widely recognized priority. Fluid resuscitation in TBI has been the focus of much discussion because of the possible development of cerebral edema after administration of large volumes of resuscitative fluids. The goal of fluid resuscitation in TBI should always be euvolemia to optimize cerebral perfusion pressure without contributing to cerebral edema. The blood–brain barrier has peculiar features being freely permeable to water, but nearly impermeable to larger, colloid-sized molecules, and minimally permeable to most ions. The osmotic gradient between blood and brain regulates water flux across the blood–brain barrier. The colloid osmotic pressure does not influence greatly fluid flux across the blood–brain barrier because plasma colloids account for a small fraction of the total number of particles in solution. Serum osmolality is the major determinant of fluid flux across the normal blood–brain barrier. However, TBI and hemorrhagic shock are associated with proinflammatory mediator production that alters capillary permeability in the brain. If the blood–brain barrier becomes permeable to ions but not to larger colloid particles, choice of fluid for resuscitation in TBI could be important. If the blood–brain barrier is disrupted, however, permeability to both ions and colloidal particles may occur, so fluid selection would be inconsequential. Patient with TBI not associated with hemodynamic instability may be treated with fluid restriction and brain dehydrating agents, but whenever traumatic shock occurs, large volumes of fluids are necessary to restore hemodynamic stability. There is a lack of evidence so far as to the choice of fluid in this scenario. Serum osmolarity has an established importance in the development of cerebral edema, and hypertonic crystalloids alone or in combination with colloids have theoretic advantages in terms of small-volume resuscitation with beneficial effects on cerebral blood flow and cerebral edema. Although invasive monitoring must not delay volume resuscitation, early invasive blood pressure monitoring and central venous pressure monitoring may guide more objectively hypotension treatment and fluid resuscitation. Especially when sedatives or opioids are used, inotropes like epinephrine or norepinephrine and vasopressors like metaraminol and phenylephrine may be necessary to control hypotension while fluid resuscitation is under way or complete.

Neurologic Evaluation

When cardiorespiratory stability has been achieved an assessment of neurologic function is important to determine the severity of TBI. An initial evaluation during resuscitation, as suggested by the ATLS guidelines, is based on response to stimulation: the patient may be awake, may respond to verbal or painful stimuli, or may be unresponsive. The neurologic evaluation in TBI is based on the GCS. GCS should be applied only after cardiopulmonary resuscitation and prior to surgical intervention. Neurologic evaluation should always assign the patient to one of the HISS categories that will guide the following management of TBI. Pupil size and reactivity should also be assessed in the initial neurologic evaluation, particularly prior to the administration of opioids, sedatives, and muscle relaxants. Anisocoria associated with unilateral mydriasis may be associated with a homolateral intracranial mass indicating compression of the third cranial nerve and impending herniation. Sometimes paralysis homolateral to the cerebral lesion is also present (Kernoan Woltman syndrome). A motor function examination deeper than that included in the GCS is suggested to find out hemiparesis, lateralizing signs, Babinski sign, and paraparesis and quadriparesis (from spinal injuries) (Box 20-16).

The Multiple Trauma Patient

TBI is often associated with other potentially fatal lesions that make the TBI patient a multiple trauma patient. Once the initial assessment is complete, a careful survey with a top to toe approach is mandatory.

Box 20-16   Neurologic Evaluation

- GCS
- HISS
- Pupils examination before administration of opioids
- Motor function examination before administration of sedatives or muscle relaxants

---

To exclude important lesions every multiple trauma patient should receive x-rays of the chest, pelvis, and cervical spine and baseline blood tests. In fact, the multiple trauma patient may have extracranial causes of hypoxia like hemo- or pneumothorax that need prompt, life-saving treatment. Hemorrhages from major vascular disruption or visceral injuries necessitate aggressive treatment because of life-threatening cardiovascular instability. In TBI hypotension may trigger secondary damage so a target mean arterial pressure equal to the patient's usual blood pressure must be reached even with inotropes or vasopressors. Fractures and lacerations may also cause significant blood loss that must be interrupted. Diagnosis and treatment of these problems minimize secondary damage.

CLINICAL CAVEAT

Every multiple trauma patient should receive:
- X-rays of the chest
- X-rays of the pelvis
- X-rays of the cervical spine
- Baseline blood test
  Any doubt of lesion, particularly in the cervical spine, should be clarified using CT scan.

Early Management of Intracranial Hypertension

The early treatment of intracranial hypertension based on hyperventilation and osmotherapy requires a

---

CLINICAL CAVEAT

Hyperventilation and Intracranial Pressure
- Hyperventilation is the most potent nonsurgical way to reduce intracranial pressure
- The reduction in cerebral blood flow associated with hyperventilation may precipitate cerebral ischemia
- Hyperventilation is reserved for patients with unequivocal signs of increased intracranial pressure associated with impending herniation (mydriasis, anisocoria, lateralizing signs)

diagnosis of intracranial hypertension because they may have negative side effects aggravating secondary damage. Hyperventilation is the most potent nonsurgical way of reducing intracranial pressure.

The other option used in the medical treatment of intracranial hypertension is *mannitol* (0.25–1 g/kg) that is an osmotically active agent administered to increase plasma osmolality. *Hypertonic saline* (3%) increases plasma osmolality and expands plasma volume restoring systemic and cerebral perfusion in the acute phase of TBI. Hypertonic saline has fewer side effects than mannitol. It does not induce any osmolal gap so it allows an easier titration. Hypertonic saline is the intracranial pressure-reducing agent of choice in the early phase of TBI because it reduces intracranial pressure and increases cerebral blood flow in the early hypoperfusion phase.

CLINICAL CAVEAT

Osmotic Therapy and Intracranial Hypertension
- Mannitol treatment prior to imaging is reserved for cases with unequivocal intracranial hypertension
- Hypertonic saline increases plasma osmolality and expands plasma volume with fewer side effects than mannitol in the acute phase of TBI

Early Diagnostic Workup

Every multiple trauma patient receives x-rays of the chest, pelvis, and cervical spine. Any doubt of lesion, particularly in the cervical spine, should be clarified using computed tomography (CT) scan. TBI guidelines define the role of CT scan according to the severity of TBI. In severe TBI a CT scan should be obtained as soon as cardiovascular and respiratory stability has been achieved. The patient will be then admitted to an intensive care unit (ICU). In minimal injuries the risk of complications is low and hospital admission is not necessary. The patient may be discharged with an instruction form including symptoms (severe headache, repeated vomiting, confusion, reduced level of consciousness) that should lead the patient to contact a physician. Additional risk factors in TBI are therapeutic anticoagulation, hemophilia, radiographically demonstrated skull fracture, clinical signs of depressed skull fracture or skull base fracture, post-traumatic seizures, shunt-treated hydrocephalus, and multiple injuries (Box 20-17).

If one of these risk factors is present CT scanning should be performed even in minimal TBI and the patient should be admitted to the hospital for observation. In mild TBI CT scanning should be performed and, if it is normal and additional risk factors are absent, the patient may be discharged with a copy of the instruction form. If CT scan is not normal or an additional risk factor

---

Box 20-17 Additional Risk Factors in Traumatic Brain Injury

- Therapeutic anticoagulation
- Hemophilia
- Radiographically demonstrated skull fracture
- Clinical signs of depressed skull fracture or skull base fracture
- Post-traumatic seizures
- Shunt-treated hydrocephalus
- Multiple injuries

---

is present the patient should be admitted to the hospital for observation. In moderate TBI the patient should always receive CT scanning and hospital admission for observation. In-hospital observation has a sensitivity for detection of intracranial hematoma lower than early CT scan and is dependent on strict observation including assessment of GCS, pupillary responses, motor responses, blood pressure, and heart rate. This assessment should occur every 15 minutes for the first 2 hours after admission and thereafter every hour until at least 12 hours after injury. If admitted patients deteriorate during observation developing focal neurological deficits or a reduction of the GCS of ≥2 points, urgent CT scan should be performed. CT scanning is the most useful radiologic evaluation in TBI. It allows a prompt detection of mass lesions such as extradural or subdural hematomas. CT scanning should be performed, using both parenchymal and bone windows, with 5 mm thick axial slices from the foramen magnum through the sella, followed by 10 mm thick slices through the supratentorial region. Combative patients may require orotracheal intubation, sedation, and ventilation to facilitate CT scanning.

CLINICAL CAVEAT

Early Diagnostic Workup
- In severe TBI perform CT scan as soon as cardiopulmonary stability has been achieved
- In moderate TBI perform CT scan and admit the patient for observation
- In mild TBI perform CT scan and admit the patient if it is abnormal or there are additional risk factors; otherwise discharge the patient with an instruction form
- In minimal TBI with additional risk factors perform CT scan and admit the patient for observation
- In minimal TBI without additional risk factors discharge the patient with an instruction form

---

The degree of TBI may be quantified by radiologic criteria useful for comparison with subsequent scans,

---

Box 20-18 Marshall's Classification of CT Scans after Traumatic Brain Injury

- Diffuse injury (DI) I - no intracranial pathology visible on CT scan
- DI II - cisterns present a midline shift of 0-5 mm, lesion densities present high or mixed density <25 mm
- DI III - cisterns are compressed or absent with midline shift of 0-5 mm, high or mixed densities <25 mm
- DI IV - midline shift >5 mm, high or mixed densities <25 mm
- Nonevacuated mass lesion - high or mixed density lesion >25 mm not surgically evacuated
- Evacuated mass lesion - any lesion surgically evacuated

---

for intracranial pressure monitoring decisions, and for prognosis. The classification listed in Box 20-18 of CT scan appearance following TBI is the most popular.

TBI may be associated with a vascular injury like carotid artery dissection. In these cases cerebral angiography may be considered. The suspicion of carotid artery dissection may rise from an abnormal CT scan or from a discrepancy between the patient's clinical condition and CT scan findings. Although NMR can detect small hemorrhagic collections and contusions, usually it does not provide information significantly better than that deriving from CT scan. Limitations in placement and monitoring an acute trauma patient in an NMR scanner raise an additional risk that advises against its use in these cases.

Indications for Surgery

In TBI several primary damages may necessitate surgical treatment. Urgent surgical evacuation is the primary therapy for extradural hematoma; in these cases surgery is urgent. Surgical treatment is also the therapy of choice for subdural hematoma even if the chances of good outcome decrease when subdural hematoma is associated with a large brain laceration. A surgical approach to intracerebral hematoma is not always possible. Brain contusion and lacerations may be submitted to surgical treatment, but after evaluation of the clinical and CT scan evolution of the lesions. Among skull fractures, depressed vault fractures and growing fractures may be surgically treated (Box 20-19).

Anesthesia for the Head-Injured Patient

Anesthesia for TBI is necessary whenever indication for surgery is present. In these cases anesthesia should

---

Box 20-19 Indications for Surgery

- Extradural hematoma
- Subdural hematoma
- Some kinds of intracerebral hematoma
- Some kinds of brain contusions and lacerations
- Depressed vault fractures
- Growing fractures

---

follow the general principles of maintaining good cerebral oxygenation and appropriate cerebral perfusion pressure and controlling intracranial hypertension. Appropriate monitoring includes invasive blood pressure monitoring besides the other standard monitors. PaO_2 should always be maintained above 100 mmHg. While high FIO_2 may be necessary to achieve this target, the value of positive end-expiratory pressure (PEEP) should remain below 10 cmH_2O. The use of a higher PEEP is discouraged because of the possibility of decreases in blood arterial pressure in hypovolemic patients and of compromised cerebral venous return resulting in increased intracranial pressure. Appropriate cerebral perfusion pressure requires a systemic blood pressure maintained to the preinjury level for every patient. Elderly and hypertensive patients may require a higher systemic blood pressure to obtain an appropriate cerebral perfusion pressure. The restoration of the euvolemic state is critical to maintain arterial blood pressure during anesthesia. Overhydration should be avoided. Adjusting the depth of anesthesia to the surgical stimulation usually ensures a good cerebral perfusion pressure; sometimes it may be necessary to administer vasopressors or inotropes. The target of appropriate arterial pressure should always be achieved (Box 20-20).

Anesthetic agent choice should be based on the effects on cerebral physiology. Intravenous anesthetic agents cause parallel alterations in cerebral metabolic rate and cerebral blood flow reducing both. Ketamine is the exception increasing both cerebral metabolism and

---

Box 20-20 Targets of Anesthesia for the Head-Injured Patient

- Avoidance of hypoxia
- Maintenance of cerebral perfusion pressure
- Control of intracranial hypertension

These targets require:
- Appropriate FIO_2
- PEEP up to 10 cmH_2O
- Maintenance of systemic arterial pressure to the preinjury level

cerebral blood flow. Probably intravenous anesthetic agents preserve the coupling between cerebral metabolic rate and cerebral blood flow. The cerebral metabolic rate/cerebral blood flow ratio is different using different intravenous agents so these drugs may have direct effects on cerebral vessels. Propofol preserves autoregulation and CO_2 responsiveness. Opioids have relatively little effect on cerebral blood flow and cerebral metabolism causing modest reductions of both. Inhaled anesthetics increase cerebral blood flow/cerebral metabolic rate ratio reducing cerebral metabolism more than cerebral blood flow. This may result in increased intracranial pressure. Halothane has more vasodilating potency than isoflurane and sevoflurane and can produce reversible toxicity when administered in very high concentrations interfering with oxidative phosphorylation in the brain. Halothane should be avoided in anesthesia for TBI because other inhaled anesthetics show a better profile. Enflurane is potentially epileptogenic and should also be avoided. Isoflurane and sevoflurane can be safely used. They may increase cerebral blood flow in relation to cerebral metabolism, but a moderate hypocapnia prevents or even reverses this alteration in cerebral blood flow resulting in an unchanged intracranial pressure. Nitrous oxide increases cerebral blood flow, cerebral metabolic rate, and intracranial pressure, and so it should be avoided. Nitrous oxide effects on cerebral physiology are blunted by intravenous agents such as opioids and benzodiazepines. The most popular anesthetic technique for anesthesia in the head-injured patient is probably a balanced technique using opioids and newer inhaled anesthetics (sevoflurane, isoflurane) or intravenous agents (propofol). Sometimes the head-injured patient is placed in the sitting position for surgery. In these cases attention to the cardiovascular effects of this position and careful survey for early detection of venous air embolism are mandatory. Nitrous oxide is deleterious in case of venous air embolism (Box 20-21).

Box 20-21 Anesthetic Agents for the Head-Injured Patient

Among anesthetic agents:
- Ketamine increases intracranial pressure
- Propofol preserves autoregulation and CO_2 responsiveness
- Opioids have little effect on intracranial pressure
- Inhaled anesthetics increase cerebral blood flow/cerebral metabolic rate ratio
- Halothane and enflurane should be avoided
- Nitrous oxide should be avoided when intracranial hypertension is a concern

---

INTENSIVE CARE UNIT CARE

The intensive care for TBI still presents controversies deriving from the progressive change in the pathophysiology of brain injury over the time following trauma. Controversies about the targets of intensive care in brain injury still exist. These targets may be cerebral oxygenation, intracranial pressure, cerebral perfusion pressure, or transcapillary filtration factors. It is possible that intensive care for TBI should have different targets at different points of development of its pathophysiology. If this is the case neuromonitoring methods are the way to direct therapy against the pathophysiologic target of choice. The use of neuromonitoring should be encouraged whenever doubts exist about intracranial pressure, cerebral blood flow, and cerebral oxygenation (Box 20-22).

Neuromonitoring

Following TBI the most accurate monitor of brain function is a complete neurologic clinical examination performed in the absence of the effects of sedatives or muscle relaxants. This is not always possible. In any case the ICU care of TBI should include the regular assessment of GCS and pupillary and motor responses. This clinical assessment should occur every hour initially. When the patient becomes more stable a less frequent assessment may be sufficient. A deterioration in clinical assessment requires prompt CT scan. Besides this clinical evaluation, there are a lot of neuromonitoring tools that provide information about intracranial pressure, intracranial pressure/volume relationship, cerebral perfusion, and cerebral function.

Intracranial Pressure Monitoring
TBI is often associated with intracranial hypertension that reduces cerebral perfusion pressure and cerebral blood flow resulting in cerebral ischemia. Hence intracranial pressure monitoring is very important. According to the Brain Trauma Foundation guidelines, intracranial pressure should be monitored in severe brain injury associated with an abnormal CT scan (diffuse

---

Box 20-22 Targets of Intensive Care Unit Care for Traumatic Brain Injury

- Cerebral oxygenation
- Cerebral perfusion pressure
- Intracranial pressure
- Transcapillary filtration factors

injury II–IV or high–mixed density lesions larger than 25 mm), with age greater than 40 years, with unilateral or bilateral motor posturing, or with extracranial trauma with hypotension. Intracranial pressure may be monitored using fluid-coupled intraventricular catheters, fluid-coupled surface devices, or solid-state devices. Intraventricular catheterization with fluid-couple catheters allows the most accurate measures of intracranial pressure and can also be used therapeutically to drain cerebrospinal fluid in the case of intracranial hypertension. They require to be zeroed at a reference point represented by the external auditory meatus or the Lundberg point (1.5 cm below the uppermost part of the head). Air, blood, and debris can interfere with fluid-coupled catheter function. Fluid-coupled surface devices measure intracranial pressure at the surface of the hemisphere. Pressure gradients between intracranial compartments result in inaccurate monitoring of intracranial pressure and should be considered if the patient's clinical condition does not agree with intracranial pressure measurements. Blood, debris, and brain swelling may also interfere with fluid-coupled surface devices. Solid-state devices include fiber optic and strain-gauge-tipped catheters. They are devoid of fluid coupling for pressure transduction, resulting in fewer artifacts. The transducer is not zeroed once it has been inserted, but a baseline drift requiring transducer replacement occurs after a few days (Box 20-23).

Complications of intracranial pressure monitoring include infection, parenchymal hemorrhage, and subdural hemorrhage subsequent to catheter placement (Box 20-24). Infections such as meningitis are more frequent with the irrigation of the catheter or the drainage system and with prolonged catheter insertion (>5 days). Solid-state devices seem to be associated with fewer complications. Coagulopathy is the main contraindication to intracranial pressure monitoring because of the risk of parenchymal and subdural hemorrhage.

Box 20-23   Indications for Intracranial Pressure Monitoring

Indications for intracranial pressure monitoring include severe TBI associated with:
- Diffuse injury II–IV on CT scan
- High–mixed density lesions larger than 25 mm on CT scan
- Age greater than 40 years
- Unilateral or bilateral motor posturing
- Extracranial trauma with hypotension

Methods for intracranial pressure monitoring:
- Fluid-coupled intraventricular catheters
- Fluid-coupled surface devices
- Solid-state devices

Box 20-24   Complications of Intracranial Pressure Monitoring

- Infection
- Parenchymal hemorrhage
- Subdural hemorrhage

Intracranial pressure monitoring allows the calculation of cerebral perfusion pressure resulting from mean arterial blood pressure minus intracranial pressure. For this calculation both pressures should be referenced to the external auditory meatus. Usually intracranial pressure monitoring is stopped when cerebral edema is resolved on CT scan or when intracranial pressure stability below 25 cmH_2O occurs. Intracranial pressure monitoring for periods longer than 7 days is often associated with baseline drift (solid-state devices), infection (intraventricular fluid-coupled devices), or occlusion (fluid-coupled surface devices). Intracranial pressure monitoring may provide information about brain elastance if the relationship between intracranial volume and intracranial pressure is explored. Pressure–volume index is the response in intracranial pressure following the injection of fluid into an intraventricular catheter over 1 second. If intracranial pressure increases more than 3 mmHg for each milliliter of fluid injected intracranial elastance is considered reduced and surgical decompression should be considered.

Cerebral Blood Flow Monitoring

Methods to monitor directly cerebral blood flow are lacking. Laser Doppler flowmetry, thermal diffusion flow measurement, and the use of labeled xenon to estimate cerebral blood flow under CT are methods resulting in an intermittent evaluation of cerebral blood flow. An indirect evaluation is more practical and actually is a useful parameter to guide therapy in association with intracranial pressure monitoring and CT scanning.

Jugular Oxygen Saturation Monitoring

Cerebral blood flow may be indirectly assessed by monitoring oxygen saturation in the jugular bulb. The brain should have homogeneity in perfusion and metabolism for the jugular oxygen saturation to monitor usefully the relationship between cerebral oxygen delivery and cerebral oxygen demand. Unfortunately TBI is associated with heterogeneity in perfusion and metabolism and in this case jugular oxygen saturation will represent the global average between the lower oxygen saturations derived from areas where oxygen metabolism outstrips oxygen demand and the higher oxygen saturations derived from areas with poor metabolism but high perfusion. Jugular oxygen saturation monitoring requires barbiturate coma should be reserved for intracranial hypertension refractory to all the previous treatments in patients hemodynamically stable. Body position is a determinant of intracranial pressure: a 30-45° elevation with the head kept in the neutral position improves venous flow and intracranial pressure control.

CLINICAL CAVEAT

A stair-step approach for the treatment of intracranial hypertension:

- Appropriate body position with 30-45° head elevation with the head in the neutral position
- Sedation and analgesia
- Neuromuscular block in patients competing with mechanical ventilation
- Cerebrospinal fluid drainage
- Osmotic agents
- Barbiturate coma

Sedation, Analgesia, and Neuromuscular Block

In TBI sedation and analgesia should be titrated according to hemodynamic stability, intracranial pressure, and the trauma-related disorder of consciousness. A general rule is to maintain a level of sedation deep enough to facilitate mechanical ventilation and light enough to allow frequent clinical neurologic evaluations. During the initial hypoperfusion phase sedation should be carefully titrated in order to avoid systemic arterial hypotension. For this purpose short-acting opioids are useful because they ensure cardiovascular stability and blunt sympathetic discharge. However pupillary examination should be performed before opioids are administered. Prolonged administrations of benzodiazepines may delay the return of consciousness because these drugs tend to accumulate. Benzodiazepines may also cause an emergence delirium state. Among opioids, sufentanyl and especially remifentanyl should probably be preferred for prolonged administrations because they have a good profile of the context-sensitive half-life curve. Propofol has attractive properties for sedation in TBI. Even used as the sole sedating agent, it ensures deep levels of sedation resulting in the control of intracranial hypertension and sympathetic discharges. Propofol has a short context-sensitive half-life. This property allows frequent clinical neurologic evaluations that are so important to monitor neurologic function in TBI. Propofol has the advantage that it does not interfere with pupillary responses and the disadvantage that it has a higher cardiovascular impact because of its negative inotrope effect. Therefore, even if propofol remains an option in hemodynamically unstable patients, it requires careful titration in these cases. Vasopressors or inotropes may be necessary to maintain an appropriate systemic arterial pressure, which is a primary target in TBI.

Ventricular Drainage

Intracranial hypertension may be treated by draining cerebrospinal fluid through a fluid-coupled intraventricular catheter placed for intracranial pressure monitoring. The catheter may be placed 5-10 cm above the head and opened every 2-4 hours. Although ventricular drainage may increase transcapillary filtration of fluid, this method is effective in the treatment of intracranial pressure and should be used if appropriate sedation and analgesia, eventually associated with muscle relaxation, fail to reduce intracranial hypertension.

Osmotic Diuresis: Mannitol

If appropriate sedation and analgesia associated with intermittent ventricular drainage fail to control intracranial hypertension, osmotic diuresis using mannitol can be used. Mannitol (0.25-1 g/kg) is an osmotically active agent administered to increase plasma osmolality causing an efflux of fluid from edematous areas of the brain that results in the reduction of intracranial pressure (if the blood-brain barrier is intact enough to be still impermeable to mannitol). Mannitol also causes a plasma expanding effect that increases cerebral blood flow. This may contribute to the reduction of intracranial pressure. Mannitol increases diuresis with an osmotic mechanism. Hypertonic saline (3%) increases plasma osmolality and expands plasma volume restoring systemic and cerebral perfusion. Hypertonic saline has fewer side effects than mannitol, and it does not induce any osmolal gap so it allows an easier titration. Hypertonic saline is particularly beneficial in the early hypoperfusion phase because it improves cerebral blood flow. However, mannitol and hypertonic saline should be used in patients with unequivocal intracranial hypertension unresponsive to appropriate sedation and ventricular drainage. Hemodynamic instability and hypovolemia contraindicate osmotic diuresis as does a serum osmolality greater than 320 mosm/l.

Hyperventilation

Hyperventilation decreases intracranial pressure because a reduction in $PaCO_2$ determines cerebral alkalosis that results in cerebral vasoconstriction with a decrease in cerebral blood flow and cerebral blood volume. The effect of hyperventilation on cerebral blood flow is transient because readjustment of brain pH occurs within 6-24 hours and thereafter the normalization of retrograde placement of a fiber optic catheter into the jugular bulb that should be confirmed by radiologic imaging. If cerebral metabolic rate remains stable, an increase in cerebral blood flow results in an increased jugular oxygen saturation. If jugular oxygen saturation decreases below 55%, cerebral hypoperfusion is under way because of intracranial hypertension, hypocapnia, or systemic hypoperfusion. Decreased jugular oxygen saturation may occur independently of increases in intracranial pressure. Cerebral hyperemia or depressed neuronal metabolism may cause a jugular oxygen saturation higher than 85%. Both jugular oxygen saturations above 85% and below 55% are associated with poor outcome. Jugular oxygen saturation monitoring is useful if hemodynamic instability poses the patient at risk of cerebral hypoperfusion. In this case vasopressor infusion may be titrated with a target jugular oxygen saturation above 55%. Jugular oxygen saturation monitoring should be considered also to titrate other therapeutic strategies such as hyperventilation, hypothermia, and barbiturate coma, always aiming to a jugular oxygen saturation of between 55% and 85%.

Tissue Oxygen Monitoring

Tissue oxymetry probes allow one to monitor directly brain tissue oxygen content. The insertion technique for tissue oximetry probes is similar to that for intra-parenchymal pressure monitoring. These probes measure brain tissue oxygen content in a small volume of tissue. These results may be extrapolated to apply at least regionally. Tissue oximetry probes provide continuous, real-time measurements of brain tissue oxygen saturation. These data are very useful to titrate cerebral perfusion pressure manipulation, hyperventilation, and intracranial hypertension management.

Transcranial Doppler

Blood flow through large cerebral vessels may be evaluated with transcranial Doppler ultrasonography. This is a noninvasive method that provides an intermittent evaluation. The transtemporal area is a natural acoustic window that allows the pulsed Doppler probe to assess the anterior, middle, and posterior cerebral arteries and anterior and posterior communicating arteries. Systolic, mean, and diastolic flow velocities are usually considered indices of flow. Hyperemic, normal, vasospastic, and absent flow may be differentiated using derived indices such as the Gosling pulsatility index and the Lindegaard ratio. Transcranial Doppler should be used in association with other techniques because it provides intermittent measures.

Near Infrared Spectroscopy

Near infrared spectroscopy monitors regional oxygen saturation in the brain. A scalp sensor emits light of wavelengths in the rang... the light reflected to t... venous, and capillary l... average oxygen saturatio... hemoglobin is evaluated l... and should be around 7... interfere with near infrared... a noninvasive monitor of... jugular oxygen saturation... monitor of cerebral blood flo...

Electrophysiologic Monito...

Electrophysiologic monitori... toring methods such as elect... active monitoring methods s... evoked potentials. In ICUs monit... interfere with electroencephalog... to titrate barbiturate therapy and... may contribute to brain injury. Bisp... recommended for barbiturate thera... its role in TBI is the object of stu... evoked potentials assess sensorial a... and may provide diagnostic and prog... Initial bilaterally absent cortical som... potentials indicate high probability... normal evoked potentials predict... Electrophysiologic recovery often p... recovery.

Temperature Monitoring

TBI may be associated with hyperther... to the damage of thermoregulatory cente... the brain are worsened by hyperthermi... cause of secondary damage in TBI. Core... monitoring may underestimate brain tem... 1–2°C, but it is a useful method for temper... toring. Every effort should be made to ma... temperature below 37.5°C.

TREATMENT OF INTRACRANIAL HYPERTENSION

TBI has been traditionally treated with early s... treatment of intracranial mass lesions and careful... care treatment to avoid secondary damage and min... intracranial hypertension. When intracranial press... monitored a stair-step approach is used to treat intr... nial hypertension. Methods to reduce intracranial p... sure are added considering the complications associa... with each therapy. Usually the first step is sedation, an... gesia, and neuromuscular block; then cerebrospinal flu... drainage may be added if intracranial hypertension... poorly controlled. If these treatments still fail to contro... intracranial hypertension, osmotic agents may be added,

$PaCO_2$ can dramatically increase intracranial pressure. Thus it does not make sense to use prophylactic hyperventilation resulting in a $PaCO_2$ below 35 mmHg, especially in the first 24 hours after brain injury, when cerebral blood flow is already reduced as much as 50% (hypoperfusion phase). Prolonged hyperventilation therapy resulting in a $PaCO_2$ below 25 mmHg should be avoided in the absence of elevated intracranial pressure. Although hyperventilation still has a role in the treatment of intracranial hypertension unresponsive to conventional intracranial pressure-lowering therapies, its use requires an appropriate cerebral oxygenation monitor such as jugular oxygen saturation monitoring or tissue oxygen monitoring because hyperventilation may precipitate cerebral ischemia. Ischemia related to hyperventilation may aggravate the pre-existing brain injury. Cerebral vasoreactivity after TBI increases over time. In particular cerebral vessels show a decreased responsiveness the first day after injury, and a progressive increase in $PaCO_2$ reactivity between the second and the fifth day after injury. Intracranial hypertension is often difficult to treat just three to five days after injury. Therefore hyperventilation therapy is likely to be performed just when cerebral vessels are more sensitive to hypocapnia and the brain is more susceptible to the hyperventilation-related ischemia. When jugular oxygen saturation demonstrates that cerebral oxygen delivery significantly outstrips cerebral oxygen demand, hyperventilation may be beneficial in decreasing cerebral blood volume and intracranial pressure without inducing ischemia.

Cerebral Perfusion Pressure Manipulation (Vasoconstriction and Vasodilatation Cascades)

In the early hypoperfusion phase of TBI the maintenance of a high cerebral perfusion pressure could trigger a vasoconstriction cascade leading to a reduction in intracranial hypertension. The target for cerebral perfusion pressure should be 60 mmHg, although sometimes cerebral perfusion pressure should be higher than 70–80 mmHg to remain in the autoregulatory range. If cerebral perfusion pressure management may be useful to treat intracranial hypertension in the early hypoperfusion phase, it could be less effective or even deleterious in the late hyperaemic phase.

High-Dose Barbiturate Therapy

In intracranial hypertension unresponsive to traditional therapies high-dose barbiturate may be useful. Barbiturates at high doses reduce cerebral metabolic rate and intracranial pressure. Barbiturate dose should be titrated using electroencephalography. The target should be burst suppression. At the high doses used for intracranial hypertension treatment barbiturates may cause reductions in systemic arterial blood pressure and cerebral blood flow. This could be deleterious in the hypoperfusion phase of TBI when cerebral blood flow is already reduced. In this case the use of vasopressors should be considered. The use of barbiturates impairs a frequent clinical neurologic evaluation and delays awakening of patients.

Hypothermia

In TBI the lesions to the brain are temperature dependent. Fever may worsen TBI, and an aggressive treatment of fever is mandatory. Hypothermia reduces cerebral metabolism and may have a beneficial effect on intracranial hypertension. In several experiments hypothermia resulted in a decreased intracranial hypertension when used immediately after brain injury. Some clinical trials failed to demonstrate an improvement in outcome with the use of hypothermia in TBI. Hypothermia to temperatures of 30–33°C prolongs ventilation and increases the risk of nosocomial infections. These side effects could lead to increased morbidity and mortality in TBI, even though hypothermia shows beneficial effects on cerebral metabolic rate and intracranial hypertension.

Steroids

Glucocorticoids may reduce intracranial inflammation. Inflammatory mechanisms underlie blood–brain barrier alterations resulting in vasogenic cerebral edema and may be involved in excitotoxicity that may contribute to cytotoxic edema. Although steroids at high doses for 24 hours are useful in the treatment of acute spinal cord injury if treatment is initiated within eight hours, they have shown no beneficial effect in the outcome of TBI. Moreover, steroids increase the risk of infection.

Cranial Decompression

When intracranial hypertension is unresponsive to all therapies wide bilateral frontoparietal craniectomies may result in a dramatic reduction of intracranial hypertension. Preemptive decompressive craniectomy may have a role in high-risk patients.

Current Controversies

There are still several controversies regarding the treatment of TBI. In this setting the strategies proposed are essentially three: intracranial pressure-directed therapy, cerebral perfusion pressure-directed therapy, and the Lund approach.

CURRENT CONTROVERSY

Controversy in the treatment of TBI includes:
- Intracranial pressure-directed therapy
- Cerebral perfusion pressure-directed therapy
- The Lund approach

Intracranial pressure-directed therapy includes intracranial pressure monitoring and a stair-step approach to treat intracranial hypertension.

Cerebral perfusion pressure-directed therapy aims at an appropriately high mean arterial pressure to trigger the vasoconstriction cascade.

The goals of the Lund approach are to preserve a normal colloid osmotic pressure in cerebral vessels with infusion of albumin and erythrocytes, to reduce cerebral capillary hydrostatic pressures by reducing arterial blood pressure, and to reduce cerebral blood volume by vasoconstriction of precapillary resistance vessels achieved with low-dose thiopental or dihydroergotamine (Box 20-25). The Lund approach discourages treatments that could result in an increased transcapillary filtration of fluids including cerebrospinal fluid drainage, high-dose barbiturates, osmotic diuresis, and high cerebral perfusion pressures.

GENERAL CARE

General intensive care is fundamental in TBI. It includes electrolytes and fluid management, nutritional support, prevention and treatment of post-traumatic seizures, prevention and treatment of deep venous thrombosis and pulmonary embolism, and prevention and treatment of gastrointestinal bleeding (Box 20-26).

Electrolytes and Fluid Management

Primary targets of electrolytes and fluid management in TBI are the maintenance of euvolemia and of a relatively high serum osmolality (Box 20-27).

Box 20-25   Goals of the Lund Approach

- To preserve a normal osmotic pressure in cerebral vessels using infusions of albumin and erythrocytes
- To reduce cerebral capillary hydrostatic pressures reducing arterial blood pressure
- To reduce cerebral blood volume by vasoconstriction of precapillary vessels achieved with low-dose thiopental or dihydroergotamine

Box 20-26   General Care of TBI

General care of TBI includes:
- Electrolytes and fluid management
- Nutritional support
- Prevention and treatment of post-traumatic seizures
- Prevention and treatment of infectious complications
- Prevention and treatment of deep venous thrombosis and pulmonary embolism
- Prevention and treatment of gastrointestinal bleeding

Since hypervolemia may be implicated in increases in cerebral edema and hypovolemia may reduce cerebral blood flow, euvolemia should be maintained to allow an appropriate cerebral blood flow without increasing cerebral edema. The volume of fluids administered should be titrated considering pulse rate, mean arterial pressure, central venous pressure, and urine output. A hematocrit of 30% offers the best rheology to cerebral circulation; therefore red cell transfusions should be used in case of active bleeding to keep a hemoglobin concentration around 10 g/dl. Regarding the quality of fluids administered in TBI, no evidence supports the use of either colloids or crystalloids. The osmotic gradient between blood and brain regulates water flux across the blood–brain barrier. Serum osmolality is the major determinant of fluid flux across the normal blood–brain barrier. However, TBI is associated with alterations of the blood–brain barrier. If it becomes permeable to ions but not to larger colloid particles, the choice between colloids and crystalloids could be important. If the blood–brain barrier is disrupted, however, permeability to both ions and colloidal particles may occur and fluid selection is inconsequential. Serum osmolarity has an established importance in the development of cerebral edema and should be kept at the higher values of normality. In this regard the use of hypo-osmolar solutions such as 5% dextrose in water is discouraged and may be required only if patients become hyperosmolar (>320 mosm/l). Normal saline has an osmolarity slightly higher than plasma and is the preferred fluid in TBI. When using normal saline for fluid management, also other ions such as potassium, magnesium, and calcium should be administered to maintain normal electrolyte homeostasis.

Box 20-27   Targets of Electrolyte and Fluid Management in Traumatic Brain Injury

- Euvolemia
- Relatively high serum osmolality

CLINICAL CAVEAT

What Fluid in Traumatic Brain Injury?

- Normal saline has an osmolarity slightly higher than plasma and is the preferred fluid in TBI
- Other ions such as potassium, magnesium, and calcium should be administered to maintain normal electrolyte homeostasis
- 5% dextrose in water is discouraged and may be required only if patients become hyperosmolar (>320 mosm/l)

Fluid management may be particularly challenging in head-injured patients because TBI is often associated with the syndrome of inappropriate antidiuretic hormone secretion and with diabetes insipidus. Sometimes even when fluid management has achieved euvolemia, cerebral perfusion pressure is still inadequate. Particularly if these cases occur in the early hypoperfusion phase of TBI, vasopressors and inotropes should be used because cerebral perfusion pressure is the major determinant of cerebral blood flow and is the priority when cerebral hypoperfusion is underway.

CLINICAL CAVEAT

TBI is often associated with:

- Syndrome of inappropriate antidiuretic hormone secretion (SIADH)
- Diabetes insipidus

Nutritional Support

In TBI early enteral nutrition should be performed to meet the caloric needs of head-injured patients. Nutritional support should provide calories corresponding to 140% of the resting energy expenditure in nonparalyzed patients and 100% of the resting energy expenditure in paralyzed patients. At least 15% of calories should derive from proteins. Orogastric or oroenteral tubes are inserted in TBI because of the possible fracture of the cribriform plate. In any case once cribriform plate fracture has been excluded, nasopostpyloric tubes are used because TBI may be associated with gastroparesis. Hyperglycemia may complicate nutritional support. Glycemia should be strictly maintained in the normal range because either hyperglycemia or hypoglycemia may induce secondary damage to the brain. Insulin is very useful in the case of hyperglycemia.

Prevention and Treatment of Post-traumatic Seizures

Short-term prophylactic use of anticonvulsants does not prevent late post-traumatic seizures. TBI is rarely associated with seizures that usually are present at the time of injury. When seizures occur, benzodiazepines and other anticonvulsants are used. Prophylaxis with phenytoin may be useful only in patients with significant parenchymal lesions evident on CT scan and should be prolonged for ten days after injury.

Prevention and Treatment of Infectious Complications

TBI patients who receive prolonged mechanical ventilation show an increased risk of nosocomial pneumonia that is associated with an increased mortality. Stress ulcer prophylaxis, hypothermia, and barbiturates increase the risk further. Penetrating injuries and intracranial pressure monitoring, especially using fluid-coupled devices, increase the risk of meningitides and other neurologic infections. The risk is low if intracranial pressure monitoring lasts less than 5–7 days. The frequent use of intravascular catheters for arterial pressure monitoring, central venous pressure monitoring, jugular oxygen saturation monitoring, and fluid and drug infusions increases the risk of bloodstream infections. The frequent use of bladder catheters put the head-injured patient at risk of urinary tract infection. The use of antibiotics should follow the accepted microbiological principles. Cultures of cerebrospinal fluid, blood, fluid from BAL, and urine should guide antibiotic therapy.

Prevention and Treatment of Deep Venous Thrombosis and Pulmonary Embolism

Brain-injured patients who require prolonged immobility are at increased risk of thromboembolism. Prevention of deep venous thrombosis and pulmonary embolism is particularly challenging in TBI patients because anticoagulants such as fractionated and low molecular weight heparins are contraindicated because of intracranial hemorrhage. Until CT scan demonstrates resolution of intracranial hemorrhages and significant brain lesions anticoagulants should be avoided. Therefore prevention of deep venous thrombosis and pulmonary embolism in TBI patients is entrusted to nonpharmacologic methods such as elastic stockings, pneumatic calf compressors, and physiotherapy. If pelvic fractures increase the patient's risk of deep venous thrombosis, frequent Doppler ultrasound of the iliofemoral veins is recommended. If brain-injured patients develop a deep vein thrombosis and anticoagulants are contraindicated by an intracranial hemorrhage, inferior vena caval filters are useful to prevent pulmonary embolism. If pulmonary embolism occurs in TBI patients the use of anticoagulants should be considered if there is a real risk of death.

<table>
<tr><td colspan="1">Box 20-28　Extended Glasgow Outcome Scale</td></tr>
</table>

Score 6: Death
Score 7: Persistent vegetative state
Score 8: Severe disability
Score 9: Moderate disability
Score 10: Good recovery

Prevention and Treatment of Gastrointestinal Bleeding

An appropriate resuscitation and an early enteral feeding are the best methods for gastrointestinal bleeding prevention. Sucralphate, H_2 antagonists, and proton pump inhibitors are useful to prevent gastrointestinal bleeding and are usually administered during the whole ICU stay, although they may be avoided once enteral feeding starts at least in patients without a previous history of peptic ulceration.

OUTCOME

Outcome from TBI is influenced by the severity of primary and secondary damages. Patient-related factors such as age, comorbidities, and sex also influence outcome. In particular, age greater than 60 years worsens outcome. Time may result in significant neurological improvements and outcome is difficult to predict. The extended Glasgow Outcome Scale is a very useful tool to quantify objectively functional outcome after TBI and should be used 6 and 12 months after injury (Box 20-28).

SELECTED READING

Bath PMW: Optimising homeostasis. Br Med Bull 56:422-435, 2000.

Brain Trauma Foundation, American Association of Neurological Surgeons, Joint Section on Neurotrauma and Critical Care: Guidelines for the management of severe head injury. J Neurotrauma 13:641-734, 1996.

Brain Trauma Foundation, American Association of Neurological Surgeons, Joint Section on Neurotrauma and Critical Care: Hyperventilation. J Neurotrauma 17:513-520, 2000.

Brain Trauma Foundation, American Association of Neurological Surgeons, Joint Section on Neurotrauma and Critical Care: Hypotension. J Neurotrauma 17:591-595, 2000.

Brain Trauma Foundation, American Association of Neurological Surgeons, Joint Section on Neurotrauma and Critical Care: Initial management. J Neurotrauma 17:463-470, 2000.

Bruns J Jr, Hauser WA: The epidemiology of traumatic brain injury: a review. Epilepsia 44(Suppl 10):2-10, 2003.

Chesnut MR: Hyperventilation versus cerebral perfusion pressure management time to change the question. Crit Care Med 26:210-212, 1998.

Chesnut RM: Avoidance of hypotension: condition sine qua non of successful severe head-injury management. J Trauma 42:S4-S9, 1997.

Chesnut RM, Marshall LF, Klauber MR et al: The role of secondary brain injury in determining outcome from severe head injury. J Trauma 34:216-222, 1993.

Cruz J: The first decade of continuous monitoring of jugular bulb oxyhemoglobin saturation: management strategies and clinical outcome. Crit Care Med 26:344-351, 1998.

Eker C, Asgeirsson B, Grande PO et al: Improved outcome after severe head injury with a new therapy based on principles for brain volume regulation and preserved microcirculation. Crit Care Med 26:1881-1886, 1998.

Ingerbrigtsen T, Rommer B, Kock-Jensen C: Scandinavian guidelines for initial management of minimal, mild, and moderate head injuries. J Trauma 48:760-766, 2000.

Kiening KL, Hartl R, Uterberg AW, Schneider GH et al: Brain tissue pO_2 monitoring in comatose patients: implications for therapy. Neurol Res 19:233-240, 1997.

Marshall LF, Bowers-Marshall S, Klauber MR et al: A new classification of head injury based on computerized tomography. J Neurosurg 75:S14-S20, 1991.

Martin NA, Patwardhan RV, Alexander MJ et al: Characterization of cerebral haemodynamic phases following severe head trauma: hypoperfusion, hyperemia and vasospasm. J Neurosurg 87:9-19, 1997.

McKeating EG, Andrews PJ: Cytokines and adhesion molecules in acute brain injury. Br J Anaesth 80:77-84, 1998.

Qureshi AI, Suarez JI: Use of hypertonic saline solutions in treatment of cerebral edema and intracranial hypertension. Crit Care Med 28:3301-3313, 2000.

Robertson CS, Valadka AB, Hannay HJ et al: Prevention of secondary insults after severe head injury. Crit Care Med 27:2086-2095, 1999.

Robertson CS: Management of cerebral perfusion pressure after traumatic brain injury. Anesthesiology 95:1513-1517, 2001.

Rosner MJ, Rosner SD, Johnson AH: Cerebral perfusion pressure: management protocol and clinical results. J Neurosurg 83:949-962, 1995.

Stein SC, Spettel C: The Head Injury Severity Scale (HISS): a practical classification of closed-head injury. Brain Inj 9:437-444, 1995.

Strebel S, Lam AM, Matta BF, Newell DW: Impaired cerebral autoregulation after mild brain injury. Surg Neurol 47:128-131, 1997.

Struchen MA, Hannay HJ, Contant CF, Robertson CS: The relation between acute physiological variables and outcome on the GOS and DRS following severe traumatic brain injury. J Neurotrauma 18:115-125, 2001.

Thees C, Scholz M, Schaller C et al: Relationship between intracranial pressure and critical closing pressure in patients with neurotrauma. Anesthesiology 96:595-599, 2002.

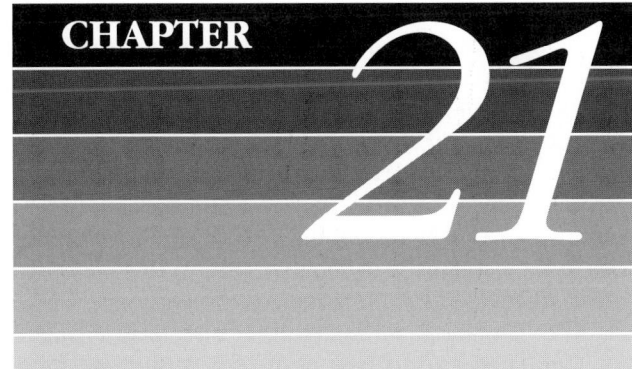

CHAPTER 21

Neurologic Monitoring

JOSEPH DOOLEY, M.D.

Neurologic Examination
Intracranial Pressure
Electroencephalogram and Bispectral Analysis
Conclusion

Assessing a patient's neurologic status is an important component of critical care. Clearly patients with brain or spinal cord pathology require their neurologic status to be monitored in order to determine the progression of the pathologic process. Decisions about further evaluation and treatment are dependent upon this assessment. Critically ill patients with a variety of problems are prone to neurologic abnormalities. These include ischemic and hemorrhagic strokes, traumatic brain and spinal cord injuries, central nervous system (CNS) tumors, neuropathies, and CNS infections. This chapter focuses on the methods to assess a patient's neurologic status in the intensive care unit (ICU). The neurologic examination is the mainstay of neurologic monitoring. Intracranial pressure monitoring is the next most common tool for following a patient's status. The electroencephalogram (EEG) is used for patients with suspected seizures and to assess cortical function. In addition, many institutions are using the Bispectral Index Scale (BIS) monitor to assess patients' level of sedation in the operating room. The use of the BIS to monitor progression of neurologic disease in the ICU is less clear.

NEUROLOGIC EXAMINATION

The neurologic examination is an important component in the daily assessment of the critically ill patient. Many patients are sedated and some are chemically paralyzed. This should be noted in the patient's evaluation. Ideally, the patient's sedation should be titrated, so that they are comfortable but easily arousable and as interactive as possible.

The neurologic examination has several components. These include the mental status examination, cranial nerve examination, motor examination, sensory examination, cerebellar examination, and assessing reflexes. The examination of the critically ill patient is less detailed than a neurologist's formal examination but should be detailed enough to diagnose significant abnormalities and assess changes in the patient's neurologic status. The mental status examination includes orientation (to person, place, and time), speech, ability to follow commands, and the ability to interact appropriately. Purposeful movement indicates the presence of some cortical function. Examination of the cranial nerves includes pupil examination (size and reactivity), presence or absence of conjugate gaze, facial symmetry, and gag reflex. These tests evaluate CN II, III, IV, VI, VII, IX, and X, and thus a significant portion of the brainstem. On motor examination, symmetry of extremity movement and, if possible, individual muscle group strength should be assessed. The sensory examination should include response to stimuli at each extremity. The cerebellar examination would mainly be significant for patients with cerebellar lesions and includes evaluation for ataxia (finger to nose test and heel-shin test). The gait examination is rarely practical in the ICU. Deep tendon reflexes should be assessed in patients with suspected spinal cord lesions. The examination described can be accomplished rapidly and provide quick assessment of the patient's neurologic status.

A neurologic scoring system often used for trauma patients in the ICU is the Glasgow Coma Scale (GCS). Patients are assigned a score, based on three components. The responses assessed are verbal response, eye opening, and motor response. The responses are scored as follows:

Verbal response. Oriented speech (5), confused conversation (4), inappropriate speech (3), incomprehensible speech (2), and no speech (1).

Eye opening. Spontaneous (4), response to verbal stimuli (3), response to noxious stimuli (2), and no eye opening (1).

Motor response. Follows commands (6), localizes to noxious stimuli (5), withdraws to noxious stimuli/normal flexion (4), abnormal flexion/decorticate posturing (3), abnormal extension/decerebrate posturing (2), and no movement to noxious stimuli (1).

The GCS is a useful, rapid screen of head injury severity. Mild head injury usually produces a score of 13 to 15, moderate head injury produces a score of 9 to 12, and severe head injury generally carries a score of 8 or less. If the patient is intubated, the score is qualified with an "I."

The GCS is a useful screening tool for the initial assessment but is less reliable for assessing subtle changes in a patient's status while in the ICU. A detailed neurologic examination should be done for the initial presentation followed by more focused examinations concentrating on known deficits for subsequent evaluations.

INTRACRANIAL PRESSURE

Intracranial pressure (ICP) monitors are used primarily for patients with known or suspected intracranial hypertension, and those with head injuries where a neurologic examination is not possible. Patients who cannot be followed with a neurologic examination include those under general anesthesia, or those who are chemically paralyzed or heavily sedated in the ICU. The use of an ICP monitor alerts the clinician to an elevation of ICP, which can then be treated.

An understanding of ICP is important when making decisions about treatment. The intracranial vault can be considered a fixed volume, which is about 1500 ml in the adult. The intracranial vault contains three broad categories of substances. These are the brain and its support structures, cerebrospinal fluid (CSF), and blood. The brain and its supporting structures account for about 85% of the volume. CSF and blood account for 10% and 5%, respectively, of the remainder. If any one of these components is increased, intracranial hypertension can result. Processes that increase the volume of the brain and its support structures include brain edema (cytotoxic edema due to ischemic strokes and vasogenic edema around tumors and abscesses) and the mass of tumors. Elevated volumes of CSF occur in various clinical scenarios and is known as hydrocephalus. Elevated volumes of intracranial blood can occur either extravascularly or intravascularly. Intracranial hemorrhages (such as epidural hematomas, subdural hematomas, and intracerebral hematomas) can lead to critical elevations of ICP.

Etiologies of increased intravascular blood volume include hypercarbia, hypoxia, and volatile anesthetics.

Studies looking at the relationship between intracranial volume and pressure have been performed by gradually increasing the volume of an intracranial balloon in animals. The ICP increases at a relatively slow rate with increased balloon volume. At a certain point (at an ICP of approximately 20 torr) the ICP increases dramatically with small increases in balloon volume. At this point the system changes from a relatively compliant system to a relatively noncompliant system. Because small changes in volume can lead to large increases of ICP and then cerebral herniation at this pressure, an ICP of 20 torr and above is considered to be intracranial hypertension.

Another important physiologic parameter is cerebral perfusion pressure (CPP). This can be calculated by subtracting the ICP from the mean arterial pressure (CPP = MAP – ICP). Most authorities advocate maintaining a CPP of 50 torr or greater. This ensures adequate cerebral blood flow (CBF). Insufficient CBF results in brain ischemia and cerebral injury. Therefore, it is important to know the CPP and ICP in critically ill patients with neurologic injury. The MAP is best measured using an intra-arterial catheter. This allows continuous assessment of the MAP, which is not possible with noninvasive blood pressure monitoring. If the patient is felt to have elevated ICP (usually predicted by evaluation of the head computed tomography (CT) scan), an ICP monitor should be placed.

CLINICAL CAVEAT

CPP = MAP – ICP
Maintain ICP < 20 torr, CPP > 50 torr
Intraventricular catheters:
- Most reliable means of measuring ICP
- Allows drainage of CSF in order to lower ICP
- More prone to complications

Intraparenchymal, subdural, and epidural monitors:
- More easily placed
- Less associated complications
- Less reliable ICP measurement

ICP monitors include ventricular catheters connected to an external strain gauge transducer or catheter-tip pressure transducer devices, parenchymal catheter-tip pressure transducer devices, subarachnoid or subdural fluid-coupled devices, and epidural devices. External strain gauge transducers are located at the bedside and are coupled to the patient's intracranial space through fluid-filled lines. The catheter-tip transducers are either strain gauges or fiberoptic technologies and are placed intracranially.

The fluid-filled lines connected to the external strain gauges can become obstructed or have an air bubble in the line, which can lead to inaccurate pressures. The external devices can be recalibrated after insertion. The transducer has to be positioned at the level of the patient's head and therefore has to be moved if the height of the patient's bed is moved. Intracranial transducers are calibrated prior to insertion and cannot be recalibrated once in place. Therefore, there is the potential for measurement drift. The intracranial transducer devices give ICP measurements that are independent of head elevation.

The ICP monitors can be placed in the epidural space, subdural space, subarachnoid space, brain parenchyma, or intraventricular space. Intraventricular catheters have been used as the reference standard for ICP measurement. Intraventricular catheters can be used to treat intracranial hypertension by draining CSF. The intraventricular catheters are usually connected to an external strain gauge transducer, but some incorporate intracranial, fiberoptic transducers. This allows simultaneous drainage and ICP measurement. When using the external transducer, ICP measurements cannot be obtained while CSF is drained. There is potential for significant complications when using intraventricular catheters. These devices are usually placed through the nondominant hemisphere away from the motor strip and the sagittal sinus. The catheter has to travel through a significant amount of brain parenchyma to reach the lateral ventricle. There is the potential for bleeding, CNS injury, infection, catheter misplacement, and obstruction.

The other devices (parenchymal, subarachnoid, subdural, and epidural catheters) are less likely to cause a complication. The parenchymal catheters are placed a short distance into the parenchyma. These devices cannot be used therapeutically to drain CSF. Many studies support the accuracy of these devices for measuring ICP. However, other studies have shown significant discrepancies when compared to ventricular ICP. The decision as to which device to use is multifactorial. Clearly, if the head CT shows significant fluid in the ventricles, drainage via an intraventricular catheter would be beneficial. Patients who are coagulopathic are at increased risk for developing intracerebral hemorrhage as a complication of intraventricular catheter placement. Patients with fulminant hepatic failure and high-grade encephalopathy have a high mortality often as a result of uncal and tonsillar herniation. A retrospective study by Blei and colleagues showed fewer complications with epidural catheters (3.8%) compared to subdural (20%) and intraparenchymal (22%) catheters. The intraparenchymal catheters included intraventricular catheters. In fact, fatal hemorrhage occurred with 5% of the subdural catheters and 4% of the intraparenchymal catheters.

Fatal hemorrhage occurred in 1% of the patients with epidural catheters.

Occasionally, lumbar subarachnoid catheters (lumbar drains) are used in the ICU. These drains are used for some neurosurgical procedures (primarily cerebrovascular procedures) in order to "decompress" the brain and facilitate the surgical dissection. They are also used for some vascular surgery procedures (such as thoracoabdominal aneurysm resections). In these cases, there is a significant risk of spinal cord ischemia due to resection of anterior spinal arteries (most significantly the artery of Adamkeiwicz). The catheters are used to drain CSF and thus lower the ICP. This optimizes spinal cord perfusion and, theoretically, minimizes the risk of cord ischemia. Postoperatively, ICP is not measured directly, but the catheters are drained at a predetermined level (highest point of catheter) above the supine patient. Generally, the catheter height is placed at approximately 10 cm ($10 cmH_2O/CSF$) above the patient. This will be the ICP as long as the catheter drains freely. It is important not to "overdrain" the catheter by placing it at or below the level of the patient. This could lead to complications. The most severe complication is a subdural hematoma. Typically, the time patients are most at risk for overdraining is during transport. It is suggested that the catheter be clamped during these periods. The ICP will rise only minimally if the catheter is clamped for a short period (i.e., less than 30 minutes).

ICP can be measured using a variety of devices. The intraventricular catheters are probably the most accurate and can be used therapeutically. Unfortunately, these catheters have the highest risk for complications. The decision about which device to use should be made in conjunction with the neurosurgical team and should be based on the patient's comorbidities.

ELECTROENCEPHALOGRAM AND BISPECTRAL ANALYSIS

The EEG is another neurologic monitor of some use in the ICU. A complex discussion of the EEG is well beyond the scope of this chapter. Briefly, neurons generate electric fields when ions move between the intra- and extracellular spaces. Neurotransmitter interactions with postsynaptic receptors affect ion channel permeability of the neuron, which allows movement of the ions. This results in changes in its transmembrane voltage. This is known as the postsynaptic potential (PSP). If the membrane potential of a neuron is depolarized beyond its threshold value, an action potential (AP) is generated which then propagates rapidly along the neuron's membrane. The electric fields generated by the neurons result in electrical potential differences at the skin's surface. Electrodes at the skin's surface act as transducers, which convert the physiologic current at the skin to an electrical current which is then processed by the EEG monitor. This principle applies to the electrocardiogram where the synchronous depolarization of all cells of the atria followed by depolarization and repolarization of all cells of the ventricles produce the classic normal EKG with its P waves, QRS complex, and T waves.

Under normal circumstances the PSPs and APs generated by neurons are not synchronous. The normal EEG signal has no obvious repetitive pattern or any morphology that correlates with underlying neurologic function. Indeed, "spikes" or "sharp waves" due to synchronous neuronal activity is diagnostic of seizure activity. Due to its complexity, interpreting raw EEG data is extremely difficult. Methods to compress and simplify the raw EEG data require complex and intensive mathematical computations. These processed EEGs are used in the operating room to detect cerebral ischemia (e.g., during carotid surgery) and to determine if drug therapy causes burst suppression (e.g., during aneurysm surgery). Examples of processed EEGs include the compressed spectral array (CSA) and the density spectral array (DSA). The primary use of the EEG in the ICU is to make the diagnosis of status epilepticus in the patient suspected of this disorder. Sometimes, the diagnosis is not obvious on observation of the patient. The EEG is also used in the ICU as a confirmatory test when brain death is suspected. Beyond these indications, there is not much use for the EEG in the ICU. Certainly, it is not a very useful monitor for following the patient's neurologic status and correcting abnormalities. In the operating room there has been much work to use the EEG to determine depth of anesthesia. Similarly, in the ICU it would be desirable to have a measure of sedation. Often this is difficult to determine. For example, it is very difficult to assess the adequacy of sedation of patients who are chemically paralyzed or extremely edematous. Often, the patient's eyes are swollen shut. They are weak and unable to move their extremities well. The desire to obtain useful information about anesthetic and sedation depth has led to the development of the bispectral index.

Bispectral analysis represents a different type of mathematical analysis of the raw EEG data from the analysis performed by the processed EEG. The analysis is extremely complex and only became possible with the advent of fast microprocessors. The bispectral index monitor is a device manufactured by Aspect Medical Systems. It uses one- or two-channel EEG signal acquisition. The analysis creates a dimensionless number known as the Bispectral Index Scale (BIS). The number is scaled from 100 to 0 with 100 indicating an awake EEG and 0 representing complete electrical silence. BIS values are then correlated against clinical endpoints to sedation (movement to noxious stimuli, hemodynamic response to stimuli, level of consciousness, etc.). The BIS has been through multiple versions with improved clinical correlation in each. In the operating room the BIS indicates the potential for awareness and hypnotic overdose. It cannot determine exactly when consciousness returns. It does not predict unconsciousness when ketamine or nitrous oxide is used.

It would be desirable to use the BIS to monitor the level of sedation in the ICU. This could ensure patient comfort and prevent oversedation. It is not clear that conclusions about BIS values obtained from healthy patients undergoing anesthesia/sedation would be applicable to critically ill patients in the ICU. Studies to address this issue are problematic, since it is difficult to determine awareness and recall in ICU patients. In addition, the electrical environment of the ICU can interfere with the monitor. Studies in the ICU are ongoing. More studies are needed.

CONCLUSION

Neurologic monitoring is an important part of the care of patients in the ICU. While patients with known CNS pathology clearly require this monitoring, a large number of ICU patients are at risk to develop neurologic injury. The neurologic examination, performed by physicians and nurses, is the main component of this monitoring. When indicated, monitoring ICP directly with either a ventriculostomy or other intracranial device can be very useful in diagnosing and treating intracranial hypertension. The EEG is an important tool in diagnosing seizures and brain death. The role of the BIS monitor to measure the level of sedation of critically ill patients is yet to be determined.

SELECTED READING

Chestnut RM: Medical management of severe head injury: present and future. New Horizons 3(3):581–593, 1995.

Ghajar J: Intracranial pressure monitoring techniques. New Horizons 3(3):395–399, 1995.

Johansen JW, Sebel PS: Development and clinical application of electroencephalographic bispectrum monitoring. Anesthesiology 93(5):1336–1344, 2000.

Lang EW, Chestnut RM: Intracranial pressure and cerebral perfusion pressure in severe head injury. New Horizons 3(3):400–409, 1995.

Rampil IJ: A primer for EEG signal processing in anesthesia. Anesthesiology 89(4):980–1002, 1998.

Todd MM: EEGs, EEG processing, and the bispectral index (Editorial View). Anesthesiology 89(4):815–817, 1998.

CHAPTER 22

Endocrine Dysfunction

CARLOS J. LOPEZ III, M.D.

Endocrine dysfunction in the critically ill patient poses frequent and challenging situations for the clinician. They are as pervasive as glycemic control, and as relatively rare as pheochromocytoma. In this chapter several pathologies are reviewed, their clinical manifestations discussed, and approaches established to managing them.

THYROID DYSFUNCTION

The thyroid gland is responsible for the production of thyroxine (T_4) which is converted peripherally to the more potent triiodothyronine (T_3). Thyrotropin-releasing hormone (TRH) from the hypothalamus stimulates the release of thyroid-stimulating hormone (TSH) from the anterior pituitary. TSH then stimulates the release of T_4 by the thyroid. A negative feedback loop involving T_4 then helps modulate the release of TSH from the pituitary gland. Both T_3 and T_4 are bound reversibly to plasma proteins, primarily thyroxine binding globulin (TBG). It is the free fraction of T_3 and T_4 that produces the biological effect. They are responsible for maintaining metabolism in tissues at an optimal level. They alter the rate of cellular metabolism, oxygen consumption, and heat production, and facilitate mobilization of free fatty acids. Alterations in the production of T_4 and its subsequent conversion to T_3 are responsible for many of the clinical syndromes we see.

Hypothyroidism

Hypothyroidism results from a decrease in the production of T_4 and T_3. The symptoms and signs are due chiefly to a decrease in metabolism. Etiologies include Hashimoto's thyroiditis which is the most common cause in adults, thyroidectomy, radioactive iodine, antithyroid medications, amiodarone, iodine insufficiency, and secondary hypothyroidism. The signs can be subtle. The patient may complain of weight gain, cold intolerance, muscle fatigue, or lethargy. Physical examination may reveal dull facial expression, depression, and hypoactive reflexes. In the elderly subclinical disease may be present and difficult to identify. A high TSH level establishes the diagnosis of primary hypothyroidism when TSH > 20 μU/ml. When levels are moderately elevated, but < 20 μU/ml, a low plasma free T_4 is used to confirm the diagnosis. This is the case with secondary hypothyroidism (Box 22-1).

Myxedema

Myxedema is a severe, potentially life-threatening form of hypothyroidism. It tends to occur more commonly in the elderly and women. Patients often have preexisting moderate or unrecognized hypothyroidism. It is typically associated with a precipitant such as infection,

---

Box 22-1 Diagnosing Hypothyroidism

- Cold intolerance, lethargy, weight gain, hypoactive reflexes, and dull facial expression
- TSH is best test
  - TSH > 20 μU/ml, primary hypothyroidism
  - TSH < 20 μU/ml, low free T_4, secondary hypothyroidism

---

trauma, surgery, sedative, gastrointestinal bleed, and hypothermia.

The clinical manifestations are more severe. Signs and symptoms include those seen in hypothyroidism and also nonpitting edema, loss of eyebrow and scalp hair, hypothermia, severe lethargy leading to coma, macroglossia with possible airway obstruction, hypotension, and cardiac and respiratory failure. The presence of coma associated with bradycardia, hypoventilation, and hypothermia is life threatening. Associated findings on laboratory workup include hypoxemia, hypercapnia, and respiratory failure. The chest x-ray may disclose a large cardiac silhouette, pericardial effusion, or pleural effusion. The EKG may show bradycardia with low voltage. Although an elevated TSH level greater than 60 μU/ml establishes the diagnosis, high-dose glucocorticoids or high-dose dopamine may blunt the level of TSH seen in the critically ill hypothyroid patient. Additional thyroid function tests including a free T_4 may be useful. The clinical picture as in all thyroid illnesses still remains the most useful diagnostic tool (Box 22-2).

Mild hypothyroidism is treated with T_4, in single daily doses of 50 to 200 μg. The treatment of myxedema typically is started, however, with T_3 because of the decreased conversion of T_4 to T_3 in the critically ill patient. A treatment regimen is 12.5 to 25 μg q 6 h IV for the first 24 hours followed by 25 to 50 μg/day. As the patient improves T_3 is replaced with T_4. T_4, and especially T_3, stimulates metabolism and increase in oxygen consumption so care must be taken with the elderly and patients with coronary artery disease. In these patients, half a starting dose is typically instituted and increased gradually. If angina occurs while on T_4 it must be considered as unstable since the half-life of T_4 is greater than 1 week. The half-life of T_3 on the other hand is approximately one day. Replacement of hormone takes time and so there is no indication for frequent TSH or free T_4 or T_3 levels. One does not check levels more frequently than once a week. Clinical status is a more reliable gauge of response to therapy.

DRUG INTERACTIONS

T_4 and T_3
- T_4 and especially T_3 may precipitate ischemia in patients with CAD
- In CAD start with half the dose and monitor closely
- T_3 should be reserved for severe myxedema due to its cardiac effects
- T_4, however, has a longer half-life therefore continues to be a problem longer

---

Adrenalitis with decreased cortisol production may occur in myxedema. Treatment of myxedema may therefore unmask adrenal insufficiency and result in hypotension. The pituitary axis should be checked upon the diagnosis of myxedema and consideration should be given to starting dexamethasone until the diagnosis of adrenal insufficiency is excluded or continuing with hydrocortisone if it is not.

CLINICAL CAVEAT

Myxedema and Adrenal Insufficiency
- Adrenalitis with decreased cortisol production may occur
- Treatment with T_4 or T_3 may unmask adrenal insufficiency
- Consider dexamethasone replacement while pituitary–adrenal axis is checked
- If diagnosis confirmed begin hydrocortisone at 100 mg q 8 hours

---

Box 22-2 Diagnosing Myxedema

- Severe lethargy, loss of eyebrow hair, nonpitting edema, macroglossia, hypothermia, bradycardia, and hypercapnia
- Typically TSH > 60 μU/ml
  - But lower with high-dose steroids or dopamine
  - May need free T_4 level

Supportive care during this time may include correcting the core temperature by warming the patient; considering mechanical ventilation if mental status, hypoventilation, or acidosis are at a critical stage; and searching for precipitating causes. Myxedema can be fatal and hypercapnia and hypothermia are poor prognosticators. However, early recognition, hormone replacement, evaluation of pituitary–adrenal axis, and supportive care will improve outcome.

Hyperthyroidism

Hyperthyroidism results from an excess of T_4 and T_3 production. Graves' disease is the most common cause followed by toxic multinodular goiter, thyroiditis, TSH-secreting pituitary tumors, thyroid adenomas, excess hormone replacement, and amiodarone. The symptoms are the result of a hypermetabolic state. The patient may present with weight loss, heat intolerance, muscle weakness, diarrhea, and nervousness. Signs may include tachycardia, atrial fibrillation, tremor, hyperactive reflexes, goiter, and exophthalmos. The diagnosis is confirmed by high free T_4 and free T_3 and low TSH. Total T_4 and T_3 levels may not be helpful in critical illness (Box 22-3).

Thyroid Storm

Thyroid storm is an extreme form of hyperthyroidism in long-standing uncontrolled or poorly controlled hyperthyroidism. It may be related with a precipitating illness or event such as thyroid surgery, infection, trauma, acute abdominal problem, or anesthesia. Along with the hypermetabolic crisis there is a breakdown in the body's thermoregulatory mechanism resulting in hyperthermia. Signs and symptoms include tachycardia and atrial fibrillation; tremor, agitation, confusion, psychosis, and even coma; congestive heart failure (CHF), hypotension, and shock; nausea, vomiting, diarrhea, weight loss, and cachexia; moist, warm, flushed, velvety skin; and goiter in patients with Graves' disease. The clinical diagnosis is confirmed by a high total and free T_4 and T_3 and reduced TSH, but T_3 and T_4 may be distorted acutely (Box 22-4).

Urgent treatment is necessary in the presence of fever, delirium, exacerbation of CHF, and coronary artery disease (CAD). Cardiovascular resuscitation with volume repletion is an immediate priority in the treatment. Reduction of thyroid hormone synthesis is then undertaken. Thyroid hormone synthesis is reduced with propylthiouracil (PTU) with a loading dose of 600 to 1200 mg PO, followed by 200–300 mg PO q 6. Two hours after PTU is initiated, potassium iodide, SSKI, 5 drops q 6 hours can be started. To control heart rate and help prevent T_4 to T_3 conversion, propranolol 40 mg PO q 6 hours (or 1–2 IV q 15 minutes to a total dose of 10 mg)

Box 22-3 Diagnosing Hyperthyroidism

- Weight loss, heat intolerance, nervousness, tachycardia, hyperactive reflexes, goiter, and exophthalmos
- High free T_3 and free T_4, low TSH
- Total T_4 and T_3 may be normal

Box 22-4 Diagnosing Thyroid Storm

- Tachycardia, atrial fibrillation, agitation, psychosis, coma; if left untreated vascular collapse and shock
- High free T_3 and free T_4, low TSH
- Total T_3 and T_4 may be distorted acutely

or esmolol IV drip can be started. Glucocorticoids (dexamethasone 4 mg IV q 6 hours or hydrocortisone 100 mg IV q 8 hours) which also prevent T_4 to T_3 conversion are given due to the relative adrenal insufficiency which occurs due to the physiologic stress and increased glucocorticoid metabolism caused by the hypermetabolic state. Supportive measures include the treatment of hyperpyrexia with acetaminophen, fluid and electrolyte replacement as needed, and identifying and treating the underlying cause. These patients require observation and treatment in a monitored setting such as an intensive care unit (ICU). Left untreated survival is poor.

CLINICAL CAVEAT

Treatment of Thyroid Storm
- Volume resuscitation
- PTU and SSKI to decrease thyroid hormone synthesis
- Propranolol or other beta-blockade for tachycardia and to decrease T_4 to T_3 conversion
- Glucocorticoids to decrease T_4 to T_3 conversion and for relative adrenal insufficiency
- Acetaminophen for fever
- Aggressive supportive care

Sick Euthyroid Syndrome

Many illnesses and conditions alter thyroid studies without being due to thyroid disease. Patients with starvation, mild illnesses, surgery, and trauma can have a decrease in peripheral conversion of T_4 to T_3 resulting in a low total T_3 level. They typically will have a normal TSH level. In more acutely ill patients there may be a central suppression in the thyroid axis and T_4 may also fall to low levels. The TSH levels will thus be low despite the low serum hormone levels. These conditions are referred to as the *sick euthyroid syndrome*. It is believed not to represent true thyroid illness, as these patients do not manifest clinical signs of hypothyroidism. However, there are some who believe this may more accurately represent a form of hypothyroidism and use the term *nonthyroidal illness syndrome*. While the critical illness gets worse and T_4 becomes involved there is the development of a more complex syndrome.

As T_4 serum levels decrease below 4 μg/dl the probability of death increases in these patients. A T_4 level < 2 μg/dl is in fact associated with an 80% mortality. Whether this represents a treatable condition or a marker for severe illness is unclear. Some clinicians advocate the use of T_3 replacement in the setting of significant cardiac depression. However, the use of T_3 or T_4 in these patients has not been associated with improved outcomes.

CURRENT CONTROVERSY

Sick Euthyroid Syndrome
- Occurs in critically ill patients
- Low T_3, normal TSH; the more acutely ill have low T_4, low TSH
- Many believe it does not represent thyroid disease
- However, low levels of T_4 associated with high mortality
- Some clinicians recommend T_3 replacement in severely ill patients
- But no evidence of improved outcomes with T_3 use

PARATHYROID DYSFUNCTION

The four parathyroid glands produce parathyroid hormone (PTH). PTH along with vitamin D (1,25-dihydroxy-vitamin D) are responsible for the regulation of ionized calcium in serum. Ionized calcium is the physiologically active form of calcium; total serum calcium as commonly measured is not. Total serum calcium is dependent on albumin level, acid–base status, and chelators. A low total serum calcium which commonly occurs in critically ill patients due to a low albumin is generally associated with a normal ionized calcium level. These patients are not truly hypocalcemic. An ionized calcium level should be measured instead. The clinical manifestations of hypo- and hyperparathyroidism are therefore due to a decrease or increase in ionized calcium level. The diagnoses of these conditions are made by evaluating ionized calcium and PTH level. The etiologies and clinical manifestations are discussed below but the management of both hypo- and hyperparathyroidism are covered elsewhere in this text.

CLINICAL CAVEAT

Calcium Level
- Ionized calcium is the physiologically active form of calcium
- Ionized calcium is altered by albumin level, acid–base status, and chelators

---

Hypoparathyroidism

Hypoparathyroidism can occur postoperatively following surgery on the parathyroid glands and on the thyroid gland if all four parathyroid glands are removed. Other conditions that result in hypoparathyroidism are severe and acute hyperphosphatemia, hypomagnesemia, and sepsis. The symptoms and signs associated with hypocalcemia are paresthesia, weakness, spasm, tetany, laryngospasm, apnea; anxiety, irritability, confusion, depression; hypotension, bradycardia, QT prolongation, arrhythmias, and cardiac arrest. On clinical examination hyperreflexia and Chvostek's and Trousseau's signs may be elicited.

Hyperparathyroidism

Primary hyperparathyroidism is the most common cause of hypercalcemia in the outpatient setting. Solitary adenoma accounts for 80% to 85% of cases, followed by hyperplasia of all four glands, parathyroid cancer, and multiple adenomas. Multiple endocrine neoplasia (MEN) types I and II represent a particularly important subgroup due to their associated endocrinopathies. Secondary hyperparathyroidism is due to a compensation in PTH secretion because of chronic low serum calcium. Chronic renal failure accounts for most of this group, followed by malabsorption, rickets, and osteomalacia. Tertiary hyperparathyroidism occurs when hypercalcemia develops in secondary hyperparathyroidism. The symptoms of hyperparathyroidism and its resultant hypercalcemia are often described by the constellation of symptoms referred to as "bones, stones, psychic moans, and abdominal groans." The symptoms and signs include weakness, hypotonia, and hyporeflexia; confusion, psychosis, coma, and seizures; constipation, polyuria, and anorexia; fractures, osteopenia, and ectopic calcification; and QT shortening, cardiac arrhythmias, hypertension, and heart block.

ADRENAL DYSFUNCTION

The adrenal gland is responsible for the production of glucocorticoids, mineralocorticoids, sex hormones, and catecholamines. The adrenocorticotropic hormone (ACTH) secreted by the anterior pituitary stimulates the release of cortisol, the principal glucocorticoid produced by the adrenal cortex. This is done in a diurnal pattern and is increased during periods of stress. Cortisol has effects on protein, fat, and carbohydrate metabolism. It is essential for proper carbohydrate–protein metabolism, norepinephrine to epinephrine conversion in the adrenal medulla, adrenergic receptors function, cardiac contractility, vascular tone, endothelial integrity, immune function, and numerous other functions.

Deficiency of cortisol has various clinical manifestations which depend on the extent and acuteness of onset.

Acute Adrenal Insufficiency

Adrenal insufficiency can result from primary, secondary, or tertiary causes. Primary adrenal insufficiency, or Addison's disease, is due to the destruction of the adrenal cortex. Autoimmune diseases account for a large percentage of cases. Other causes include chronic infections besides tuberculosis like AIDS-related infections such as cytomegalovirus (CMV), or fungal infections; Gram-negative bacterial infections; invasion of the adrenal by cancer cells that have spread from another part of the body, especially the breast; rarely, hemorrhage into the adrenals during shock; abdominal trauma; and the surgical removal of both adrenals. Drugs such as ketoconazole and etomidate have also been implicated. It can be chronic, but can develop into acute addisonian crisis during periods of stress. The signs and symptoms are of both mineralocorticoid deficiency - hyperpigmentation, vitiligo, hyperkalemia, hyponatremia, and hypovolemia - and glucocorticoid deficiency - weakness, fatigue, hypoglycemia, and hypotension.

Secondary adrenal insufficiency is most commonly due to previous glucocorticoid use which suppresses the pituitary–adrenal axis. The subsequent ability of the adrenal gland to increase cortisol production in periods of stress is decreased. In fact adrenal recovery may take 9 to 12 months following the discontinuation of steroid use. These patients should be considered to be at risk for secondary adrenal insufficiency. Other causes are post-partum pituitary necrosis, pituitary tumors, pituitary surgery, brain tumors, head trauma, radiation therapy, and anoxic encephalopathy. Some clinicians believe that sepsis itself may suppress adrenal function, which returns once sepsis resolves. Patients typically manifest signs and symptoms of glucocorticoid deficiency.

Tertiary adrenal insufficiency refers to tissue glucocorticoid deficiency typically from sepsis or multiple organ dysfunction. These patients in effect have relative tissue resistance to cortisol. These patients may have high levels of circulating cortisol, which may make the diagnosis of adrenal insufficiency difficult to make.

The diagnosis can be made by demonstrating a decreased clearance of cortisol.

Acute adrenal insufficiency results from either addisonian crisis due to acute hemorrhage into the adrenal cortex or during periods of stress in patients with secondary and tertiary adrenal insufficiency. This is usually associated with a concurrent illness such as sepsis, trauma, or surgery. Along with the signs of glucocorticoid and mineralocorticoid deficiency, signs of cardiovascular collapse are pronounced. Hypotension, relatively unresponsive to volume resuscitation, will predominate. It can progress to cardiovascular collapse and death. Hyperpigmentation seen in primary adrenal insufficiency is not seen in secondary adrenal insufficiency.

Diagnosis (Box 22-5) requires a high index of suspicion. While an insulin tolerance test would be the most sensitive diagnostic test it is not practical in the critically ill patient. A random cortisol level is obtained instead. Normal patients with an intact hypothalamic–pituitary–adrenal (HPA) axis during periods of stress will have a random cortisol >18 µg/dl and generally >25 µg/dl. However, a low random cortisol level does not make the diagnosis of adrenal insufficiency. The HPA axis needs to be checked. Traditional diagnosis requires a 250 µg bolus of cosyntropin (ACTH). By convention this dose is thought to exclude adrenal insufficiency if the post-stimulation level at 60 minutes increases the cortisol level by >8 µg/dl or if the level is >18 µg/dl. However, the precise diagnostic criteria for adrenal suppression are unclear. We know that levels of up to 25 µg/dl may represent an inadequate response. Moreover, the standard test dose of 250 µg of ACTH is in fact several hundred-fold greater than the stress ACTH response. This supraphysiologic dose may in fact cause the adrenal to respond when it would not otherwise. One may therefore fail to diagnose patients with partial or relative adrenal insufficiency. Many clinicians are concerned that the standard testing is not sensitive enough. Therefore a lower dose cosyntropin test of 1 µg is advocated by some. Under a protocol advocated by Marik and Zaloga, a hypotensive

---

CLINICAL CAVEAT

AIDS and Adrenal Insufficiency
- AIDS has a high association with primary adrenal insufficiency
- Infections, especially CMV and fungal, are implicated
- Consider acute adrenal insufficiency in the hypotensive, critically ill AIDS patient

---

Box 22-5 Diagnosing Acute Adrenal Insufficiency

- Mineralocorticoid deficiency - vitiligo, hyperkalemia, hyponatremia, and hypovolemia
  - Hyperpigmentation only in primary adrenal insufficiency
- Glucocorticoid deficiency - weakness, fatigue, hypoglycemia, and hypotension
  - Hypotension with cardiovascular collapse; unresponsive to fluids and pressors
- Cortisol assay

patient with a random cortisol of <25 μg/dl undergoes a 1 μg ACTH stimulation test. An appropriate response is considered to be a subsequent cortisol level >25 μg/dl at 30 minutes. They follow this up with a 250 μg dose to differentiate between primary adrenal failure, HPA axis failure, and ACTH resistance. More experience, however, is needed before conclusions can be made. We are currently assessing the use of a 1 μg dose of ACTH followed by a 250 μg dose which is injected at the time the 60 minute sample is obtained. When in doubt we treat with a short course of steroids and observe.

CURRENT CONTROVERSY

ACTH Stimulation Test
- Precise diagnostic criteria for acute adrenal insufficiency using cortisol assays are unavailable
- Standard ACTH stimulation test with 250 μg is supraphysiologic
- May mask partial or relative adrenal insufficiency
- Low dose with 1 μg is advocated by some
- What cortisol level to use is still unclear

Treatment is with stress doses of hydrocortisone IV at 100 mg q 8 hours in patients with an established diagnosis. In patients with a possible diagnosis, emergent treatment can be started with dexamethasone IV 4 mg q 6 hours. Dexamethasone does not interfere with the cortisol assay. Treatment can therefore be started while testing is in progress. However, it has no mineralocorticoid activity so it should be changed to hydrocortisone once the cosyntropin test is complete or diagnosis is made. Emergent treatment should also include D5NS to treat the associated hypoglycemia and volume depletion.

DRUG INTERACTIONS

Dexamethasone
- Dexamethasone does not interfere with cortisol assay
- Little mineralocorticoid activity
- Switch to hydrocortisone once diagnosis is made
- If must continue dexamethasone add flucortisone

Perioperative stress dose steroid replacement has traditionally required full replacement of hydrocortisone IV at 100 mg q 8 initiated at the time of surgery and subsequent tapering over the next several days. This was regardless of the planned surgery in any patient who has received steroids over the last 9 to 12 months. The normal basal production of cortisol, however, is 30 mg/day. A more tempered approach appears to be gradually developing assessing the type of surgery planned and the preoperative steroid dose. Generally those patients who are on a low-dose prednisone ≤5 mg/day or are getting minor or peripheral surgery receive that dose. This is tailored upwards with full replacement reserved for patients on a high preoperative regimen or those scheduled to receive major surgery.

DIABETES INSIPIDUS

Diabetes insipidus (DI) is a disorder of water imbalance due to a lack of production of or response to antidiuretic hormone (ADH). ADH is secreted by the pituitary and is responsible for the absorption of water in the collecting tubules. There are neurogenic and nephrogenic causes. Neurogenic (central) DI may be idiopathic in one-third of cases or caused by the destruction of hypophysis due to trauma, surgery, granulomatous disease, vascular accidents, neoplasms, or infections. Nephrogenic DI can be caused by drugs, amphotericin B, democycline, and lithium; renal failure including correction of post-obstructive uropathy, systemic diseases such as amyloidosis, multiple myeloma, and sarcoidosis; and pregnancy.

Central DI tends to be more severe. These patients present with polyuria, polydipsia if alert, hypernatremia with high serum osmolarity and low urine osmolarity <300 mOsm/kg. In the ICU these patients can have very large urine outputs of ~1 l/hour up to 20 l/day. They will be hypovolemic and may even be in shock. While a water deprivation test and desmopressin challenge test may be useful in differentiating a central from nephrogenic cause of DI, the most useful test in the critically ill patient is urine specific gravity. A urine specific gravity of <1.004, or a urine osmolarity <300 mOsm/kg, in the face of hypernatremia and large urine output is diagnostic for DI (Box 22-6).

Treatment for central DI is with the use of desmopressin (DDAVP) IV or SC at 1–4 μg q 6 to 24 hours depending on severity or intranasally at 5–20 μg q 12 hours if mild. Free water deficits must be calculated and replaced (Box 22-7).

Initial fluids may include normal saline (NS) for volume expansion but is soon switched to D_5W and PO replacements. Potassium, magnesium, and phosphorus losses are replaced simultaneously. In severe nephrogenic DI, thiazide diuretics are administered. DI may be masked in patients with adrenal insufficiency, so care must be taken when initiating steroid treatment.

Box 22-6 Diagnosing Central Diabetes Insipidus

- Polyuria, polydipsia if alert; hypernatremia
- Urine specific gravity < 1.004
- Urine osmolarity <300 mOsm/kg

> **Box 22-7   Calculating Free Water Deficit**
>
> Water deficit = 0.6 × (wt in kg) × (([Na] − 140)/140)

GLYCEMIC DYSFUNCTION

Disorders of glycemic control are extremely common in the ICU.

Hypoglycemia

Hypoglycemia as defined by Whipple's triad is a serum glucose < 50 mg/dl, associated with central nervous system symptoms, which resolves with glucose administration. Initial symptoms and signs include nervousness, diaphoresis, blurred vision, and tachycardia. Failure to treat hypoglycemia can lead to lethargy, seizures, coma, and irreversible brain damage. In the critically ill patients symptoms can be easily masked by the underlying disease process and by sedation. Therefore the clinician needs to have a high index of suspicion and monitor serum glucose closely in at-risk patients. Conditions associated with hypoglycemia are liver disease, alcoholism, adrenal failure, myxedema, insulinomas, and medications such as insulin, sulfonylureas, and pentamidine. Iatrogenic causes account for most cases in the hospitalized patient. They include excessive insulin, decreased caloric intake, and treatment of hyperkalemia with insulin; conditions such as sepsis, shock, acute renal failure, and acute fulminant hepatic failure can result in hypoglycemia. The treatment is with 50 cm^3 IV D$_{50}$W. If hypoglycemia is particularly resistant to treatment continuous infusions can be used. Glucagon 0.5 to 1.0 mg IV, PO or SC, can also be used if hypoglycemia is persistent or there is no IV access. Those patients who are alcoholic or malnourished should get 100 mg IV thiamine before the administration of glucose to prevent the onset of Wernicke's encephalopathy. Specific treatment with steroid for acute adrenal insufficiency, thyroxine for myxedema, and activated charcoal for overdoses of oral hypoglycemic agents should be given.

> **CLINICAL CAVEAT**
>
> **Treatment of Hypoglycemia**
> - D$_{50}$W 50 cm^3 IV
> - D$_{10}$W 100 IV 100 to 200 cm^3/hour
> - Glucagon 0.5 mg to 1.0 mg IV, PO or SC
> - Steroids if adrenal insufficiency, thyroxine for myxedema, and activated charcoal for oral hypoglycemic agents

Hyperglycemia

Stress-induced hyperglycemia is common in critically ill patients. This occurs not only in patients with known diabetes, but can also occur in patients with no previous history. There are various etiologies aside from insulin deficiency and resistance. Stress itself with the release of cytokines, and hormones such as catecholamines, cortisol, and growth hormone can play a role. Dextrose-containing IV fluids, total parenteral nutrition (TPN), and drugs such as steroids can also contribute.

Hyperglycemia in critically ill patients is known to be associated with an increased morbidity especially due to infections in surgical patients. The control of glucose has subsequently been shown to decrease the infection rate. Traditionally hyperglycemia is handled with either subcutaneous insulin or an IV insulin drip when the glucose level is more difficult to manage. The goal had been to maintain a blood glucose < 180–200 mg/dl. Tighter control was avoided by many because of its perceived unclear efficacy and concern for hypoglycemia. This is in spite of various studies suggesting continued improvement in morbidity as the blood glucose target level was decreased. Recently a study showed an almost 50% reduction in mortality in patients who were on mechanical ventilation more than 5 days when their blood glucose levels were kept between 80 and 110 mg/dl vs. traditional goals of <180–200 mg/dl. While these patients had a slightly higher number of hypoglycemic episodes it was neither statistically significant nor was it associated with any residual effects. Although we await further confirmation from other centers we insist on the same tight control with close monitoring.

> **CURRENT CONTROVERSY**
>
> **Blood Glucose Target**
> - Traditional goal is <180 mg/dl to 200 mg/dl
> - Concerns about further efficacy and hypoglycemia with tighter control
> - Evidence, however, that further decreases improve morbidity
> - Evidence that a goal of 80 mg/dl to 110 mg/dl decreases mortality
> - No significant hypoglycemic effects
> - Our goal is 80 mg/dl to 110 mg/dl

Diabetic Ketoacidosis

Diabetic ketoacidosis (DKA) is a potentially fatal consequence of uncontrolled diabetes occurring almost exclusively in type I diabetes mellitus (DM). It commonly occurs in children and young adults due to new-onset diabetes, noncompliance of insulin therapy, or concurrent conditions such as infections, trauma, myocardial ischemia, and emotional stress. On rare occasions it occurs in severely stressed older patients with type II DM. Its pathogenesis is due to a complete or relative deficiency of insulin during periods of stress. This, coupled with a secondary counter regulatory hormone excess of glucagon and catecholamines, results in the overproduction and underutilization of glucose and lipolysis. The clinical picture is due to these metabolic disturbances.

In DKA hyperglycemia results typically with a blood glucose of 400–800 mg/dl. This is accompanied by an osmotic diuresis, an anion gap metabolic acidosis due to the increased production of acetoacetic acid and β-hydroxybutyric acid, and the accumulation of ketones due to acetone and acetoacetic acid. Patients may present with polyuria, mild dyspnea, nausea, vomiting, vague abdominal discomfort, lethargy, and occasionally an altered mental status. Findings on physical examination may include tachypnea, tachycardia, and a weak thready pulse consistent with hypotension. The diagnosis is established in a hyperglycemic patient by a serum sample revealing an anion gap metabolic acidosis and positive for ketones. Urine for ketones which can be analyzed rapidly at the bedside may also be useful. Hyperkalemia due to lack of insulin and acidosis is typically present in spite of large potassium deficits due to the osmotic diuresis. The diuresis may also cause hypomagnesemia and hypophosphatemia. Free water loss at the expense of sodium occurs readily. However, a low or normal sodium is often seen on laboratory tests. This is due to the dilutional effect of hyperglycemia and hypertriglyceridemia on serum sodium concentrations. This "psuedohyponatremia" underestimates the true total body sodium level. A correction formula adding 1.6 mg/dl Na$^+$ to the measured Na$^+$ concentration for every 100 mg/dl of glucose over 100 mg/dl is generally used (Box 22-8). True total sodium levels may actually be normal or high. The osmotic diuresis causes volume depletion and dehydration as evidenced by the increased urea nitrogen, creatinine, and osmolarity. Increased plasma amylase without evidence of pancreatits and hypertriglyceridemia can also be seen.

Insulin, volume resuscitation, and electrolyte replacement are crucial in the treatment of DKA. Insulin is needed to decrease hepatic production of glucose and ketones and to increase glucose utilization and ketone clearance. A bolus of insulin is given at 0.1 units/kg and a drip is started at 0.1–0.2 units/kg/hour. Blood glucose should be monitored q 1 hour at first and a reasonable goal should be a decrease of 100–150 mg/dl/hour initially. Fluid deficits, typically of the order of 5–8 liters, are replaced aggressively with NS. Although patients may actually be hypernatremic, the correction of volume status initially with NS is more important than the risk of increasing sodium content. Infusion of 500 to 1000 cm^3/hour for the first 1 to 2 hours is followed by 250 to 500 cm^3/hour for the next 2 to 4 hours depending on the extent of dehydration. Although care should be taken in patients with cardiac dysfunction, volume resuscitation should be started early and continued until after the resolution of ketoacidosis. When blood glucose approaches 250 mg/dl the fluid is changed to D$_5$W or D$_5$W1/2NS in order to prevent hypoglycemia while continuing to give insulin. Insulin is maintained until the ketoacidosis resolves. Potassium replacement must be initiated early. In fact patients with normal and especially with low potassium should have their potassium replacement begun prior to insulin administration. Magnesium and phosphate replacement will also need to be addressed. Although a pH <7.2 or even <7.1 with a serum HCO$_3$ <10 is not uncommon, the use of NaHCO$_3$ should be avoided. We reserve its use for a persistent pH <7.0 after several hours of treatment. Underlying precipitants are searched for and treated.

CLINICAL CAVEAT

Treatment of Diabetic Ketoacidosis
- Volume – NS at 500 to 1000 cm^3/hour then D$_5$W or D$_5$W1/2NS
- Insulin drip – continue <250 mg/dl until ketoacidosis resolves
- Potassium, magnesium, and phosphorus replacements early
- Treat precipitating illness

Nonketotic Hyperosmolar Syndrome

Nonketotic hyperosmolar syndrome (NKHS) is a condition that occurs in older, type II diabetics and rarely in type I diabetics. These patients typically secrete enough insulin to prevent lipolysis and ketogenesis and the subsequent DKA from occurring, but not enough to prevent hyperglycemia. An altered mental status along with renal insufficiency or prerenal azotemia appear to be important in the development of the hyperglycemia. Typical precipitating factors are infections, stroke, myocardial

---

Box 22-8   Correction of Serum Sodium Concentration

Corrected [Na$^+$] = 1.6 × [([Glucose]−100)/ 100] mg/dl + [Na$^+$]

ischemia, and noncompliance. The clinical picture is due mostly to hyperglycemia and dehydration.

As in DKA, polyuria and polydipsia (if the patient is able) are common, but a more severely depressed mental status occurs. Hyperglycemia is generally in the 800 to 1200 mg/dl range, and severe dehydration and lack of significant acidosis tends to be the rule. Although ketosis and even mild ketoacidosis are sometimes seen, typically acidosis when present is from lactic acidosis or renal insufficiency. Electrolyte loss due to osmotic diuresis is present, especially potassium and magnesium, but the pseudohyponatremia that occurs is more pronounced than in DKA owing to the greater hyperglycemia. Other evidence of dehydration is also found in laboratory tests.

The treatment approach to NKHS is similar to that of DKA. Volume resuscitation, insulin, and electrolyte replacement are also crucial but with a greater emphasis on volume replacement. Fluid deficits are greater and in the range 5–10 liters. Initial replacement is with NS at 1000 cm^3/hour for the first 1 to 2 hours and subsequently 250 to 500 cm^3/hour for the next 2 to 4 hours. After the initial resuscitation to restore intravascular volume, consideration can be given to using a less hypotonic fluid such as 1/2NS, LR, or D$_5$W in cases of severe hypernatremia. D$_5$W is started when the blood glucose approaches 250 mg/dl. Although blood glucose rapidly decreases just by the dilution effect of the initial resuscitation, insulin, however, remains a crucial part of the treatment. A bolus of insulin is given at 0.1 units/kg and a drip is started at 0.1 to 0.2 units/kg/hour. Blood glucose should be monitored q 1 hour at first. Once the blood glucose is around 250 mg/dl the drip can be decreased to 1 to 2 units/hour. Hypokalemia and hypomagnesemia are addressed shortly after initiation of volume resuscitation. As in DKA, an aggressive search and treatment of all precipitating causes is undertaken.

CLINICAL CAVEAT

Diabetic Ketoacidosis vs. Nonketotic Hyperosmolar Syndrome
- Age: typically younger vs. typically older
- BG: 400 mg/dl to 800 mg/dl vs. 800 mg/dl to 1200 mg/dl
- Acidosis: ketoacidosis vs. none but lactic or renal insufficiency occurs
- Volume loss: 5 to 8 liters vs. 5 to 10 liters
- DKA associated with symptoms and signs of acidosis
- NKHS associated with altered mental status and renal insufficiency
- Both need aggressive insulin administration
- Both need aggressive electrolyte replacement

PHEOCHROMOCYTOMA

Pheochromocytomas are usually benign tumors of the adrenal medulla with unregulated growth and secretion of catecholamines. The adrenal medullae account for 90% of presentations. The rest are extra-adrenal with the organ of Zuckerkandl at the aortic bifurcation being a common intra-abdominal site. Associations with MEN IIA and IIB and Von Recklinghausen syndrome do occur.

The signs and symptoms are related to catecholamine excess. Pheochromocytomas account for 0.1% of all cases of hypertension. Paroxysmal changes in blood pressure, a "hallmark" of pheochromocytomas, occur in only a third of patients, and sustained hypertension occurs in about half. Patients classically experience spells characterized by headaches, palpitations, and diaphoresis in association with severe hypertension. These four characteristics together have a sensitivity of 91% and are strongly suggestive of pheochromocytoma. Other signs and symptoms include anxiety, cutaneous flushing, chest pain, abdominal pain, orthostatic pressure fluctuations, CHF, and changes related to chronic hypertension. Paroxysmal changes can be precipitated by trauma, induction of anesthesia, surgery, and certain medications such as opioids, histamine, beta-blockers, glucagon, and dopamine antagonists.

The diagnosis requires a high index of suspicion which may be supported in the ICU by hypertension poorly responsive to therapy. It is made by measuring an increase in 24-hour urinary collection of catecholamines and their byproducts such as metanephrines and vanillymandelic acid (VMA). Plasma catecholamines which are more difficult to measure can help with borderline cases. However, there are acute physiologic changes that occur in the critically ill that may make it difficult to differentiate them from patients with pheochromocytomas. Provocative testing such as the clonidine suppression test can also be used but has little role in ICU patients. The definitive diagnosis therefore often awaits resolution of the acute illness. Once the diagnosis is made, localizing the tumor is done by computed tomography (CT) or preferably magnetic resonance imaging (MRI). A scan with iodine-131 (^{131}I)-labeled meta iodobenzylguanidine (MIBG) is used when CT scan or MRI fails to localize the tumor.

CLINICAL CAVEAT

Diagnosing Pheochromocytoma
- Classic triad of headaches, palpitations, and diaphoresis in the presence of severe hypertension has a 91% sensitivity
- Testing is difficult in the critically ill due to assay interference
- Definitive diagnosis often awaits resolution of critical illness
- Imaging studies locate tumor once diagnosis is made

Alpha-adrenergic blockade is the cornerstone of hypertension control in these patients, and in fact needs to occur before beta-blockade is introduced. Beta-blockade without adequate alpha-blockade can result in unopposed alpha-mediated vasoconstriction and severe hypertension. Labetolol because of its combined alpha- and beta-blockade has been promoted as a first-line agent. However, there are reports of worsening hypertension in some patients presumably due to inadequate alpha-blockade.

DRUG INTERACTIONS

Beta-Blockade and Pheochromocytomas
- Beta-blockade before adequate alpha-blockade results in unopposed alpha-mediated vasoconstriction and hypertension
- Labetolol may not provide adequate alpha-blockade

Acute hypertensive episodes requiring immediate management can be treated with phentolamine a short-acting alpha-adrenergic blocker at 2–5 mg IV q 5 minutes until the blood pressure is controlled. Prazosin, another alpha-blocker, can also be used at a starting dose of 1–2 mg PO q 6 hours. A nitroprusside infusion may be useful during the acute management of the hypertensive episode. Definitive treatment is with surgical removal of the tumor. However, prior to surgery, adrenergic blockade, blood pressure control, and volume resuscitation need to take place. Phenoxybenzamine, a noncompetitive alpha-adrenergic receptor blocker, is started at a dose of 10 mg PO q 12 hours for 7 to 10 days before surgery. Expansion of intravascular volume is also undertaken during this time. Subsequent to adequate alpha-blockade, beta-blockers are sometimes used for the management of tachyarrhythmias. Nitroprusside, phentalomine, and beta-blockers are sometimes needed intraoperatively. Immediately postoperatively a short course of phenylephrine may be needed to maintain vascular tone. If both adrenals are removed steroid replacement therapy must be started.

SUMMARY

Endocrinopathies have an impact on the critically ill patient in many ways. These conditions can be as rare as pheochromocytoma or as ubiquitous as hyperglycemia. The apparent affects may be extraordinary and life threatening or subtle and seemingly trivial. While the need to have approaches to diagnosing and aggressively managing the more serious complications are well appreciated, those subtle and trivial effects warrant careful consideration. Recent data for instance supporting the concept of partial or incomplete adrenal insufficiency and that tight blood glucose control improves mortality in mechanically ventilated patients forces us to view these "subtle or trivial" effects in a new light. So while we must manage life-threatening situations without delay, we cannot forget that other abnormalities which are thought to be minor may have a detrimental impact on our patients.

CASE STUDY

A 47-year-old female with a history of poorly controlled hypertension and a recent diagnosis of medullary carcinoma of the thyroid is admitted to the ICU for uncontrolled hypertension immediately postoperatively after a thyroidectomy. Examination in the ICU reveals an extubated, thin, anxious diaphoretic female. Her blood pressure is 176/94, heart rate is 142 regular, respiratory rate is 22, and temperature is 38.2°C. Her examination other than the dressing on her neck which is clean and dry is otherwise unremarkable. She is noted to be on nitroprusside drip at 3.5 µg/kg/minute.

QUESTIONS
1. What is your differential diagnosis?
2. How can you explain her presentation?
3. What other abnormalities may be present?
4. What medications would you use for her blood pressure control?
5. How would you make the diagnosis?

SELECTED READING

Braunwald E, editor: *Harrison's Principles of Internal Medicine*, ed 15, New York: McGraw-Hill, 2001.

Broide J, Soferman R, Kivity S et al: Low-dose adrenocorticotropin test reveals impaired adrenal function in patients taking inhaled corticosteroids. J Clin Endocrinol Metab 80:1243–1246, 1995.

Farwell AF: Sick euthyroid syndrome in the intensive care unit. In Irwin RS, Cerra FB, Rippe JM, editors: *Intensive Care Medicine*, ed 4, Philadelphia: Lippincott Williams and Wilkins, 1999.

Farwell AP: Sick euthyroid syndrome. J Intensive Care Med 12:249–260, 1997.

Goldman L et al, editors: *Cecil Textbook of Medicine*, ed 21, Philadelphia: WB Saunders, 2000.

Hamilton BP, Landsberg L, Levine RJ: Measurement of urinary epinephrine in screening for pheochromocytoma in multiple endocrine neoplasia Type II. Am J Med 65:1027–1032, 1978.

Larsen PR et al, editors: *Williams Textbook of Endocrinology*, ed 10, Philadelphia: WB Saunders, 2002.

Longnecker D et al, editors: *Principles and Practice of Anesthesiology*, ed 2, Philadelphia: Mosby, 1998.

Marik PE, Kiminyo K, Zaloga GP: Adrenal insufficiency in critically ill HIV infected patients. Crit Care Med 30:1267-1273, 2002.

Marik PE, Zaloga GP: Adrenal insufficiency during septic shock. Crit Care Med 31:141-145, 2003.

Marik PE, Zaloga GP: Adrenal insufficiency in the critically ill: a new look at an old problem. Chest 122(5):1784-1796, 2002.

Murray M et al; ASCCA, editors: *Critical Care Medicine: Perioperative Management*, ed 2, Philadelphia: Lippincott Williams and Wilkins, 2002.

Van den Berghe GW et al: Intensive insulin therapy in the critically ill patients. N Engl J Med 345(19):1359-1367, 2001.

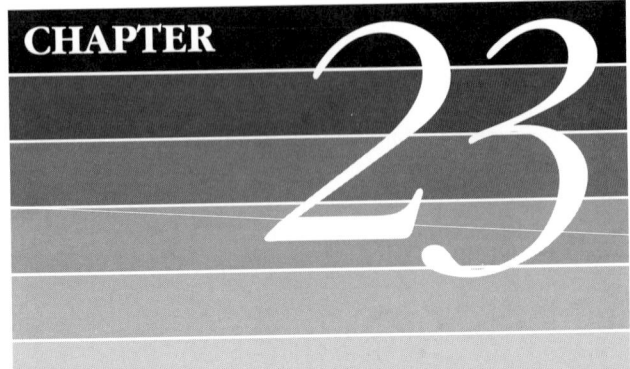

CHAPTER 23

Critical Care in Pregnancy

SUSAN E. DANTONI, M.D., F.A.C.O.G.

PHYSIOLOGY

Intensive care of the pregnant patient involves the simultaneous care of two individual patients. Critical decisions made for maternal well-being can profoundly affect the fetus. A basic understanding of the physiologic changes associated with pregnancy is necessary to provide proper care to the critically ill gravida. The following is a brief review of the major physiologic changes seen in pregnancy (Box 23-1).

Cardiorespiratory Systems

The following increase significantly during pregnancy: respiratory rate, oxygen consumption, minute ventilation, tidal volume, and PaO_2. Functional residual capacity and $PaCO_2$ decrease but there is also a compensatory decrease in plasma bicarbonate concentration thereby avoiding a marked respiratory alkalosis. As the uterus enlarges, the diaphragm is elevated and thoracic breathing is favored over abdominal breathing. During periods of apnea, there is rapid oxygen desaturation due to a decreased functional residual capacity and increased oxygen consumption. It is especially important to presaturate pregnant patients to avoid hypoxemia during induction of general anesthesia. Maintaining a maternal PO_2 above 60 mmHg will help ensure adequate fetal oxygenation. Uptake of inhalation agents is accelerated due to the increase in minute ventilation. Respiratory mucosa becomes engorged and prone to bleeding due to hormonal changes so special care must be rendered during intubation.

Maternal blood volume increases by up to 50% at term. Cardiac output increases significantly to accommodate the increased maternal and fetal demands by an increase in both heart rate and stroke volume. Cardiac output is greatest during delivery and immediately thereafter. There is generally about a 400 cm^3 and 800 cm^3 blood loss during vaginal and cesarean deliveries, respectively, but this is usually well accommodated by the increased blood volume. Blood volume as well as cardiac output generally return to normal one to two weeks postpartum.

The supine position causes decreases in cardiac output due to compression of the great vessels. This aortocaval compression is a significant and easily correctable cause of fetal distress due to the hypotension causing a significant uterine hypoperfusion. Gravidas in the third trimester especially should be placed in a tilt if they need to lie down in order to displace the enlarged uterus. It is also important to note that during the second trimester, there is a decrease in systemic vascular resistance lowering the maternal blood pressure, which gradually rises back to normal at term. Maternal systolic blood pressure should be maintained at 90 mmHg to ensure adequate placental perfusion.

EKG changes are common including a left axis deviation and chest x-rays can give the appearance of an enlarged heart due to elevation of the diaphragm. Finally, systolic flow murmurs are commonly appreciated due to increased blood volume.

Box 23-1 Physiologic Changes of Pregnancy

- Increased oxygen consumption
- Increased minute ventilation
- Increased respiratory rate
- Increased PaO_2
- Decreased functional residual capacity
- Decreased $PaCO_2$
- Increased maternal blood volume
- Increased cardiac output
- Left axis deviation of EKG
- Increased glomerular filtration rate
- Decreased BUN and creatinine
- Increased gastroesophageal reflux
- Hypersecretion of gastric acid
- Delayed gastric emptying
- Hypercoagulable state: increased risk of DVT

Renal and Gastrointestinal Systems

Glomerular filtration rate increases significantly in pregnancy by as much as 50% causing decreases in blood urea nitrogen (BUN) as well as creatinine. There is a decrease in renal tubular threshold for both glucose and amino acids causing glycosuria as well as proteinuria (less than 300 mg/dl). Disease processes such as preeclampsia can affect the renal system significantly causing profound proteinuria and even renal failure.

Gastroesophageal reflux and delayed emptying of the stomach are significant causes of maternal morbidity and mortality. This is due to a combination of factors including progesterone effect as well as upward displacement of the stomach by the gravid uterus. There is generally hypersecretion of gastric acid causing a gastric pH under 2.5 placing gravidas at risk for severe aspiration pneumonitis.

Hematologic

Pregnancy is considered a hypercoagulable state that increases the risk for deep venous thrombosis (DVT) and pulmonary embolism but is protective against maternal hemorrhage. Mild leukocytosis and a 20% decrease in platelet count are also seen. Finally, a physiologic anemia caused by a nonconcordant increase in red blood cell mass versus plasma volume is seen commonly.

BASIC FETAL MONITORING

When a pregnant patient is admitted to the intensive care unit, a team approach will optimize outcomes.

A qualified obstetrician should be consulted at the onset of care due to the necessity of providing proper monitoring of not only the mother but also the fetus.

The most commonly used modalities in fetal monitoring include ultrasound, the nonstress test (NST), the contraction stress test (CST), and the biophysical profile. Ultrasound can be used to assess fetal viability, position, placenta location and possible abruption status, amniotic fluid volume, and uterine artery blood flow, all of which are helpful in assessing fetal well-being. The NST is used to assess fetal heart rate variability and accelerations in relation to fetal movement as well as uterine activity. In term pregnancies, an NST is considered reactive when the fetal heart rate rises for 15 beats over a 15-second time period. In preterm pregnancies, a 10 by 10 criterion is sometimes used. When an NST is determined to be nonreactive, further testing is usually warranted, either by a CST or a biophysical profile. The CST is used to determine fetal tolerance of the intrauterine environment. Contractions are induced generally with the use of oxytocin and the fetal heart rate response is assessed. If there are three late decelerations within a 10-minute period, the test is considered positive and intervention needs to be considered. Fetal heart rate decelerations are important to identify as they have different physiologic meanings. Briefly, early decelerations signify head compression, essentially a brief vagal response to uterine contractions. Variable decelerations signify cord compression and are generally benign unless they start to show atypical signs. Late decelerations are generally considered a sign of uteroplacental insufficiency and warrant prompt attention. It is important to consider the maternal condition when interpreting fetal tracing prior to intervening, as some maternal conditions such as hypotension and hypoxemia can sometimes be quickly corrected with a subsequent improvement in the fetal testing results. The biophysical profile is another useful test to assess fetal well-being. This test involves factors such as fetal movement, fetal tone, fetal breathing, as well as amniotic fluid measurement and results of NSTs. Each category is given 0 or 2 points. A score of 8 or 10 is generally reassuring. Anything below that requires either additional testing or intervention based on the circumstances.

OBSTETRIC COMPLICATIONS

Pregnancy can result in serious complications requiring the expertise of an intensive care team. The most common problems generally stem from massive blood loss, hypertensive diseases of pregnancy, and amniotic fluid/pulmonary embolus.

Massive Blood Loss

Obstetric hemorrhage is the leading cause of maternal death worldwide. It is generally caused by uterine atony, although other causes include retained placental fragments, abnormal placentation (placenta previa, accreta, percreta, increta), placental abruption, genital lacerations, uterine inversion, uterine rupture, coagulopathy, and hematoma. Postpartum hemorrhage is defined as more than 500 cm³ and 1000 cm³ losses during vaginal and cesarean deliveries, respectively; a decrease in hematocrit by more than 10%; or a need for transfusion after delivery secondary to blood loss. Management of hypovolemic shock includes maintaining systolic blood pressure above 90 mmHg, maintaining urine output above 25 ml/hour, and maintaining normal mental status. Volume replacement is especially important, but overaggressive replacement may contribute to the development of pulmonary edema.

Hypertensive Disorders

Pregnancy-induced hypertension (PIH), preeclampsia, eclampsia, and HELLP (hemolysis, elevated liver enzymes, and low platelets) syndrome are all part of a spectrum of hypertensive diseases of pregnancy. There can be pathophysiologic changes seen in the cardiovascular, hematological, renal, hepatic, and neurologic systems. Hallmarks of preeclampsia and its related diseases include hypertension (generally readings of 140/90), proteinuria (generally >300 mg/dl), and edema (although this may be absent). When present, the edema is commonly seen in the periorbital region. Eclampsia is the addition of tonic-clonic seizures with preeclampsia. There are several variations of HELLP syndrome, which can manifest with hepatic involvement without thrombocytopenia. Other serious sequelae of hepatic involvement can include acute fatty liver of pregnancy as well as development of a subscapular hematoma of the liver leading to rupture of the liver. Delivery is the only known cure although there have been reports of preeclampsia developing up to two weeks postpartum. Management can often be difficult especially in the face of prematurity as delivery may be devastating for the fetus while beneficial for the mother. There is a fine balance needed to obtain the best outcome, and with proper surveillance delivery can often be delayed to allow the fetus to become more mature without undo harm to the mother. The hallmarks of management involve early identification, consideration of delivery, prevention of seizures with the use of magnesium sulfate (4–7 mEq/l), management of hypertension (hydralazine, labetolol, nicardipine), management of oliguria, prevention of renal failure, and prevention of the serious sequelae of hepatic involvement (Box 23-2).

Box 23-2 Criteria for Severe Preeclampsia

- Blood pressure greater than 160/110
- Greater than 5 g/24 hours proteinuria
- Oliguria
- Cerebral changes such as altered mentation, blurred vision, seizure activity
- Severe right upper quadrant or epigastric pain (hepatic involvement)
- Thrombocytopenia (nonhematologic such as ITP)
- Fetal growth restriction

Amniotic Fluid Embolus

Amniotic fluid embolus (AFE) is a devastating complication of pregnancy with mortality rates as high as 80%. It is rare, unpredictable, and unpreventable. In the USA this in combination with pulmonary embolus are the leading causes of maternal mortality. AFE results from entry of amniotic fluid into the maternal circulation and results in sudden onset of severe dyspnea, tachypnea, and profound hypoxia. In addition, there is abrupt onset of disseminated intravascular coagulation as well as complete cardiovascular collapse. The differential of AFE includes pulmonary embolism, air embolism, aspirations of gastric contents, acute heart failure, and hemorrhagic shock with its associated causes. Management involves supportive measures including cardiopulmonary resuscitation, volume replacement, and correction of coagulopathy.

Pulmonary Embolus

There is a wide range of reported incidence of thrombotic events during pregnancy. Incidence of DVT ranges from 0.18% to 0.25%. In patients with untreated DVT, 15–25% develop pulmonary emboli versus 5% in treated patients. Etiologies for DVT are vessel wall trauma, venous stasis, and alterations in coagulation (Virchow's triad). Risk factors include advanced maternal age and increased parity, obesity, prolonged bedrest, and antithrombin III deficiency. Presenting signs for DVT include pain, tenderness, edema, change in limb color, and/or a palpable cord in the back of the leg. Diagnosis can be confirmed with Doppler ultrasound, ascending venography, and/or magnetic resonance imaging (when pelvic or ovarian vein thrombosis is suspected). Treatment involves the use of heparin and careful monitoring.

Pulmonary embolus (PE) is defined as an occlusion of a pulmonary vessel secondary to an intravascular clot from another location of the body. Signs of PE include dyspnea, tachypnea, and pleuritic chest pain. Diagnosis is made from clinical presentation, arterial blood gases, EKG, chest x-ray,

V/Q scan, spiral computed tomography, and/or pulmonary arteriography. Pulmonary arteriography is generally reserved for patients in whom lung scanning results are indeterminate or do not coincide with a patient's clinical symptoms or when heparin therapy is considered high risk.

CLINICAL CAVEAT

Pulmonary Embolus in Pregnancy

Pulmonary embolus is a common complication in pregnancy and needs close monitoring and prevention in the critically ill pregnant patient.

SELECTED READING

Cheek TG, Samuels P: Pregnancy-induced hypertension. In Datta S, editor: *Anesthetic and Obstetric Management of High-Risk Pregnancy*, ed 2, St Louis: Mosby, 1996.

Clark SL, Cotton DB, Hankins GDV, Phelan JP, editors: *Handbook of Critical Care Obstetrics*, London: Blackwell Science, 1995.

Dantoni S: Toxic shock syndrome. In Kruse JA, Fink MP, Carlson RW, editors: *Saunders Manual of Critical Care*, Philadelphia: Saunders, 2002.

Mason BA: Obstetric crises. In Kruse JA, Fink MP, Carlson RW, editors: *Saunders Manual of Critical Care*, Philadelphia: Saunders, 2002.

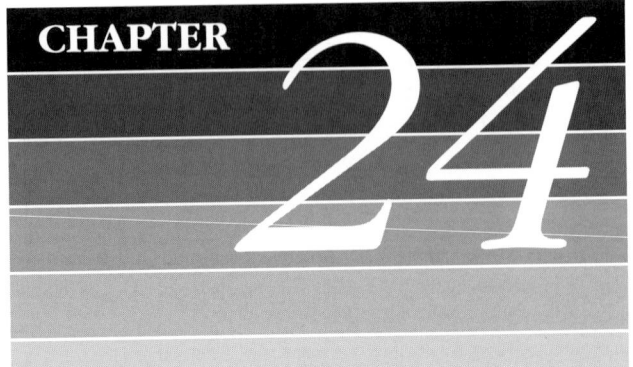

CHAPTER 24

The Immune-Compromised Host and the HIV patient

CARLOS J. LOPEZ III, M.D.

Host defense mechanisms are either nonspecific, nonimmune-mediated or specific, immune-mediated. Intact physical barriers are in part responsible for the nonimmune-mediated defense mechanism. Conversely, the various immune components with their complex interrelationships provide the immune-mediated response. The immune-compromised host can be defective in any part of the host defense system, while the immune-suppressed host refers only to the immune defective group.

NONSPECIFIC HOST DEFENSES

The skin and mucosal surfaces are responsible for the primary defense due to physical barriers. The breakdown of skin and mucosa due to trauma, either inadvertently or iatrogenically, results in the introduction of pathogens. Infections at the various sites are due to pathogens that either normally colonize the site or are introduced by contamination. Instrumentation with IV lines, dialysis catheters, and surgical procedures are common insults. The introduction of an endotracheal tube for mechanical ventilation will result in both the loss of protective airway mechanisms and allow a direct conduit for pathogens to the lungs. Obstruction or injury to the genitourinary mucosa due to instrumentation, calculi, and cytotoxic agents may result in infections.

Breakdown of the gastrointestinal mucosal barrier commonly results from cytotoxic agents during treatment for malignancies. The neutropenic patient may have a subtle, not easily apparent gastrointestinal source, or may present with an acutely ill fulminant picture. These patients often have polymicrobial infections. A high index of suspicion is necessary.

The normal flora should be considered as a host defense mechanism. It competes with nonindigenous pathogens that are introduced, and generally inhibits their growth. Disruption of normal flora may allow the propagation of nonindigenous pathogens. Patients who have been institutionalized, have received broad-spectrum antibiotics, or who are neutropenic have altered flora.

Other nonspecific defense mechanisms include the normal flow of secretions from either drainage, as in the biliary tract, or the ciliary action of the respiratory mucosa; and the gastric acidity of the stomach, which kills bacteria. Adequate nutritional status is crucial in providing substrates for metabolic needs and protein synthesis.

SPECIFIC HOST DEFENSES

Specific host defenses are immune-mediated, and are categorized into four different components. They are the polymorphonuclear leukocytes (PMNs), cell-mediated, humoral, and complement arms of the immune response. The immune-suppressed host is susceptible to indigenous, common community-acquired and nosocomial pathogens, along with unusual or opportunistic ones. Community-acquired and nosocomial infections that typically occur in hosts with intact immune systems present in a more virulent and fulminant fashion.

Unusual or opportunistic organisms, not generally virulent, or otherwise found as normal flora or as inconsequential colonizers, may result in severe, life-threatening infections. The initial presentation of these infections may be subtle and atypical. A delay in recognition, diagnosis, and treatment is therefore more likely. Although there is significant interrelationship between the immune components, the different types of immune deficiency are associated with characteristic infections. An understanding of the pathology associated with the specific immune deficiency will allow the clinician to more accurately diagnose, and choose aggressive, targeted therapy.

Polymorphonuclear Leukocytes

PMNs are also called neutrophils or granulocytes, and are responsible for phagocytosis and killing of extracellular microbes. The microbes are phagocytozed by PMNs subsequent to being opsonized by antibodies and complement. PMNs can be defective due to both congenital deficiencies and qualitative defects towards chemotaxis and killing. Chediak–Higashi syndrome is an example of a congenital defect to chemotaxis. The most common causes of impaired PMN dysfunction, however, are related to acquired deficiencies. Neutropenia defined by an absolute neutrophil count (ANC) < 500 cells/mm^3 is associated with a significant increase in bacterial infections. Counts below 100 cells/mm^3 have an even higher risk and are associated with the most severe infections. Neutropenia is most commonly associated with malignant diseases and their treatment with cytotoxic agents. Bone marrow infiltration by hematologic malignancies and lymphomas may result in bone marrow failure. Treatment with cancer chemotherapy (adriamycin, ARA-C, and cyclophosphamide) along with affecting bone marrow activity also results in damage to mucosal membranes and therefore significantly increases the risk to infections. Other causes of neutropenia include total body radiation, aplastic anemia, β-lactam antibiotics, and idiopathic drug reactions (Box 24-1).

Neutropenic patients most often develop infections from endogenous bacteria and fungal flora. Traditionally infections were due to Gram-negative aerobic bacteria such as *Escherichia coli*, *Klebsiella pneumoniae*, and *Pseudomonas aeruginosa* with occasional Gram-positive bacteria from the staphylococcal and streptococcal species. More recently, Gram-positive bacteria have become the most commonly isolated pathogens. Although the most severe infections are still Gram-negative infections, severe life-threatening α-hemolytic streptococcal (*Streptococcus viridans*) infections have emerged. Nosocomial infections clearly play a role and occur in a significant proportion of neutropenic patients. They tend to be associated with prolonged duration of neutropenia and physical exposure to these organisms. Fever with neutropenia of

---

Box 24-1   Characteristics of Polymorphonuclear Leukocyte Dysfunction

- Associated with malignant diseases and their treatment with cytotoxic agents
- Decreases phagocytosis and killing of extracellular organisms
- Neutropenia
  - ANC < 500 cells/mm^3 has an increase in infections
  - ANC < 100 cells/mm^3 higher risk and more severe
- Typically from endogenous bacteria and fungal flora

---

less than 1 week is associated with Gram-positive cocci, between 1 and 2 weeks with Gram-negative bacilli, and greater than 3 weeks with opportunistic infections, especially with *Candida* spp. and *Aspergillus* spp.

Different sites are associated with specific pathogens. Pneumonias may be due to enteric Gram-negative bacilli *P. aeruginosa*, *Staphylococcus aureus*, and *Aspergillus fumigatus*. Central nervous system (CNS) infections include enteric Gram-negative bacilli *Aspergillus* spp. and *Mucormycosis* spp. Skin and line infections may result from *S. epidermis*, *S. aureus*, *P. aeruginosa*, *Bacillus* spp., *Corynebacterium jeikeium*, and fungal pathogens. Perirectal infections result in *P. aeruginosa* and polymicrobial infections. Typhilitis may be due to *P. aeruginosa*, *Bacteroides fragilis*, and *Clostridium septicum*. Severe life-threatening infections associated with septic shock are associated with enteric Gram-negative bacilli *P. aeruginosa*, *S. aureus*, *Candida* spp., *Aspergillus* spp., and α-hemolytic streptococcus.

A febrile (temperature > 38.5°C) neutropenic patient may have a subtle, atypical infection. Although a source may be apparent, a definitive site is not found in 60–70% of patients. In fact, microbiological identification of pathogen occurs in only 30% of cases. There is the potential for a delay in determining whether an infection is truly present and initiating treatment. The use of empiric therapy has fortunately been shown to decrease mortality during neutropenic fever. Therefore, the use of empiric antibiotic therapy is the key to treating these patients.

CLINICAL CAVEAT

Neutropenic Fever
- ANC < 500 cells/mm^3 and temperature > 38.5°C
- Subtle, atypical infections may progress to life-threatening ones
- No site identified in up to 60–70%, or organism in 30% of patients
- Empiric therapy, however, decreases mortality

Empiric broad-spectrum therapy should be chosen with an understanding of the local microbiological flora. Local sensitivity patterns of likely infections may alter the specific choices. Treatment will include coverage against Gram-negative bacteria including *P. aeruginosa* and Gram-positive organisms. In noncritically ill patients monotherapy with imipenem-cilastatin, or an antipseudomonal third-generation cephalosporin may be sufficient. In critically ill patients combination therapy is used. Coverage against nosocomial antibiotic-resistant organisms and *Serratia, Citrobacter,* and *Enterobacter* spp., which become rapidly resistant to β-lactams, is essential. Possible combinations include an antipseudomonal third-generation cephalosporin or an antipseudomonal penicillin plus an aminoglycoside or a fluoroquinolone (especially ciprofloxacin). Vancomycin can be added if a Gram-positive infection due to methicillin-resistant *S. aureus* (MRSA) is suspected, or if patients become hemodynamically unstable. If fever persists after 4 to 7 days, or there is rapid clinical deterioration, empiric coverage for fungal infections with amphotericin B should be started. The broad-spectrum antibiotics should be continued for a minimum of 10 to 14 days or longer until the ANC is >500 cells/mm^3.

CLINICAL CAVEAT

Empiric Neutropenic Therapy
- Noncritically ill – monotherapy may be sufficient
  - Imipenem-cilastatin, or an antipseudomonal third-generation cephalosporin
- Critically ill – combination therapy is needed
  - Antipseudomonal third-generation cephalosporin or an antipseudomonal penicillin plus an aminoglycoside or a fluoroquinolone
  - Add vancomycin if MRSA or hemodynamically unstable
  - Add amphotericin B if fever > 4 to 7 days or decompensates
- Know local microbiological sensitivities
- Continue for 10 to 14 days or until ANC > 500 cells/mm^3

Cell-Mediated Immunity

The components of cell-mediated immunity are macrophages and T-lymphocytes. Macrophages perform phagocytosis, while T-lymphocytes are important in the initiation of the immune response and include CD$_4$ helper lymphocytes and CD$_8$ suppressor lymphocytes. T-lymphocytes also include the "natural killer cells." Cell-mediated immunity is responsible for eliminating obligate intracellular pathogens, virus-infected cells, and

malignant cells. Acquired defects are the most common while congenital ones are rare. Human immunodeficiency virus (HIV) infections, lymphoreticular malignancies, and cytotoxic and immunosuppressive chemotherapy with azathioprine, vincristine, bleomycin, cyclosporine, tacrolimus, OKT3, and high-dose corticosteroids result in the majority of acquired cell-mediated deficiencies in the developed world. HIV and severe protein malnutrition are the most common cause in developing nations.

Defects in cell-mediated immunity are associated with infections due to bacteria, fungi, viruses, and protozoa. These infections can be indigenous, community acquired, or nosocomial in origin. Unusual infections due to cell-mediated infections may occur in various organs. Lungs can develop pneumonias due to *Pneumocystis carinii, Legionella pneumophilia,* cytomegalovirus (CMV), herpes simplex virus (HSV), varicella zoster virus (VZV), adenovirus, coccidiomycosis, and *Cryptococcus neoformans.* The CNS can be infected with *C. neoformans, Toxoplasma gondii,* and *Listeria monocytogenes.* Mucocutaneous infections can occur due to *Candida* spp., HSV, VZV, and CMV. Unusual disseminated infections with *Mycobacterium avium intracellulare* (MAI), CMV, and VZV can occur (Box 24-2).

Factors determining the pathogen and site of infection include the CD4 count, which reflects the progressive decline of cell-mediated immune function; the duration of immune suppression; and, if an organ was transplanted, the time since the transplant and the organ transplanted. As the CD4 site decreases opportunistic infections particularly *Pneumocystis carinii* and CMV become more prevalent. As time progresses from 0 to 6 months from organ transplantation, typical postsurgical or nosocomial infections are replaced by opportunistic infections. After 6 months the infections depend on level of immune suppression and environmental factors. They are similar to those in immune-competent individuals. The treatment which is individualized on the basis of the

---

Box 24-2 Characteristics of Cellular-Mediated Dysfunction

- HIV, lymphoreticular malignancies, chemotherapy, and malnutrition are causes
- Macrophage and T lymphocytes (along with CD$_4$ and CD$_8$) function poorly
- Affects phagocytosis and initiation of the immune response
- Poor removal of obligate intracellular organisms, virus-infected cells, and malignant cells
- CD$_4$ count is useful in predicting the organism and the site affected

nature of the immune defect and the above factors, is discussed elsewhere in this chapter.

Humoral Immunity

Humoral immunity is mediated through antibodies (immunoglobulins) produced by B lymphocytes. Immunoglobulins generally assume one of two roles. They may act as plasma membrane-bound antigen receptors on the surface of a B-cell or as antibodies free in cellular fluids functioning to intercept and eliminate antigenic determinants. These antibodies activate complement and go on to destroy microorganisms by promoting phagocytosis via opsonization, toxin neutralization, and lysis of susceptible organisms. Similar to complement immunity, humoral immunity is responsible for the clearance of extracellular bacteria. For practical purposes humoral and complement deficiencies can be considered together. Multiple myeloma (MM), chronic lymphatic leukemia (CLL), and Waldenström's macroglobulinemia are common causes of disease states associated with impaired humoral defects. Several cytotoxic chemotherapeutic agents, including azathioprine, cyclophosphamide, and methotrexate, suppress humoral function along with other effects on the immune system (Box 24-3).

Pathogens frequently found include encapsulated pyogenic bacteria such as *Streptococcus pneumoniae*, *Haemophilus influenzae*, and rarely *Neisseria meningitidis*. Pneumonias tend to predominate with *S. pneumoniae*, *Haemophilus influenzae*, and occasionally *K. pneumoniae*. CNS infections include *S. pneumoniae*, *H. influenzae*, and *N. meningitidis*. Overwhelming sepsis can occur with *S. pneumoniae*, *H. influenzae*, and *N. meningitidis*. CNS infections are predominantly caused by these organisms.

Asplenia, either anatomic or functional, results in immune defects which have properties of both humoral and complement deficiencies. The spleen contains many antibody-producing B-lymphocytes, and is involved in T-cell independent immune responses. Specific complement deficiencies also result if asplenia occurs. The spleen is therefore important in the clearance of nonopsonized and opsonized bacteria. Overwhelming septicemia may occur in asplenic patients. *Streptococcus pneumoniae* and *Haemophilus influenzae* infections predominate, although *Neisseria meningitidis* has been described. Mortality approaches 80%; and multiple amputations are frequent in survivors. Due to the rapid progression of illness, febrile, splenectomized patients require treatment with high-dose antipneumococcal antibiotics. The incidence of penicillin-resistant *S. pneumoniae* has been increasing, and so initial therapy with ceftriaxone and vancomycin is wise. All splenectomized patients require immunization with pneumococcal, meningococcal A and C, and haemophilus influenza B vaccines. Uncommon infections with intraerythrocyte protozoa such as *Plasmodium malariae* and *Babesia* can also occur in splenectomized patients.

CLINICAL CAVEAT

Asplenia
- Has both humoral and complement deficiencies
- Loss of both antibody-producing B-lymphocytes and complement proteins
- Overwhelming sepsis can occur, mortality approaches 80%
- Encapsulated organisms: *S. pneumoniae*, *H. influenzae*, and *N. meningitidis*
- Immunization crucial, acutely treat with antipneumococcal antibiotics

---

Complement System

The complement cascade is involved in regulating the immune response. Complement are proteins, C3 and C5 being the most crucial, which form complexes that interact with specific cell receptors or directly with cell membranes. They facilitate phagocytosis, may independently kill extracellular organisms, and mediate acute inflammatory reactions. Acquired deficiencies in complement are the most common and occur in systemic lupus erythematosus (SLE) and MM, while congenital deficiencies are rare.

The pathogens are similar to those present during humoral defects, and can present with overwhelming infections due to encapsulated organisms. Infections with *Neisseria meningitidis*, *Streptococcus pneumoniae*, and less commonly *N. gonorrheae* occur. Infections of the CNS and joints may occur along life-threatening disseminated infections (Box 24-4).

Box 24-3   Characteristics of Humoral Dysfunction

- MM, CLL, Waldenström's macroglobulinemia, and cytotoxic agents are causes
- Immunoglobulin function and activation of complement is decreased
- Poor phagocytosis by opsonization, toxin neutralization, and lysis of organisms
- Failure to clear extracellular organisms and encapsulated pyogenic bacteria
- Humoral and complement deficiencies are considered together

Box 24-4   Characteristics of Complement Dysfunction

- Acquired deficiencies most common, SLE, MM
- Congenital deficiencies rare
- C3 and C5 the most crucial
- Affects phagocytosis, extracellular killing, and inflammatory response
- Encapsulated organisms: *S. pneumoniae*, *H. influenzae*, and *N. meningitidis*
- Humoral and complement deficiencies are considered together

IMMUNOSUPPRESSION AND TRANSPLANT PATIENTS

Solid Organ Transplant Patients

These patients are primarily faced with the immune-related complications of allograft rejection and infections. The need to prevent rejection is juxtaposed with the infectious consequences of immunosuppression.

Rejection is defined as an acute deterioration of function associated with specific pathologic changes. Allograft rejection is common in transplant patients. It occurs in up to 30% of kidney transplants, 50–80% of heart transplants, and 60% of liver transplants. Most episodes occur in the first 6 months. Allograft rejection is classified as hyperacute rejection, accelerated acute rejection, acute rejection, and chronic rejection.

Hyperacute rejection is due to cytotoxic antibodies, anti-HLA, antivascular endothelium, and isohemagglutinins against ABO antigens. These antibodies cause platelets and fibrin to aggregate, and result in thrombosis of the graft. Onset is within 48 hours of transplant, and can occur immediately after unclamping of vessels. Diagnosis is made by ultrasound, which reveals thrombosis of the graft. Kidney and heart transplants are often involved.

Accelerated acute rejection occurs within 7–10 days. Cellular and humoral-mediated components play a role. There is both antibody involvement with anti-HLA and increased T-lymphocyte activity due to previous sensitization. The rate of allograft loss is high.

Acute rejection generally occurs between 7 and 90 days after transplant. It can be seen, however, any time after discontinuing immunosuppression. Both humoral and cellular mechanisms are involved with antibodies and T-lymphocytes playing a role. There are common symptoms and signs such as graft pain, swelling, warmth, fever, malaise, and fatigue. However, there are specific abnormalities dependent on the organ transplanted. Renal transplant patients will have hypertension, edema, and weight gain. Liver transplant patients have ascites,

hepatosplenomegaly, and elevated transaminases. Cardiac transplant patients may complain of dyspnea, be hypotensive, and develop arrhythmias. Diagnosis is by ultrasound and biopsy; severity is graded on the basis of specific histopathologic findings. Treatment for acute rejections is generally directed by the transplant team but options include corticosteroids, monoclonal anti-T-cell antibody (OKT3), antithymocyte globulin, and plasmapheresis.

Chronic rejection is a slowly progressive decline in function of the allograft and occurs months to years after transplant. The etiology is controversial, but it is characterized by gradual vascular and ductal obliteration, parenchymal atrophy, and interstitial fibrosis. Clinical presentation depends on the organ involved. Kidney transplant patients have hypertension, proteinuria, and elevated creatinine. Lung transplant patients will present with dyspnea, hypoxemia, and abnormal PFTs. Chronic rejection of the liver is associated with jaundice and hyperbilirubinemia. Pancreatic rejection will reveal decreased urinary amylase and hyperglycemia on laboratory studies. Diagnosis is again made by biopsy. There is no effective treatment for chronic rejection.

The improvement in success rate of organ transplant has been possible through the use of cytotoxic chemotherapeutic agents. Many of these primarily induce defects in cell-mediated immunity. Although cell-mediated immunity is responsible for eliminating intracellular pathogens including viruses, these patients are also at risk for a variety of infections from normal flora, community-acquired, and nosocomial organisms. Dividing solid organ transplant on the basis of time since transplant allows us to better predict the pathogens involved.

Susceptibility to life-threatening infections is greatest in the first 6 months after the transplant. During the first month infections are due to bacteria and fungi that typically cause infections in the immunocompetent postsurgical patient. They may be secondary to perioperative illness, IV catheters, endotracheal tube, and infections originating at the surgical site. They tend to be nosocomial, and reflect local sensitivity patterns. Reactivation of latent or subclinical infections of HSV and *M. tuberculosis* can also occur. Between 1 and 6 months pathogens specific to cell-mediated defects play a large role. Viral and opportunistic infections are most common. CMV, EBV, *Pneumocystis carinii*, aspergillosis, *Listeria monocytogenes*, *Toxoplasma gondii*, *Cryptococcus* spp., and others may occur. After 6 months the infections tend to reflect the immunosuppressant state. Those patients on minimal immunosuppression develop infections similar to immunocompetent patients. Those who remain on high-dose immunosuppression continue to be at risk for opportunistic infections. *P. carinii*, *L. monocytogenes*, aspergillosis, *Cryptococcus neoformans*, and various viral infections may play a role (Box 24-5).

is often used. Foscarnet is reserved for the sickest patients because of its nephrotoxicity.

Box 24-5 Pattern of Infections in Solid Organ Transplants

- First 30 days – infections typical of the immuno-competent patient
  - Nosocomial, and reflect local sensitivity patterns
- 30 to 180 days – infections from cell-mediated deficiency play a larger role
  - Viral and opportunistic infections are most common
- After 180 days – reflect immunosuppressant state
  - If on high-dose immunosuppressants then opportunistic infections

---

Treatment strategies consider possible site of infection, pathogen if identified, local sensitivity patterns, and time since transplant. Signs and symptoms of infections should be pursued aggressively. Prevention of viral infections through the use of pretransplant immunization with pneumococcal and hepatitis, and yearly influenza A vaccines should be done. Prophylaxis against opportunistic infections with trimethoprim-sulfamethoxazole (TMP/SMX) for *P. carinii* and nocardia, acyclovir for HSV, ganciclovir for CMV, and flucanazole or ketoconazole for fungal infections is also performed.

CMV infections pose a very common problem in transplant patients. It typically occurs from reactivation of CMV in a seropositive patient, but can be due to a new infection from a CMV-positive organ. It is the most common cause of fever in the post-transplant patient. CMV infections can cause isolated fever, hypotension, hepatitis, pneumonitis, encephalitis, enterocolitis, and glomerulonephritis. Involvement of the transplanted organ occurs frequently. The diagnosis is difficult. Shell vial culture of the buffy coat is useful when prepared less than 24 hours after obtaining a sample. Intranuclear inclusion bodies in cells from biopsied tissue are useful if seen. New techniques using polymerase chain reaction (PCR) are becoming more common. Treatment is with ganciclovir. When organ involvement occurs hyperimmune globulin

---

CLINICAL CAVEAT

Cytomegalovirus Infection
- Most common cause of fever in the post-transplant patient
- Also may have hypotension, hepatitis, pneumonitis, encephalitis, enterocolitis, and glomerulonephritis
- Involvement of transplanted organ frequent
- Diagnose with buffy coat, intranuclear inclusion bodies on biopsy or PCR
- Treat with ganciclovir, occasionally hyperimmune globulin and foscarnet

---

Bone Marrow Transplant Patients

Bone marrow transplants are performed for acute and chronic leukemias, lymphomas, solid tumors, multiple myeloma, and severe aplastic anemia. These patients have a combined alteration in immune function due to both early ablative chemotherapy with its severe neutropenia, and the depression in cell-mediated and humoral immunity mostly from immunosuppressive therapy. After a preparative regimen with ablative chemotherapy and possibly radiation therapy, a profound pancytopenia, ANC < 100 cells/mm^3, for 7–10 days occurs in all patients. The granulocytopenia generally resolves within 30 days, although some phagocytic dysfunction remains. At this point, cell-mediated and humoral dysfunction becomes important. The pattern of infectious complications reflects the sequence and is characterized by three broad time periods (Box 24-6).

The preengraftment period lasts from bone marrow ablation until 30 days post-transplant. It is characterized by ongoing neutropenia and mucositis. Bacterial, fungal, and viral infections similar to other neutropenic patients are common. Treatment is aggressive, with empiric broad-spectrum antibiotic regiments similar to those used for other febrile neutropenic patients. Nearly all patients experience fever during this period, and require empiric antibiotic coverage. Prophylaxis with acyclovir, for HSV and VZV, along with TMP/SMX, for *P. carinii*, is given during this time.

The postengraftment period lasts from 30 to 100 days post-transplant. Neutropenia has recovered, and infections are due mostly to cell-mediated and, to a lesser

---

Box 24-6 Pattern of Infectious Complications in Bone Marrow Transplant Patients

- Preengraftment period – 0 to 30 days: neutropenia and mucositis
  - Bacterial, fungal, and viral – similar to other neutropenic patients
- Postengraftment period – 30 to 100 days: cellular and humoral dysfunction
  - Become susceptible to viral, especially CMV, opportunistic infections
- Late post-transplant period – more than 100 days: persistent cellular and waning humoral dysfunction
  - VZV reactivation and viral respiratory tract infections
  - Susceptibility to encapsulated pathogens remains

degree, humoral defects resulting from the antirejection immunosuppressive therapy. Patients become susceptible to viral infections, especially CMV, other opportunistic infections such as *P. carinii*, *T. gondii*, and aspergillosis, along with other bacterial infections. Treatment requires an aggressive search for a pathogen while broad empiric coverage, including opportunistic coverage, is instituted.

The late post-transplant period occurs after 100 days. Cellular-mediated immune dysfunction is present and late infections due to VZV reactivation and viral respiratory tract infections such as respiratory syncytial virus (RSV), and parainfluenza virus may occur. A humoral defect characterized by a decrease in opsonizing antibodies also persists for years, and predisposes patients to infections with encapsulated pathogens.

Graft versus host disease (GVHD) is an immunologic response by the donor to recipient antigens, and is the major complication of allogenic bone marrow transplants. Acute GVHD occurs within the first 100 days and results in a skin rash that appears first in the hands, feet, and face; large amounts of watery or bloody diarrhea; and liver dysfunction. Chronic GVHD occurs more than 100 days after transplantation and resembles an autoimmune disorder. A dry, itchy rash of the skin with involvement of the face with the mouth and eyes is common. Chronic GVHD substantially increases susceptibility to infections.

Human Immunodeficiency Virus Patients

It is estimated that as of 2002 about 42 million people worldwide and over 1 million people in the USA are infected with HIV. Although the median incubation period appears to be around 10 years, the progression from HIV infection to acquired immunodeficiency syndrome (AIDS) can vary from months to years. Fortunately since the implementation of highly active antiretroviral therapy (HAART) in the USA in 1996, the number of persons diagnosed with AIDS and the number of deaths among persons with AIDS have declined substantially. Not only has the progression of disease been altered, but the mortality of AIDS patients admitted to the intensive care unit (ICU) has also improved. During the early phases of the AIDS epidemic, admission to the ICU for patients with AIDS was associated with very high mortality approaching 90%. Over the years this has improved significantly, with recent survival rates of better than 50%. This improvement in ICU mortality appears to be due to the improved and aggressive use of antiretroviral therapy, prophylaxis, and treatment of opportunistic infections and malignancies and supportive care.

HIV infections and AIDS are caused by the human retrovirus HIV type I. HIV type I infects lymphocytes and other cells carrying the CD_4 surface protein. Screening is performed with an enzyme-linked immunosorbent assay

(ELISA). A positive test is then confirmed by a repeat positive ELISA and a Western blot test. Once a patient is infected with the virus, through either parenteral or sexual transmission, viral replication soon begins. If viral replication is not suppressed, it progressively results in lymphopenia and CD_4 T-cell reduction with impaired cell-mediated immunity. The cell-mediated defects result in the classic picture of opportunistic infections and malignancies. HIV infections, however, may also cause a reduction in immunoglobulin production by B-lymphocytes and cause humoral immune defects. These humoral defects lead to an increased susceptibility to encapsulated organisms such as *S. pneumoniae* and *H. influenzae*. AIDS can subsequently result if the HIV infection advances. AIDS is defined as the presence of an opportunistic infection, malignancy, HIV-related syndrome, or depletion of CD_4 counts (<200 cells/mm^3 or <14% total) in a patient with evidence of HIV infection.

The CD_4 count correlates well with type and site of infections and malignancies found in patients with HIV. PCR assays for HIV type I RNA viral load are also useful to assess clinically the degree of immunosuppression, but are less frequently used. Normal CD_4 count has a wide range, typically considered to be from 500 to 1500 cells/mm^3. In general, the CD_4 count goes down as HIV disease progresses. However, any single CD_4 count value may differ from the last one even though the health status has not changed. Patients with a CD_4 count > 500 cells/mm^3 will have infections from community-acquired organisms. On close examination these patients may have a generalized lymphadenopathy. An increase in the incidence of tuberculosis has also been reported. As the CD_4 count decreases below 500 cells/mm^3 opportunistic infections with esophageal candidiasis, reactivation of HSV and VZV, and bacterial pneumonias such as *S. pneumoniae* appear along with a wasting syndrome comprising of low-grade fever associated with unexplained weight loss. When the count goes below 200 cells/mm^3 the likelihood of *P. carinii* pneumonia (PCP) increases significantly, along with the reactivation of coccidioidomycosis and histoplasmosis leading to disseminated infections. At 50–100 cells/mm^3 CNS infections from *C. neoformans* and *T. gondii* and disseminated *M. tuberculosis* occur. Lymphomas, primarily non-Hodgkin's lymphomas (NHL), can be anticipated as the CD_4 counts decrease and primary CNS lymphomas are increasingly more common as the count decreases to less then 100 cells/mm^3. With CD_4 counts below 50 cells/mm^3, disseminated infections with *M. avium intracellulare*, CMV, cryptosporidia, microsporidia, isospora, and progressive multifocal leukoencephalopathy (PML) from the Jakob Creutzfeldt virus (JCV) can occur.

Pulmonary and CNS infections comprise two of the most common causes of ICU admissions. Pneumonias with

CLINICAL CAVEAT

CD$_4$ Count
- Correlates with type and site of infection in HIV/AIDS patients
- Normal 500 to 1500, although individual variations exist
- As CD$_4$ < 500 – opportunistic infections
  - Esophageal candidiasis, reactivation of HSV, VZV
  - *S. pneumoniae*
  - Wasting syndrome
- As CD$_4$ < 200
  - PCP increases significantly
  - Reactivation of coccidioidomycosis and histoplasmosis
- As CD$_4$ < 50 disseminated infections
  - MAI, CMV, cryptosporidia, microsporidia, isospora
  - PML from JCV

CLINICAL CAVEAT

***Pneumocystis carinii* Pneumonia**
- Most common infection and the leading cause of death in AIDS
- Progressive, nonproductive cough with dyspnea and hypoxemia
- Interstitial pneumonia and CD$_4$ < 200 cells/mm^3
- Induced sputum or BAL
- Treatment:
  - TMP/SMX or pentamidine
  - Steroids with PaO$_2$ < 70 mmHg or a PAO$_2$-PaO$_2$ gradient > 35 mmHg; steroids improve survival
  - Aggressive supportive care

S. pneumoniae are common in HIV-positive patients. Opportunistic infections with *M. tuberculosis*, histoplasmosis, coccidioidomycosis, CMV (with CD$_4$ count < 50 cells/mm^3), and *P. carinii* in particular become increasingly common as the CD$_4$ decreases. PCP is the leading cause of death in AIDS patients. As a result prophylaxis typically with TMP/SMX or pentamidine for PCP is instituted when the CD$_4$ count is <200 cells/mm^3. Progressive respiratory failure with fever, hypoxemia, and diffuse pulmonary infiltrates requires an aggressive assessment. Induced sputum has a 70–90% sensitivity for *P. carinii*. A bronchiolar lavage (BAL) is indicated if a sample does not yield a diagnosis. Empiric antibiotic coverage on the basis of a CD$_4$ count should be started. Treatment with TMP/SMX with pentamidine as an alternative is indicated for 21 days. Prednisone or an equivalent should be started at 40 mg bid and tapered over the 21 days of treatment in patients with PaO$_2$ < 70 mmHg or a PAO$_2$-PaO$_2$ gradient > 35 mmHg. This regimen has been shown to improve survival in patients with severe PCP. The lung can also be affected by lymphoid interstitial pneumonitis which is believed to be due to direct HIV infection to the lung. It is a nonspecific interstitial pneumonitis that resembles PCP, but the CD$_4$ is between 200 and 500 cells/mm^3 and the BAL is negative for PCP. Treatment is with HAART and steroids are added by many if symptoms progress. Some patients become oxygen dependent.

CNS infections such as brain abscess, meningitis, and encephalitis along with primary CNS lymphomas and NHL involvement of the brain may result in admission to the ICU. Patients at risk or known to have HIV disease who present with altered mental status require an aggressive evaluation including computed tomography (CT) scan or magnetic resonance imaging (MRI) of the brain, and lumbar puncture for cerebrospinal fluid analysis. Empiric antibiotic coverage is initiated on the basis of the clinical picture while awaiting results. *C. neoformans* will require amphotericin B, *T. gondii* is treated with sulfadiazine/pyrimethamine along with leucovorin (to prevent hematologic toxicity), and *M. tuberculosis* is treated with various evolving regimens. PML from the JCV can occur, and results in a clinical picture of mental status changes, weakness, and disorders of gait. A characteristic picture of white matter lesions is present on MRI. Antiretroviral therapy has improved the outcome of PML. CNS lymphomas are treated with chemotherapy and radiation therapy. Although not the cause of ICU admissions, CMV retinitis occurs in 85% of AIDS patients and can lead to significant morbidity. It is treated with ganciclovir which may lead to neutropenia. Other drugs such as AZT may similarly be myelotoxic. Treatment with neupogen (G-CSF) may be beneficial.

DRUG INTERACTIONS

Gancyclovir
- Commonly used in AIDS patients
- Causes neutropenia which exacerbates that caused by AZT and HIV itself
- Treat with neupogen to maintain ANC of 1000-2000/mm^3

There are several other organs that may be involved with HIV/AIDS that may have an impact on the care of the critically ill patient. While some of these are a direct result of secondary opportunistic infections, the mechanisms for others are not known. Cardiomyopathy is well described and in fact 8% of HIV patients have a dilated cardiomyopathy on echocardiogram. Subclinical cardiac abnormalities are common and correlate with the degree of immune suppression. Treatment with angiotensin converting enzyme (ACE) inhibitors is often prescribed and diuretics and digitalis can be added for symptomatic left ventricular disease. Nephropathy can occur and is commonly characterized on biopsy as a focal segmental glomerulosclerosis. Patients present with nephrosis and can have a rapid course to end-stage renal disease in 1 to 4 months. Response to antiretroviral therapy HAART has been reported by clinical and biopsy data. ACE inhibitors are useful and the response to steroids is variable. Adrenal gland involvement appears to occur commonly. It has been documented in up to two-thirds of HIV patients on postmortem studies with CMV infection found in up to 80% of cases. The frequent incidence of adrenal gland involvement is reinforced by studies examining the hypothalamus–pituitary–adrenal (HPA) axis in HIV/AIDS patients. Although many of these patients are typically asymptomatic, unexplained hypotension or hypotension out of proportion to the clinical picture should warrant an examination of the HPA axis. Treatment with supplemental or replacement steroids during periods of stress may be warranted. Some of the other organs involved include the gastrointestinal tract with mouth ulcers, gingivitis, esophagitis, anorexia, nausea/vomiting, and profuse diarrhea; hepatobiliary tract with papillary strictures, papillary stenosis, pancreatitis, and hepatitis B and C; hematologic system with anemia, neutropenia, idiopathic thrombocytopenic purpura (ITP), and thrombotic thrombocytopenic purpura (TTP); and the nervous system with peripheral neuropathy, myopathy, and HIV-associated dementia.

SUMMARY

An understanding of the pathophysiology involved in the immune-compromised patient is crucial in not only anticipating the clinical course of the disease process but also in diagnosing infections and noninfectious complications and choosing appropriate therapy. These patients may present with subtle, atypical signs and symptoms which may progress rapidly to life-threatening situations. Yet there are patterns related to the specific deficiency, the time since onset, the time since transplant, and even specific "markers" such as ANC and CD_4 count which gives the clinician information to better choose treatment. By understanding these diseases with their particular patterns we may thus be able to choose timely, aggressive treatment and improve outcome.

CASE STUDY

A 51-year-old patient is referred to you for management and admission to the ICU because of hypotension unresponsive to volume resuscitation. The patient is now 11 days post a stem cell transplant for acute myeloid leukemia. The patient previously had undergone induction chemotherapy with ara-c and daunorubicin and was in remission prior to the transplant. On examination the patient is anxious, diaphoretic, febrile to 39.9°C, tachycardic with a heart rate of 130 regular, and a hypotensive at 83/49. Physical examination aside from disclosing mild cachexia and mucositis with mouth ulcers is otherwise unremarkable.

QUESTIONS

1. What laboratory workup would you request?
2. What would you expect to find?
3. What are the possible causes of hypotension in this patient?
4. How likely are you to find the organism and definitive site of infection?
5. What antibiotic coverage would you chose?

SELECTED READING

Barbaro G et al: Incidence of dilated cardiomyopathy and detection of HIV in myocardial cells of HIV-positive patients. N Eng J Med 339:1093–1099, 1998.

Braunwald E et al, editors: *Harrison's Principles of Internal Medicine*, ed 15, New York: McGraw-Hill, 2001.

CDC: HIV Infection and AIDS in the United States. Semi Annual HIV/AIDS Surveillance Report. Vol 15, 2003.

CDC: Update: The AIDS epidemic in the United States. MMWR. 51:592–595, 2002.

Goldman L et al, editors: *Cecil Textbook of Medicine*, ed 21, Philadelphia: WB Saunders, 2000.

Humphreys MH et al: Human immunodeficiency virus-associated glomerulosclerosis. Kidney Int 48:311–320, 1995.

Mayo J et al: Adrenal function in the human immunodeficiency virus-infected patient. Arch Intern Med 162:1095–1098, 2002.

Murray M et al; ASCCA, editors: *Critical Care Medicine: Perioperative Management*, ed 2, Philadelphia: Lippincott Williams and Wilkins, 2002.

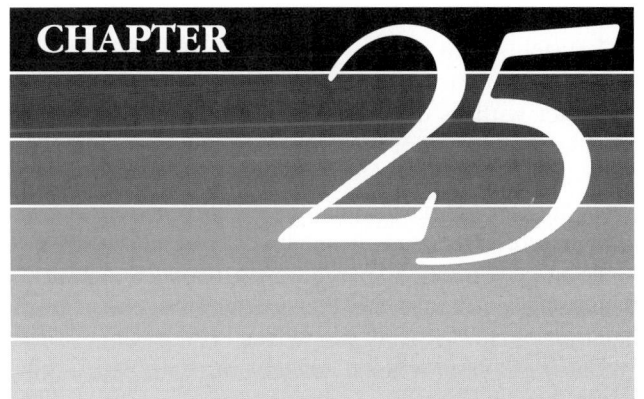

CHAPTER 25

Coagulation and Disseminated Intravascular Coagulation

PER A. J. THORBORG, M.D., Ph.D.

LYNN K. BOSHKOV, M.D.

PHYSIOLOGY AND DEVELOPMENT OF THE COAGULATION

Hemostasis is achieved through a three-phase process: primary hemostasis (minutes) where activated platelets form a platelet plug, secondary hemostasis (hours) reinforces the frail platelet plug with fibrin strands, and fibrinolysis (days) dissolves the clot after vascular wall repair. This system is volume controlled by several modulators such as antithrombin (AT), the thrombomodulin (TM)/protein C (PC) and protein S (PS) system, and tissue factor pathway inhibitor (TFPI).

In the last ten years a revised coagulation concept, based on new understanding of secondary hemostasis and its modulation, has replaced the in vitro-based "coagulation cascade" concept presented in 1964 by Davie, Ratnoff, and MacFarlane. These new insights include the regulatory role of the vascular endothelium as well as the links between inflammation and coagulation. Loss of the normal modulation of the coagulation in, for example, sepsis, is now believed to contribute to multisystem organ

failure (MSOF), the most common cause of death in the intensive care unit (ICU).

Endothelial cells are normally antiadhesive (by release of nitric oxide (NO), prostacycline (PGI$_2$), adenosine, and interleukin-10 (IL-10)), antithrombotic (due to expression of TM, heparans, and TFPI), and fibrinolytic (by secretion of tissue plasminogen activator (tPA)). The underlying smooth muscle tone is predominantly relaxed due to release of vasodilators such as NO and PGI$_2$ opposing endothelin (ET-1), a polypeptide that is predominantly vasoconstrictive. The damaged endothelium exhibits the opposite characteristics. Vasoconstriction by serotonin (5-HT) and thromboxane (TxA$_2$) from activated platelets serves to limit local blood loss after trauma. Primary hemostasis is primed due to release of von Willebrand factor (vWF), activation of platelet-activating factor (PAF), and release of IL-8 and P-selectins. Secondary hemostasis is promoted by release of tissue factor (TF) and by exposure of phosphatidylserine (from lipids in cell membranes), which can mimic the activated platelet surface (platelet factor 3, PF3). Endothelium released plasminogen activator inhibitor (PAI-1) will inhibit tPA, which promotes deposits of fibrin. The activated endothelium allows adhesion molecules to bind and activated white blood cells (WBCs), attracted by inflammatory mediators, migrate out into the tissues and eventually set the stage for tissue repair. It has become clear that the endothelium itself is a crucial regulator of the different stages of hemostasis, and also that inflammation is a necessary component of tissue repair.

The primary hemostasis is initiated by activation of platelets that undergo a conformational change from discoid shape to irregular shape with multiple pseudopods, release of secretions (containing vWF, FV, FVIII, Ca^{2+}, 5-HT, fibrinogen, ADP, TxA$_2$) from granules, and extrusion of several types of domains with glycoprotein receptors, as the Ib (GPIb) and IIb/IIIa (GPIIb/IIIa) receptors. ADP as well as TxA$_2$ promote platelet activation. Other strong

261

activators are thrombin, PAF, and immune complexes. Exposed collagen permits the platelet to attach to the site of injury using its GPIb receptor and an intermediary vWF molecule that allows binding to the site of injury. Activated platelets form a three-dimensional plug using their GPIIb/IIIa receptors and intermediary fibrinogen molecules. The activated platelets expose a phospholipid surface, PF3, which will become the catalytic center for the secondary hemostasis.

The secondary hemostasis is most commonly triggered by appearance of TF in the blood, normally a membrane-bound small protein not in direct contact with blood, that when combined with circulating FVIIa can activate FIX and FX in the extrinsic tenase complex, enough to form a small amount of thrombin. This initial thrombin formation serves to activate the platelet, but is too small for substantial fibrin formation. On the activated platelets, the prothrombinase complex is the catalytic center where FXa and FVa generate the first thrombin. Further thrombin feedback by activation of FVIII, FIX, and FXI in the intrinsic tenase complex serves to produce larger amounts of thrombin required for fibrin production. It appears that a substantial "thrombin burst" is required to form enough fibrin to stabilize the platelet clot, the more thrombin the more stable the clot. Formed fibrin is then cross-linked by FXIII, increasing clot strength. In this process the activated FVIII sheds its carrier protein vWF that is used in the initial platelet adhesion.

The major new understanding is the role of thrombin, which, once formed, maintains its own production for the prothrombinase complex, and the extrinsic tenase complex is no longer needed. Note that calcium is needed as a bridge to anchor the activated prothrombinase complex and intrinsic tenase complex to the PF3 surface in order to reach critical concentration of activated factors for reactions to occur. In patients treated with Coumadine, the calcium-binding site is no longer exposed on factors II, VII, IX, and X, so calcium cannot anchor these factors to the catalytic site. Secondly, phospholipid membranes are necessary for these catalytic reactions to take place, either normally on activated platelets (PF3) or after endothelial injury as phosphatidylserine sites appear on cell membranes of damaged endothelial cells.

Several important modulating systems control secondary hemostasis. First, TFPI rapidly inactivates the extrinsic tenase complex after it activates FX. In disseminated intravascular coagulation (DIC), however, this does not appear to be an effective pathway to neutralize large amounts of TF. New data indicate that heparin stimulates the release of TFPI and that a significant part (1/3) of the heparin effect is mediated through this pathway. The second important modulator is AT, formerly called ATIII, which inactivates thrombin as well as FXa, FIXa, and FXIa. Heparan, a naturally occurring glucosaminoglycan, is the physiologic stimulant of this system, increasing the

speed of inactivation. The third modulating system is the PC system, activated by the large cell surface-bound molecule TM after TM is activated by thrombin. PC then together with its cofactor PS inactivate FVa and FVIIIa. Deficiencies in any of these three modulating systems, as by consumption in DIC, or as a genetic predisposition, can contribute to prothrombotic states of varying severity.

Fibrinolysis occurs normally several hours to days later by activation of plasminogen to plasmin by tPA. Plasmin then degrades fibrin (and fibrinogen) to fibrin split products (FSP), also known as FDP. Plasmin's physiologic modulator is alpha$_2$-antiplasmin with high affinity for its catalytic site (when not occupied by fibrin). PAI-1 inactivates tPA and thereby controls the degree of activation of fibrinolysis. A distinction is sometimes made between normal (secondary) plasma-activated fibrinolysis (by tPA) and abnormal (primary) clot-activated fibrinolysis that may appear after burns and prostate and neurosurgery, and after streptokinase or urokinase therapy. When plasmin lyses a clot with cross-linked fibrin, small segments that can be analyzed with the D-dimer test are formed. Of historical interest is that activation of the contact system with FXII will also induce fibrinolysis through activation of pre-kallikrein to kallikrein and eventually plasminogen to plasmin.

The development of the coagulation system in vertebrates has occurred over the last 1.5 billion years. In pre-vertebrates there was only an antibacterial system where intruders were marked for phagocytosis by coagulation of an early version of fibrinogen on their surface. With the development of a closed vascular system in the first vertebrates, separate immune and coagulant systems eventually developed, initially the contact system with FXII. Studies have revealed that genes coding for coagulation factors are derived from cytokine genes. With the development of vertebrates, three main families of serine proteases have undergone 10–12 generations of change, the last 8 generations in vertebrates. The first family was the ancestors to FXII, TPA, PC, thrombin, TF, and the complement system. The second family was factors VII, IX, X, XI, and kallikrein. The third family stems from the development of an ancestor to ceruloplasmin that led to FVIII and FV. The clinical interest this has today is that it explains the commonly observed problem of cross-activation of systems such that many mediators of inflammation cause activation of the coagulation and vice versa.

PATHOPHYSIOLOGY OF DISSEMINATED INTRAVASCULAR COAGULATION

In DIC increased TF exposure will induce a prothrombotic state with initially normal fibrinogen and platelet levels, sometimes referred to as compensated DIC.

Increased fibrinolysis lyzes the increased fibrin clot load until increasing levels of PAI-1 inhibits plasmin. If the speed of consumption of coagulation products progresses beyond liver (coagulation products) and bone marrow (platelets) production capacity, the patient becomes hypocoagulable, sometimes referred to as decompensated DIC. Platelet counts and fibrinogen levels are then decreased below normal levels. It is believed that large deposition of fibrin in the microvasculature leads to local hypoperfusion (patchy ischemia), MSOF, and, ultimately, organ failure and death. DIC can present with differing speed varying from explosive (acute) to slow (chronic) onset.

One of the most common causes for acute DIC is sepsis, where it occurs in 30–50% of patients, regardless of the cause for sepsis (Box 25-1). Delayed resuscitation from shock can lead to endothelial cell injury making the patient procoagulant. In extensive crush injury, particularly in head injury with release of thromboplastin, and in fat embolism 50–70% can be shown to have DIC. Acute leukemias (particularly acute promyelocytic leukemia) and metastatic prostatic carcinomas are frequently (15%) associated with DIC development. In abruptio placenta, abortion, amniotic fluid embolism, hemorrhage, and shocked obstetric patients 50% develop DIC. In contrast, only 7% of preeclamptic patients have DIC. Many immunologic disorders develop DIC, including thrombotic thrombocytopenic purpura (TTP), HELLP (hemolysis, elevated liver enzymes, and low platelets) syndrome, and transfusion and transplant reactions. In newborns with a congenital homozygous PC deficiency, purpura fulminans with DIC can be life-threatening. Reactions to toxins, either drugs or snake or spider bites, can lead to DIC. Prothrombin complex solutions formerly used in life-threatening emergencies to stop a catastrophic bleeding can induce DIC, as opposed to rVIIa.

In contrast, chronic DIC occurs predominantly in some types of cancer, aortic aneurysms, and giant cavernous hemangiomas (Kasabach–Merritt syndrome), dead fetus in utero, and in chronic infections such as tuberculosis, abscess, and osteomyelitis. Chronic DIC can be asymptomatic or present as prothrombotic state with deep venous thrombosis (DVT) and pulmonary embolism (PE). Chronic inflammatory bowel disease such as Crohn's disease and ulcerative colitis can be associated with slow-onset DIC. Cancers can express either TF or a direct activator of FX (Box 25-2).

In sepsis and systemic inflammatory response syndrome (SIRS) release of IL-6 has been shown to up-regulate TF while release of tumor necrosis factor-α (TNF-α) down-regulates TM as well as up-regulates PAI-1. This produces a procoagulant state while at the same time the modulators through the PC/PS system are down-regulated and fibrinolysis is suppressed through release of PAI-1. This common inflammatory response pattern produces the compensated DIC state described above. Several prospective studies have shown that DIC with sepsis or trauma doubles the risk of death.

Box 25-1   Key Etiologies in Acute Disseminated Intravascular Coagulation

- Sepsis
- Delayed shock resuscitation
- Trauma
- Certain cancers
- Obstetric complications
- Preeclampsia
- Immunologic disorders
- Extensive burns
- Vasculitis
- Certain blood products
- Newborn purpura fulminans
- Toxins

Box 25-2   Key Etiologies in Chronic Disseminated Intravascular Coagulation

- Cancer
- Vascular
- Obstetric
- Chronic infections
- Inflammatory bowel disease

CONGENITAL HYPOCOAGULABLE STATES

The most common congenital hypocoagulable state (1% of the population, autosomal dominant) is von Willebrand's disease (vWD), of which three major types exist. Type I, present in >70%, has a quantitative decrease in normally shaped vWF molecules. Many patients are unaware of their mild disease until trauma or surgery. The levels of vWF are sensitive to the estrogen level, and some female patients present with perimenopausal bleeding problems. Complicating genetic workup in these patients is the variability of the disease penetrance. Type II has several subtypes with variable structural abnormalities of the vWF, e.g., type 2N resembles type II with low FVIII levels. Type III is much rarer but severe with undetectable levels of vWF in plasma. Since vWF is the carrier protein for FVIII, this group of patients may clinically appear to have hemophilia A and are usually detected earlier in life. Detection is usually by long BT, workup is with FVIII levels, vW antigen, Ristocetin cofactor activity, while immunoelectropheresis helps subtype vWD (Box 25-3).

Box 25-3   Congenital Hypocoagulable States

- vWD (types I, II, and III)
- Hemophilia A, B, and C
- Bernard–Soulier syndrome and Glanzmann's thrombasthenia
- Inborn platelet abnormalities
- Isolated coagulation factor deficiency
- Dysfibrinogenemias
- Alpha$_2$-antiplasmin deficiency

Treatment modalities vary by type. In pregnancy, levels of vWF increase dramatically, and type I patients do not require therapy at delivery. In general, 1-deamino-8-D-arginine vasopressin (DDAVP) (0.3 µg/kg over 30 minutes) is the mainstay therapy for Type I. Most of the Type IIs and Type III require FVIII (virally inactivated Humate-P), based on FVIII levels.

Patients with hemophilia A, B, and C have a variable deficiency in FVIII, FIX, and FXI, respectively. Of the hemophiliac types, 85% are type A, 14% type B, and 1% type C. Mild deficiency is present when the patient has factor levels above 5%, moderate at 1–5%, and severe at <1%. Hemophilia A and B are X chromosome-linked diseases that affect 1 in 10,000 males, while C is an autosomal recessive disease. These problems are usually detected early in life. Activated partial thromboplastin time (APTT) is typically prolonged while prothrombin time (PT) and thrombin time (TT) are normal. Diagnosis is established by measuring plasma levels of factors VIII, IX, or XI.

Preoperative treatment of hemophilia A consists of FVIII level-driven replacement every 12 hours (levels kept >50% first postoperative week), hemophilia B requires FIX concentrate every 24 hours, and hemophilia C requires fresh frozen plasma (FFP). Approximately 10% of hemophilia A patients have developed antibodies to FVIII, and may require rFVIIa that bypasses the FVIII step on the activated platelet. Mild hemophilia A may also respond well to DDAVP. Recombinant FVIII decreases the risk for viral transmission to these patients, but is more expensive at this time. A significant number of these patients have contracted hepatitis B and/or C and/or HIV from repeated transfusions in the past.

Two congenital forms of thrombocytopathy are Bernard–Soulier syndrome (defective GPIb receptor) and Glanzmann's thrombasthenia (defective GPIIb/IIIa receptor). They are both uncommon and can be identified by platelet aggregation studies. Some of these patients respond to DDAVP, and may require platelets for ongoing bleeding.

Other rare inherited types include other inborn platelet abnormalities conferring platelet dysfunction (but normal numbers) or congenital thrombocytopenia with large, small, or normally sized platelets. Isolated factor deficiencies as well as alpha$_2$-antiplasmin deficiency are also rare. Dysfibrinogenemias may be hereditary or acquired, and can be associated with either a bleeding or a thrombotic propensity.

ACQUIRED HYPOCOAGULABLE STATES

Continuous activation of coagulation and/or down-regulation of its modulation or fibrinolysis can lead to a hypocoagulable state. Acquired states are more common in the older population (Box 25-4).

Acquired thrombocytopenia (<150,000/µl) can be the result of impaired production, increased destruction (immune or nonimmune causes), or sequestration. Impaired production is found in aplastic and myeloproliferative disorders, as a result of drugs or toxins (chemotherapy, radiation), in viral illness (HIV, AIDS), and also in vitamin B$_{12}$ and folate deficiency. Increased destruction from immune causes includes TTP and hemolytic-uremic syndrome (TTP-HUS; lack of protease activity cleaving large vWF multimers, producing fever, schistocytes, tissue ischemia, anemia, ARF, fluctuating mental state), idiopathic thrombocytopenic purpura (ITP; afebrile, autoAb to GPIIb/IIIa receptor), isoantibodies in post-transfusion purpura (in women sensitized during pregnancy, lacking the PL-A1 Ag), other immune complex disorders (systemic lupus erythematosus, SLE), as well as in drug-induced thrombocytopenia (heparin: 3% heparin-induced

---

Box 25-4   Acquired Hypocoagulable States

- DIC
- Acquired thrombocytopenia
- Acquired platelet dysfunction
- Drug induced
- Uremia
- Hepatic dysfunction
- Massive transfusion
- Transfusion reaction
- Cardiopulmonary bypass
- Vitamin K deficiency
- Hypocalcemia
- Inhibitors to clotting factors (II, V, VII, VIII, X)
- Lupus-type inhibitors
- Primary fibrinolysis
- Hypothermia
- Dilutional
- Leukemia
- Polycythemia vera

thrombocytopenia (HIT)/1% HIT with thrombosis (HITT); quinidine, cimetidine, ranitidine, sulfa, vancomycin).

Nonimmune-related mechanisms occur in DIC, cardio-pulmonary bypass, and hypersplenism.

Massive transfusion (>10 U/24 hours) can lead to thrombocytopenia from blood loss and failure to replace platelets as well as from dilution (platelets and coagulation factors) associated with massive fluid resuscitation.

Thrombocytopenia in acquired thrombocytopenia can be treated with platelet infusions if there is a bleeding problem except in the contraindicated states of TTP-HUS, HIT/HITT, and the presence of platelet antibodies. Drugs known to induce thrombocytopenia should be discontinued.

Dysfunctional platelets (thrombocytopathy) are less common than low platelet count but may be present with normal platelet count or with thrombocytopenia. Acquired forms are uremia, postcardiopulmonary bypass, malignant paraproteinemia (Waldenstrom, multiple myeloma), hypothermia, after antiplatelet therapy (ticlopidine, clopidogrel, abciximab, tirofiban, eptifibatide), or after other drugs (COX and TxA_2 inhibitors, CCB, H_2-receptor antagonists, PCN, cephalosporin, dextran, starch, gelatins, NTP, NTG). Treatment is to identify and deal with the underlying condition or drug. DDAVP may be helpful. Platelet transfusion into a toxic environment may make the platelets rapidly dysfunctional.

Drug-induced hypocoagulable states can be found in patients on various types of anticoagulants, after rat poison intoxication, and in patients on fibrinolytic drugs. See also under acquired thrombocytopenia and thrombocytopathy for drug-induced problems. The drug should be stopped, and correction carried out with blood products and high doses of vitamin K in the case of rat poison intoxication.

In liver failure variable impairment of the production of coagulation factors is often associated with hypersplenism, low platelet counts, and decreased clearing of FDPs and PAI leading to platelet dysfunction and impaired fibrinolysis. Fibrinogen production is usually well maintained until end-stage liver disease. FFP may be required, and vitamin K should always be given. Anemia may be present when bleeding varices. When exposed to trauma or extensive surgery, massive transfusion scenarios often ensue. Release of thromboplastin can cause DIC. One should plan for good venous access and frequent laboratory findings to guide replacement therapy.

The patient with renal failure may have associated bone marrow failure leading to thrombocytopenia, and this type of patient often additionally has a chronic anemia. Uremia confers a platelet dysfunction that is reversible with dialysis. Acute renal failure frequently has a component of associated low-grade DIC. Heparin overdosing is common for dialysis patients, and heparin may need to be neutralized with protamine or with FFP. DDAVP can temporarily (day)

improve platelet function by release of vWF. Conjugated estrogens (dose 0.6 mg/kg for 5 days) have a longer duration of action (weeks) but the response comes slower than after DDAVP. Erythropoietin is frequently used to raise hemoglobin in this type of patient.

Massive transfusion is defined as transfusion of >10 U blood/24 hours. Coagulation problems are usually rare with loss of less than one blood volume unless the patient has a preexisting coagulation problem. After loss of more than one blood volume thrombocytopenia and coagulation factor deficiencies are common. Risks include hypothermia, under-resuscitation leads to hypovolemia, while over-resuscitation may lead to dilution of coagulation factors and platelets. Hypocalcemia results from chelation by ACD (citrate) in blood bags. Blood products replacement must be based on frequent laboratory findings, possibly thromboelastograph (TEG). All fluids except platelets should go through high-capacity fluid warmers. The blood bank should be contacted early. Damage control is an alternative procedure for the patient where surgical hemostasis is difficult or impossible.

In hypothermia a reversible platelet dysfunction occurs due to decreased TxA_2 and other platelet enzymatic activities. Hypothermia is also associated with enhanced fibrinolytic activity. Acidosis depresses platelet aggregation, fibrinogen levels fall, and FDP increases. The triad of hypothermia, coagulopathy, and acidosis has been called "the triangle of death." All these changes are reversible with correction of hypothermia. The patient should be warmed actively with a warmed air convection blanket, in addition to fluid warmers.

In cardiopulmonary bypass platelet dysfunction from degranulation, loss of GP receptors, hypothermia, and heparin- and protamin-induced malfunction add to consumptive dysfunction of primary and secondary hemostasis. Additionally, cytokine-activated TF expression and increased primary fibrinolysis and decreased alpha$_2$-antiplasmin add to the scenario to create a complex state. Basically, all three steps of the hemostatic response are affected. This may explain why 29% of patients on cardiopulmonary bypass bleed excessively, part of which is due to platelet dysfunction. In addition to perioperative heparinization there is sometimes need for inhibition of a primary fibrinolysis as well as for fresh platelets. This is particularly indicated when risk for bleeding is higher as in repeat cardiac surgery, underlying coagulation abnormality, or after aspirin ingestion the last week.

Antifibrinolytic therapy may be required in a variety of situations including cardiopulmonary bypass, and after tonsillectomy and gynecological and prostate surgery. Both FDP and D-dimers will be high, while other laboratory findings depend on the extent of the bleeding. Two groups of fibrinolytics are available. The lysine derivates (aminocaproic acid 5 g bolus followed by a 1 g/hour infusion; tranexamic acid 10–15 mg/kg every 8 hours) prevent plasminogen binding to fibrin(ogen) at the lysine site and activation to plasmin. They have been shown to reduce postoperative blood loss after prostate surgery, after dental extraction in hemophiliacs and anticoagulated patients, and reduce blood loss in cardiopulmonary bypass by 30–40%. Aminocaproic acid has also been shown to reduce blood loss in liver transplantation. The main complication with this type of drug is thrombosis. Aminocaproic acid is also US FDA approved for hereditary angioneurotic edema.

The second group of antifibrinolytics is the serine protease inhibitor aprotinin which inhibits TF, FXII, and kallikrein, in addition to plasmin. In high dose the concern has been that it may also inhibit PC and make the patient hypercoagulable. Aprotinin (low dose 1 million KIU bolus plus 1 million in pump prime and 250,000 KIU/hour) has been shown to be more effective in reducing blood loss (than lysine derivates) in coronary artery bypass grafting, valves, endocarditis, and heart transplantation, as well as in patients who took aspirin before surgery. Extracted from bovine lung, there has been some concern in Italy of transmission of bovine spongiform encephalopathy and Creutzfeldt–Jakob disease to humans.

INCREASED RISK FOR THROMBOSIS (THROMBOPHILIA)

This is a larger problem from a hospital perspective than bleeding since it affects a large part of the patient population and the consequences are longstanding and expensive. A patient with a DVT or PE may be on warfarin medication for 6 months.

There are a number of both acquired and inherited states that increase the risk for DVT and PE. The most common inherited disorders include PC deficiency, PS deficiency, AT deficiency, FV Leiden, prothrombin mutation, dysfibrinogenemia, and elevated homocystein levels. The most common acquired hypercoagulable states are extensive trauma (particularly the first 24 hours), head trauma, surgery and immobilization, vasculitis (SLE), lupus anticoagulants, DIC (sepsis), cancer, TTP-HUS, drugs (antifibrinolytics, iatrogenic hyperfibrinogenemia, heparin (HIT/HITT), warfarin (if PC/PS deficient), oral contraceptives, chemotherapy) (Box 25-5).

Immune-type HIT occurs in 3% of heparin-treated patients, and one-third of these patients go on to develop HITT, sometimes with life-threatening consequences. This has been shown to be caused by the formation of an IgG type antibody (some patients have IgA or IgM antibodies) against a heparin–platelet factor 4 complex. There is a small cross-reactivity with low molecular weight heparin (LMWH), which should not be used in these patients.

Box 25-5   Inherited and Acquired States that Increase the Risk for DVT and PE

CONGENITAL HYPERCOAGULABLE STATE
- Factor V Leiden
- PC deficiency
- PS deficiency
- AT deficiency
- Prothrombin mutation
- Dysfribrinogenemia
- Elevated homocystein level

ACQUIRED HYPERCOAGULABLE STATE
- Trauma
- Surgery
- Immobilization
- Vasculitis
- APLA syndrome
- Sepsis with DIC
- Cancer
- TTP-HUS
- Drugs

Direct thrombin antagonists like hirudin (0.4 mg/bolus, infusion 0.15 mg/kg/hour), recombinant hirudin (lepirudin dose 0.4 mg/kg max. 44 mg then 0.15 mg/kg/hour max. 16.5 mg/hour), or synthetic AT (argatroban dose 2 µg/kg/minute) appear to be effective and safe but should be managed by a hematologist. Dosing is usually checked by APTT.

Antiphospholipid antibody (APLA) syndrome consists of the presence of antibodies against certain phospholipids associated with a hypercoagulable state, sometimes thrombocytopenia, repeated fetal loss, stroke, and dementia. A detailed knowledge of the underlying pathology is lacking. Primary APLA syndrome is the diagnosis when SLE is not a patient diagnosis, otherwise called lupus anticoagulant or lupus inhibitor. Chlorpromazine, dilantin, and quinidine are also known to induce APLA. They can develop both venous and arterial thrombosis already at young age. These patients have an elevated APTT and sometimes PT. Heparin treatment appears more effective than warfarin. Anticoagulation with heparin or LMWH is necessary for surgery, problematic after trauma.

Practice guidelines for management of these patients have been published recently (see Selected Reading). Management options include sequential compression devices, aspirin, LMWH (prophylaxis: enoxaparin 30 mg q 12 hours; therapeutically 1 mg/kg q 12 hours: anti-Xa 0.3–0.6), heparin (prophylaxis: 5000 sq q 8 hours; therapeutically 80 U/kg bolus and then infusion to keep APTT 1.5-2.5 times normal), and warfarin (prophylaxis: 1-5 mg po qd; therapeutically 5-10 mg/day: international normalized ratio (INR) 2-3 use heparin initially), as well as inferior vena cava (IVC) filter for those patients where anticoagulation is perceived as too high of a risk. IVC filter may actually increase the risk for DVT (if no anticoagulation) but should decrease the risk for PE from lower parts of the body.

Thrombolytic therapy may be indicated in patients experiencing DVT, hemodynamically unstable PE, acute myocardial infarction (MI), peripheral arterial occlusion, and ischemic stroke. The alternatives include tPA (bolus plus infusion: dose by indication), streptokinase (250,000 U for 24-72 hours by indication), and urokinase (4400 U/kg loading plus 4400 U/kg/hour for 12 hours) all followed by heparin. Contraindications for their use are recent surgery, head trauma, hemorrhagic stroke, and active bleeding. A major complication is bleeding, particularly intracranial bleeding.

CLINICAL FINDINGS IN COAGULOPATHY

Petechia on skin and mucous membranes or spontaneous gingival or epistaxial bleeding suggest an abnormal primary hemostasis, most commonly due to low platelet number or abnormal platelet function. It can also be associated with hypofibrinogenemia due to slow platelet plug formation. Patients with Type I vWD typically present with these symptoms, or with a large postoperative hematoma. Type II and III may present with a hemophiliac-type bleeding.

Overt bleeding as in hematochezia, melena, hematemesis, blood in NGT, bleeding from previously dry surgical incisions or wounds, hematuria, hemoptysis, bleeding from vascular catheter sites, hemarthrosis, and muscle, brain, or subcutaneous bleeding suggest a defect in the secondary hemostasis. Hemophiliacs typically present with hemarthrosis and muscle or brain bleeding.

Acute DIC patients bleed from multiple sites, display skin and mucous membrane ecchymoses, and signs of tissue ischemia. Petechia are commonly seen in thrombocytopenia accompanying decompensated DIC, the first usually found under the blood pressure cuff. The dead fetus situation in chronic DIC may show the signs of acute DIC.

Commonly, occult bleeding manifests with hemodynamic instability and falling hematocrit, such as in retroperitoneal bleeding, postoperative bleeding with clotted drains, hemothorax, intra-abdominal bleeding, and pelvic or femoral hemorrhage.

Fibrinolysis-associated bleeding occurs mostly in specific settings (see above), but also in liver failure. See also under DIC.

Trousseau described the association between cancer and DVT, but half of his patients also had tuberculosis. Chronic DIC patients usually present with DVT, PE, or arterial embolism, sometimes recurring and in multiple locations.

LABORATORY FINDINGS IN COAGULOPATHY

A particular laboratory may have established reference values that may be slightly different from the values cited below. The reference values of a local laboratory should be used when in doubt. In general a laboratory should be able to provide a complete blood count (including a platelet count), PT INR, partial thromboplastin time (PTT), and fibrinogen within 20-30 minutes. Table 25-1 lists some common causes of abnormal coagulation parameters and typical patterns of associated coagulation abnormalities.

Low platelet count (normal 150,000-400,000) is more common than platelet dysfunction. Bleeding is rare when the count is >50,000, unless the platelets are dysfunctional. High platelet counts in polycythemia vera or essential thrombocythemia are associated with thrombosis or bleeding. A number of commonly used drugs are associated with thrombocytopenia, including amiodarone, diltiazem, heparin, quinidine, cimetidine, ranitidine, sulfa, gentamycin, and vancomycin. Three percent of all heparin-treated patients develop HIT and a third of them go on to develop HITT, also known as white clot syndrome. This immune type of thrombocytopenia develops typically after 5-7 days of heparin therapy and is different from the nonimmune transient drop in platelet counts commonly seen after heparin initiation. Platelet count should therefore always be checked twice a week for all heparinized patients.

Bleeding time (BT): a function test (Ivy 3-6 minutes). In GPIb receptor failure (postcardiopulmonary bypass, old bank platelets), blockage by dextran, and congenital absence (Bernard-Soulier syndrome) platelets cannot bind to vWF. BT is also prolonged in vWD and certain connective tissue diseases (scurvy, Ehler-Danlos) where collagen has abnormal structure and vWF cannot bind normally. Inhibition of cyclooxygenase (COX) by ASA (irreversibly) prevents normal activation of the GPIIb/IIIa receptor by TxA$_2$. Other drugs like nonsteroidal anti-inflammatory drugs (NSAIDs), carbenicillin, ampicillin, piperacillin, heparin, nitroprusside, and dextran can also affect platelet metabolic function but usually less pronounced than ASA. Patients with severe anemia, myeloma, and uremia also may have prolonged BT.

PFA-100 (Platelet Function Analyser-100): an "in vitro bleeding time" that has replaced the BT at

Table 25-1   Coagulation Findings in Conditions Commonly Seen in Clinical Practice

	Platelet Count	PT INR	PTT	Fibrinogen	Comment
Vitamin K deficiency/ OACs	Normal	Prolonged (major prolongation in severe deficiency)	Prolonged (severe deficiency)	Normal	PTT normally not prolonged at therapeutic doses of OACs
SH	Normal	Mildly prolonged (massive doses)	Prolonged	Normal	PT INR usually not prolonged at therapeutic SH doses
LMWH	Normal	Normal	Normal (or slightly prolonged)	Normal	PTT cannot be used to monitor anticoagulation on LMWHs. Routine monitoring is usually unnecessary. If assessment of coagulation is necessary do a heparin level
Acute DIC	Decreased	Prolonged	Prolonged	Decreased	
Chronic DIC	Decreased or normal	Prolonged (rarely normal)	Prolonged (rarely normal)	Decreased or normal	
Liver disease	Mildly to moderately decreased	More prolonged	Prolonged	Normal (decreased in end-stage liver disease)	In early liver disease the PT INR will be prolonged and the PTT normal, reflecting the short half-life of FVII
Circulating anticoagulant "acquired factor inhibitor"	Normal	Normal or prolonged	Prolonged	Normal	1:1 mix that does not correct is supportive of diagnosis. Clinical problem is excess bleeding. Lupus inhibitor should be excluded
LAC	Normal (sometimes decreased if antiphospholipid syndrome)	Normal or prolonged	Often prolonged (depends on reagent sensitivity)	Normal	1:1 mix that does not correct is supportive of diagnosis. Clinical problem is excess thrombosis. Specific LAC testing indicated

DIC, disseminated intravascular coagulation; INR, international normalized ratio; LAC, "lupus anticoagulent/lupus inhibitor"; LMWH, low molecular weight heparin; OAC, oral anticoagulant; PT, prothrombin time; PTT, partial thromboplastin time; SH, standard heparin.

many institutions. Citrated whole blood is forced under high shear over a grid impregnated with the platelet agonist pairs collagen/epinephrine or collagen/EDTA, with the readout being time to occlusion of flow through tubing on the other side of the grid. Prolonged closure times (range for each agonist pair is institution specific) indicate platelet dysfunction. Prolongation to collagen/epinephrine alone is highly characteristic of drug effects (ASA, NSAIDs). Like the BT, the PFA-100 will also become abnormal if the platelet count is <80,000 or if the hematocrit is low (<28). Because platelet adhesion to collagen under high shear conditions is dependent on vWF, the PFA-100 is often abnormal (closure times prolonged) in patients with vWD, although normal values do not absolutely exclude this diagnosis.

PT (normal 11–13 seconds) has largely been replaced by INR due to quality variability in the tissue phospholipid used to activate the extrinsic tenase complex in the PT test. The INR test uses human brain thromboplastin as a reference substance that permits calculation of an International Sensitivity Index (ISI). The local ISI value permits calculation of the INR: INR = $PT^{(ISI)}$, a logarithmic relationship. INR is the recommended way to monitor warfarin anticoagulation therapy with recommended range 2–3 for all conditions except bileaflet prosthetic valves and recent MI (2.5–3.5).

APTT (normal 21–35 seconds): kaolin is used to surface activate FXII as well as FXI in the intrinsic tenase complex. As it is sensitive even to lower factor levels, a normal APTT does not rule out mild factor deficiency. In systemic heparin therapy (DVT, PE) the target APTT is 60–85 seconds.

1:1 mixing studies. These may be done for the PT or the PTT and can be helpful in distinguishing whether a prolonged PT or PTT is due to factor deficiency or due to the presence of a circulating inhibitor (either to a factor called an "acquired inhibitor" or to phospholipids in the test system called the "lupus anticoagulant" or "lupus inhibitor"). In the 1:1 mix patient plasma is mixed in equal proportion with normal plasma (assuring at least

50% of any given factor is present) and the test is repeated. Full correction is seen in factor deficiencies, as even with sensitive reagents, the PT and PTT do not begin to "pull out" unless factor levels are <40%. Lack of correction suggests the presence of either an acquired inhibitor (most commonly anti-FVIII or anti-vWF – these patients have a bleeding diathesis) or a lupus anticoagulant (these patients have a thrombotic propensity). Distinction between these two is often suggested by the clinical presentation but can be clarified by a lupus inhibitor panel (see below). It is important, especially in the case of acquired factor inhibitors, to look not only for immediate correction of the test in question, but also for correction at 60 minutes after mixing, as many antifactor antibodies show complex kinetics and the mix may only be abnormal at 60 minutes.

Lupus inhibitor panel and anticardiolipin antibodies. There is no single "gold standard" test for the lupus anticoagulant/lupus inhibitor. In accordance with international standards most laboratories do three different tests (such as a sensitive PTT, dilute Russell's viper venom time, hexagonal PTT, dilute PT, or other tests). Presence of a lupus inhibitor is suggested by prolongation of a clot-based assay and its correction with the addition of phospholipids. Making this diagnosis implies the patient has a thrombotic propensity. Anticardiolipin antibodies are another part of the "antiphospholipid" spectrum. These antibodies do not prolong clot-based assays but are detected by separate enzyme-linked immunosorbent assay (ELISA) testing. Their presence also implies a thrombotic propensity.

Reptilase is a thrombin-like enzyme that is not sensitive to heparin (unlike APTT), and is used to diagnose heparin effect.

TT (normal 7–12 seconds) monitors fibrinogen transformation to fibrin after addition of thrombin, a qualitative test (as opposed to fibrinogen level, a quantitative test). TT is prolonged in fibrinolysis and at low fibrinogen levels (<90 mg/100 cm^3). It is sometimes used in DIC diagnosis, as well as to monitor heparin or thrombolytic therapy.

Activated clotting time (ACT; normal 94–120 seconds, therapeutic level 400–600 seconds) is used for monitoring of intraoperative heparinization. Activation of the intrinsic tenase complex is achieved by using celite (diatomaceous earth) to activate FXII. Platelet quantity, quality, hemodilution, as well as hypothermia all affect the ACT. When there is discrepancy between the clinical status and the ACT result, it usually means the patient is hypothermic, since the test cuvette is heated to 37°C. It is insensitive to coagulation abnormalities. It does not correlate well with microvascular bleeding after cardiopulmonary bypass.

Fibrinogen level (normal 175–350 mg/100 ml) is usually low in consumptive processes such as DIC, in severe liver disease, or in massive transfusion by consumption and/or dilution. The most common reason for elevated PT/INR and PTT is hypofibrinogenemia. Required level is 50–100% for effective hemostasis. It is common practice to give cryoprecipitate to the bleeding patient if the fibrinogen level is below normal range, while this is not true for a stable nonbleeding patient. Iatrogenic hyperfibrinogenemia should be avoided, which can trigger thrombotic events.

Factor assays are sometimes measured in hemophilia patients to guide replacement therapy before or after surgery. In hemophilia A a FVIII level > 50% is recommended, and since the half-life is 6–12 hours replenishment twice daily is required. In massive transfusions, FV and FVIII drop off quickly ("labile factors") since their activity is lost rapidly in stored blood. DDAVP will induce transient release of vWF and also of FVIII, since vWF is the carrying molecule for FVIII. LMWH in higher dosage is sometimes monitored by anti-Xa activity assays according to patient weight.

AT (also known as ATIII; normal 70–130%) is usually low in DIC by consumption in the thrombin inactivation as well as breakdown by elastase (from polymorphonuclear leukocytes). Congenital AT deficiency is more uncommon. AT inhibits thrombin, FIXa, FXa, and FXIa but its activity is enhanced 100 times by heparin, or physiologically heparan. Low AT levels are responsible for "heparin resistance." Since it is produced by the liver, advanced liver disease may lead to deficiency. Children with nephritic syndrome may also exhibit low AT levels and heparin resistance. Rapid consumption of AT in DIC and sepsis may lead to low AT levels. Low AT levels in DIC make patients heparin resistant.

Calcium (normal 8.9–10.1 mg/100 ml) is required to hold coagulation factors down to catalytic centers on platelets via a calcium bridge. Calcium activity is better monitored with ionized (or free) calcium (normal 1–1.25 mmol/l) since it is protein bound in the normal state. Excess ACD in massive transfusion can rapidly produce hypocalcemia, which needs to be corrected in massive transfusion scenarios.

Magnesium level can affect coagulation in that substituting subnormal magnesium levels will improve the clotting ability of FIX.

D-dimers (normal < 250 μg/ml) and FSPs (or FDPs) (normal < 10 μg/ml) are both indicative of plasmin activity on fibrin, but the presence of D-dimers is specific for cross-linked fibrin. FSPs are elevated in both primary and secondary fibrinolysis, whereas elevated D-dimer implies that there has been clot formation with secondary fibrinolysis. Moderately to strongly positive D-dimers are present in DIC. Elevated D-dimers are also seen in DVT and PE as well as in any clinical setting where there is widespread secondary fibrinolysis (postoperative major surgery, trauma). Weakly positive D-dimers are frequent in line draws and in sick hospitalized patients. FSPs are normally cleared by the reticuloendothelial system (normal half-life 9 hours), as are other activated coagulation products. High FSP titers inhibit thrombin, prevent cross-linking of fibrin, and disrupt platelet function. High FSP levels (>100 μg/ml) are also seen in active renal disease and renal transplant rejection.

Fibrinopeptide A is a breakdown product of fibrinogen by thrombin, elevated in DIC.

Euglobulin lysis time (normal >2 hours at 37°C) is elevated in states with high circulating plasmin levels, but normal in clot-bound fibrinolysis.

High *PAI-1 levels* (normal < 50 ng/ml) can be seen in sepsis and DIC, and indicate a suppressed fibrinolysis. The patient is at risk for microthrombi and MSOF.

Schistocytes (fragmented red blood cells) are high in microangiopathic hemolytic anemia (MHA) but may also be present in DIC from other causes.

Thromboelastograph (TEG) is a whole blood, in vitro point-of-care system, for assessment of the tensile strength of the developing clot, as well as for disappearing clot strength in fibrinolysis. It can give directions in blood component therapy and also test drugs in vitro before administration to the patient. It has been shown to save blood products in massive bleeding scenarios and liver transplantation. Additionally, it is very useful in evaluations for hypercoagulability.

HIT test: ELISA platelet aggregation test or serotonin release test (not available everywhere). Laboratory testing for HIT can be frustrating and HIT is still largely a clinical diagnosis. ELISA tests are sensitive but often falsely positive. Functional HIT tests (aggregation, serotonin release) are less sensitive but more specific.

KEY LABORATORY FINDINGS IN DISSEMINATED INTRAVASCULAR COAGULATION

Traditionally, in acute DIC serial assays of platelet count (90%), fibrinogen (sensitivity < 50% but high specificity of 80%), APTT (sensitivity 50%), PT/INR (sensitivity 68%), FDP (sensitivity 87%), and D-dimers (sensitivity 95%) have been used. More recently, thrombin–AT complex (TAT; sensitivity 98%), plasmin–plasmin inhibitor complex (PPIC; sensitivity 95% but low specificity of 35%), and soluble fibrin monomer (sFM; sensitivity 81%) have been shown to be more specific for DIC but are not used in routine clinical practice yet. There is not a single parameter but a group of markers that accurately predict DIC and these are a combination of TAT, PPIC, and sFM. High plasma TM levels are common in DIC patients with organ failure indicating endothelial injury. AT levels fall with rapid consumption. IL-6 and TNF-α levels are both high.

In chronic DIC FDP is usually increased, but the other laboratory diagnostics discussed above are unreliable. A shortened APTT is sometimes seen in chronic DIC.

Box 25-6 Differential Diagnosis to Disseminated Intravascular Coagulation

- Severe liver failure
- Vitamin K deficiency
- Primary fibrinolysis
- HITT
- Idiopathic purpura fulminans

DIAGNOSIS OF DISSEMINATED INTRAVASCULAR COAGULATION

The combination of test results (low platelet count or its rapid decline; prolonged PT/APTT; elevated FDP or D-dimers; low AT or/and PC) and the presence of a clinical condition known to be associated with DIC will be required for diagnosis. If uncertainty remains, soluble fibrin monomer or TAT complexes should be measured in a specialty laboratory (Box 25-6).

TREATMENT OF COAGULOPATHY AND DISSEMINATED INTRAVASCULAR COAGULATION

It is very important to move the patient to an ICU where monitoring of vital signs as well as frequent blood draws can enable the team to follow the course and the effect of treatment. Depending on the situation, the most common approach is to reverse coagulopathy with blood products prior to insertion of devices for central monitoring. In massive transfusions, all fluids except platelets are given through a fluid warmer. Normal blood volume is maintained as guided with central monitoring and urine output using LR, saline, and colloids. Hematology consult will be particularly helpful when speed of bleeding high (can expedite transfer of blood products from blood bank) particularly in a massive transfusion situation, and when the patient does not stop bleeding with standard therapy.

Red blood cells should be replaced to restore oxygen carrying capacity. In overt bleeding if hematocrit < 30, otherwise if hematocrit < 23 in a young and otherwise healthy patient. It is advisable to keep hematocrit = 30 in patients with coronary artery disease and with age over 70.

FFP: if INR > 2.0 or PTT > 1.5 times normal and fibrinogen is normal. Also consider FFP in hemodynamic instability if coagulation results are not immediately available. 4 FFP is a common initial dose.

Cryoprecipitate: in a bleeding patient with fibrinogen lower than 125 g/dl; avoid hyperfibrinogenemia. A 5 pack will raise a moderately decreased fibrinogen level into the lower normal range.

Platelets should be transfused in a bleeding patient if <50,000. In stable patients not due for surgery, transfusion is not recommended unless platelet count is <10,000. Transfusion should be started when necessary with platelets from five donors, or alternatively pheresis platelets from one donor. Platelet transfusion is contraindicated in TTP, HIT/HITT, and in the case of platelet autoantibodies. ITP: prednisone, immunoglobulin, possible splenectomy; TTP: prednisone, plasma exchange 5 days; HIT/HITT: discontinue heparin and heparin-coated central venous catheters, and if anticoagulation is required argatroban or recombinant hirudin (leprudin) should be used, not LMWH. Post-transfusion purpura patients may require immunoglobulin, plasmapheresis, and corticosteroids.

Dysfunctional platelets: drug list should be checked (penicillins, cephalosporins, H_2 receptor antagonists, dextran, hetastarch, heparin, warfarin, antiplatelet drugs, NSAIDs) if abnormal PFA-100 or prolonged bleeding time and platelet count in normal range. Central core temperature should be kept above 36°C. Keeping the hematocrit around 30 probably facilitates platelet adhesion. DDAVP (0.3 µg/kg) or conjugated estrogens (0.6 mg/kg/day for 1-5 days) are recommended for uremic platelets.

Pathologic primary fibrinolysis can occur in the postoperative cardiac bypass patient (aprotinin), after tonsillectomy, in obstetric or gynecological bleeding, and after prostate surgery. Antifibrinolytic therapy (drug and dose) should be considered.

Surgical hemostasis should be considered in postoperative patients if bleeding is from drains or surgical sites only. If perioperative uncontrolled diffuse bleeding and coagulopathy is present, packing the patient should be considered, and they should be taken to an ICU for correction of coagulopathy and later second look ("damage control"). Small series of trauma patients with uncontrollable bleeding have received rFVIIa (Novo7®: 90 µg/kg q 2 hours) with rapid cessation of bleeding, but the expense limits its use. Also used successfully in patients on warfarin after head trauma, it stops bleeding rapidly. If surgical hemostasis not possible, angiographic localization and embolization should be considered.

DIC. Identification and elimination of the underlying factor(s) is the essential part. If the triggering factor can be dealt with the DIC state gradually subsides over the next few days. Acute DIC is usually treated with blood components (platelets, FFP, cryoprecipitate, PRBC) that control bleeding if necessary. Prophylactic administration of FFP or other blood products have not been shown to confer advantage to these patients. The heparin dose is 300-500 U/hour as infusion. LMWH can also be used as an alternative to heparin. Direct inhibitors of thrombin (AT independent) have not undergone controlled trials

---

Box 25-7 Drug Side Effects
• Heparin: HIT/HITT; osteoporosis, hyperlipidemia from lipase release, PLA_2 stimulation causes cytokine release
• LMWH: small risk for cross-reaction in HIT patients
• Hirudin-type anticoagulants: no reversal
• Warfarin: if heparin is not used initially, certain categories with inborn PC or PS deficiency or PC resistance (FV Leiden) may become hypercoagulable before they become fully anticoagulated. Warfarin-induced skin necrosis
• Thrombolytics: bleeding
• Antifibrinolytics: DVT and PE
• DDAVP: transient hypotension, tachyphylaxis; hyponatremia

for DIC yet, but are known to be associated with a higher risk of bleeding and cannot be reversed. Heparin is most frequently used for DIC associated with thromboembolism (Box 25-7).

AT concentrates have in trials been shown to reduce mortality slightly (but not statistically significantly) in sepsis. A meta-analysis showed a mortality reduction from 56 to 44%, but the costs are substantial. A recent large multicenter trial of more than 2300 patients failed to show survival advantage at 28, 56, or 90 days. TFPI has failed in large multicenter trials to show survival benefit in sepsis-induced DIC.

While antifibrinolytics may be effective in some bleeding patients, they are contraindicated in DIC, except if the bleeding can be shown to result from hyperfibrinolysis, as in promyelocytic leukemia.

Activated PC has been shown to decrease sepsis-induced mortality in patients with the highest Apache II scores, but has been associated with bleeding in patients with lower Apache scores. It has not been tested for DIC associated with conditions other than severe sepsis.

Site-inactivated rFVIIai may theoretically be an attractive way to block increased TF activity known to precipitate DIC, but no human trials support this approach yet.

CURRENT CONTROVERSIES

When is it safe to use heparin in DIC? Even though controlled trials have not shown benefit for heparinization, it appears reasonable to anticoagulate DIC patients with heparin if there are signs of ischemia from gut, or acral ischemia (fingertips, nose, ears). On the other hand, heparin does not appear to increase the risk for bleeding in the DIC patient. In chronic DIC long-term therapy with LMWH appears to be a reasonable choice until the underlying factor is brought under control. Warfarin therapy is often ineffective for long-term control.

SELECTED READING

Colman RW, Hirsh J, Marder VJ, Clowes AW, George JN, editors: *Hemostasis and Thrombosis*, ed 4, Philadelphia: Lippincott Williams & Wilkins, 2001.

DeLoughery TG: *Hemostasis and Thrombosis*. Austin, TX: Landes Bioscience, 1999.

Geerts WH, Heit JA, Clagett GP et al: Prevention of venous thromboembolism. 6th ACCP consensus conference on antithrombotic therapy. Chest 119:132S-175S, 2001.

Levi M, Cate HT: Disseminated intravascular coagulation. N Engl J Med 341:586-592, 1999.

Shimura M, Wada H, Wakita Y et al: Plasma tissue factor and tissue factor pathway inhibitor levels in patients with disseminated intravascular coagulation. Am J Hematol 52:165-170, 1996.

Wada H, Nakese T, Nakaya R et al: Elevated plasma tissue factor antigen levels in patients with disseminated intravascular coagulation. Am J Hematol 45:232-236, 1994.

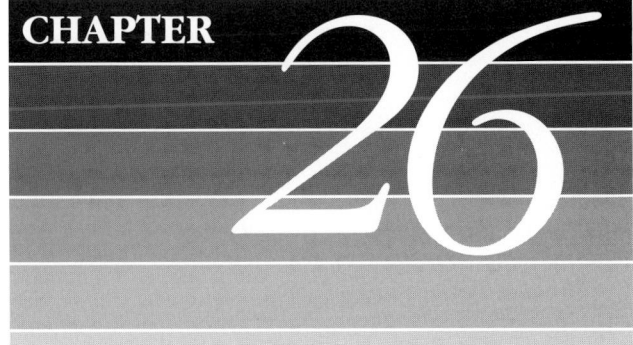

CHAPTER 26

Blood and Blood Component Therapy

LYNN K. BOSHKOV, M.D.

PER A. J. THORBORG, M.D., Ph.D.

PREPARATION AND COMPOSITION OF BLOOD AND BLOOD COMPONENTS AND DERIVATIVES

Blood products in North America are normally donated by volunteers, either as whole blood or by apheresis. Over 11 million units of whole blood are collected annually in the USA. In whole blood donation a 450 ml unit (U) is collected into citrate-based anticoagulant. Autologous units (donated by a person for their own later use) are stored as whole blood. Other whole blood units are separated into two or three components: into 1 U of red blood cells (RBCs), 1 U of plasma, and sometimes into 1 U of "random donor" platelets. The plasma may be further separated into 1 U of cryoprecipitate (a small-volume product rich in fibrinogen) and 1 U of cryosupernatant plasma. Platelets are most commonly not made from whole blood but are collected by apheresis harvest of donor platelet-rich plasma. One apheresis platelet unit is equivalent to 5–6 "random donor" platelet units. Apheresis can also be used to harvest RBCs and plasma, although these products are not yet available in most areas of North America. Plasma derivatives (albumin, plasma-derived clotting factor concentrates, intravenous gammaglobulin, etc.) are made by subfractionation of pooled plasma or cryopsupernatant plasma from large numbers of donors (up to 20,000). Also, specialized hyperimmune gammaglobulins (rhesus (Rh)-immune globulin, cytomegalovirus (CMV)-immune globulin, etc.) can be made from plasma of special donors with high titers of the desired antibody. The composition, shelf life, and postissue storage conditions for red cells, plasma, cryoprecipitate, and platelets are given in Table 26-1. Note that most RBC units currently have an additive solution added to them, which improves viability and increases their shelf life. All blood components should be administered through a standard blood filter ("170–260 micron") to remove any aggregates that may have formed during storage.

SPECIAL TRANSFUSION NEEDS: LEUKOREDUCTION, "CMV SAFE," IRRADIATION, WASHING

Contaminating leukocytes in whole blood preparations in North America partition about 80% into the red cell component. Leukoreduction of red cells and platelets can remove 3–4 log of these leukocytes. This is usually done

Table 26-1 Blood Products, Contents, and Storage

Blood Component	Contents	Approx. Volume	Shelf Life	Comments
Whole blood (autologous predonation)	RBCs and plasma. 450 ml blood and 63 ml CPDA-1 anticoagulant. Hct ~ 35	520 ml	35 days at 4°C. Transfuse within 4 hours at room temperature	WBCs and platelets not viable after 24 hours. Factors V and VIII significantly decreased after 2 days
Red cell concentrate (additive solution red cells – AS-1, AS-3, AS-5)	RBCs with about 25 ml plasma and 100 ml of additive solution (saline, adenine, dextrose). Hct 55–60	340 ml	42 days at 4°C. Transfuse within 4 hours at room temperature	"Packed cells" (Hct 70) lack the additive solution and are not usually provided
Platelet "random donor"	Platelets (5.5 × 10^{10}); some WBCs; 50 ml plasma; few RBCs (Hct < 0.005)	50 ml	5 days at 20°C with agitation	Refrigeration results in echinocytic transformation and dysfunction
Platelet "apheresis"	Platelets (3.5 × 10^{11}); fewer WBCs and RBCs than "randoms"; 300 ml plasma	300 ml	5 days at 20°C with agitation	1 apheresis U = 5–6 "random donors." Do not refrigerate
FFP; FP	Normal levels all coagulation factors, natural inhibitors (AT, protein C, protein S) and plasma proteins. No significant difference between FFP and FP	250 ml	1 year frozen at −18°C; post-thaw: 4°C × 24 hours	~30 minutes to thaw. Post-thaw: major decreases in factors V and VIII after 24 hours
Solvent detergent plasma	All coagulation factors. Plasma proteins. Significant decreases in proteins C and S vs. FFP and FP	200 ml	1 year frozen at −18°C; post-thaw: room temperature × 24 hours	~30 minutes to thaw. Storage at 4°C may activate factor VII. Possibly prothrombotic vs. FFP and FP
Cryoprecipitate	~150 mg fibrinogen, at least 80 U factor VIII, von Willebrand factor, factor XIII	15 ml/U. Note: also comes in 5 U pools	1 year frozen at −18°C; post-thaw: room temperature × 4 hours	~15 minutes to thaw. Refrigeration may re-precipitate proteins – warm to room temperature

AS-1, AS-3, AS-5, RBC additive solutions; AT, antithrombin III; CPDA-1, citrate phosphate dextrose-1 anticoagulant; FFP, fresh frozen plasma; FP, frozen plasma; Hct, hematocrit; RBC, red blood cell; WBC, white blood cell.

by filtration or by sophisticated apheresis technology at the blood center at the time of collection (prestorage leukoreduction). It may also be done using special leukoreduction filters in the hospital transfusion service or at the bedside. Leukoreduced products are more costly but are less likely to cause febrile transfusion reactions and human leukocyte antigen (HLA) alloimmunization. They are also considered by the American Association of Blood Banks to be the equivalent of "CMV seronegative" units in being "CMV safe," and many hospitals no longer specifically provide "CMV negative" products. Leukoreduced products are routinely given to hematology/oncology patients, solid organ transplant candidates/recipients, neonates, and patients who have had previous febrile reactions. Flow rates for bedside leukoreduction are often slow and for surgery prestorage leukoreduced products are preferred.

Irradiation of red cells and platelets with 2500 centigrays abrogates blastogenesis of contaminating lymphocytes and prevents transfusion-associated graft versus host disease (TA-GVHD). Frozen plasma and cryoprecipitate do not need irradiation. Prestorage leukoreduction alone is inadequate to prevent TA-GVHD. Irradiated products are needed by patients who have undergone bone marrow transplant, who have congenital immunodeficiency, or who are receiving directed donations from a blood relative. In addition irradiated products are given to many patients with hematologic malignancy and to some solid tumor patients. Solid organ transplant patients and AIDS patients do not require irradiated products. Irradiation increases potassium leak from RBCs and should ideally be done at the time of product issue from the hospital transfusion service.

Washing of RBCs and platelets is rarely needed. It is used in prevention of recurrent refractory major allergic reactions, to remove potassium (K$^+$) where K$^+$ toxicity is an issue (RBCs < 5 days old may be substituted in most cases), and to prepare frozen deglycerolized RBCs (rare blood groups). Washing of RBCs normally takes 1–2 hours, and washing of platelets 2–3 hours. Once washed the RBCs must be used within 24 hours and platelets within 4 hours.

Box 26-1   ABO Incompatibility

ABO incompatibility is the leading cause of preventable transfusion fatalities.

- Meticulous attention to specimen and recipient identification would have prevented most of these deaths

Box 26-2   Basic Principles of Blood Component Therapy

- Replace what is needed – red cells for anemia, platelets for thrombocytopenia, plasma for coagulopathies, etc.
- Transfuse only if the defect is clinically significant.
- Weigh the risks, benefits, and alternatives to transfusion

COMPATIBILITY ISSUES

ABO Compatibility

ABO compatibility of donor and recipient is critically important for RBCs and plasma. There are four basic blood groups: O, A, B, and AB. The A and B genes code for glycosyltransferases that add A or B substance onto a base H substance on all red cells. Anyone who *lacks* A or B on their red cells *always* has the corresponding naturally occurring antibody in their plasma. Anti-A and anti-B are complement-fixing antibodies that are active at body temperature and cause nasty or fatal acute intravascular hemolytic reactions (Box 26-1).

Basic donor/recipient ABO compatibility of RBCs and plasma can be found in Table 26-2. When in doubt one should use O red cells and AB plasma (O red cells can be used for all blood groups because there is very little O plasma in red cells).

CLINICAL CAVEAT

Blood Component Compatibility with Solutions and Drugs

- Compatible with isotonic crystalloid and with 5% albumin
- Do *not* mix with drugs (acidic pH, protein binding), calcium-containing solutions (may clot), or hypotonic solutions (lysis of RBCs and platelets)

Replacement of the Total Blood Volume of an Adult

The total blood volume (TBV) of an adult is about 70 cm^3/kg, or for a 70 kg individual about 5 liters. If the hematocrit is 0.40, about 2 liters of this TBV is red cells, and about 3 liters is plasma. Using the product volumes and composition in Table 26-1 one can calculate that, roughly, to replace the TBV of a 70 kg person would require about 10 U of red cells, 10–12 U of plasma, and 10–12 U "random donor" platelets = 2 U apheresis platelets. Keeping this in mind one can roughly estimate the number of units of a particular product needed to correct a given level of deficiency (Box 26-2).

RED BLOOD CELLS AND ANEMIA

More than 11 million red cell units are transfused annually in the USA to more than 3 million recipients.

Physiologic Response to Acute and Chronic Anemia

Normal physiologic response to anemia consists of cardiac and peripheral tissue adaptations as well as changes in RBC 2,3-diphosphoglycerate (2,3-DPG). Cardiac output is increased by increasing heart rate or stroke volume. As the heart normally extracts ~80% of O_2 delivered, increased cardiac O_2 extraction is largely

Table 26-2   Recipient and Donor ABO Groups and RBC and Plasma Compatibilities

Recipient Blood Group	Antigens on RBCs	Antibodies in Plasma	Donor RBC Compatibility	Donor Plasma Compatibility
O	None	Anti-A and anti-B	O only	O, A, B, AB
A	A	Anti-B	A, O	A, AB
B	B	Anti-A	B, O	B, AB
AB	A and B	None	AB, A, B, O	AB only
Unknown or undeterminable	Unknown	Unknown	O	AB

achieved by increasing coronary artery flow by coronary artery vasodilatation. As demand escalates in excess of compensatory increases in heart rate and vasodilatation, the heart shifts from aerobic to anaerobic metabolism and blood flow is shifted from the subendocardium to the epicardium, placing the subendocardium at ischemic risk. Clearly patients with impaired ability to increase their heart rate (intrinsic disease, pharmacologic blockade) or to increase coronary flow through vasodilatation (stenotic lesions) are at increased risk for ischemia. Animal studies suggest the lower limit of cardiac tolerance for anemia in the presence of a normal cardiovascular system is a hemoglobin (Hb) of ~3-5 g/dl, and in the presence of coronary stenosis is in the range 7-10 g/dl.

Peripheral tissue compensation for anemia is to increase O_2 delivery by increasing blood flow through vascular beds, to recruit more capillaries, or in the case of supply-dependent tissues to increase oxygen extraction. However, these compensatory mechanisms may be limited and dependent on circulating intravascular volume as well as on red cell mass in the case of the splanchnic bed, muscles, and skin. With chronic anemia, RBC intracellular 2,3-DPG concentrations also increase, shifting the oxyhemoglobin dissociation curve to the right, thereby facilitating tissue off-loading of O_2 (Box 26-3).

Serologic Safety of Uncrossmatched Red Blood Cells

Once a blood sample reaches the hospital transfusion service it takes about 10 minutes to do an ABO and Rh type, about 30 minutes to do an antibody screen, and about 45 minutes to issue crossmatched RBCs if no irregular antibodies are identified (in most hospitals 2-5% of patients will have such antibodies). If RBC transfusion is needed more urgently than this, uncrossmatched O or group-specific uncrossmatched RBCs may be issued on request of appropriate personnel. Statistically, if a unit of RBCs is randomly selected with no effort to ensure serologic compatibility with the recipient (ABO, Rh, or other clinically significant anti-RBC antibodies) it will serendipitously be compatible ~64% of the time. This is fortunate as available data show ~1 in 30,000 to 1 in 40,000 patients get the wrong blood! If ABO compatibility is assured (as it

can be by giving group O RBCs) serologic safety rises to 99.4%; for ABO and Rh compatibility to 99.8%; and for ABO and Rh compatibility with a negative antibody screen to 99.94%. Also even if irregular antibodies are present titers are often low, and the clinical sequelae are usually not immediate but delayed in the form of a delayed hemolytic transfusion reaction. Therefore, when faced with an exsanguinating patient the clinical risk/benefit is usually overwhelmingly in favor of using uncrossmatched blood.

Choice of the Perioperative Red Blood Cell "Transfusion Trigger"

There is little to justify a specific Hb or hematocrit, such as the former "10/30" Hb/hematocrit rule, in making decisions regarding perioperative RBC transfusion, and withholding transfusion unless a patient is symptomatic has been advocated by some expert groups. Adults with Hb of <7 g/dl are more likely to manifest hemodynamic symptoms than are children, who more often become dyspneic or show impaired levels of consciousness. However, multiple studies indicate that signs and symptoms of anemia are unreliable especially in the surgical setting, and that myocardial ischemia is often silent, particularly postoperatively. Complicating this is the fact that estimates of intraoperative blood loss are often difficult, and estimates of intraoperative blood volume indirect (inferred from arterial, central venous, and pulmonary capillary wedge pressures). Even when invasive monitoring is used to measure whole-body O_2 consumption, or O_2 extraction ratios, such measurements are global and have not been verified as predictive of ischemia. The real issue of interest is the adequacy of O_2 delivery to specific organs and regions within these organs, and unfortunately it is not possible to measure this directly in the routine clinical setting. The dynamic nature of surgical hemorrhage and the anticipation of major blood loss are also frequent factors in the decision to transfuse intraoperatively.

It should also be noted that a Hb/hematocrit that is adequate in the stable intraoperative setting (where the patient is paralyzed and the ventilation and FIO_2 controlled) may no longer be adequate in the same patient in the postoperative setting, breathing room air and with exertional demands for increased O_2 delivery. A recent study in Jehovah's Witnesses indicates that postoperative morbidity and mortality begin to rise when the Hb is <5 g/dl in patients without cardiovascular compromise and when it is <6 g/dl in patients with cardiovascular compromise (Box 26-4).

Choice of "Transfusion Trigger" in the Critical Care Setting

One recent randomized trial in which adult patients were randomized to a hemoglobin (Hb) of 7-9 g/dl vs. a Hb

---

Box 26-3 Increment Expected per RBC Unit Transfused in Nonbleeding Patients

- In an adult 1 U RBCs will increase the hematocrit by ~3 % and the hemoglobin by ~1 g/dl
- In the pediatric patient the roughly equivalent dose is 10–15 ml RBCs/kg

Box 26-4   Recommended Perisurgical Red Blood Cell "Transfusion Trigger"

- None firm – need for transfusion needs to be individualized for any given patient in any given clinical setting
- Transfusion is frequently indicated when the hemoglobin/hematocrit are <6 g/dl/18% and rarely indicated when they are >10 g/dl/30% (exception is acute blood loss)
- Postoperatively hemoglobins <5 g/dl in patients without cardiovascular compromise and <6 g/dl in patients with cardiovascular compromise appear to carry increased morbidity and mortality

Table 26-3   Coagulation Factor Characteristics in Plasma

Coagulation Factor	$t^1/_2$ Postinfusion (hours)*
Fibrinogen	96
II	60
V	24
VII	4–6
VIII	11–12
IX	22
X	35
XI	60
XIII	144
vWF	8–12

* $t^1/_2$ = half-disappearance time of the clotting factor in the absence of accelerated consumption.

of 10–12 g/dl suggested a trend to decreased 30-day mortality in the former group. Subgroup analysis showed younger (age < 55 years), less critically ill patients (Acute Physiology and Chronic Health Evaluation II score ≤ 20) were half as likely to die in the Hb 7–9 g/dl group as in the 10–12 g/dl group. Conversely a large retrospective study showed that in patients with myocardial infarction, anemia below a hematocrit of 33 was associated with increased mortality in patients over the age of 65.

CURRENT CONTROVERSY

Red Blood Cell "Transfusion Trigger" in the Critical Care Setting

Optimal hemoglobin/hematocrit in the critical care setting is unclear and likely dependent on clinical setting, patient age, and underlying cardiovascular status.

PLASMA, CRYOPRECIPITATE, AND COAGULOPATHY

More than 2 million U of plasma and almost 1 million U of cryoprecipitate are transfused annually in the USA. The basic composition, volume, shelf life, and postissue storage conditions for plasma and cryoprecipitate are given in Table 26-1. Specific coagulation factor characteristics of plasma are given in Table 26-3.

Clinically, spontaneous bleeding is rare in isolated factor deficiencies unless levels are below 5% of normal. Under conditions of stress (surgery, invasive procedures) bleeding often occurs when factor levels are below 30%, particularly in the case of multifactorial coagulopathies. Monitoring of individual factor levels (except for fibrinogen) is not feasible in routine clinical settings, and more global measures of coagulation (prothrombin time

international normalized ratio (PT INR), partial thromboplastin time (PTT)) are normally used for clinical assessment (see Chapter 25). Although sensitivity to factor deficiencies is reagent specific, in general the PT INR and PTT do not prolong until factors are <40% of normal.

Plasma

The major indications for plasma use are given in Box 26-5 and the usual dosing in Box 26-6.

Box 26-5   Major Indications for Use of Plasma

- Urgent clinical correction of a multifactorial coagulopathy (vitamin K deficiency, warfarin reversal, severe liver disease, DIC, dilutional coagulopathy) when the PT INR is >1.5*or the PTT is >1.5 times normal
- Factor replacement for known factor deficiencies for which specific plasma-derived or recombinant factor concentrates are unavailable (factor II, V, VII**, X, XI**, and XIII** deficiencies; protein C** and protein S deficiencies)
- Correction of microvascular bleeding when the PT INR is >1.5 or the PTT is >1.5 times normal (or when the PT and PTT are not available in a timely fashion)
- Plasmapheresis or plasma infusion in TTP

* The choice of a PT INR of >1.5 as predictive of clinical bleeding is quite conservative. Some groups have in fact argued that the literature does not really support this and that a PT INR of >2.0 is more appropriate.
** Specific replacement products available in some geographical areas.

Box 26-6   Plasma Dosing

- ~20/ml/kg will achieve coagulation factor concentrations of ~30% of normal in nonbleeding, otherwise stable adults and children
- A minimum of 2–4 U (500–1000 ml) is generally required to have an impact on a clinically significant coagulopathy in an adult

---

Plasma should not be used as a volume expander, as a nutritional supplement, or for nonurgent correction of vitamin K deficiency (pharmaceutic preparations of vitamin K will usually reverse this in 6–12 hours). Hypofibrinogenemia (massive transfusion, disseminated intravascular coagulation (DIC)) is best corrected with cryoprecipitate (see below).

Although plasma is frequently used to correct mild prolongations of the PT INR (1.2–1.5) and the PTT (<1.5 times normal) prior to invasive procedures (line placements, biopsies, paracentesis), there is little evidence to support this, practice and the skill of the operator doing the procedure is more predictive of bleeding. It should also be noted that increasing coagulation factor levels by 10% will have a significant effect on the PT and PTT when they are prolonged more than twice mid-range normal but will have only a minimal effect on more modest prolongations. It is difficult or impossible to correct the coagulopathy of severe liver disease with plasma because the short half-life of factor VII (4–6 hours) makes it difficult to infuse the product fast enough. In this setting 1-deamino-8-D-arginine vasopressin (DDAVP) (for the platelet function defect), plasma exchange (to correct the factor defect), and more recently recombinant factor VIIa (if available) may be helpful.

Cryoprecipitate

Cryoprecipitate (cryo) is supplied as individual "bags" or units (each made from 1 U of plasma) or as 5 U pools.

Table 26-4   Major Plasma Proteins in a Single 10–15 ml Bag (U) of Cryo

Constituent	Amount per Bag	Half-life (hours)
Fibrinogen	150–250 mg	100–150
Von Willebrand factor (normal multimeric pattern)	100–150 U (40–70% of original plasma)	12
Factor VIII	80–150 U	12
Factor XIII	50–75 U	150–300

The major plasma proteins contained in cryoprecipitate are given in Table 26-4 and dosing guidelines in Table 26-5. Cryo is used in congenital and acquired hypofibrinogenemia (fibrinogen < 100 mg/dl – DIC, obstetrical catastrophe, fulminant hepatic failure). It is also used in dysfibrinogenemias with microvascular bleeding. Although used in the past for treatment of both hemophilia A and von Willebrand's disease (vWD), cryo is no longer the first-line treatment for either as factor concentrates (now treated to inactivate viruses or made by recombinant technology) and DDAVP (which carries no risk of transfusion-transmitted disease) carry less risk. Cryo is suitable for treatment of vWD unresponsive to DDAVP if von Willebrand concentrates are unavailable, as well as for treatment of moderate to severe factor VIII deficiency where DDAVP is ineffective and factor concentrates are unavailable. Factor XIII deficiency is usually treated with plasma, although cryo can also be used. Other uses for cryo, although not confirmed by randomized clinical trials, include treatment of platelet dysfunction unresponsive to DDAVP (uremia, drug-induced). Cryo is ineffective and contraindicated for treatment of multiple organ failure.

Cryo can also be used as a source of fibrinogen in making "homemade" fibrin glue, where it is mixed with a source of thrombin (usually bovine) at the time of use.

Table 26-5   Dosing Guidelines for Cryo

Clinical Condition	Usual Dose	Minimal Hemostatic Level
Fibrinogen replacement	Adult: 10 U (two 5-pools); child: 1 U/10 kg (will increase fibrinogen by 60–100 mg/dl)	Fibrinogen of 75–100 mg/dl (measure postinfusion – dosing frequency can vary from hours in active DIC to days)
Von Willebrand's disease (second-line therapy – see text)	Adult: 10–12 U q 12 hours; child: 1 U/6 kg q 12 hours	This dose will usually ensure hemostasis
Hemophilia A (factor VIII deficiency) (second-line therapy – see text)	Assume 1 U contains 100 U factor VIII; 1 U/6 kg will usually give a factor VIII level of ~35%	Factor VIII levels of 35–100% depending on clinical setting
Factor XIII deficiency	1 U/10 kg q 7–14 days	2–3% levels of factor XIII are hemostatic

Fibrin glue is used most commonly in cardiothoracic and vascular surgery, neurosurgery, and maxillofacial surgery to provide local control of slow venous bleeding, diffuse ooze, and lymphatic leaks. Commercial fibrin sealant preparations, which use human thrombin, may be preferred as bovine thrombin may rarely be associated with formation of antifactor V antibodies.

PLASMA DERIVATIVES

Albumin

Albumin, unlike other blood products, comes in glass bottles and must be vented for IV administration. The 5% solution is isotonic and the 25% solution hypertonic. Albumin and other colloids are often used to restore intravascular volume in patients with hypovolemia.

CURRENT CONTROVERSY

Albumin (Colloid) vs. Crystalloid in Acute Resuscitation
- Two controversial recent meta-analyses of randomized trials comparing albumin and nonalbumin volume expanders with crystalloid for resuscitation found a 4–6% excess of deaths in the colloid group
- Caution may be warranted in the use of albumin and other colloids for acute resuscitation

---

Rhesus Immune Globulin

Rh immune globulin (RhIg) is used to prevent formation of anti-D anti-RBC antibodies by Rh-negative women (about 15% of Caucasians) exposed to Rh-positive blood. If anti-D is formed, hemolytic disease of the newborn may result. The source of the sensitizing Rh-positive blood is usually exposure to fetal red cells as the result of abdominal trauma or invasive procedures, or during delivery. Usual preventative dose is 300 μg, best given within three days of exposure.

Other Plasma Derivatives

A detailed discussion of the use of plasma derivatives, including the use of specialized plasma-derived and recombinant factors for treating hemophilia (factor VIII and IX concentrates, prothrombin complex concentrates, FEIBA, recombinant factor VIIa), as well as the use of specialized plasma derivatives (intravenous gammaglobulin, hyperimmune globulins, antithrombin concentrates, C1 esterase inhibitor, etc.), is beyond the scope of this chapter. In dealing with the perioperative management of patients with hemophilia (particularly those with inhibitors), vWD, and complex coagulopathies including congenital and acquired prothrombotic disorders such as antithrombin (AT, formerly antithrombin III) deficiency hematological consultation should be sought. If at all possible patients with hemophilia should not be taken to surgery without being tested for the presence of inhibitors and without a trial infusion of factor to assess adequacy of factor recovery. Likewise patients with vWD should have the subtype of their vWD defined prior to surgery and a DDAVP trial, if appropriate. Patients with mild to moderate Type I vWD (where the defect is in endothelial cell release of normal von Willebrand factor (vWF)) will often respond to DDAVP. In other types of vWD an abnormal vWF is made and DDAVP should not normally be used. Table 26-6 provides some basic guidelines and caveats regarding perioperative treatment of hemophilia and vWD (and of patients with AT deficiency). Antifibrinolytic therapy (epsilon aminocaproic acid, tranexamic acid) can be a useful adjunct for oral surgery in patients with underlying coagulation disorders.

PLATELETS AND THROMBOCYTOPENIA

The basic composition, volume, shelf life, and storage conditions for "random donor" and apheresis platelets are given in Table 26-1. Platelets are given both prophylactically, to prevent bleeding, and therapeutically, to treat active bleeding or to ensure effective hemostasis during surgery or other invasive procedures (biopsies, thoracentesis, paracentesis). Spontaneous bleeding is rare at platelet counts of $>10 \times 10^9/l$ providing platelet function is normal and there is no coincident coagulation or hemostatic defect, and this is the usual prophylactic "transfusion trigger." In the absence of accelerated consumption, splenic sequestration, etc., approximately 80% of the transfused platelets will still be circulating 24 hours later. Perisurgically, as well as for invasive procedures, platelet counts of $40–50 \times 10^9/l$ functional platelets, in the absence of other coagulation defects, are usually enough to ensure hemostasis. For central nervous system and life- or limb-threatening bleeding higher target platelet counts ($75–100 \times 10^9/l$) are often used. Platelets may also be used to treat thrombocytopathy (postcardiopulmonary bypass, drug-induced, etc.). The normal dose in this situation is sufficient to raise the platelet count by $40–50 \times 10^9/l$, as normal platelets will recruit dysfunctional platelets into the hemostatic plug. Nontransfusion treatments for platelet dysfunction may be useful as alternatives or adjuncts to platelet transfusion. These include intravenous or intranasal DDAVP, keeping the hematocrit around 30, and use of conjugated estrogens (in uremia) or antifibrinolytic agents (oral bleeding).

Table 26-6   Use of Plasma Derivatives

Condition	Clinical Setting	Agent and Dose	Caveats
Hemophilia A (factor VIII deficiency): no inhibitor	Surgery or trauma	Factor VIII concentrate: • Usual goal is FVIII level of 100% initially, then 50% until wound healing begins, then 30% until healing complete (usually 7–14 days) • 1 unit/kg usually ↑s FVIII level by 2% • Usual dose: 50 U/kg initially then 25 U/kg q 8-12 hours (or by continuous infusion)	• Severe hemophiliacs (<1% factor VIII) and moderate hemophiliacs (2–5%) require factor VIII concentrates. Mild hemophilia A may be responsive to ddAVP 0.3 mg/kg - preoperative trial infusion recommended • Neurosurgery goal: 100% initial then 50–100% × 10–14 days or until complete healing • Factor levels should be monitored perioperatively
Hemophilia B (factor IX deficiency): no inhibitor	Surgery or trauma	Factor IX concentrate: • Usual goal is FVIII level of 100% initially, then 50% until wound healing begins, then 30% until healing complete (usually 7–14 days) • 1 unit/kg usually ↑s FIX level by 1% • Usual dose: 100 U/kg initially, then 50 U/kg q 8-12 hours (or by continuous infusion)	• ddAVP is *ineffective* in Factor IX deficiency • Neurosurgery goal: 100% initial then 50–100% × 10–14 days or until complete healing • Factor levels should be monitored perioperatively
Hemophilia A or B *with* inhibitors	Surgery or trauma	• Activated prothrombin complex concentrates (aPCCs): 75 U/kg or • Porcine factor VIII (if available and no antibody cross reactivity; VIII inhibitors only): 100-150 U/kg or • Recombinant factor VIIa (rVIIa): 90 µg/kg - repeat at 2–3 hour intervals (usually at least 2-3 doses needed)	• Perisurgical management of hemophiliacs with inhibitors can be very challenging. **Elective surgery should *not be* done on inhibitor patients without consultation with a hematologist** • aPCCs prothrombotic especially with repetitive doses in older patients or patients with liver disease • rVIIa: issues of cost, availability, and possible thrombogenicity
Factor XI deficiency	Surgery or trauma	• Plasma infusion q 12-24 hours to maintain factor levels of 40-60% ($t\frac{1}{2} \approx 45$-60 hours) • Factor XI concentrate unavailable in North America and thrombogenic • rVIIa (experimental): 90 µg/kg - repeat at 2-3 hour intervals (usually at least 2-3 doses needed)	• Poor correlation of hemostatic control with either PTT or measured factor levels - often a management challenge. Hematologic consultation advised
Von Willebrand's disease (vWD)	Surgery or trauma	• Mild-moderate Type I vWD may respond to ddAVP IV 0.3 µg/kg - usual rise in factor VIII and vWF is 3-5 fold • Other forms of vWD should be treated with von Willebrand concentrates (Humate-P®): 50-60 U/kg will usually ↑ plasma level in severe (Type III) vWD to 100%	• ddAVP is first-line treatment only for mild-moderate Type I vWD. Other treatment modalities should normally be used in the different Type II subtypes and in Type III • Plasma factor levels of vWF required perioperatively are similar to those required for FVIII hemophiliacs • Hematological consultation is advised in treating vWD patients
Antithrombin (AT) deficiency	Surgery or trauma	Antithrombin concentrates (Thrombate®) • 1 U/kg will ↑ AT by ~2% ($t\frac{1}{2}$ ~ 60 hours) • Dose in patients with heterozygous AT deficiency needing surgery (heparin: ↑ hemorrhagic risk): 25 U/kg (should ↑ baseline levels by 50%)	• In sick or pregnant patients higher doses (50 U/kg) should be used and $t\frac{1}{2}$ may be significantly less, so daily dosing may be necessary • Hematological consultation is advised in treating AT deficient patients perioperatively and during pregnancy

Dosages are rough guidelines for use in the perioperative setting. Hematologic consultation should normally be sought in managing patients with the above-mentioned conditions preoperatively, intraoperatively, and perioperatively.

Box 26-7   Platelet Dosing

One apheresis unit in an adult (or 1 U random donor platelets/10 kg) should raise the 15 minute to 1 hour postplatelet count by $40-50 \times 10^9/l$.

Relative contraindications to platelet transfusion include idiopathic thrombocytopenic purpura (ITP) unless there is life-threatening bleeding (half-life of transfused platelets in ITP is only ~15 minutes). There is also fairly good evidence that platelet transfusion in heparin-induced thrombocytopenia (HIT) and in thrombotic thrombocytopenic purpura/hemolytic uremic syndrome (TTP-HUS) may precipitate thrombosis, and in these situations platelet transfusion is contraindicated except in the presence of active bleeding (Box 26-7).

Refractoriness may be defined as the failure to achieve a 15 minute to 1 hour postplatelet increase of at least $10 \times 10^9/l$. Insufficient platelet dose should be excluded. The differential diagnosis of refractoriness includes clinical factors (accelerated consumption, sepsis, DIC, bleeding, splenic sequestration), infusion of a suboptimal platelet product (ABO mismatch, especially A platelets transfused to a group O recipient; product more than 48 hours old), and alloimmunization. Alloimmunization is most frequent (~75-80%) to HLA class I antigens (shared by platelets and leukocytes) but may also be to platelet-specific antigen systems. Use of leukodepleted red cell and platelet products will minimize HLA alloimmunization risk in multiply transfused patients. Approaches to diagnosing and treating alloimmunization vary from institution to institution. At the authors' institution the first intervention is to try as fresh as possible ABO-matched platelet products and to measure the 15 minute to 1 hour postplatelet count. If there is a reasonable but suboptimal rise in the platelet count and a higher count is needed, dose and/or frequency of transfusion are increased. If there is no significant rise, patient plasma is tested for the presence of anti-HLA and antiplatelet-specific antibodies and either platelet-crossmatched or HLA-matched apheresis platelet products provided as appropriate.

TRIGGERS FOR TRANSFUSION: CONSENSUS STATEMENTS

We have tried to provide a short discussion for each blood product highlighting the issue of the "transfusion trigger" indicating where there are new data, where clinical judgment is necessary, and where controversy exists. In fact there have been significant discrepancies in recommendations for blood component therapy as set forth by different expert groups within North America, among them the National Institutes of Health consensus conferences in the late 1980s, the American College of Physicians in 1992, the American Society of Anesthesiology in 1996, and the Canadian Medical Association in 1997. The interested reader is referred to these sources, which are referenced in the Selected Reading.

MASSIVE TRANSFUSION

Massive transfusion is defined as replacement of the entire circulating blood volume within a 24-hour period. As a rule in an adult this occurs when ≥ 10 U of RBCs have been transfused. Massive transfusion occurs most often in the setting of major trauma and surgery, although gastrointestinal bleeding, especially in liver disease, is another frequent cause. The coagulopathy that occurs in massively transfused patients is multifactorial and not normally due to "dilution" of factors and platelets by large volumes of crystalloid, colloid, and transfused RBCs alone. There is no simple correlation between the amount of blood lost and replaced and the incidence of coagulopathy; rather coagulopathy is strongly correlated with the incidence and duration of hypotension. In general patients with no or only brief hypotension do not develop coagulopathy despite massive transfusion, those with hypotension for more than 1 hour develop severe coagulopathy, and those with intermediate levels of hypotension develop moderate coagulopathy. Other factors that will influence the development of coagulopathy in the massive transfusion setting are the following:

- Presence of preexisting clinically evident or subclinical coagulation defects (congenital, disease-related, drug-related). For example, patients with liver disease will "pull out" dilutionally very rapidly and patients with uremia or who are on antiplatelet agents will be particularly sensitive to thrombocytopenia.
- Presence of significant tissue injury (especially crush injury and head trauma) or overwhelming sepsis, which release large amounts of tissue factor and result in a systemic procoagulant drive.
- Administration of large volumes of hetastarch (more than a liter may cause acquired vWD) or dextrans (platelet dysfunction).

Formula replacement of blood components ("give 2-4 units of plasma and 1 apheresis platelet per 10 U RBCs transfused") is wasteful and may be harmful. Decision to transfuse should be guided by clinical considerations including the presence of microvascular bleeding and by serial monitoring of the hemoglobin/hematocrit, platelet count, PT INR, PTT, and fibrinogen (see Table 26-6). Given the time required to thaw plasma (~30 minutes), if the presence of coagulopathy is clinically likely, 4 U of plasma should be thawed "on spec." If the initial dose chosen of a particular component does not satisfactorily correct the target coagulation parameter, and bleeding is ongoing, the next dose should be doubled.

Rapid transfusion of cold citrated blood products can also result in metabolic derangements. Hypothermia (body temperature 35°C) in particular is associated with platelet dysfunction and diffuse microvascular bleeding in addition to being synergistic with hypocalcemia (Ca^{2+} chelation by citrate) in potentiating arrhythmia. Table 26-7 summarizes some of the special problems surrounding massive transfusion and suggested management of these.

TRANSFUSION REACTIONS AND COMPLICATIONS

Although public preoccupation has been with viral transfusion-transmitted diseases (TTDs) such as HIV and hepatitis, viral TTD is actually a very uncommon cause of transfusion-related morbidity and mortality. Blood products in the USA are currently tested for HIV 1 and 2, for hepatitis B (HBV) and C (HCV), for human lymphotrophic virus I and II, for syphilis, and from the summer of 2003 for West Nile virus. In the case of HIV and HCV nucleic amplification testing is used and residual risk is estimated at ~1 in 2 million to 1 in 4 million per unit transfused for HIV and at ~1 in 1 million to 1 in 2 million for HCV, with some geographical variability. Many patients receive multiple blood products and overall average patient risk of TTD has been estimated as ~1 in 100,000. Although surveillance data from the United Kingdom indicate possible transfusion transmission of spongiform encephalopathy ("mad cow disease," variant Creutzfeldt-Jakob disease) in man in two cases, this appears to be very rare. Transfusion recipients are actually much more likely to have serious adverse

---

<table>
<tr><td colspan="2">**Box 26-8 The Three Leading Causes of Transfusion-Related Fatalities**</td></tr>
<tr><td>

• Acute hemolytic transfusion reactions (most due to ABO incompatibility)
• Bacterial sepsis (4–5 day old platelets)
• Transfusion-related acute lung injury (TRALI)

</td></tr>
</table>

effects from other transfusion complications, and the current leading causes of transfusion-related fatalities come as a surprise to most people (Box 26-8).

Some common and clinically important transfusion reactions, including their approximate frequency, clinical presentation, cause, prevention, and treatment, can be found in Table 26-8. All suspected transfusion reactions should be reported to the hospital transfusion service; post-transfusion blood (and sometimes urine) samples should be sent to the transfusion service along with the implicated product bag and any remaining product. An area of major controversy in transfusion medicine currently is whether blood transfusion is immunomodulatory, whether this effect is clinically significant in humans as regards postoperative infections and tumor progression, and whether leukodepletion will abrogate this effect if present. Some practitioners have gone so far as to advocate a policy of universal leuko-reduction to prevent the putative significant immuno-modulatory effects of transfusion. However, at present data are conflicting, the majority of transfusion medicine specialists are opposed to such a policy due to lack of firm evidence of benefit and cost/benefit, and major US blood suppliers are still supplying both leukoreduced and nonleukoreduced red cell and platelet products.

Table 26-7 Special Issues in Massive Transfusion

Issue	Cause	Suggested management
Coagulopathy	Multifactorial (see text)	• Obtain baseline complete blood count (hemoglobin, hematocrit, platelet count), PT INR, PTT, and fibrinogen and continue to monitor these as clinically indicated (in major bleeding every 45–60 minutes) • Transfuse RBCs to maintain a Hct > 24, platelets to keep platelet count > 50–80, plasma to keep PT INR < 1.5–2.0, and cryoprecipitate to keep fibrinogen > 100
Hypothermia	Transfusion of cold blood; clinical causes (trauma, etc.)	Use of a validated blood warmer is helpful in massive transfusion settings and most rapid infusion devices have blood warmers. Platelets should not be given through blood warmers
Hypocalcemia	Infusion of citrate	• Check Ca^{2+} after transfusion of about 10 U RBCs in an adult and give Ca^{2+} as necessary to correct the Ca^{2+}. Formula administration may be harmful and should be avoided • In truly massive transfusion (>2 blood volumes) Mg^{2+} should also be checked
Hyperkalemia	K^+ load in RBCs	• Depending on their age RBCs may contain from 10 to 60 mEq/l of K^+. This is usually not a problem in adults, but rarely may be in neonates and small children receiving large volumes of RBCs rapidly, especially in the presence of renal failure and acidosis • K^+ should be monitored and if necessary RBCs < 5 days old or washed RBCs used

Table 26-8   Transfusion Reactions

Reaction Type	Usual Urgency	Approximate incidence	Signs and Symptoms	Cause	Treatment and Prevention
Acute hemolytic	+++++	1:12,000–1:35,000; ~50–75% of fatalities (1:100,000–1:600,000)	Fever, rigors, IV site pain, hypotension, hematuria, renal failure, DIC	Serological incompatibility (ABO) due to specimen/recipient misidentification	Meticulous specimen/ recipient identification is preventative. Maintain blood pressure, treat DIC and metabolic derangements
Delayed hemolytic	+	1:1000–1:12,000; severe symptomatic hemolysis: 1:250,000; death rare	Fever, jaundice 2–3 days to 2–3 weeks post-transfusion	Recipient has antibody to antigen on donor RBCs	No treatment usually required. Antigen negative RBCs needed for subsequent transfusion
Febrile non-hemolytic	+/– to ++	0.5–1.4%, 15% recur; 43–75% of reactions	Temp. rise of >1°C	Contaminating leukocytes; cytokines generated during product storage	If recurrent reactions use leukoreduced RBCs and platelets and premedicate with acetaminophen
Allergic		• Minor (rash, urticaria) – 1–3% • Generalized (confluent urticaria, bronchospasm, anaphylactoid) – 1:1000–1:5000 • Anaphylactic: 1:20,000–1:50,000		Idiosyncratic IgA-mediated reaction to a plasma component	Diphendyramine (minor); hemodynamic and respiratory support, corticosteroids (major). If severe rule out IgA deficiency. Premedication with benadryl +/– corticosteroids +/– H1 and H2 blockers
Bacterial sepsis	++++	Platelets: 1:54,000; RBCs: 1:1.4 million	Fever, rigors, hypotension	Gram-positive or Gram-negative contamination	Culture patient and blood bag. Treat shock. Provide "on spec" Gram-positive and Gram-negative antibiotic coverage
Volume overload	+ – ++++	? 1:100	Congestive heart failure, pulmonary edema.	Excess volume administration for cardiopulmonary reserve	Treat pulmonary edema
Transfusion-related acute lung injury (TRALI)	+++ – ++++	? 1:5000; likely under-recognized	Acute respiratory compromise; noncardiogenic pulmonary edema. Fever and hypotension may occur	Passive transfer of antileukocyte antibodies in donor plasma; neutrophil-priming activity generated during storage of RBCs and platelets	Provide respiratory support as needed. With antibody-mediated TRALI risk of recurrence is very low. With neutrophil-priming TRALI recurrence rate is higher and use of prestorage leukoreduced RBCs and apheresis and fresh-as-possible platelets may prevent recurrence

ALTERNATIVES TO BLOOD COMPONENT THERAPY

Alternatives to blood component therapy are numerous, and a number have been touched upon in the discussions above on plasma, cryo, and coagulopathy and platelets. Unfortunately, for many of these alternatives the risks, benefits, and cost-effectiveness are unclear, and there may also be associated reimbursement issues. General blood conservation measures include minimizing blood draws, use of pediatric tubes, stopping aspirin at least four days prior to surgery, correction of coagulopathies and nutritional anemias (iron, folate, B_{12}) preoperatively, and use of an experienced surgeon and anesthesiologist. If the estimated blood loss is >750–1000 ml and/or the hemoglobin is <14 g/dl consideration should be given to increasing the preoperative hemoglobin with erythropoietin (see below). Autologous predonation (donation of whole blood by a patient for their own later use – donations are generally given 1 week apart beginning 3 weeks prior to surgery) avoids TTD but has other risks: it results in preoperative anemia and increases overall chance of transfusion; the risks of patient/specimen misidentification, volume overload, and bacterial contamination remain; and it is significantly more costly than allogeneic blood due to nonutilization of collected units. In addition about 1 in 17,000 standard risk donors are hospitalized as a direct result of complications of the autologous donation. Autologous predonation of high-risk patients (stable cardiac disease, on pharmacologic agents that block compensatory response) should be done only under conditions of close monitoring and isovolemic fluid replacement.

CURRENT CONTROVERSY

Autologous Predonation

Once considered the "standard of care" for some surgeries (orthopedic) recent studies have suggested that, with declining transmissible disease risks, the risks of autologous predonation in many cases appear to outweigh the benefits.

Isovolemic hemodilution appears to be safe and effective, and considerably more cost-effective than autologous predonation in selected surgeries (radical prostatectomy). However, the technique is poorly standardized, data are conflicting, operating room time may be necessary, and meticulous attention to volume is crucial in borderline cases. Intraoperative blood salvage (cell saver, etc.) is suitable for high-volume "clean" losses (vascular surgery). If large-volume (>500–1000 ml) salvage is done, the device should "wash" the salvaged blood and return only the RBCs to the patient. Postoperative blood salvage (mediastinal drainage, knee and hip drains) is more controversial. In general such salvage is costly and little blood is salvaged; there may also be issues of sterility and of inducing coagulopathy. In selected surgical settings and patients, particularly in bloodless medicine and surgery programs, hypotensive anesthesia may be used.

A variety of pharmacologic agents can be useful as adjuncts or alternatives to blood products. Erythropoietin can be useful to increase the hematocrit preoperatively (see above) and is approved for this purpose in noncardiovascular surgery. The dose is 600 U/kg/week for 3 weeks prior to surgery (days –21, –14, and –7) or 300 U/kg given 10 consecutive days before surgery and 4 days postoperatively. It usually takes a minimum of 10–14 days to get any meaningful increase in hematocrit. Adequate iron repletion should be ensured. Postoperatively there is resistance to the action of erythropoietin and it is less effective. DDAVP is first-line therapy in treatment of mild to moderate hemophilia A and mild to moderate Type I vWD and may be given both IV and intranasally. IV dose is 0.3 µg/kg. A preoperative trial is recommended to ensure hemostatic levels. DDAVP may also be useful in correction of platelet dysfunction (uremia, drug-induced). Fibrinolytic inhibitors (aprotinin, tranexamic acid, epsilon aminocaproic acid) can be useful in attenuating blood loss in cardiac surgery (especially reoperative surgery) and in oral surgery and perhaps in other settings. Dose optimization is unclear, cost can be an issue, and there are questions regarding possible prothrombotic risk. Fibrin glues have been discussed above. Recombinant factor VIIa is a new pharmacologic hemostatic agent whose therapeutic role is evolving. It is extremely costly and not readily available. It is probably now the established first-line therapeutic agent in congenital hemophiliacs with inhibitors and in acquired hemophilia. Its role and cost/benefit in correction of other hemostatic abnormalities (urgent warfarin reversal, refractory coagulopathy of hepatic dysfunction, severe congenital platelet abnormalities, microvascular bleeding in trauma, etc.) remains to be established.

There are currently no "red cell substitutes" licensed in North America, although a bovine hemoglobin-based O_2 carrier (HBOC), Hemopure, was recently licensed in South Africa. Three HBOCs have now completed or are undergoing US FDA phase 3 trials in the USA: Hemopure (bovine hemoglobin glutamer, Biopure Corp.), PolyHeme (human pyridoxilated polymerized hemoglobin, Northfield Laboratories), and Hemolink (human hemoglobin raffimer, Hemosol Inc., although this trial was halted prematurely). The products are being investigated primarily in the perioperative setting, although acute resuscitation studies are planned. An earlier human diasporin-linked HBOC (Hemassist, Baxter) has been discontinued. All the HBOCs have short plasma half-lives (days), and it is not clear that they are equivalent in efficacy or side effects. Their clinical roles remain to be established, and rather than "red cell substitutes" discussion is now turning to their potential broader role in "oxygen therapeutics." Their presence in the plasma may also interfere with certain laboratory tests (including optically based tests of coagulation and O_2 determination by pulse oximetry). Perfluorocarbon solutions are also capable of carrying O_2 dissolved in solution, although like HBOCs they have short plasma half-lives and a variety of side effects reported. One of them, Perflubron (Alliance Pharmaceuticals), was being used in a phase 3 trial in perioperative hemodilution, but this was recently halted. Potential platelet substitutes are being developed (infusible platelet membranes, fibrinogen-coated albumin microspheres).

Jehovah's Witnesses refuse whole blood and all of its primary components (RBCs, platelets, and plasma) and pose special challenges in the perioperative setting. However, plasma derivatives (cryo, albumin, fibrin glues) are considered "matters of conscience" and are accepted by some Jehovah's Witnesses but not others. Autologous predonation is unacceptable to Jehovah's Witnesses but perioperative hemodilution and intraoperative salvage procedures where the blood is kept in a continuous circuit with the body are "matters of conscience."

Erythropoietin (stabilized with traces of albumin) is acceptable to most Jehovah's Witnesses, as are all pharmacologic blood-sparing agents. HBOCs, when available, will be "matters of conscience." The Jehovah's Witness community has a hospital liaison network which can provide information and put practitioners in contact with physicians experienced in managing Jehovah's Witness patients who can provide advice.

SELECTED READING

Expert Group Recommendations

American College of Physicians: Practice strategies for elective red blood cell transfusion. Ann Int Med 116:403–406, 1992.

Expert Working Group: Guidelines for red blood cell and plasma transfusions for adults and children. Can Med Assoc J 156(Suppl 11):S1–S25, 1997.

Practice guidelines for blood component therapy: a report by the American Society of Anesthesiologists Task Force on Blood Component Therapy. Anesthesiology 84:732–747, 1996.

General

Carson JL, Noveck H, Berlin J, Gould SA: Mortality and morbidity in patients with very low postoperative Hb levels who decline transfusion. Transfusion 42:812–818, 2002.

DeLoughery TG: *Hemostasis and Thrombosis*, Austin, TX: Landes Bioscience, 1999.

Dzik S: The use of blood components prior to invasive bedside procedures: a critical appraisal. In Mintz PD, editor: *Transfusion Therapy: Clinical Principles and Practice*, Bethesda, MD: AABB Press, 1999, pp 151–169.

Goodnight SH Jr, Hathaway WE, editors: *Disorders of Hemostasis and Thrombosis: A Clinical Guide*, ed 2, McGraw-Hill: New York, 2001.

Goodnough LT, Bach RG: Anemia, transfusion and mortality [editorial]. New Engl J Med 345:1272–1274, 2001.

Goodnough LT, Brecher ME, Kanter MH, AuBuchon JP: Transfusion medicine: I. Blood transfusion. New Engl J Med 340:438–447, 1999.

Goodnough LT, Brecher ME, Kanter MH, AuBuchon JP: Transfusion medicine: II. Blood conservation. New Engl J Med 340:525–533, 1999.

Hebert PC, Wells G, Blajchman MA, Marshall J et al; Transfusion Requirements in Critical Care Investigators for the Canadian Critical Care Trials Group: A multicenter, randomized controlled clinical trial of transfusion requirements in critical care. New Engl J Med 340:409–417, 1999.

Jahr JS, Nesargi SB, Lewis K, Johnson C: Blood substitutes and oxygen therapeutics: an overview and current status. Am J Therapeut 9:437–443, 2002.

Spence RK, Jeter EK, Mintz PD: Transfusion in surgery and trauma. In Mintz PD, editor: *Transfusion Therapy: Clinical Principles and Practice*, Bethesda, MD: AABB Press, 1999, pp 171–197.

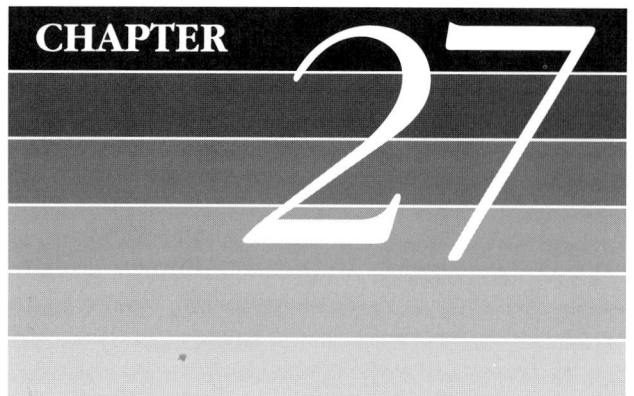

CHAPTER 27

Cirrhosis, Fulminant Hepatic Failure, and Liver Transplantation

JASON DZIAK, M.D.

ASHWANI CHHIBBER, M.D.

Cirrhosis is an irreversible process of fibrosis and nodular regeneration that occurs throughout the liver. This represents the end stage of hepatocellular injury in which viable hepatocytes are replaced primarily by connective tissue due to a chronic disease process, e.g., longstanding alcohol use or chronic viral infection, usually occurring over decades. Cirrhosis can be classified histologically as micro- or macronodular depending on the stage of liver disease, and its natural history can also be divided into compensated and decompensated states. Decompensation is characterized by the development of jaundice, ascites, gastrointestinal (GI) bleeding, or hepatic encephalopathy.

Fulminant hepatic failure (FHF) is defined as development of hepatic encephalopathy within eight weeks of the clinical onset of acute hepatic disease without a previous history of liver disease. This hepatic dysfunction is due to either massive hepatocellular necrosis or, less commonly, replacement of hepatocytes with malignant tissue.

CURRENT CONTROVERSY

New classifications of FHF have been proposed by many clinicians. One modification suggests that the term FHF be reserved for encephalopathy that occurs within 2 weeks of the onset of acute liver disease, and that the term subfulminant hepatic failure be used when encephalopathy occurs between 2 weeks and 3 months after the onset of jaundice or other clinically apparent liver disease, i.e., coagulopathy or jaundice.

ETIOLOGY

The causes of cirrhosis can be broadly divided into two major categories: (1) parenchymal liver disease and (2) cholestasis with or without extrahepatic biliary obstruction. The pathophysiology of cholestatic liver disease is thought to be secondary to bile acid accumulation in viable hepatocytes that leads to apoptosis in these cells. Most cirrhotic patients in the USA today are likely to have multiple parenchymal hepatic insults, most commonly chronic hepatitis C, alcohol abuse, and fatty liver of obesity, also known as nonalcoholic steatohepatitis (NASH). The presence of any two of these three etiologies has been shown to be synergistic in causing cirrhosis. Since 1990, when obesity was convincingly shown to be a causative factor for cirrhosis, the diagnosis of cryptogenic cirrhosis has decreased dramatically. The pathophysiology of NASH has been linked to coexisting insulin resistance with subsequent development of dysfunctional fatty acid metabolism. This is thought to result in excess free fatty acids that lead to oxidative

Table 27-1 Etiologies of Cirrhosis

Parenchymal Disease	Cholestatic Disease
Chronic hepatitis C*	Primary biliary cirrhosis
Ethanol or Leannec's cirrhosis*	Primary sclerosing cholangitis
Nonalcoholic steatohepatitis (NASH)*	Neoplasm of bile ducts or pancreas
Chronic hepatitis B	Chronic biliary obstruction due to stone/stricture
Other drugs or toxins, e.g., methotrexate and isoniazid	Cystic fibrosis
Hemochromatosis	
Wilson's disease	
Alpha-1-antitrypsin deficiency	
Chronic congestive heart failure or pericarditis with hepatic venous congestion	
Cryptogenic	
Autoimmune	
Polycystic liver disease	

* These three etiologies comprise 80% of all causes of cirrhosis.

stress and direct hepatotoxicity. The etiologies for cirrhosis are shown in Table 27-1.

The etiologies for FHF are listed in Table 27-2. Hepatitis A and B (HAV and HBV) are the two most common viral etiologies for FHF. Although hepatitis C (HCV) is also a rare cause of FHF, recent studies have shown that patients with chronic HCV are particularly prone to develop FHF when superinfected with HAV. Hepatitis D is an uncommon etiology unless present concomitantly with HBV. Hepatitis E has been associated with cases of FHF outside of the USA. Of note, chronic viral infection with either hepatitis B or C can predispose to the development of hepatocellular carcinoma.

There are multiple potential mechanisms for drug-induced FHF. They are listed in Table 27-3.

Acetaminophen-induced FHF involves a dose-related mechanism. It is initially metabolized via glucuronide and sulfate conjugation, and at higher doses this pathway becomes saturated. The metabolism is then shifted to an alternative cytochrome p450 system that is dependent on glutathione. With excessive dosing, glutathione stores become depleted. This results in an accumulation of the hepatotoxic metabolite N-acetyl-p-benzoquinone. N-acetylcysteine, a glutathione donor, is commonly used in the setting of acetaminophen overdose to prevent further hepatotoxicity. The risk for acetaminophen toxicity has been shown to be higher in chronic alcoholics wherein lower doses can result in FHF. The associated morbidity and mortality of acetaminophen-related FHF is also higher in this patient population. Halothane hepatitis is an example of an immunoallergic drug reaction. Metabolites of halothane, an inhalational anesthetic agent, are recognized as antigenic, and an autoimmune response occurs that results in cross-reactivity with hepatic tissue. This is a rare but severe reaction. More commonly, mild postoperative increases in hepatic transaminases can be seen with the use of halothane and other inhaled agents such as isoflurane. This reaction is less severe, self-limited, and is the result of indirect toxicity due to decreased hepatic blood flow that occurs with inhaled anesthetics. Isoniazid and tricyclic antidepressants are classic examples of drugs whose metabolites are hepatotoxic. They are potentially dangerous to administer in combination with drugs that induce the cytochrome p450 system.

CLINICAL CAVEAT

Acetaminophen serum levels do not reliably indicate the degree or severity of hepatotoxicity. If an overdose is suspected, N-acetylcysteine should be administered immediately.

Table 27-2 Etiologies of Fulminant Hepatic Failure

Predominant Causes*	Other Causes	
Viral hepatitis	Acute fatty liver of pregnancy	Reye's syndrome
Acetaminophen toxicity (attempted suicide, intentional/unintentional overdose)	Autoimmune hepatitis (initial presentation)	Primary graft nonfunction following liver transplantation
Other drug reactions/toxicities	Vascular abnormalities (Budd Chiari or other hepatic veno-occlusive disease)	Other infectious cause (other viruses, tuberculosis)
	Cardiac failure; eclampsia; ischemia (hypotension, heat stroke)	Toxins: *Amanita phylloides*, organic solvents, herbal medications (ginseng,
	Lecithin-cholesterol acyl transferase deficiency	pennyroyal oil), bacterial toxins
	Malignant infiltration (primary or metastatic)	(*B. cereus*, cyanobacteria), Ecstasy
	Wilson's disease (initial presentation)	(methyldioxymethamphetamine), cocaine

* Approximately 15–20% of causes are indeterminate.

Table 27-3   Mechanisms of Drug Toxicity*

Direct toxicity (dose related)
Drug metabolite toxicity
Immunoallergic
Idiosyncratic reactions (sporadic and not dose related)

* Idiosyncratic reactions are most common.

DRUG INTERACTION

- Isoniazid and rifampin: rifampin is a potent p450 induction agent and greatly increases the quantity of hepatotoxic metabolites generated by isoniazid.
- Barbiturates and tricyclic antidepressants (TCAs), e.g., Amitryptilline: barbiturates such as sodium thiopental are potent inducers of cytochrome p450 and greatly increase the metabolism of TCAs with a subsequent increase in hepatotoxic TCA metabolites.

The list of drugs that can result in hepatotoxicity is an exhaustive one that will not be covered here. There are, however, certain clinical indicators that are helpful to consider when assessing whether or not drug toxicity is the etiology of hepatic failure. These include the presence of an acute process (drug toxicity is rarely chronic in nature), ruling out other etiologies of liver disease and specific chronological parameters. The time interval between use of the drug and the onset of hepatic toxicity is generally 1 week to 3 months. Resolution or improvement of liver disease after withdrawal of the suspected agent or worsening of disease after accidental use of the drug are also suggestive chronologic markers. Table 27-4 lists the remainder of commonly observed positive clinical criteria associated with drug-induced hepatotoxicity.

CLASSIFICATION OF SEVERITY OF CIRRHOSIS AND FULMINANT HEPATIC FAILURE

Cirrhosis

The Child-Pugh score (CPS) is the most commonly used classification scale for cirrhotic patients. Survival has been shown to be inversely related to the CPS. Patients with 10 points usually require frequent medical checkups. Patients with 12 points regularly require hospitalization for management of decompensated liver disease. Patients with 13–14 points generally require management in the intensive care unit (see Table 27-5).

Table 27-4   Positive Clinical Criteria for Drug-Induced Hepatotoxicity

Age > 50 years
Polypharmacy
Use of known hepatotoxic drugs or toxins
Drug serum levels (e.g., acetaminophen)
Specific serum autoantibodies
Specific liver biopsy findings (e.g., drug deposits, eosinophilic infiltration)

The Model End Stage Liver Disease or MELD score has currently been adopted by the United Network for Organ Sharing (UNOS) as an alternative to the CPS system. UNOS is the national organization that assigns listing status for organ allocation to recipients based on disease severity. The MELD is calculated using a formula with three primary variables which include serum creatinine, total bilirubin, and international normalized ratio (INR). The formula for the MELD score and its correlation with the former CPS-based UNOS listing criteria are shown in Table 27-6.

Fulminant Hepatic Failure

Table 27-7 shows prognostic indicators that are associated with adverse outcomes in patients with FHF. These variables were obtained from King's College Hospital in London, UK, and since their introduction in 1989 they are the most widely utilized FHF criteria. In patients with acetaminophen toxicity the presence of a single indicator is associated with a mortality rate of at least 55%. The presence of severe acidosis in acetaminophen patients carries a mortality rate of 95%. The presence of a single indicator in nonacetaminophen patients is associated with an 80% mortality rate, and the presence of three indicators carries a mortality rate of greater than 95%. All of these respective mortality rates, however, vastly exceed perioperative mortality rates associated with liver transplantation.

Table 27-5   Child-Pugh Scoring System

	1 Point	2 Points	3 Points
Serum albumin (g/dl)	>3.5	2.8–3.5	<2.8
INR	<1.7	1.7–2.3	>2.3
Ascites	None	Slight or diuretic controlled	Moderate or severe
Encephalopathy	None	Mild or moderate	Severe

Table 27-6		MELD Score and UNOS Status
MELD*	**UNOS Status**	**Comments**
< 24	3	CPS > 7 and requires continuous medical surveillance
24–29	2b	CPS > 10 or CPS > 7 with at least one of the following criteria: significant variceal hemorrhage, hepatorenal syndrome, SBP, or refractory ascites
> 30	2a	End-stage chronic liver disease with CPS > 10 and life expectancy < 7 days
	1	FHF with life expectancy < 7 days, primary nonfunction of liver transplant within 7 days, hepatic artery thrombosis within 7 days of liver transplant

* Maximum MELD score is 40. MELD score formula: $10[0.957(Cr) + 0.378(Tbili) + 1.12(INR) + 0.643]$.

CURRENT CONTROVERSY

Some clinicians advocate the use of CT-guided hepatic volumetry and liver histology, i.e., parenchymal necrosis of greater than 50% as prognostic indicators for FHF. The practicality of these measures has been questioned due to bleeding risk with hepatic biopsy and the difficulty of transporting critically ill patients for CT evaluation.

DIAGNOSTIC STUDIES

Laboratory Testing

Specific laboratory tests are ordered routinely for patients with suspected or documented cirrhosis and/or FHF. Certain results can detect treatable chronic liver disease before significant decompensation occurs. These tests also facilitate care of FHF patients and help rule out specific FHF etiologies. A complete blood count can reveal anemia secondary to splenic sequestration, GI hemorrhage, or decreased erythropoietin production in the setting of hepatorenal syndrome. Thrombocytopenia may present secondary to splenic sequestration, bone marrow suppression, disseminated intravascular coagulation, or massive hemorrhage. Elevated white blood cell count (WBC) can present with infectious processes such as spontaneous bacterial peritonitis (SBP). A full liver panel is routinely obtained with subsequent serial measurements. It is important to note that serum AST and ALT levels may not be elevated in cirrhotic patients due to extensive hepatocyte destruction and subsequent decrease of transaminase production. Prolonged prothrombin time (PT)/INR and partial thromboplastin time

Table 27-7	King's College Hospital Criteria
Acetaminophen Patients	**Nonacetaminophen Patients**
pH < 7.30 INR > 6.50 Serum creatinine > 3.4 mg/dl in patients with stage 3 or 4 encephalopathy	Age <10 years or >40 years INR > 3.5 Etiology: non-A and non-B hepatitis, halothane hepatitis, drug/toxin mediated Duration of jaundice > 1 week before the development of encephalopathy Serum bilirubin > 18 mg/dl

(PTT) generally result from decreased synthesis of clotting factors by the liver. Poor absorption of fat-soluble vitamin K due to altered bilirubin excretion and poor nutritional intake of vitamin K are other factors to consider when evaluating for a coagulopathy. The degree of PTT abnormalities tends to parallel PT/INR abnormalities in patients with acute or chronic liver disease.

CLINICAL CAVEAT

Chronically cirrhotic patients are unlikely to respond to vitamin K administration for the treatment of coagulopathy secondary to nonfunctioning hepatocytes with impaired synthetic ability.

Serologic testing for viral hepatitis is routine for patients with evidence of chronic or acute hepatic disease. Quantitative DNA and RNA tests for hepatitis B and C, respectively, are now commonly obtained if antigen or antibody tests are positive. Hepatitis B quantitative DNA testing has largely replaced the e antigen test. Serial measurements of serum electrolytes and glucose levels are also routinely obtained. Cirrhotic patients may present with decreased serum potassium and magnesium levels secondary to chronic diuresis. Hypocalcemia may be present with advanced renal dysfunction due to hepatorenal syndrome or in the setting of citrate toxicity secondary to blood product administration. Hypoglycemia can occur with malnourishment or with impaired gluconeogenesis and glycogenolysis at the hepatocyte level. Hyperglycemia can be seen in patients with cirrhosis secondary to NASH who often exhibit insulin resistance. Hyponatremia is a common clinical entity in cirrhotic patients due to either chronic diuresis or an overall total body hypervolemic state. Table 27-8 outlines the remainder of standard laboratory screening tests obtained in the setting of acute or chronic liver disease.

Table 27-8 Laboratory Screening Tests

Laboratory Test	Etiology
Serum iron, ferritin, iron saturation	Elevated with hemachromatosis
Antinuclear and smooth muscle antibodies	Present with autoimmune hepatic disease
Antimitochondrial antibodies	Present with primary biliary cirrhosis
Ceruloplasmin levels	Elevated with Wilson's disease
Alpha-1-antitrypsin phenotype	Present with alpha-1-antitrypsin deficiency
Alpha-fetoprotein	Increased with hepatocellular carcinoma

CLINICAL CAVEAT

Some degree of hyponatremia should be tolerated in cirrhotic patients. Aggressive replacement of sodium with excessive fluids can precipitate central pontine myelinolysis or volume overload with pulmonary edema.

Imaging Studies

Ultrasonography is the least invasive, least expensive, and most widely utilized imaging modality in the management of acute and chronic liver disease. Assessing the size of both the spleen and portal vein and the presence of ascites or tumor are the primary concerns when performing abdominal ultrasonography. Maximum spleen dimension greater than 12 cm or a portal vein diameter greater than 13 mm are suggestive of portal hypertension. Doppler scanning is also used to observe vascular flow and can detect thromboses. Although cholelithiasis is detected in approximately one-third of cirrhotic patients, they are generally asymptomatic.

CLINICAL CAVEAT

Cholecystectomy is to be avoided in cirrhotic patients. Mortality rates associated with this procedure in the cirrhotic patient population have been reported as high as 80% in some studies.

CLINICAL CAVEAT

The use of a contrast agent should be avoided if the serum creatinine is 2 mg/dl or greater.

Computed tomography (CT) scans are also commonly obtained for cirrhotic patients. This modality involves radiation and usually the addition of an intravenous contrast agent. It is also more expensive. Spiral CT is currently the preferred method due to its superior scanning speed and decreased artifact.

Esophagogastroduodenoscopy (EGD) is used as both a diagnostic tool and treatment modality in the management of esophageal varices. This is discussed in more detail later in this chapter. Colonoscopy is commonly performed as a part of the pretransplantation evaluation. It is generally not performed in nontransplantation candidates.

CURRENT CONTROVERSY

The practice of performing colonoscopy in hepatic transplant candidates is controversial and not supported by some data. Polypectomy in the presence of ascites can lead to an increased risk of colonic perforation.

Imaging-guided liver biopsy can be performed to document the presence of cirrhosis, to assess the etiology of hepatic disease, and to evaluate the severity of hepatic injury. Percutaneous approaches are associated with higher morbidity in the setting of ascites or coagulopathy. Transjugular biopsy can be performed if the biopsy is required, and the patient is in a high-risk category.

CLINICAL MANIFESTATIONS OF CIRRHOSIS AND FULMINANT HEPATIC FAILURE

Encephalopathy

Hepatic encephalopathy or portasystemic encephalopathy (PSE) is the second most common complication of cirrhosis, developing in approximately 28% of patients within 10 years after the diagnosis of decompensated disease. It can also be present in FHF and becomes clinically apparent as liver function progressively worsens. Encephalopathy is due primarily to shunting of toxins past the liver and into the systemic circulation. In the setting of FHF, however, the greater concern is that many patients develop cerebral edema with the potential for increased intracranial pressure, cerebral herniation, and subsequent brain death. The pathogenesis of this cerebral edema has not been completely elucidated, but both vasogenic and cytokine-mediated mechanisms have been proposed. In general, vasogenic edema results from a breakdown in the blood–brain barrier that allows passage of plasma contents into the brain parenchyma.

CLINICAL CAVEAT

Although cerebral edema has been implicated primarily in FHF, there have been a significant number of reports concerning cerebral edema in cirrhotic patients with severe PSE.

The grades of hepatic encephalopathy are listed in Table 27-9. Grades I and II have a better prognosis compared to grades III and IV with respect to progression to cerebral edema, especially in patients with FHF. Elective intubation and mechanical ventilation is often performed in patients who progress to grade III encephalopathy.

In cirrhotic patients encephalopathy can develop spontaneously as liver disease progressively worsens or it can be unmasked by certain medications such as sedatives or narcotics, polysubstance abuse, or other precipitating factors. These factors include infections (e.g., spontaneous bacterial peritonitis), GI bleeding, dehydration, or hypokalemia. The treatment of these underlying disturbances or the removal of the offending factor usually rapidly reverses PSE symptoms.

CLINICAL CAVEAT

Sedatives and/or narcotics should be specifically avoided or minimized in cirrhotic patients with the exception of advanced hepatocellular carcinoma or the perioperative setting.

The primary therapy for PSE is lactulose. Approximately 90% of patients with PSE will respond to lactulose in combination with the correction of a coexisting precipitating factor. Patients who are refractory to lactulose therapy can be treated with oral neomycin in combination with lactulose. Serial serum ammonia levels

Table 27-9	Grades of Portasystemic Encephalopathy

Grade	Mental Status
I	Restless, mild confusion
II	Lethargic, inappropriate behavior
III	Somnolent but rousable, incoherent speech
IV	Comatose

and dietary protein restriction are also commonly initiated in the treatment of PSE.

CLINICAL CAVEAT

Overdosing of lactulose via oral route, nasogastric tube, or enema can lead to complications such as hypernatremia, central nervous system demyelination with rapid increases in serum sodium levels, or permanent coma. It is important for clinicians to be patient in assessing response to lactulose administration.

CURRENT CONTROVERSY

Recent literature has shown that cirrhotic patients are at times inappropriately hospitalized or experience longer hospital stays due to asymptomatic elevated serum ammonia levels. Other clinicians have shown that protein restriction can actually worsen PSE symptoms due to aggravation of malnutrition in cirrhotic patients.

As stated previously, patients with grades III and IV encephalopathy, especially those with FHF, are at higher risk for the development of cerebral edema. A prolonged intracranial pressure (ICP) greater than 40 mmHg or a prolonged cerebral perfusion pressure (CPP) less than 50 mmHg have been associated with poor neurological recovery.

CURRENT CONTROVERSY

Some clinicians consider a CPP below 40 mmHg for longer than 1 hour a contraindication for liver transplantation. However, there have been multiple case reports of patients making full neurologic recoveries following prolonged episodes (24-38 hours) of severely impaired CPP.

Treatment of elevated ICP is managed primarily with mannitol, although no single agent has been shown to benefit all patients. Corticosteroids have not been shown to have clinical efficacy. N-acetylcysteine has been shown to improve neurological outcome in patients with acetaminophen toxicity. Some clinicians advocate the use of pentobarbital with continuous EEG monitoring for burst suppression. However, the use of this agent is controversial due to the risk of barbiturate-induced leukocyte suppression and hypotension.

Propofol has been proposed as an alternative to barbiturates, but there has been associated hypotension, increased cost, and no discernible clinical advantage with this agent. Hyperventilation is in general currently avoided due to critical decreases in cerebral blood flow seen with this intervention. There are also now new data to support the institution of mild hypothermia (35°C) in this patient population. Mild hypothermia significantly decreases cerebral metabolic rate and can be utilized as a bridge to transplantation or in the intraoperative transplant setting to improve neurological outcome. Hyperthermia and hyperglycemia should be specifically avoided because of poorer neurological outcomes associated with these specific clinical factors.

> ## CURRENT CONTROVERSY
>
> Monitoring of ICP in the setting of advanced encephalopathy is controversial, although many clinicians advocate its use. Identifying patients with severely elevated ICP and decreased CPP allows the rejection of transplant candidates who are higher risk of intraoperative brain death. The use of CT scanning and clinical signs such as papilledema are also much less sensitive for detecting increased ICP in this patient population. Some clinicians avoid ICP monitoring due to the increased risk of intracranial hemorrhage, especially with ventriculostomies.

Cardiovascular Manifestations

A hyperdynamic circulation with elevated cardiac output and decreased systemic vascular resistance (SVR) develops in 30-60% of all patients with cirrhosis. A similar circulatory disturbance with concomitant hypotension is also common in the setting of FHF. Ultimately, this circulatory state makes hemodynamic parameters difficult to evaluate. Elevated levels of circulating vasopressors and vasodilators with the balance in favor of vasodilation is thought to be the mechanism of the hyperdynamic circulation and pressor resistance seen in both the cirrhotic and FHF population. Cirrhotic patients tend to have impaired contractility in response to physiologic stress, and those with ascites have been shown to manifest small degrees of diastolic dysfunction. Cardiac dysrhythmias, decreases in tissue oxygen uptake, and development of arteriovenous shunts may also develop. Intravascular volume depletion is also a common finding in both chronic and acute liver disease due to GI hemorrhage, production and replacement of protein-rich ascites, and/or chronic diuresis.

> ## CLINICAL CAVEAT
>
> The incidence of coronary artery disease in transplant recipient patients older than 50 years has been shown to be in the range 5-27%. These patients require aggressive initial and subsequent continued cardiac evaluation.

Pulmonary Manifestations

Pulmonary dysfunction is common in the setting of FHF and cirrhosis. Pneumonia and acute respiratory distress syndrome (ARDS) are the most common pulmonary manifestations in the FHF population. Some studies have reported rates of ARDS as high as 33% in cases of acetaminophen toxicity. The development of ARDS in the setting of FHF is also associated with high mortality rates. Chronically debilitated cirrhotic patients are prone to pulmonary dysfunction due to atelectasis, obstructive airway disease, aspiration, and pleural effusions. In addition, severe ascites with abdominal distention predisposes these patients to early airway closure and a restrictive pattern of lung disease. Cirrhotic patients also manifest vascular pulmonary disease in the form of intrapulmonary vasodilations (IPVDs), true shunting, and potentially portopulmonary hypertension. Hepatopulmonary syndrome is defined as hypoxemia that is caused by IPVDs or intrapulmonary shunts. This hypoxemia is often the result of impaired diffusion of oxygen across the significantly dilated capillary. Oxygen does not effectively penetrate this widened stream of blood, and thus part of the stream circulates through deoxygenated and is essentially shunted. True anatomic shunts are much less common and are usually portopulmonary. Treatment with 100% oxygen increases the driving force of oxygen through the capillary bed and usually is effective therapy. The supine position is also surprisingly helpful due to the shifting of blood to the apices where IPVDs and shunting are less common. The pathophysiology of hepatopulmonary syndrome is thought to be due to vasodilatory vasoactive mediators, most likely nitric oxide and endothelin, which are shunted into the systemic circulation secondary to portal hypertension.

Portopulmonary hypertension secondary to or in conjunction with hepatopulmonary syndrome is a concerning condition in patients with end-stage liver disease. This population experiences much higher perioperative mortality rates when undergoing hepatic transplantation. Pulmonary hypertension is defined as a mean pulmonary artery pressure of 25 mmHg or greater with a pulmonary capillary wedge pressure less than 15 mmHg or, as an alternative, a pulmonary vascular resistance (PVR) of greater than 120 dynes/cm/s^5. In general, transplant candidates with mean pulmonary arterial pressures greater than 35–50 mmHg are rejected on the basis of significantly increased risk of perioperative death.

CURRENT CONTROVERSY

Some clinicians argue that patients with mean pulmonary artery pressures in the range 35–50 mmHg should be risk stratified between PVR values of greater or less than 250 dynes. There are data to support proceeding with transplantation in patients who have resistance of less 250 dynes in this population. Certain clinicians also advocate a pharmacologic challenge in this setting with agents such as nitric oxide or prostaglandin E1 to assess responsiveness of the pulmonary vasculature. A decrease in mean pressure or PVR by 20% or greater is cited as a favorable response. Patients with mean pulmonary arterial pressures of greater than 50 mmHg and a PVR of greater than 250 dynes are usually not accepted as hepatic transplant candidates.

There is also debate regarding whether or not portopulmonary syndrome and hepatopulmonary syndrome are completely separate entities. Some clinicians argue that pulmonary hypertension develops as a result of chronic hypoxemia in the setting of hepatopulmonary syndrome. Others claim that portopulmonary hypertension develops independently due to a pulmonary vasoconstrictive process, whereas hepatopulmonary syndrome is exclusively a pulmonary vasodilatory phenomenon.

Gastrointestinal Manifestations

Ascites is a common GI manifestation of cirrhosis, and it occurs secondary to elevated portal pressures and volume overload with subsequent leakage of excess fluid across the liver capsule. The two-year survival rate in cirrhotic patients who develop ascites is approximately 50%. The cornerstones of treatment are dietary sodium restriction and diuresis. Diuretics increase urine sodium excretion which is generally reduced in cirrhotic patients. A combination of potassium sparing and wasting diuretics is often chosen to maintain normokalemia. In addition, cirrhotic patients usually have significantly elevated aldosterone levels, and spironolactone is generally thought of as the single best diuretic in this population because of its antialdosterone activity. If ascites becomes diuretic resistant, the patient is often given a diagnosis of prehepatorenal syndrome which carries a mortality rate of approximately 50% within 6 months of onset.

DRUG INTERACTION

Due to the intravascular volume depletion seen with these agents, diuretics can often potentiate hypotension that occurs with the use of both inhaled and intravenous anesthetic agents, e.g., isoflurane and propofol. Hyperkalemia can also be seen with the use of spironolactone, and serum potassium levels should be checked prior to administration of succinylcholine. The transient increase of serum potassium seen with succinylcholine use may be dangerously high with this drug combination.

If ascites is diuretic resistant, large-volume paracentesis is generally performed. Many studies have now demonstrated the safety of this technique, and it can generally be performed every 2 weeks. It should, however, be reserved for those patients who are truly diuretic resistant.

CURRENT CONTROVERSY

Some clinicians advocate albumin infusions following large-volume paracentesis due to removal of proteins that cannot be easily synthesized and replaced by the cirrhotic liver. Many studies, however, have not shown a difference in mortality rates with this approach. Other studies that show a benefit have been criticized as regards their design.

The transjugular intrahepatic portosystemic shunt (TIPS) is also utilized in the management of intractable ascites. This procedure is performed by an interventional radiologist and is generally indicated for diuretic-resistant ascites, variceal bleeding not responsive to other forms of therapy, and hepatorenal syndrome.

CURRENT CONTROVERSY

TIPS has been criticized by some clinicians because of poorer survival rates shown to be associated with this intervention. Although it is less invasive than an open surgical shunt, there is also a relatively high risk of complications with the procedure. These include hemorrhage, shunt obstruction, and a 25% incidence of encephalopathy. The mortality rate directly related to this procedure has also been quoted as high as 10%. TIPS is, however, preferred by some clinicians who utilize it as a bridge to liver transplantation, and some studies have shown that TIPS improves outcomes in decompensated cirrhotic patients who undergo nontransplant surgical procedures. New stent grafts have also been used with lower complication rates in some studies.

Variceal bleeding is the third most common complication of cirrhosis, and the distal esophagus is the usual site of variceal hemorrhage. Interestingly, more than 50% of patients with known liver disease develop hemorrhage from lesions other than varices such as portal hypertensive gastropathy. Variceal bleeding carries a high mortality rate and emergency treatment is crucial. Fluid resuscitation with crystalloid and blood products is essential for initial treatment; however, over-transfusion, i.e., hemoglobin greater than 10 g/dl or excessive use of plasma expanders may increase portal pressures and exacerbate variceal bleeding and/or ascites. Orogastric lavage is also performed to confirm GI source of bleeding and to clear clots and frank blood in preparation for endoscopy. Endoscopic management of variceal hemorrhage is now done primarily with band ligation, and this approach has been shown to be superior to sclerotherapy. Balloon tamponade is usually reserved for massive bleeding that cannot be seen well enough to treat directly. Reducing portal pressure with agents such as octreotide and somatostatin is also routinely carried out. These agents are generally used in combination with endoscopic therapy because of high re-hemorrhage rates when they are used as sole therapy.

CLINICAL CAVEAT

Placement of an orogastric tube may initially worsen variceal bleeding or rupture additional varices with passage through the esophagus. These tubes should generally be softened with warm water and lubricated to minimize this risk. If the tube is placed through the nose, a vasoconstrictive agent should also be added through the nares to minimize potential trauma and additional hemorrhage.

In contrast to cirrhotic patients, GI bleeding in the setting of FHF is due primarily to stress ulceration and coagulopathy. H2 antagonists are commonly administered to prevent and treat this clinical entity. Somatostatin and octreotide are usually avoided in this setting to prevent additional decrease in portal blood flow to the acutely failing liver. Pancreatitis can also occur with FHF but is not generally a contraindication to transplantation unless there is a necrotizing component.

Approximately 50% of cirrhotic patients who present with variceal bleeding will experience a repeat hemorrhage. Secondary prevention of rebleeding involves weekly endoscopic banding until varices are obliterated. Surveillance endoscopy is then performed every 3 months.

As noted earlier, TIPS is utilized by some clinicians for the management of variceal hemorrhage that is refractory to endoscopic treatment. This again is a controversial

CLINICAL CAVEAT

Nonsteroidal anti-inflammatory drugs should be strictly avoided in cirrhotic patients. Even a single aspirin can trigger a fatal GI bleed in this patient population. Many clinicians advocate the use of acetaminophen as long as the total daily dose does not exceed 3000 mg.

procedure primarily because of its relatively high complication rate. Newer shunts are being investigated for this indication.

CURRENT CONTROVERSY

Beta-blockers, with their ability to reduce portal hypertension, have been convincingly shown to prevent a first bleeding episode in patients who have documented varices. Their use in rebleeding prevention is controversial. Although these medications have been shown to reduce repeat hemorrhage, compliance with these drugs is an issue due to exacerbation of fatigue and hypotension seen in cirrhotic patients. There are also data to suggest that beta-blockade does not reduce overall mortality rates in patients at risk for rebleeding. New studies looking at rebleed rates have shown that certain subsets of patients may respond to combination drug therapy consisting of beta-blockade and isosorbide mononitrate. These responders were identified by significant reductions in hepatic venous pressure gradients while taking combination therapy.

DRUG INTERACTION

Beta-blockers can potentiate the cardiovascular instability seen with most anesthetic agents, especially in the relatively hypotensive and vasodilated cirrhotic patient. Beta-blockade can also compromise hemodynamic compensatory mechanisms that are critical for patients undergoing liver transplantation.

SBP is a common and potentially fatal complication of cirrhosis. It is defined as the abrupt onset of bacterial peritonitis without any external or intra-abdominal source of infection. Colonization is thought to be precipitated by decreased immune-mediated opsonization of organisms in the ascitic fluid or by bacterial translocation across the intestinal wall. Cirrhotic patients with GI bleeding, FHF, recent history of invasive procedure, or severely elevated bilirubin concentrations have been shown to be at a higher risk for this condition. SBP presents without abdominal symptoms in approximately one-third of patients. GI bleeding, encephalopathy, and worsening renal insufficiency may be the only symptoms present. Diagnosis of SBP is confirmed by an ascitic fluid cell count of greater than 250 PMN/mm^3 or a pure growth positive bacterial culture. Cultures are positive in approximately 50–75% of patients. The most common organisms (70%) are aerobic Gram negatives with *E. coli* and klebsiella predominating. The remaining 30% are Gram-positive cocci with *S. pneumonia* predominating. The recommended treatment is appropriate intravenous antibiotic therapy.

> ### CLINICAL CAVEAT
>
> Although the Gram stain of ascitic fluid is positive in 30% of cases, the result of the Gram stain does not correlate with culture growth in about one-third of those cases.

Renal Manifestations

Hepatorenal syndrome (HRS) is the most common manifestation of renal disease in cirrhotic patients and can also be seen in the setting of FHF. Other etiologies of renal dysfunction can also be seen in both chronic and acute liver disease. Simultaneous hepatic and renal damage can occur due to systemic conditions such as collagen vascular disease or amyloidosis. Acute tubular necrosis can be seen with acetaminophen toxicity and in the setting of FHF. Prerenal azotemia is common in cirrhotic patients secondary to chronic diuresis or multiple large-volume peritoneal taps. Intrinsic renal disorders can also be seen with certain liver diseases such as the association between IgA nephropathy and alcohol-induced cirrhosis and the link between glomerulonephritis and hepatitis B and C.

HRS is a diagnosis of exclusion and other clinical entities including GI bleed, SBP, nephrotoxic agents, and hypovolemia must be ruled out before assigning the diagnosis. There are two distinct clinical patterns of HRS that are generally recognized. Type 1 HRS is usually seen in the FHF population or in cirrhotic patients who acutely decompensate. It is characterized by a doubling of the initial serum creatinine to a level greater than 2.5 mg/dl or a 50% reduction in the 24-hour creatinine clearance to a level lower than 20 ml/minute in less than 2 weeks. Type 2 HRS is recognized as the more chronic form of the disease and occurs in relatively compensated patients with refractory ascites. Renal function generally worsens over months. Urinary parameters of HRS include urine volume of less than 500 cm^3/day and urine sodium of less than 10 mEq/day. However, there are well-documented cases of nonoliguric forms of HRS and cases with significantly increased urine sodium excretion.

Although the pathophysiology of HRS is complex and controversial, it is generally thought to be due to renal vasoconstriction that occurs in response to splanchnic vasodilation and increased intra-abdominal pressure from ascites. Activation of the renin–angiotensin–aldosterone system with simultaneous decreases in renal prostaglandin production results in the observed renal vasoconstriction. Some clinicians have hypothesized a hepatorenal sympathetic reflex that occurs secondary to portal hypertension as the initiating factor. The mechanism of systemic and splanchnic vasodilation has multiple hypotheses that include increased levels of nitric oxide (NO), endotoxins, and bilirubin, and elevated levels of cytokines such as tumor necrosis factor and interleukin (IL)-1 and IL-6. Others have proposed the hypothesis of elevated NO levels in the splanchnic circulation with concomitantly low levels of NO present in the portal circulation.

> ### CLINICAL CAVEAT
>
> Nonsteroidal anti-inflammatory drugs should be strictly avoided in any patient with acute or chronic liver disease due to concerns of impaired renal function. These medications can decrease already significantly reduced levels of vasodilating prostaglandins and promote additional renal vasoconstriction.

Treatment of HRS focuses initially on treatment of refractory ascites, especially in type 2. This can be done by large-volume paracentesis, although smaller volumes have been advocated due to potential intravascular volume depletion. The use of selective renal prostaglandins has shown no direct benefit. The use of vasopressin analogues such as ornipressin for splanchnic vasoconstriction with or without intravascular volume loading has shown some positive results when used over a period of time greater than 1 week. A TIPS procedure is advocated by some clinicians, but, as noted previously, this intervention is controversial and has a significant complication rate. Hemodialysis or continuous veno-veno hemofiltration (CVVH) can be used as a bridge to transplant. CVVH offers more hemodynamic stability in this setting and also has been shown to reduce vasopressor requirements. Liver transplantation is the definitive therapy for HRS. The diagnosis of HRS, however, carries with it a significant increase in perioperative hepatic transplant mortality rates, especially in patients with a serum creatinine > 2 mg/dl. Renal function may not return to normal after transplantation in the setting of HRS, especially with the use of nephrotoxic immunosuppressive medications in the postoperative setting.

Coagulation Manifestations

There are multiple mechanisms of coagulopathy in the setting of acute and chronic liver disease. Thrombocytopenia can occur due to blood loss, sequestration in liver and spleen, disseminated intravascular coagulation (DIC), or autoimmune destruction. Platelet dysfunction is also common. Vitamin K-dependent factors are often depleted secondary to malnutrition, decreased synthesis, impaired fat absorption, or blood loss. Essentially all of the factors, both pro- and anticoagulant, involved in the clotting cascade are produced by the liver with the exception of factor VIII and tissue plasminogen activator (TpA). Because the liver is also the primary site of TpA metabolism, some degree of fibrinolysis is always present in this patient population and does contribute to coagulopathy.

Immunologic Manifestations

Infectious processes other than SBP are common in patients with cirrhosis and FHF due to immunosuppression. The source of infections in both groups is most commonly the respiratory or urinary tract. These infections predominate in FHF patients with one study finding an 80% incidence. Bacteremia is also more common in the FHF population and has been cited as high as 20%. Defects in both humoral and cell-mediated immunity have been seen in both populations. There is often decreased complement production by liver in advanced disease which results in impaired opsonization of bacteria. These patients demonstrate decreased IgM activity against Gram-negative organisms, and also develop reticuloendothelial dysfunction. The macrophages in the reticuloendothelial system represent a critical filtering mechanism for blood-borne pathogens that becomes compromised. Bacterial translocation of viable bacteria and endotoxins into mesenteric lymph nodes also occurs in the setting of splanchnic hypoperfusion. This is thought to initiate the release of multiple inflammatory mediators.

LIVER TRANSPLANTATION

Orthotopic liver transplantation (OLT) has evolved from an experimental treatment to the standard of care for patients with end-stage liver disease and FHF. The mortality rate of FHF, for example, approaches 80% for cases in which liver transplant is not available. The UNOS listing criteria for transplant recipients was noted earlier in this chapter. Contraindications for liver transplantation are listed in Table 27-10.

CURRENT CONTROVERSY

The presence of severely elevated ICP with prolonged episodes of decreased CPP is a relative contraindication to orthotopic liver transplantation. In the past, HIV positive status represented an absolute contraindication to liver transplantation. However, with the increasing acceptance of HIV infection as a chronic disease state, some transplant centers will consider these patients as potential organ recipients.

Recognized factors have emerged that are associated with increased graft failure rates and increased recipient mortality rates in the setting of OLT. Increasing patient age, elevated serum creatinine, worsening UNOS status, and female gender of the donor have all been shown to be associated with lower recipient survival rates. Prolonged warm ischemic times, poor clinical status of the recipient, and female gender of the donor have been shown to be independent risk factors for graft failure following transplantation.

OLT is commonly divided into three intraoperative phases, which include the preanhepatic phase, the anhepatic phase, and the postreperfusion or neohepatic phase. The preanhepatic phase involves induction and maintenance of anesthesia, endotracheal intubation with mechanical ventilation, line placement, and ultimately surgical dissection of the liver with removal of the organ. Anesthetic induction generally involves a rapid-sequence induction and intubation. Barbiturates or propofol can be used as induction agents unless gross hemodynamic instability is evident, and succinylcholine is also used regularly. Despite the potential for significant decreases in pseudocholinesterase synthesis in the setting of advanced liver disease, metabolism of succinylcholine has not been shown to be affected clinically with a single intubating dose. Inhaled agents such as isoflurane or desflurane, narcotics, and intermediate- to long-acting muscle relaxants are the standard maintenance anesthetic agents of choice. Muscle relaxants that require renal excretion are generally avoided in the setting of HRS.

Table 27-10 Contraindications for Orthotopic Liver Transplantation

1. Advanced cardiac or pulmonary disease including severe pulmonary hypertension
2. Well-compensated cirrhosis without complications such as ascites or variceal hemorrhage
3. Alcohol use in previous six months
4. Illicit drug use in previous six months
5. Extrahepatic malignancy other than skin cancer
6. Uncontrolled systemic sepsis
7. HIV positive status (controversial)

Nitrous oxide is avoided due to associated bowel expansion and the risk of potentiating air embolic events that can occur in the setting of veno-veno bypass or vena cava manipulation. Line placement generally consists of at least one arterial line, pulmonary artery catheter, and multiple large-bore access sites including a central venous access port.

Adequate venous access is critical for all portions of the case due to the potential for large fluid shifts, large shifts in SVR, acute blood loss, and augmentation of preload with surgical caval manipulation. Immediate availability of blood products is standard throughout the procedure. Serial arterial blood gases are monitored throughout the case to assess acid–base and pulmonary status. Serial complete blood counts, PT/INR, PTT, fibrinogen levels, glucose levels, and electrolyte levels, including calcium and magnesium, are also routinely obtained. Thromboelastography (TEG) is variably utilized in transplant centers and is advocated by some clinicians. Continuous cardiac output pulmonary artery catheters with SvO_2 capability are also commonly used for management in this patient population.

CURRENT CONTROVERSY

There have been some data to suggest that desflurane is associated with a lesser decrease in splanchnic and hepatic blood flow compared to isoflurane. Certain clinicians who advocate extubation in the operating room at the conclusion of the case also note that emergence time from anesthesia is shortened with desflurane use.

The use of transesophageal echocardiography (TEE) is used variably in transplant centers. Many practitioners avoid this monitor due to the potential presence and rupture of esophageal varices.

Removal of the organ in the preanhepatic phase can be facilitated by veno-veno bypass (VVB) or by partial caval clamping near the hepatic vein(s) insertions also known as "piggy backing." There have been no data to support the use of either technique, and this is an area of controversy. VVB is generally performed initially from the femoral vein to the axillary vein with subsequent addition of the portal vein circulation. The liver is then completely removed. VVB is not routinely performed by some clinicians because of a higher risk of vascular injury, hemorrhage, thrombotic complications, and air embolus. If the partial caval clamping technique is chosen, a test clamp is generally performed first to assess if hemodynamics can be corrected with volume loading and vasopressor support. If this test is successful, many surgeons will proceed with "piggy backing" and remove the liver without the use of VVB. A perfusion team, however, is always immediately available throughout the preanhepatic and anhepatic phases whether or not VVB is utilized.

The anhepatic phase consists of surgical vascular anastamoses of the hepatic veins to the vena cava and the portal vein anastomosis. The primary anesthetic goals of this period in preparation for reperfusion of the graft are the optimization of serum potassium levels, ensuring adequate intravascular volume, administering immunosuppressives, and correction of acid–base disturbances. Serum potassium should preferably be below 4.0 mEq/l at reperfusion because of the significant rise in serum K^+ that occurs at this point in the procedure. Sodium bicarbonate, insulin, hyperventilation, calcium chloride, and potassium wasting diuretics are all commonly used to decrease serum K^+ to favorable levels. Patients with renal compromise are at particularly high risk of developing hyperkalemic complications. CVVH or dialysis can be utilized for potassium clearance prior to graft reperfusion if necessary. "Venting" through the graft prior to reperfusion has shown to decrease the degree of potassium elevation in some studies, and is practiced in some centers. This involves allowing approximately 500 cm³ of portal blood to reperfuse the liver. This blood is then discarded.

The neohepatic phase begins with reperfusion of the portal circulation through the liver, hepatic veins, and vena cava. Management is focused on treatment of postreperfusion syndrome (PRS) and any significant hyperkalemic response. PRS is generally defined as a mean arterial pressure that decreases greater than 30% from baseline or that is less than 60 mmHg. This lasts greater than 1 minute and occurs within the first 5 minutes of reperfusion. The pathophysiology of PRS is due to multiple factors including a significant decrease in SVR, relative hypovolemia, potential dysrhythmias, and acute metabolic acidosis with subsequent pulmonary hypertension and right and left ventricular depression. Treatment consists of hyperventilation with 100% inspired oxygen, volume resuscitation, and vasopressor support. Anastamoses of the hepatic artery and the biliary drainage procedure (Roux-en-y choledochojejunostomy versus choledochocholedochostomy) are the remaining surgical goals of the neohepatic phase. Anesthetic management at this point focuses on treatment of coagulopathy and monitoring for signs of function of the new graft. There are multiple mechanisms for impaired hemostasis at this juncture. These include hypothermia, hypocalcemia, metabolic acidosis, platelet consumption, hepatic dysfunction following graft reperfusion, release of heparin and heparin-like substances from the new graft, and enhanced fibrinolysis secondary to increased TpA activity with additional factor consumption.

Treatment is focused on product administration (fresh frozen plasma, packed red blood cells, platelets, cryoprecipitate), calcium replacement, correction of hypothermia, treatment of acidosis, and surgical hemostasis. Serial measurements of platelet counts, PT/INR, PTT fibrinogen levels, TEG (if utilized), and clinical reports of clot or subjective coagulopathy by the surgical team are followed. Appropriate cardiopulmonary support is provided throughout the postreperfusion phase. Continued vasopressor administration may be necessary due to delayed graft function or due to hypovolemia seen with continued blood loss. Some degree of pulmonary edema may also be present secondary to volume overload or secondary to lung injury that can occur with graft reperfusion and/or blood product administration. This pulmonary injury, when it occurs, is usually transient in nature, is often associated with an exudative edema, and generally presents within 1-2 hours after reperfusion.

CURRENT CONTROVERSY

The use of antifibrinolytics such as aprotinin or aminocaproic acid in the setting of postreperfusion coagulopathy is controversial. Many clinicians avoid the use of these agents due to concerns of initiating a hypercoagulable state with thrombotic complications. There are, however, no data to support this concern. Multiple studies have shown a decrease in overall blood product requirements with the use of antifibrinolytics without an increased incidence of thrombotic complications.

Clinical functioning of the new graft is assessed by multiple parameters including improvement of coagulopathy, decreasing vasopressor requirements, bile production, resolution of acidosis, improved calcium and magnesium homeostasis secondary to improved citrate metabolism by the new graft, and decreasing levels of serum lactate. Lactate is primarily metabolized in the liver, and lactate levels are used as a marker of graft function in some facilities. Delayed graft function may be seen in the setting of reperfusion injury with hepatic congestion. Diuresis and/or nitroglycerin have been used routinely in some centers to reduce central venous pressures and subsequently relieve congestion of the new graft.

Alternatives to Orthotopic Liver Transplantation

Adult live donor liver transplantation (aLDLT) is currently being performed in certain North American transplant centers. The number of adult recipients awaiting liver transplantation has increased significantly over the past decade. The number of adult cadaveric livers, however, has not increased proportionately, and, as a result, waiting list times and mortality rates in this adult population of recipients have risen dramatically. This procedure is being offered in response to this relative organ shortage. The use of live donor organ donation (right hepatic lobectomy) is controversial. aLDLT does offer the advantage of decreased warm and cold ischemic times for the donated graft, and it also ensures an optimally screened, healthy donor. However, the complex nature of the surgery and the potential risk to an otherwise healthy patient bring up many clinical and ethical concerns regarding live donation.

The size of the graft is crucial when performing aLDLT. This is calculated by either the graft-to-recipient weight ratio (GRWR) or the graft-to-recipient standard liver volume ratio (GSLV). It is now generally accepted that a GRWR of at least 1% and a GSLV of at least 50% are safe concerning the development of a "small for size" syndrome. However, graft congestion in the postreperfusion period can precipitate this syndrome despite adequate size, especially since the right hepatic lobe has been shown to be very susceptible to venous congestion.

There have been a significant number of biliary tract complications in the recipient population with the aLDLT procedure. These have been reported as high as 28-34% in some studies. Hepatic arterial thrombosis may also be higher in this population due to the fact that smaller vessels are used in the anastamosis. Postoperative care of these patients should involve frequent monitoring for signs of potential bile leaks or graft dysfunction and frequent Doppler examinations of the hepatic artery to ensure patency.

Artificial Liver

The use of bioartificial hybrid devices for the treatment of liver disease as a bridge to transplant has shown limited usefulness in randomized trials. Some studies using plasma exchange as the primary modality have shown increased survival times and this intervention may have some utility as a bridge to transplantation in critically ill patients.

SELECTED READING

Allen JW, Hassanein T, Bhatia SN: Advances in bioartificial liver devices. Hepatology 34(3):447-453, 2001.

Azoulay D, Buabse F, Damiano I et al: Neoadjuvant transjugular intrahepatic portosystemic shunt: a solution for extrahepatic abdominal operation in cirrhotic patients with severe portal hypertension. J Am Coll Surg 193:46-51, 2001.

Bosch J, Garcia-Pagan JC: Prevention of variceal rebleeding. Lancet 361(9361):952-954, 2003.

Butterworth RF: Mild hyperthermia prevents cerebral edema in acute liver failure. J Hepato-Biliary-Pancreatic Surg 8(1): 16-19, 2001.

Cacciarelli TV, Keeffe EB, Moore DH et al: Effect of intraoperative blood transfusion on patient outcome in hepatic transplantation. Arch Surg 134(1):25-29, 1999.

Chen C-L, Fan S-T, Lee S-G et al: Living-donor liver transplantation: 12 years of experience in Asia. Transplantation 75(Suppl):S6-11, 2003.

Chui AKK, Rao ARN, Shi LW et al: Liver transplantation in patients with transjugular intrahepatic portosystemic shunts. Transplantation Proc 32:2204-2205, 2000.

Farrell GC: Non-alcoholic steatohepatitis: what is it, and why is it important in the Asia-Pacific Region? J Gastroenterol Hepatol 18(2):124-138, 2003.

Feldman M: *Sleisenger & Fordtran's Gastrointestinal and Liver Disease*, ed 6, WB Saunders, 1998.

Fontana RJ: Management of patients with decompensated HBV cirrhosis. Semin Liver Dis 23(1):89-100, 2003.

Goldman L: *Cecil Textbook of Medicine*, ed 21, WB Saunders, 2000, Chap 153.

Gonzalez-Abraldes J, Garcia-Pagan JC, Bosch J: Nitric oxide and portal hypertension. Metab Brain Dis 17(4):311-324, 2002.

Hofmann AF: Cholestatic liver disease: pathophysiology and therapeutic options. Liver 22(Suppl 2):14-19, 2002.

Jalan R, Olde Damink SW: Hypothermia for the management of intracranial hypertension in acute liver failure. Curr Opin Crit Care 7(4):257-262, 2001.

Karasu Z, Guraker A, Kerwin B et al: Effect of transjugular intrahepatic portosystemic shunt on thrombocytopenia associated with cirrhosis. Digest Dis Sci 45(10):1971-1976, 2000.

Keeffe EB: Hepatology: a century of progress; liver transplantation at the millennium. Clin Liver Dis 4(1):241-255, 2000.

Keeffe EB: Liver transplantation: current status and novel approaches to liver replacement. Gastroenterology 120:749-762, 2001.

Kowdley KV: Motion-prophylactic banding of esophageal varices is useful: arguments against the motion. Can J Gastroenterol 16(10):693-695, 2002.

Kufner RP: Use of antifibrinolytics in orthotopic liver transplantation. Transplantation Proc 32:636-637, 2000.

Larrey D: Drug-induced liver diseases. J Hepatol 32(Suppl 1): 77-88, 2000.

Lentschener C, Ozier Y: Anesthesia for elective liver resection: some points should be revisited. Eur J Anaesthesiol 19(11):780-788, 2002.

Macintire DK, Bellhorn TL: Bacterial translocation: clinical implications and prevention. Veterinary Clin North Am Small Animal Pract 32(5):1165-1178, 2002.

McGilvray ID, Greig PD: Critical care of the liver transplant patient: an update. Curr Opin Crit Care 8(2):178-182, 2002.

O'Conner CJ, Roozeboom D, Brown R, Tuman KJ: Pulmonary thromboembolism during liver transplantation: possible association with antifibrinolytic drugs and novel treatment options. Anesth Analg 91:296-299, 2000.

Perdue PW, Balser JR, Lipsett PA, Breslow MJ: "Renal dose" dopamine in surgical patients: dogma or science? Ann Surg 227(4):470-473, 1998.

Pomfret EA, Pomposelli JJ, Jenkins RL: Live donor liver transplantation. J Hepatol 34:613-624, 2001.

Renz JF, Busuttil RW: Adult-to-adult liver transplantation: a critical analysis. Semin Liver Dis 20(4):411-424, 2000.

Rosch J, Keller FS: Transjugular intrahepatic portosystemic shunt: present status, comparison with endoscopic therapy and shunt surgery, and future prospects. World J Surg 25(3):337-345, 2001.

Rose C, Michalak A, Pannunzio M: Mild hyperthermia delays the onset of coma and prevents brain edema and extracellular brain glutamate accumulation in rats with acute liver failure. Hepatology 31(4):872-877, 2000.

Rosemurgy AS, Serafini FM, Zweibel BR: Transjugular intrahepatic shunt vs. small-diameter prosthetic H-graft portocaval shunt: extended follow-up of an expanded randomized prospective trial. J Gastrointest Surg 4(6): 589-597, 2000.

Samstein B, Emond J: Liver transplants from living related donors. Annu Rev Med 52:147-160, 2000.

Sandowski SA, Runyon BA: Hepatobiliary disease: cirrhosis. Clin Family Pract 2(1):59-77, 2000.

Scheen AJ, Luyckx FH: Obesity and liver disease. Best Pract Res Clin Endocrinol Metab 16(4):703-716, 2002.

Seaman DS: Adult living donor liver transplantation: current status. J Clin Gastroenterol 33(2):97-106, 2001.

Seeff LB, Hoofnagle JH: Appendix: National Institute of Health Consensus Development Conference Management of Hepatitis C. Clin Liver Dis 7(1):261-287, 2003.

Shakil AO, Mazariegos MD, Kramer DJ: Liver transplantation: current management; fulminant hepatic failure. Surg Clin North Am 79:1, 1999.

Vaughan RB, Chin-Dusting JP: Current pharmacotherapy in the management of cirrhosis: focus on the hyperdynamic circulation. Expert Pharmacother 4(5):625-637, 2003.

Wong F, Blendis L: Hepatology: a century of progress; hepatorenal failure. Clin Liver Dis 4:1, 2000.

Wright TL: Treatment of patients with hepatitis C and cirrhosis. Hepatology 36(5 Suppl 1):S185-194, 2002.

Zein CO, Zein NN: Advances in therapy for hepatitis C infection. Microbes Infect 4(12):1237-1246, 2002.

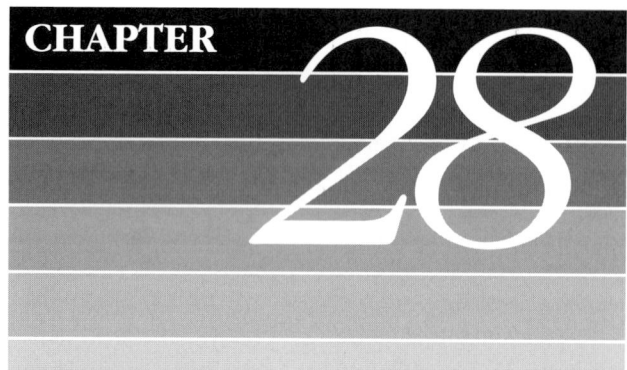

CHAPTER 28

Gastrointestinal Bleeding

CHARLES R. PHILLIPS, M.D.

PER A. J. THORBORG, M.D., Ph.D.

Acute gastrointestinal (GI) bleeding accounts for 300,000 hospital admissions every year in the USA alone. Additionally, 5% of all patients admitted to the intensive care unit (ICU) will experience clinically significant upper GI bleeding as a complication of their primary illness.

Despite advances in care and prevention, overall hospital mortality remains at 9% for those who present with bleeding as their primary complaint and over 50% for those whose bleeding complicates their primary diagnosis in the ICU.

Early recognition and diagnosis, adequate resuscitation, and proper treatment are essential in the management of acute GI hemorrhage. Prophylactic acid suppressive therapy in the ICU, in attempts to limit stress-related mucosal disease, is essential in certain subsets of patients. However, such therapy is probably being over-utilized and represents a significant cause of morbidity and cost.

In this chapter we review the causes and presentations of both upper and lower GI bleeding, the diagnostic and therapeutic modalities available, and the role of acid suppression therapy to prevent stress-related bleeding or recurrent bleeding in the ICU.

DEFINITIONS

Upper gastrointestinal (UGI) bleeding is defined as bleeding from a GI source proximal to the ligament of Treitz – a band of muscular/fibrous tissue between the fourth portion of the duodenum and the jejunum. UGI bleeding remains a significant cause of morbidity and mortality in adults despite improved practices of stress ulcer prophylaxis and treatment of *H. pylori* associated with peptic ulcer disease (PUD).

Lower GI bleeding occurs anywhere distal to the ligament of Treitz to include most of the small bowel, the colon, and anorectal area. Bleeding can present briskly with cardiovascular compromise or slowly and intermittently. Brisk bleeding typically presents with hematochezia but it is important to note that UGI bleeding remains the main cause of hematochezia and bleeding in the small bowel often presents as melena.

RESUSCITATION

Resuscitation is the first priority in treating those patients with significant GI bleeding from any source. The degree of blood loss can be assessed as per the American College of Surgeons classification scheme. Blood loss is classified into four levels of severity determined by the clinical parameters of blood pressure, urine output, and heart rate. Shock requiring aggressive hydration and blood replacement corresponds to levels II and III depending on the patient and presentation. Reversal of shock should be accomplished with rapid infusion of IV fluids. This may include blood and blood products but resuscitation should not be delayed for their arrival and crystalloid infusion should commence immediately, through a large-bore IV, ideally before hospital admission. Once admitted, consideration for placement of an introducer catheter into a central vein should be made in the event rapid large-volume fluid infusion becomes necessary. Monitoring of central venous pressure and mixed venous pO_2 can also be helpful. Adequate urine output, resolution of orthostatic blood pressure changes, pulse rate < 100, supine blood pressure > 90, and level of consciousness can all be used to assess recovery from shock (Table 28-1).

When blood is to be replaced, transfusion with packed red blood cells is preferred. Whole blood transfusion with O negative blood is rarely used and should be reserved for those patients with massive blood loss who cannot be cross-matched rapidly. Patients requiring greater than 10 units of packed red blood cells should undergo a massive transfusion protocol and should receive fresh-frozen plasma, platelets, and cryoprecipitate as needed. Timing of transfusion and goal hemoglobin, platelet counts, fibrinogen, and international normalized ratio (INR) vary with the presentation but generally hemoglobin should be kept above 8 g/dl, except in heart disease where it should be kept above 10 g/d, fibrinogen above 100 mg/dl, and INR less than 1.3–1.5. A blood warmer should be used if a patient is to receive more than 3 liters of fluid.

HISTORY AND PHYSICAL

A thorough history and physical examination can aid in determining the source of GI bleeding and its etiology. Drugs, particularly nonsteroidal anti-inflammatory drugs

Table 28-1	Classification of Hemorrhage Based on Extent of Blood Loss			
Parameter	Class I	Class II	Class III	Class IV
Loss of blood volume (%)	<15	15–30	30–40	>40
Pulse rate	<100	>100	>120	>140
Supine blood pressure	Normal	Normal	Decreased	Decreased
Urine output (ml/hour)	>30	20–30	5–15	<5
Mental status	Anxious	Agitated	Confused	Lethargic

Committee on Trauma: *Advanced Trauma Life Support Student Manual*, Chicago: American College of Surgeons, 1989, p 57.

(NSAIDs), and alcohol are associated with PUD and gastritis. NSAIDs are associated with a two-fold increase in the risk of bleeding and are felt to contribute to the development of 5–25% of all gastric ulcers. Cigarette smoking has been associated with a higher recurrence rate of PUD. A recent history of retching or vomiting prior to bleeding may be indicative of a Mallory–Weiss tear. Stigmata of liver disease and portal hypertension such as spider nevi, palmer erythema, hepatomegaly, jaundice, asterixis, or ascites should be looked for on examination with concern for a variceal source of bleeding if found. Drug-induced coagulopathies with coumadin and low-molecular-weight heparin should be evaluated for and a history of such medications sought. Recent weight loss or a change in bowel habits may be indicative of colorectal cancer. A history of diverticular disease, prior malignancy, inflammatory bowel disease, or significant vascular disease can aid in determining a diagnosis in lower GI bleeding. Crampy abdominal pain out of proportion to examination findings occurring after meals followed by hematochezia may indicate mesenteric ischemia.

UPPER GASTROINTESTINAL BLEEDING

UGI bleeding is defined as bleeding from a GI source proximal to the ligament of Treitz. It is more common than lower GI bleeding, accounting for 1–2% of all hospital admissions in the USA per year. Despite improvements in care and prevention, mortality and morbidity statistics have not improved in the last 20 years. The increased use of NSAIDs has probably contributed to an increase in the number of patients presenting with UGI bleeds, though their use has not been associated with worsening outcome.

UGI bleeding is often encountered in the critically ill complicating other primary diseases. Clinically important stress-related UGI bleeding is seen in only 1–4% of the critically ill; however, the death rate exceeds 50% in this group. Within 24 hours of admission to the ICU, 75–100% of patients will demonstrate endoscopic evidence of mucosal damage and most will have at least occult bleeding making prophylactic acid suppression a necessary part of ICU therapy. Studies have shown, however, that there is benefit with acid suppressive therapy only in patients who are mechanically ventilated for prolonged periods, have coagulopathies, recent prior bleeding from PUD, major head trauma, or significant burns. Thus acid suppressive therapy should be reserved for these subsets of patients only.

Diagnoses and Management

Presentation of Bleeding

Patients with upper GI bleeding typically present with hematemesis and melena. Nasogastric tube (NGT)

> **Box 28-1   Poor Prognostic Indicators for Acute Upper Gastrointestinal Bleed**
>
> - Age > 65 years
> - Shock on admittance: pulse > 100, SBP < 100
> - Comorbidity – renal failure, liver failure, metastatic cancer
> - Endoscopic findings: active, pulsatile hemorrhage, visible vessel, large arterial defect > 1 mm, ulcer > 2 cm, adherent clot
> - Rebleeding
> - GI malignancy
> - Bleeding complicating other critical illness

aspiration often shows "coffee-ground" material or bright red blood. If reflux through the pylorus is absent gastric aspiration can be negative, despite significant bleeding in the duodenum. Patients with massive UGI bleeding can also present with hematochezia, given the speed blood can transit the GI tract.

During the initial assessment defining factors that have prognostic value is important. Factors that predict mortality include age greater than 65 years, comorbid conditions, the presence of shock, and endoscopic findings. Comorbid conditions such as renal failure, liver failure, and metastatic malignancy have a very poor prognosis. Patients who develop significant overt bleeding as a complication of another illness while in the ICU have a greater than 50% mortality – probably indicative of overall disease severity and not necessarily attributable to the bleeding itself. Finally rebleeding carries a mortality rate ten times that of the initial cause of bleeding (Box 28-1).

> **CLINICAL CAVEAT**
>
> **Nonsteroidal Anti-inflammatory Drugs and Gastrointestinal Bleeding**
> - Cyclooxygenase II inhibitors offer lower risk for GI bleeding as compared to nonselective NSAIDs but significant risk for UGI bleeding while taking these medications still exists
> - 3–5 times increase in relative risk of UGI ulceration, twice the risk of significant bleeding with NSAIDs
> - Incidence of NSAID-induced gastric ulcers not reduced by concomitant proton pump inhibitor, H_2 blockade – has been reduced by misoprostol

Management

After adequate resuscitation has been accomplished, as described above, empiric acid neutralization should be done with high-dose IV proton pump inhibitors. In those UGI bleeds suspected to be of a variceal origin infusion of IV octreotide can also be begun. Endoscopy is then undertaken once cardiovascular stability has been achieved.

Typically endoscopy can be done electively but should be done within 24 hours of admission. If endoscopy cannot identify the source of blood, and bleeding continues, angiography with or without embolization can then be attempted. A technetium-labeled red blood cell scan can be done for gross localization of bleeding for both upper and lower GI sources but active bleeding at rates greater than 0.05 to 0.1 ml/minute is necessary at the time of the examination – and results can be difficult to interpret.

> **CLINICAL CAVEAT**
>
> **Octreotide for Esophageal Varices**
> - Infusion: 50 µg × 1 then 25–50 µg/hour IV gtt
> - Caution: impaired renal function, liver function, cardiac disease, thyroid disease, diabetes mellitus
> - Interaction with beta-blockers, calcium channel blockers may cause hypotension, bradycardia, and conduction abnormalities
> - Pancreatic hormone effects may cause hyper-/hypoglycemia

Treatment

Drugs

An algorithm for the treatment of acute UGI bleeding is shown in Figure 28-1.

For nonvariceal bleeding IV proton pump inhibitors have been shown to reduce rebleeding and the need for surgery. Patients infected with *H. pylori* should undergo eradication with triple antibiotic therapy, although this therapy has not been shown to reduce rebleeding during initial hospitalization.

If variceal bleeding is suspected, octreotide should be begun. Although rarely used, if bleeding does not stop and surgery and endoscopy are not immediately available, a Sengstaken-Blakemore (Minnesota) tube may be inserted to control massive bleeding until definitive therapy is available.

Endoscopic Therapy

Nonvariceal bleeding can be treated with a wide range and combination of therapies. However, injection with a vasoconstricting agent combined with cautery may be the best.

With regards to variceal bleeding, band ligation stops bleeding and obliterates varices with the fewest complications, but can be difficult to do in actively bleeding patients.

Angiography

Attempts at localizing bleeding and subsequent embolization can be attempted if endoscopy is unsuccessful at locating the source and stopping the bleeding. A transjugular intrahepatic portosystemic shunt (TIPS) procedure can be attempted in bleeding caused from portal hypertension – and has been highly successful at stopping variceal bleeding in the acute setting.

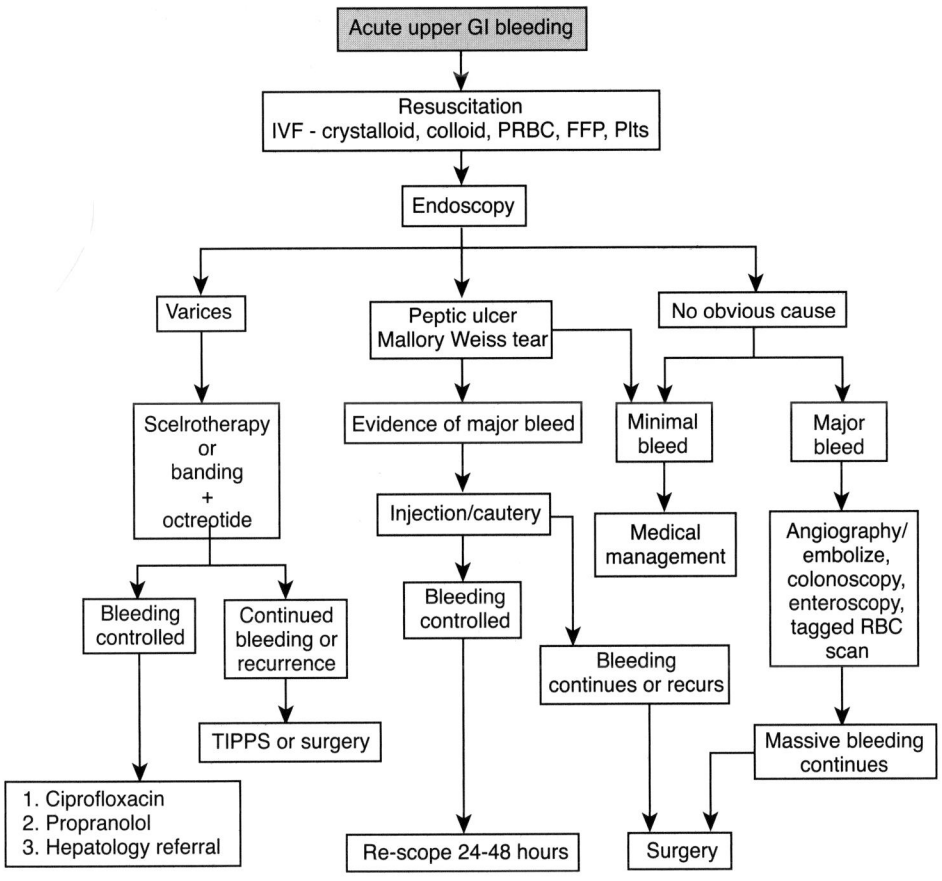

Figure 28-1 Algorithm for the treatment of acute upper GI bleeding.

Surgery

Surgical treatment is, for the most part, reserved for cases in which endoscopy, angiography, and/or TIPPS have failed (Box 28-2).

CURRENT CONTROVERSY

Acid Suppression Therapy in the Intensive Care Unit

- Probably only effective in patients with prolonged mechanical ventilation (MV), coagulopathy, and head trauma, burn victims, or to prevent rebleeding in known PUD
- H$_2$ antagonist Rx as effective in MV patients as proton pump inhibitor Rx
- Continuous IV proton pump inhibitor better to prevent UGI rebleed from PUD than intermittent bolus proton pump inhibitor and IV H$_2$ blockers
- Suppressive therapy may be associated with increased risk of aspiration pneumonia
- Suppressive therapy may be associated with higher incidence of bacterial translocation from the gut to the blood in the critically ill

---

Box 28-2 Differential Diagnosis of Upper Gastrointestinal Bleeding

Esophageal
- Mallory–Weiss tear
- Varices
- Esophagitis
- Malignancy

Gastric
- PUD
- Zollinger–Ellison syndrome
- Gastritis or stress ulcer
- Varices
- Malignancy

Duodenal
- PUD
- Malignancy

Other
- Angiodysplasia
- Coagulopathy
- Ischemia

LOWER GASTROINTESTINAL BLEEDING

Lower GI bleeding is defined as bleeding from a GI source distal to the ligament of Treitz. Bleeding typically occurs in the colorectal area but can occur in the small bowel. Despite significant advances in diagnostic methods over the last 20 years, localizing the source of bleeding can be difficult. As many as 8–12% of patients with lower GI bleeding fail to have their source identified prior to surgery. While not as prevalent as UGI bleeding, the annual incident rate of lower GI bleeding in the USA exceeds 20.5/100,000 with a mortality rate of 2.4% for those who present with bleeding and 23.1% for those whose bleeding complicates other critical illness. The most common diagnoses for massive lower GI bleeding in patients older than 50 years of age are diverticulosis, which accounts for 30–40% of all cases, followed by colorectal cancer, ischemic colitis, and angiodysplasias. For those patients younger than 50 years the most common causes are infectious colitis, anorectal disease, and inflammatory bowel disease.

Diagnoses and Management

Presentation of Bleeding

Bleeding can be occult, slow, moderate, or massive and life threatening. Episodic bleeding is more common in the lower GI tract than in the UGI tract. Bleeding typically presents as hematochezia but it is important to note that small bowel bleeding can present as melena, and massive UGI bleeding is the most common cause of hematochezia. Thus localization of bleeding to the lower GI tract begins with placement of an NGT (Box 28-3; Figure 28-2).

Specific Causes

Diverticulosis

Diverticulosis is responsible for 30–40% of all cases of lower GI bleeding and is the leading cause in patients over 50 years. Colonic diverticuli occur where major branches of the vasa recta penetrate the colonic wall. These points of penetration occur through connective tissue between sections of muscle and represent relatively weak areas in the colon wall. With increased pressure colonic tissue may herniate through these areas and may then over time erode into the arteries resulting in bleeding. The bleeding can be large volume and is usually painless, presenting typically as hematochezia, but can present as melena. This is due to the fact that whereas diverticuli occur more frequently in the left colon, bleeding from diverticuli occurs more often in the right colon. Frequent recurrent bleeding or massive life-threatening bleeding from diverticuli is an indication for hemicolectomy, which is curative.

Box 28-3 Differential Diagnosis of Lower Gastrointestinal Bleeding

UGI source
Small intestine
- Angiodysplasia
- Malignancy
- Inflammatory bowel disease
- Ischemia
- Trauma
- Meckel's diverticulum

Colon
- TICs
- Inflammatory bowel disease
- Neoplasm
- Infectious colitis
- Ischemia
- Angiodysplasia
- Radiation
- Trauma

Rectal
- Hemorrhoids
- Fissures
- Malignancy
- Trauma

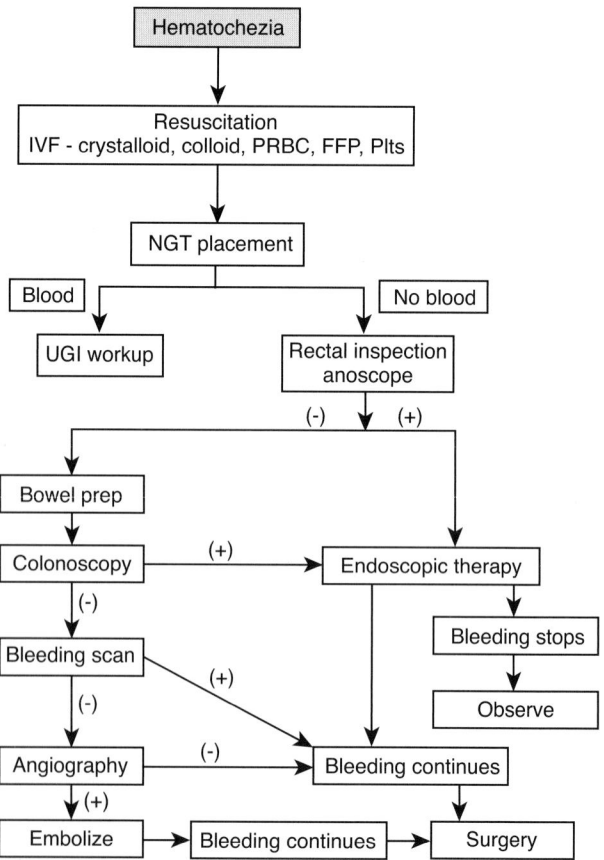

Figure 28-2 Algorithm for the treatment of hematochezia.

Ischemic Colitis

The second leading cause of lower GI bleeding in patients over 50 years is ischemic colitis. It typically presents as crampy abdominal pain out of proportion to examination findings followed by bleeding for one to two days. It can occur anytime but is often precipitated by meals. The bleeding is usually mild and self-limiting but occasionally can present as massive bleeding. Over 90% of patients with mesenteric ischemia have underlying atherosclerotic disease. Ischemia is felt to be caused by a relatively low flow state through diseased blood vessels supplying the bowel. Abdominal angina is a term sometimes used to describe the pain experienced after meals when demand for blood exceeds available supply due to atherosclerotic lesions.

Colorectal Cancer

Malignancies in the lower GI tract rarely present with massive bleeding but when they do there is a very poor prognosis. Therapy is surgical resection to control bleeding.

Angiodysplasias

Vascular malformations and anomalies in the lower GI tract are typically located in the cecum and right colon. Their cause is unclear but it is felt that most of these are acquired with age. Bleeding is usually intermittent and small volume presenting with signs and symptoms of blood loss anemia, but they can present with brisk bleeding. They are usually easily seen on endoscopy and are amenable to cautery. If refractory to endoscopic and/or medical therapy, surgery is then indicated.

Inflammatory Bowel Disease

Inflammatory bowel disease to include Crohn's disease and ulcerative colitis are the most common causes of lower GI bleeding in patients less than 50 years. It rarely presents with life-threatening hemorrhage, instead usually presenting with moderate bleeding, with blood mixed with stool and associated with crampy abdominal pain and sometimes fever. Occasionally an ulcer can erode into a major vessel and these patients will present with massive bleeding.

Infectious Colitis

Invasive infectious pathogens can cause a hemorrhagic colitis and present as hematochezia. Salmonella, yersinia, shigella, *Campylobacter jejuni*, *Clostridium difficile*, *Escherichia coli*, *Vibrio parahaemolyticus*, *Entamoeba histolytica*, and schistosomatidae are the most common of the pathogens responsible. Fever, diarrhea, crampy abdominal pain, recent travel, and recent contact or family illness are important clues in a patient's history pointing to an infectious etiology.

Meckel's Diverticulum

Meckel's diverticulum is a congenital abnormality in the terminal ileum. The diverticulum is lined with ectopic gastric cells and acid secreted from these cells can cause ulceration into the adjacent bowel wall and blood vessels supplying the bowel. It typically presents in childhood or early adult as painless hematochezia or melena, and can cause massive bleeding.

SUMMARY

GI bleeding remains a significant cause of morbidity and mortality, especially in those patients who develop bleeding while in hospital. Early recognition and prompt resuscitation is essential in the management of these patients to minimize complications associated with shock and anemia. Prompt therapy guided by early diagnostic evaluation aimed at determining the site and cause of bleeding should follow a formulation of a differential diagnoses based on bleeding characteristics, patient age, history and physical examination, and laboratory results. Early referral to gastroenterology should be made.

H_2 blockers have no role in the acute management of UGI bleeding, whereas proton pump inhibitors reduce rebleeding in PUD and gastritis. Empiric use of octreotide for suspected portal hypertension related bleeding should be done.

Stress ulcer prophylaxis in the ICU is important in select patients but indiscriminant use of such therapy with either H_2 blockers or proton pump inhibitors should be avoided.

CASE STUDY

A 63-year-old male is admitted to the ICU with community-acquired pneumonia. Medical history is significant for type II diabetes and moderate emphysema with ongoing tobacco use. Chest x-ray reveals an area of dense consolidation in the left upper lobe superimposed with changes consistent on chronic obstructive pulmonary disease. Examination reveals mild distress on 4 liters nasal oxygen, a blood pressure of 115/65, a respiratory rate of 24 with mild accessory muscle use, febrile to 38.7°C, and decreased breath sounds were appreciated on the left with rare expiratory wheezes in all lung fields. Patient was only taking minimal PO fluids, refusing to eat.

QUESTIONS

1. Should acid suppression therapy be initiated at this time?
2. What are the risks/benefits associated with acid suppression?

Patient's respiratory status deteriorated and he was subsequently intubated. Shortly thereafter he became septic requiring vasopressors despite aggressive hydration with IV crystalloid and colloid.

QUESTIONS

1. Should acid suppression therapy be initiated if not already done?
2. If yes which agent/s would you use? And why?

The next day the patient's nurse notices a large volume of bright red blood in his orogastric tube aspirate and a short time later he develops melena.

CASE STUDY—cont'd

Aggressive resuscitation with IV crystalloid and 4 units of packed red blood cells enacted cardiovascular stability.

QUESTIONS

1. What are the next steps in evaluating and treating this patient's bleeding?
2. What are the likely causes of his bleeding, and what therapies could be employed to control bleeding caused by them?
3. If not on acid suppression therapy would you now start? If on therapy would you change therapy given this new bleeding? Which treatment would you use?
4. What is this patient's estimated mortality based solely on his bleeding episode in the ICU?

SELECTED READING

Abraham J, Fennerty B, Piesegna J et al: Acid suppression in a critical care environment: state of the art and beyond. Crit Care Med 30(6 Suppl):S349-S350, 2002.

Feldman M: Gastrointestinal bleeding. In Sleisenger & Fordtran's *Gastrointestinal and Liver Disease*, ed 7, 2002, Chap 13.

Navab F, Lindenauer P, Higgins T et al: Management of upper gastrointestinal bleeding. Baystate Health System Clinical Practice Guideline, 2000.

Sharara A, Rockey D: Gastroesophageal variceal hemorrhage. N Engl J Med 345(9):669-681, 2001.

Vernava A, Moore B, Longo W, Johnson F: Lower gastrointestinal bleeding. Dis Colon Rectum 40(7):846-858, 1997.

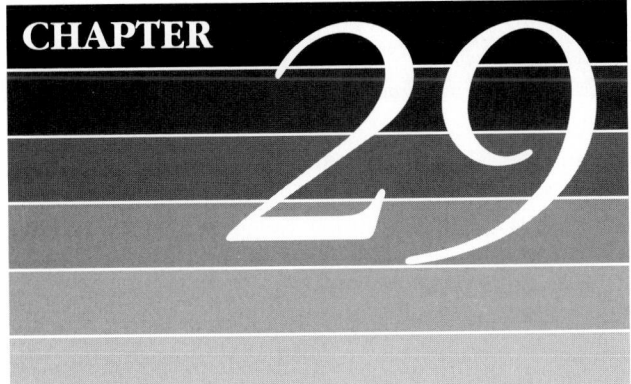
Renal Failure and Support

RINALDO BELLOMO, M.D., F.R.A.C.P., F.C.C.P

CLAUDIO RONCO, M.D., Ph.D.

Acute renal failure (ARF) remains one of the major therapeutic challenges for the critical care physician. The term describes a syndrome characterized by a rapid (hours to days) decrease in the kidney's ability to eliminate waste products. Such loss of excretory function is clinically manifested by the accumulation of end products of nitrogen metabolism (urea and creatinine) which are routinely measured in intensive care unit (ICU) patients. Other typical clinical manifestations include decreased urine output (not always present), accumulation of nonvolatile acids, and an increased potassium concentration.

Depending on the criteria used to define its presence, ARF has been reported to occur in 15-20% of ICU patients. Acute renal injury (albuminuria, loss of small tubular proteins, inability to excrete a water load or a sodium load or amino acid load) is almost ubiquitous in critically ill patients. There is some evidence, however,

that, when dialysis becomes necessary, mortality is increased. The incidence of such severe ARF has been recently reported at approximately 11 cases/100,000 people/year. It is important to realize that, unlike acute respiratory distress syndrome (ARDS) or sepsis, there is no consensus definition of ARF. Although such a definition has been suggested, the matter remains controversial. The lack of a consensus definition is holding back research in the area when compared to ARDS and sepsis.

There is limited evidence that another frequently used term, "acute tubular necrosis"(ATN), has any clinical implications or that it describes the histopathology of what is now seen in a modern ICU. The term ATN comes from animal models that poorly reflect clinical situations and from old biopsy data. Even in such cases, tubular "necrosis" is patchy and mostly isolated to the thick ascending loop of Henle. Furthermore, cells found in the urinary "tubular casts" of such patients are viable on staining studies, thus partly invalidating the term "necrosis."

ASSESSMENT OF RENAL FUNCTION

Renal function is complex (control of calcium and phosphate, acid-base balance, water balance, erythropoiesis. etc.). In the clinical context monitoring of renal function is reduced to assessment of glomerular filtration rate (GFR) by the measurement of urea and creatinine in blood. These waste products are insensitive markers of GFR and are heavily modified by nutrition, the use of steroids, the presence of gastrointestinal blood, or muscle injury. Furthermore, they become abnormal only when more than 50% of GFR is lost, they do not reflect dynamic changes in GFR, and are grossly modified by aggressive fluid resuscitation. The use of creatinine clearance (2 or 4 hour collections) or of calculated clearance by means of formulae increases accuracy but rarely if ever changes clinical management. The use of more sophisticated radionuclide-based tests is cumbersome in the ICU and only useful for research purposes.

DIAGNOSIS AND CLINICAL CLASSIFICATION

The most practically useful approach to the etiologic diagnosis of ARF is to divide its causes according to the probable source of renal injury: prerenal, renal (parenchymal), and postrenal.

So-called prerenal ARF is by far the most common in ICU. The term indicates that the kidney malfunctions predominantly because of systemic factors that diminish renal blood flow and decrease GFR or alter intraglomerular hemodynamics and thereby also decrease GFR. Renal blood flow can be diminished because of decreased cardiac output, hypotension, or raised intra-abdominal pressure. Such raised intra-abdominal pressure can be suspected on clinical grounds and confirmed by measuring bladder pressure with a urinary catheter. A pressure of >25–30 mmHg above the pubis should prompt consideration of decompression.

CLINICAL CAVEAT

Intra-abdominal Hypertension
- If intra-abdominal hypertension is suspected, such pressure must be measured
- If intra-abdominal hypertension is not relieved, there is no hope of restoring renal function

If the systemic cause of renal failure is rapidly removed or corrected, renal function improves and relatively rapidly returns to near normal levels. However, if intervention is delayed or unsuccessful, renal injury becomes established and several days or weeks are then necessary for recovery. Several tests have been used to help clinicians identify the development of such "established" ARF (Table 29-1). The clinical utility of these tests in ICU patients who receive vasopressors, massive fluid resuscitation, and, increasingly, loop diuretic infusions is untested and questionable. Furthermore, it is important to observe that prerenal ARF and established ARF are part of a continuum, and their separation has limited clinical implications. The treatment is the same: treatment of the cause while promptly resuscitating the patient using invasive hemodynamic monitoring to guide therapy.

The term parenchymal renal failure is used to define a syndrome where the principal source of damage is within the kidney and where typical structural changes can be seen on microscopy. Disorders that affect the glomerulus or the tubule can be responsible (Box 29-1).

Table 29-1 Laboratory Tests Used to Help Diagnose "Established" Acute Renal Failure

Test	Prerenal ARF	Established ARF
Urine microscopy	Normal	Epithelial casts
Specific gravity	High: >1.020	Low: <1.020
Urine sodium	Low	High
U/P creatinine ratio	High: >40	Low: <10
P urea/creatinine ratio	High	Normal

U, urine; P, plasma.

Among these, nephrotoxins are particularly important, especially in hospitalized patients. The most common nephrotoxic drugs affecting ICU patients are listed in Box 29-2. Many cases of drug-induced ARF rapidly improve upon removal of the offending agent. Accordingly, a careful history of drug administration is mandatory in all patients with ARF. In some cases of parenchymal ARF a correct working diagnosis can be obtained from history, physical examination, and radiological and laboratory investigations. In such patients one can proceed to a therapeutic trial without the need to resort to renal biopsy. However, prior to aggressive immunosuppressive therapy, renal biopsy is recommended to allow histological confirmation of the etiology of ARF. Renal biopsy in ventilated patients under ultrasound guidance does not carry additional risks compared to standard conditions.

More than a third of patients who develop ARF have chronic renal dysfunction due to factors such as age-related changes, long-standing hypertension, diabetes, or atheromatous disease of the renal vessels. They may have a raised serum creatinine. However, this is not always the case. Often, what may seem to the clinician to be a relatively trivial insult, which does not fully explain the onset of ARF in a normal patient, is sufficient to unmask lack of renal functional reserve in another.

Box 29-1 Causes of Parenchymal Acute Renal Failure

- Glomerulonephritis
- Vasculitis
- Interstitial nephropathy
- Malignant hypertension
- Pelvicaliceal infection
- Bilateral cortical necrosis
- Amyloidosis

Box 29-2   Drugs That May Cause Acute Renal Failure in the Intensive Care Unit or Operating Room

- Radiocontrast agents
- Aminoglycosides
- Amphotericin
- Nonsteroidal anti-inflammatory drugs
- β-Lactam antibiotics (interstitial nephropathy)
- Methotrexate
- Cisplatin
- Cyclosporin A
- FK-506 (Tacrolimus)

Hepatorenal Syndrome

This condition is a form of ARF, which occurs in the setting of severe liver dysfunction in the absence of other known causes of ARF. Typically, it presents as progressive oliguria with a very low urinary sodium concentration (<10 mmol/l). Its pathogenesis is not well understood but appears to involve severe renal vasoconstriction. However, in patients with severe liver disease other causes of ARF are much more common. They include sepsis, paracentesis-induced hypovolemia, raised intra-abdominal pressure due to tense ascites, diuretic-induced hypovolemia, lactulose-induced hypovolemia, alcoholic cardiomyopathy, and any combination of these.

CLINICAL CAVEAT

Hepatorenal Syndrome
- Hepatorenal syndrome is a diagnosis of exclusion
- A low urinary sodium may simply reflect sodium retention caused by inadequate intravascular volume
- Fluid resuscitation must take place under invasive monitoring and other causes of renal failure must be excluded
- Primary bacterial peritonitis must always be suspected. The clinical signs of such infection may be completely absent and an ascitic tap is needed to make the diagnosis

The avoidance of hypovolemia by albumin administration in patients with spontaneous bacterial peritonitis has been shown to decrease the incidence of renal failure in a recent randomized controlled trial. These causes must be looked for and promptly treated. Recent uncontrolled studies suggest that vasopressin derivatives

(orinipressin) may improve GFR in this condition. The use of such agents remains controversial.

Rhabdomyolysis-Associated Acute Renal Failure

This condition accounts for close to 5–10% of cases of ARF in ICUs depending on the setting. Its pathogenesis involves prerenal, renal, and postrenal factors. It is now typically seen following major trauma, drug overdose with narcotics, vascular embolism, and in response to a variety of agents that can induce major muscle injury. The principles of treatment are based on retrospective data, small series, and multivariate logistic regression analysis, because no randomized controlled trials have been conducted. Treatment includes prompt and aggressive fluid resuscitation, elimination of causative agents, and correction of compartment syndromes.

CURRENT CONTROVERSY

Role of Bicarbonate and Mannitol in Rhabdomyolysis
- The alkalinization of urine (pH > 6.5) with bicarbonate is not sustained by controlled studies. Neither is the maintenance of polyuria (>300 ml/hour)
- However, both are relatively easy to perform and are safe when done with invasive hemodynamic monitoring
- The role of mannitol is untested, but unlikely to cause harm

Obstruction to urine outflow causes so-called postrenal renal failure, which is the most common cause of functional renal impairment in the community. Typical causes of obstructive ARF include bladder neck obstruction from an enlarged prostate, ureteric obstruction from pelvic tumors or retroperitoneal fibrosis, papillary necrosis, or large calculi. The clinical presentation of obstruction may be acute or acute-on-chronic in patients with longstanding renal calculi. It may not always be associated with oliguria. If obstruction is suspected, ultrasonography can be easily performed at the bedside. However, not all cases of acute obstruction have an abnormal ultrasound and, in many cases, obstruction occurs in conjunction with other renal insults (e.g., staghorn calculi and severe sepsis of renal origin).

PATHOGENESIS OF ACUTE RENAL FAILURE

The pathogenesis of obstructive ARF involves several humoral responses as well as mechanical factors.

The pathogenesis of parenchymal renal failure is typically immunologic. It varies from vasculitis to interstitial nephropathy and involves an extraordinary complexity of immunologic mechanisms. The pathogenesis of prerenal ARF is of greater direct relevance to the intensivist. Several mechanisms appear to play a major role in the development of renal injury:

- Ischemia of outer medulla with activation of the tubuloglomerular feedback
- Tubular obstruction from casts of exfoliated cells
- Interstitial edema secondary to back diffusion of fluid
- Humorally mediated afferent arteriolar renal vasoconstriction
- Inflammatory response to cell injury and local release of mediators
- Disruption of normal cellular adhesion to the basement membrane
- Radical oxygen species-induced apoptosis
- Phospholipase A2-induced cell membrane injury

In septic patients with hyperdynamic circulations there may be adequate global blood flow to the kidney but intrarenal shunting away from the medulla causing medullary ischemia or efferent arteriolar vasodilatation causing decreased intraglomerular pressure and thus decreased GFR.

CLINICAL PICTURE

The most common clinical picture of ARF is that of a patient who has sustained a major systemic insult. When the patient arrives in the operating room or ICU resuscitation is well under way. Despite such efforts, the patient is often anuric or profoundly oliguric, the serum creatinine is rising, and metabolic acidosis is developing. Potassium and phosphate levels may also be rapidly rising. Accompanying multiple organ dysfunction (mechanical ventilation and need for vasoactive drugs) is common. Fluid resuscitation is typically undertaken under the guidance of invasive hemodynamic monitoring. Vasoactive drugs are often used to restore mean arterial pressure (MAP) to "acceptable" levels (typically >70–75 mmHg). The patient may improve over time and urine output may return with or without the assistance of diuretic agents. If urine output does not return, however, renal replacement therapy needs to be rapidly considered.

If the cause of ARF has been removed and the patient has become physiologically stable, slow recovery occurs (from 4 to 5 days to 3 or 4 weeks). In some cases, urine output can be above normal for several days. If the cause of ARF has not been adequately remedied, the patient remains gravely ill, the kidneys do not recover, and death from multiple organ failure occurs.

PREVENTING ACUTE RENAL FAILURE

The fundamental principle of ARF prevention is to treat its cause. If prerenal factors contribute, these must be identified, and hemodynamic resuscitation quickly instituted. Intravascular volume must be maintained or rapidly restored, and this is often best done using invasive hemodynamic monitoring (central venous catheter, arterial cannula, and pulmonary artery catheter in some cases). Oxygenation must be maintained. An adequate hemoglobin concentration (at least 80 g/l) must be maintained or immediately restored. Once intravascular volume has been restored, some patients remain hypotensive (MAP < 75 mmHg). In these patients autoregulation of renal blood flow may be lost. Restoration of MAP to near normal levels is likely to increase GFR. Such elevations in MAP require the addition of vasopressor drugs. In patients with hypertension or renovascular disease a MAP of 75–80 mmHg may still be inadequate. The nephroprotective role of additional fluid therapy in a patient with a normal or increased cardiac output and blood pressure is questionable. Despite these measures renal failure may still develop if cardiac output is inadequate. This may require a variety of interventions from the use of inotropic drugs to the application of ventricular assist devices.

Following hemodynamic resuscitation and removal of nephrotoxins, it is unclear whether the use of additional pharmacologic measures is of further benefit to the kidneys. Renal dose dopamine is still frequently used. Evidence of the efficacy of its administration in critically ill patients is lacking. However, this agent is a tubular diuretic and occasionally increases urine output. This may be incorrectly interpreted as an increase in GFR.

CURRENT CONTROVERSY

Role of Low-Dose Dopamine
All recent studies involving low-dose dopamine have been meta-analyzed and a large double-blind randomized controlled study has been completed. Low-dose dopamine is not different from placebo in its effects on GFR.

In a patient with a low cardiac output, however, the administration of beta-dose dopamine (as would dobutamine or milrinone) may increase cardiac output, renal blood flow, and GFR. A biologic rationale exists for the use of mannitol, as is the case for dopamine. Animal experiments offer some encouraging findings. However, no controlled human data exist to support its clinical use. The effect of mannitol as a renal protective agent remains questionable. Loop diuretics may protect the loop of Henle from ischemia by decreasing its transport-related workload. Animal data are encouraging, as are ex vivo experiments. There are no double-blind randomized controlled studies of suitable size to prove that these agents reduce the incidence of renal failure. However, there are several studies that support the view that loop diuretics may decrease the need for dialysis in patients with developing ARF. They appear to achieve this by inducing polyuria, which results in the prevention or easier control of volume overload, acidosis, and hyperkalemia, the three major triggers for renal replacement therapy in the ICU. Because avoiding dialysis simplifies treatment and reduces cost of care, loop diuretics may be useful in patients with renal dysfunction especially in the form of continuous infusion. Other agents such as theophylline, urodilatin, and anaritide (a synthetic atrial natriuretic factor) have also been proposed. Studies so far, however, have been experimental, too small, or have shown no beneficial effect.

Radiocontrast Nephropathy

In patients receiving radiocontrast a randomized controlled trial (RCT) suggested that half-isotonic saline infusion to maintain intravascular fluid expansion is superior to the addition of mannitol or furosemide. A more recent RCT of similar patients demonstrated a beneficial effect of N-acetylcysteine treatment before and after radiocontrast administration. A further study of 1620 patients recently demonstrated that isotonic saline is superior to half-isotonic saline. Since these preventive interventions have minimal toxicity they should be considered whenever a patient is scheduled for the administration of intravenous radiocontrast either in or outside the operating room.

DIAGNOSTIC INVESTIGATIONS

An etiological diagnosis of ARF must always be established. Such diagnosis may be obvious on clinical grounds. However, in many patients it is best to consider all possibilities and exclude common treatable causes by simple investigations. Such investigations include the examination of urinary sediment and exclusion of a urinary tract infection (most if not all patients), the exclusion of obstruction when appropriate (some patients) and the careful exclusion of nephrotoxins (all patients).

In specific situations, other investigations are necessary to establish the diagnosis, such as creatine kinase and free myoglobin for possible rhabdomyolysis. A chest radiograph, a blood film, the measurement of nonspecific inflammatory markers, and the measurement of specific antibodies (anti-GBM, antineutrophil cytoplasm,

anti-DNA, antismooth muscle, etc.) are extremely useful screening tests to help support the diagnosis of vasculitis or of certain types of collagen disease or glomerulonephritis. If thrombotic thrombocytopenic purpura (TTP) is suspected, the additional measurement of lactic dehydrogenase, haptoglobin, unconjugated bilirubin, and free hemoglobin is needed. In some patients specific findings (cryoglobulins, Bence-Jones proteins) are almost diagnostic. In a few rare patients a renal biopsy becomes necessary.

MANAGING ACUTE RENAL FAILURE

The principles of management of established ARF are the treatment or removal of its cause and the maintenance of physiologic homeostasis while recovery takes place. Complications such as encephalopathy, pericarditis, myopathy, neuropathy, electrolyte disturbances, or other major electrolyte, fluid, or metabolic derangement should never occur in a modern ICU. Their prevention may include several measures, which vary in complexity from fluid restriction to the initiation of extracorporeal renal replacement therapy.

Nutritional support must be started early and must contain adequate calories (30–35 kcal/kg/day) as a mixture of carbohydrates and lipids. Adequate protein (about 1–2 g/kg/day) must be administered. There is no evidence that specific renal nutritional solutions are useful. Vitamins and trace elements should be administered at least according to their recommended daily allowance. The role of newer immunonutritional solutions remains controversial. The enteral route is preferred to the use of parenteral nutrition.

Hyperkalemia (>6 mmol/l) must be promptly treated with insulin and dextrose administration (exclude spurious hyperkalemia secondary to hemolysis, thrombocytosis, and a very high white cell count), the infusion of bicarbonate if acidosis is present, the administration of nebulized salbutamol, or all of these together. If the "true" serum potassium is >7 mmol/l or electrocardiographic signs of hyperkalemia appear, calcium gluconate (10 ml of 10% solution IV) should also be administered. The above measures are temporizing actions, while renal replacement therapy is being set up. The presence of hyperkalemia is a major indication for the immediate institution of renal replacement therapy.

Metabolic acidosis is almost always present but rarely requires treatment per se. Anemia requires correction to maintain a hemoglobin level > 70 g/l. More aggressive transfusion needs individual patient assessment. Drug therapy must be adjusted to take into account the effect of the decreased clearances associated with loss of renal function. Stress ulcer prophylaxis is advisable and should be based on H_2-receptor antagonists or proton pump inhibitors in selected cases. Assiduous attention should be paid to the prevention of infection.

Fluid overload can be prevented by the use of loop diuretics in polyuric patients. However, if the patient is oliguric, the only way to avoid fluid overload is to institute renal replacement therapy at an early stage (see below). Marked azotemia ([urea] > 40 mmol/l or [creatinine] > 400 mmol/l) is undesirable and should probably be treated with renal replacement therapy unless recovery is imminent or already under way and a return toward normal values is expected within 24 hours. It is recognized, however, that no RCTs exist to define the ideal time for intervention with artificial renal support.

Renal Replacement Therapy

When ARF is severe, resolution can take several days or weeks. In these patients extracorporeal techniques of blood purification must be applied to prevent complications. Such techniques, broadly named renal replacement therapy (RRT), include continuous hemofiltration, intermittent hemodialysis (IHD), and peritoneal dialysis (PD), each with its technical variations. All of these techniques rely on the principle of removing unwanted solutes and water through a semipermeable membrane. Such a membrane is either biologic (peritoneum) or artificial (hemodialysis or hemofiltration membranes) and offers several advantages, disadvantages, and limitations.

In the critically ill patient RRT should be initiated early, prior to the development of complications. Fear of early dialysis stems from the adverse effects of conventional IHD with cuprophane membranes, especially hemodynamic instability, and from the risks and limitations of continuous or intermittent PD. However, continuous renal replacement therapy (CRRT) or slow extended IHD minimize these effects. The criteria for the initiation of RRT in patients with chronic renal failure may be inappropriate in the critically ill. A set of modern criteria for the initiation of RRT in the ICU is presented in Box 29-3.

With either IHD or CRRT there are limited data on what is "adequate" intensity of dialysis. However, this should include maintenance of homeostasis at all levels, and better uremic control may translate into better survival. An appropriate target urea is 15–25 mmol/l, with a protein intake around 1.5 g/kg/day. This can be easily achieved using CRRT at urea clearances of 30–40 l/day depending on patient size and catabolic rate. If IHD is used, daily treatment and extended treatment become desirable.

There is a great deal of controversy as to which mode of RRT is "best" in the ICU, due to the lack of RCTs comparing different techniques. Trials of sufficient statistical power are difficult to conduct and may never

---

Box 29-3 Modern Criteria for the Initiation of Renal Replacement Therapy in the Intensive Care Unit*

- Oliguria (urine output < 200 ml/12 hours)
- [Blood urea nitrogen] > 80 mg/dl
- [Creatinine] > 3 mg/l
- [K+] > 6.5 mmol/l or rapidly rising
- Pulmonary edema unresponsive to diuretics
- Uncompensated metabolic acidosis (pH < 7.1)
- Temperature > 40°C
- Uremic complications (encephalopathy/myopathy/neuropathy/pericarditis)
- Overdose with a dialyzable toxin (e.g., lithium)

* If one criterion is present, RRT should be considered. If two criteria are simultaneously present, RRT is strongly recommended.

---

be performed. In their absence, techniques of RRT may be judged on the basis of the following criteria:

- Hemodynamic side effects
- Ability to control fluid status
- Biocompatibility
- Risk of infection
- Uremic control
- Avoidance of cerebral edema
- Ability to allow full nutritional support
- Ability to control acidosis
- Absence of specific side effects
- Cost

CRRT and slow low-efficiency extended dialysis (SLED) offer many advantages over PD and conventional IHD (3–4 hours/day, 3–4 times/week), and while CRRT is almost exclusively used in Europe, Japan, and Australia, a minority of American ICU patients receive CRRT. Some salient aspects of CRRT and IHD require discussion.

Continuous Renal Replacement Therapy

CRRT was initially performed as an arteriovenous therapy (continuous arteriovenous hemofiltration, CAVH) where blood flow through the hemofilter was driven by the patient's blood pressure. The need to cannulate an artery, however, is associated with 15–20% morbidity. Accordingly, double-lumen catheters and peristaltic blood pumps have come into use (continuous venovenous hemofiltration, CVVH) with or without control of ultrafiltration rate.

In a venovenous system dialysate can also be delivered countercurrent to blood flow (continuous venovenous hemodialysis/hemodiafiltration) to achieve either almost pure diffusive clearance or a mixture of diffusive and convective clearance.

No matter what technique is used, the following outcomes are predictable:

- Continuous control of fluid status
- Hemodynamic stability
- Control of acid–base status
- Ability to provide protein-rich nutrition while achieving uremic control
- Control of electrolyte balance, including phosphate and calcium balance
- Prevention of swings in intracerebral water
- Minimal risk of infection
- High level of biocompatibility

However, CRRT mandates the presence of specifically trained nursing and medical staff 24 hours a day. Small ICUs often cannot provide such level of support. If CRRT is only used 5–10 times a year, the cost of training may be unjustified and expertise may be hard to maintain. Furthermore, depending on the organization of patient care, CRRT may be more expensive that IHD. Finally, the issues of continuous circuit anticoagulation and the potential risk of bleeding have been a major concern.

Anticoagulation During Continuous Renal Replacement Therapy

Anticoagulants are frequently used during CRRT. However, circuit anticoagulation increases risk of bleeding. Therefore, the risks and benefits of more or less intense anticoagulation and alternative strategies (Box 29-4) must be considered.

In the vast majority of patients low-dose heparin (< 500 IU/hour) is sufficient to achieve adequate filter life, is easy and cheap to administer, and has almost no effect on the patient's coagulation tests. In some patients a higher dose is necessary. In others (pulmonary embolism, myocardial ischemia) full heparinization may actually be concomitantly indicated. Regional citrate

anticoagulation is very effective but requires a special dialysate or replacement fluid. Regional heparin/protamine anticoagulation is also somewhat complex but may be useful if frequent filter clotting occurs and further anticoagulation of the patient is considered dangerous. Low-molecular-weight heparin is also easy to give but more expensive. Its dose must be adjusted for the loss of renal function. This is difficult to monitor. Heparinoids and prostacyclin may be useful if the patient has developed heparin-induced thrombocytopenia and thrombosis. Finally, in perhaps 10–20% of patients anticoagulation is best avoided because of endogenous coagulopathy or recent surgery. In such patients mean filter lives of >24 hours can be achieved provided that blood flow is kept at about 200 ml/minute and vascular access is reliable.

CLINICAL CAVEAT

Anticoagulation During Continuous Renal Replacement Therapy

- Anticoagulants should not be used during CRRT within 24 hours of surgery. They are unnecessary and dangerous
- Adequate filter life can be achieved without any anticoagulation if vascular access is adequate and blood flow is kept at 200 ml/minute or above

---

Particular attention needs to be paid to the adequacy/ease of flow through the double-lumen catheter. Smaller (11.5 Fr) catheters in the subclavian position are a particular problem. Larger catheters (13.5 Fr) in the femoral position appear to function more reliably.

Box 29-4 Strategies for Circuit Anticoagulation During Continuous Renal Replacement Therapy

- No anticoagulation
- Low-dose prefilter heparin (<500 IU/hour)
- Medium-dose prefilter heparin (500–1000 IU/hour)
- Full heparinization
- Regional heparin/protamine anticoagulation
- Regional citrate anticoagulation
- Low-molecular-weight heparin
- Prostacyclin
- Heparinoids

CASE STUDY

Continuous Renal Replacement Therapy after Cardiac Surgery

A 46-year-old man undergoes pericardectomy for constrictive pericarditis. He has a renal transplant with chronic rejection, and a BUN of 70 mg/dl. The operation is complicated by severe intraoperative bleeding from the pericardial bed. Such oozing continues postoperatively at a rate of 300 ml/minute. Despite 5 units of fresh frozen plasma, 3 units of blood, and 5 units of platelets intraoperatively, his INR is 2.5, APTT is 56 seconds, HB is 7 g/dl, and platelet count is 56,000/mm^3. The surgeon does not want to take him back to the operating room because attempts at intraoperative hemostasis have already failed. A normal clotting profile must be urgently restored. However, the patient has a pulmonary artery occlusion pressure of 20 mmHg, pulmonary congestion (revealed on chest x-ray), a urine output of 20 ml/hour on a frusemide infusion at 30 mg/hour, and a PaO$_2$ of 67 mmHg on 70% FIO$_2$.

Continued

CASE STUDY—Cont'd

CLINICAL NEED

Fluid must be removed and clotting factors and blood must be given simultaneously while avoiding further pulmonary edema.

RESPONSE

Double-lumen catheter is inserted, and CVVH started without anticoagulation. Blood flow is 200 ml/minute, net fluid removal at 1000 ml/hour. Fresh frozen plasma (10 units), cryoprecipitate (10 units), platelets (20 units), and red cells (6 units) are given over 4 hours. CVVH is continued at 1000 ml/hour for 4 hours. Net fluid removal was decreased to 300 ml/hour. Filter clotted at 12 hours. Bleeding stopped at 4 hours. Gas exchange was markedly better at 12 hours. Second filter started without anticoagulation for another 16 hours. Patient was extubated at 28 hours after ICU admission and discharged from ICU at 38 hours.

CONCLUSION

CRRT without anticoagulation is safe and effective after surgery and can help save lives.

The choice of membrane is also a matter of controversy. There are several biosynthetic membranes on the market, which have excellent biocompatibility (AN69, polyamide, polysulfone, cellulose triacetate). There are no controlled studies to show that one of them confers a clinical advantage over the others.

Intermittent Hemodialysis

Vascular access is typically by double-lumen catheter as CRRT. The circuit is also the same, with venovenous blood flow driven by a peristaltic pump. Countercurrent dialysate flow is used as in CVVHD. The major differences are that standard IHD uses high dialysate flows (300–400 ml/minute), generates dialysate using purified water and concentrate, and is applied for short periods of time (3–4 hours). These differences have important implications. Firstly, volume has to be removed over a short period of time and this may be poorly tolerated by critically ill patients, with a high incidence of hypotension. Repeated hypotensive episodes may delay renal recovery. Secondly, solute removal is episodic. This translates into inferior uremic control, and acid–base control. Limited fluid and uremic control imposes unnecessary limitations on nutritional support. Furthermore, rapid solute shifts increase brain water content and raise intracranial pressure. Finally, much controversy has surrounded the issue of membrane bioincompatibility. Standard low-flux dialyzing membranes made of

cuprophane are known to trigger the activation of several inflammatory pathways when compared to high-flux synthetic membranes (also used for continuous hemofiltration). It is possible that such proinflammatory effect contributes to further renal damage and delays recovery or even affects mortality. The matter remains unresolved.

The limitations of applying "standard" IHD to the treatment of ARF has led to the development of new approaches (so-called "hybrid techniques") such as SLED and intermittent extended hemofiltration. These techniques seek to adapt IHD to the clinical circumstance and there by increase its tolerance and its clearances.

CURRENT CONTROVERSY

How Often Should Dialysis Be Done?
- A randomized controlled trial has shown that daily dialysis increases survival and improves the rate of renal recovery in ICU patients
- Second daily conventional dialysis is inadequate therapy for critically ill patients

---

The technique of peritoneal dialysis is now uncommonly used in the treatment of adult ARF in developed countries. However, it may be an adequate technique in developing countries or in children where alternatives are considered too expensive, too invasive, or are not available.

Plasmapheresis or Plasma Exchange

This technique might be applied to some critically ill patients. Plasma is removed from the patient and exchanged with fresh frozen plasma (FFP) and a mixture of colloid and crystalloid solutions. This technique can also be performed in an ICU familiar with CRRT techniques. A plasmafilter (a filter that allows the passage of molecules up to 500 kD) instead of a hemofilter is inserted in the CVVH circuit, and the filtrate (plasma) discarded. Plasmapheresis can also be performed with special machines using the principles of centrifugation. The differences, if any, between centrifugation and filtration technology are unclear. Replacement (postfilter) will occur as in CVVH using, for example, a 50/50 combination of FFP and albumin. Plasmapheresis has been shown to be effective treatment for TTP and for several diseases mediated by abnormal antibodies (Guillain-Barré syndrome, cryoglobulinemia, myasthenia gravis, Goodpasture's syndrome, etc.) in which antibody removal appears desirable. Its role in the treatment of sepsis remains uncertain.

Blood Purification Technology for Nonacute Renal Failure Indications

There is growing interest in the possibility that blood purification may provide a clinically significant benefit in patients with severe sepsis/septic shock by removing circulating "mediators." A variety of techniques including plasmapheresis, high-volume hemofiltration, very-high-volume hemofiltration, and coupled plasma filtration adsorption are being studied in animals and in phase I/II studies in humans. Initial experiments support the need to continue exploring this therapeutic option. However, no suitably powered RCTs have yet been reported. Also, blood purification technology in combination with bioreactors containing either human or porcine liver cells is under active investigations as a form of artificial liver support for patients with fulminant liver failure or for patients with acute-on-chronic liver failure. Such complex technology is beginning to show some promising results.

Drug Prescription During Dialytic Therapy

ARF and RRT profoundly affect drug clearance. A comprehensive description of changes in drug dosage according to the technique of RRT, residual creatinine clearance, and other determinants of pharmacodynamics is beyond the scope of this chapter and can be found in specialist texts. Table 29-2 provides general guidelines for the prescription of drugs that are commonly used in the ICU.

CONCLUSIONS

The areas of ARF and of RRT have undergone remarkable changes over the last five years. Major advances have been made in the prevention of radiocontrast nephropathy. No drugs, however, have been found to help in patients with ARF from other causes. CRRT is now firmly established throughout the world as perhaps the most commonly used form of RRT. Conventional dialysis, however, which was slowly losing ground, is reappearing in the form of extended, slow, low-efficiency treatment. In the meanwhile the uses of novel membranes, of sorbents, and of different intensities of treatment are being explored in the area of sepsis management and liver support. Anesthesiologists need to keep abreast of this rapid evolution if they are to offer their patients the best of care.

SELECTED READING

ANZICS Clinical Trials Group: Low-dose dopamine in patients with early renal dysfunction: a placebo-controlled randomised trial. Lancet 356:2139–2143, 2000.

Table 29-2 Drug Dosage During Dialytic Therapy

Drug	CRRT	IHD
Aminoglycosides	Normal dose q 36 hours	50% normal dose q 48 hours – 2/3 redose after IHD
Cefotaxime or ceftazidime	1 g q 8–12 hours	1 g q 12–24 hours after IHD
Imipenem	500 mg q 8 hours	250 mg q 8 hours and after IHD
Meropenem	500 mg q 8 hours	250 mg q 8 hours and after IHD
Metronidazole	500 mg q 8 hours	250 mg q 8 hours and after IHD
Co-trimoxazole	Normal dose q 18 hours	Normal dose q 24 hours after IHD
Amoxycillin	500 mg q 8 hours	500 mg daily and after IHD
Vancomycin	1 g q 24 hours	1 g q 96–120 hours
Piperacillin	3–4 g q 6 hours	3–4 g q 8 hours and after IHD
Ticarcillin	1–2 g q 8 hours	1–2 g q 12 hours and after IHD
Ciprofloxacin	200 mg q 12 hours	200 mg q 24 hours and after IHD
Fluconazole	200 mg q 24 hours	200 mg q 48 hours and after IHD
Acyclovir	3.5 mg/kg q 24 hours	2.5 mg/kg/day and after IHD
Gancyclovir	5 mg/kg/day	5 mg/kg/48 hours and after IHD
Amphotericin B	Normal dose	Normal dose
Liposomal amphotericin	Normal dose	Normal dose
Ceftriaxone	Normal dose	Normal dose
Erythomycin	Normal dose	Normal dose

The values represent approximations and should be used as a general guide only. Critically ill patients have markedly abnormal volumes of distribution for these agents which will affect dosage. CRRT is conducted at variable levels of intensity in different units also requiring adjustment. The values reported here relate to CVVH at 2 l/hour of ultrafiltration. Vancomycin is poorly removed by CVVHD. IHD may also differ from unit to unit. The values reported relate to standard IHD with low-flux membranes for 3–4 hours every second day.

Bellomo R, Kellum JA, Wisniewski SR, Pinsky MR: Effects of norepinephrine on the renal vasculature in normal and endotoxemic dogs. Am J Respir Crit Care Med 159:1186-1192, 1999.

Bellomo R, Ronco C: Adequacy of dialysis in the acute renal failure of the critically ill: the case for continuous therapies. Int J Artif Organs 19:129-142, 1996.

Bonventre JV: Mechanisms of ischemic acute renal failure. Kidney Int 43:1160-1178, 1993.

Cole L, Bellomo R, Silvester W, Reeves JH: A prospective, multicenter study of the epidemiology, management and outcome of severe acute renal failure in a "closed" ICU system. Am J Respir Crit Care Med 162:191-196, 2000.

Davenport A: The management of renal failure in patients at risk of cerebral edema/hypoxia. New Horizons 3:717-724, 1995.

Gettings LG, Reynolds HN, Scalea T: Outcome in post-traumatic acute renal failure when continuous renal replacement therapy is applied early vs. late. Intensive Care Med 25:805-881, 1999.

Marshall MR, Golper TA, Shaver MJ, Chatoth DK: Hybrid renal replacement modalities for the critically ill. Contrib Nephrol 132:252-257, 2001.

Mehta R, Dobos GJ, Ward DM: Anticoagulation procedures in continuous renal replacement. Semin Dial 5:61-68, 1992.

Ronco C, Bellomo R, Homel P et al: Effects of different doses in continuous veno-venous haemofiltration on outcomes of acute renal failure: a prospective randomized trial. Lancet 355:26-30, 2000.

Ronco C, Brendolan A, Bellomo R: Current technology for continuous renal replacement therapies. In Ronco C, Bellomo R, editors: *Critical Care Nephrology*, Dordrecht, The Netherlands: Kluwer Academic, 1998, pp 1327-1334.

Tan HK, Baldwin I, Bellomo R: Hemofiltration without anti-coagulation in high-risk patients. Intensive Care Med 26:1652-1657, 2000.

Tepel M, van der Giet M, Schwarzfeld C et al: Prevention of radiographic contrast agent-induced reductions in renal function by acetylcysteine. N Engl J Med 343:180-184, 2000.

Tetta C, Mariano F, Ronco C, Bellomo R: Removal and generation of inflammatory mediators during continuous renal replacement therapies. In Ronco C, Bellomo R, editors: *Critical Care Nephrology*, Dordrecht, The Netherlands: Kluwer Academic, 1998, pp 1239-1248.

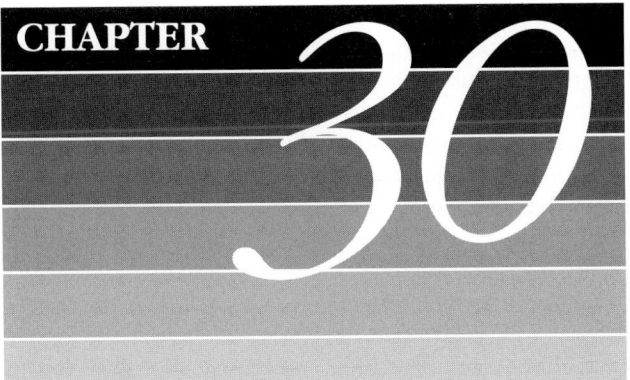

CHAPTER 30

Urologic Concerns in Critical Care

RALPH MADEB, M.D.

CRAIG NICHOLSON, M.D.

ALI BORHAN, M.D.

ERDAL ERTURK, M.D.

EDWARD M. MESSING, M.D.

The intensive care unit (ICU) represents a meeting point between the most critically ill patients receiving aggressive therapies and many specialties of medicine and surgery. Changing concepts of disease management, with more aggressive therapies being offered to the elderly patient with multiple comorbid conditions, has increased the need for urologic care in the ICU setting. Therefore the urologist's primary role in treating patients in the ICU is to expeditiously recognize and rapidly institute the appropriate medical and surgical intervention needed in coordination with the ICU team. This chapter focuses on techniques needed to treat patients with urologic problems in the ICU, diagnosis and management of emergent upper urinary tract obstruction, and nonoperative management of patients with genitourinary trauma in the ICU. Other important issues involving the genital tract such as phimosis and paraphimosis, epididymoorchitis, and pelvic abscesses can also

be present in ICU patients but will not be discussed in this chapter.

UROLOGIC PROCEDURES

Instrumentation of the upper and lower urinary tract is routinely performed in the ICU setting for diagnosis and treatment of urologic diseases. An understanding of the available instruments and procedures, and their indications, is essential for safe and successful manipulation of the urinary tract. The techniques routinely needed in patients in an ICU include:

- Urethral catheterization
- Cystourethroscopy
- Suprapubic cystotomy
- Percutaneous nephrostomy

Urethral Catheterization

Catheterization of the male and female urethra is routinely performed in the ICU for both diagnosis and therapy of urologic and medical diseases. There are numerous types of urethral catheters available for catheterization of the male and female urinary bladder (Figure 30-1). The choice of which specific catheter is to be used depends on the underlying reason for catheterization. Table 30-1 reviews the indications for urethral catheterization for diagnostic and therapeutic purposes. Common indications include collection of urine for culture, measurement of postvoid residual urine volume, and instillation of contrast agents and antibiotics into the bladder in order to diagnose and treat lower urinary tract pathologies. Therapeutic causes for urethral catheterization includes relief and management of acute urinary retention and infravesical obstruction, clot evacuation, accurate monitoring of urine output, and the need for bladder decompression after

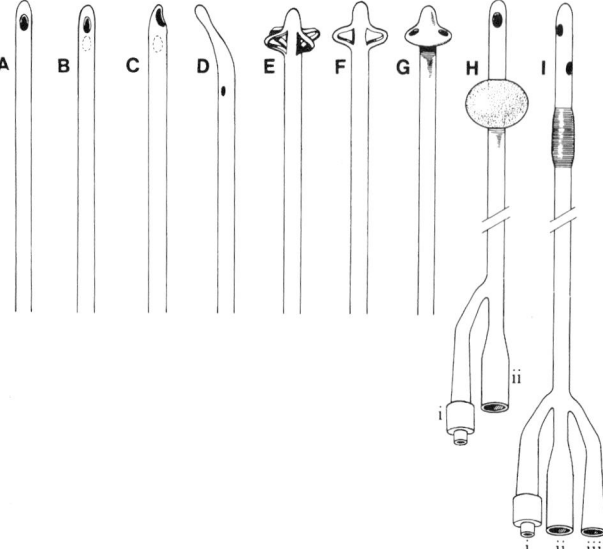

Figure 30-1 Various types of urethral catheters. A, Conical tip urethral catheter, one eye. B, Robinson urethral catheter. C, Whistle-tip urethral catheter. D, Coudé hollow olive-tip catheter. E, Malecot self-retaining four-wing urethral catheter. F, Malecot self-retaining two-wing catheter. G, Pezzer self-retaining drain open-ended head, used for cystotomy drainage. H, Foley-type balloon catheter, one limb of distal end for balloon inflation (i), one for drainage (ii). I, Foley-type three-way balloon catheter, one limb of distal end for balloon inflation (i), one for drainage (ii), and one to infuse irrigating solution to prevent clot retention within the bladder (iii). (From Carter HB: Basic instrumentation and cystoscopy. In Walsh PC, Retik AB, Vaughan D, Wein AJ, editors: *Campbell's Urology*, ed 8, Philadelphia: WB Saunders, 2002, pp 111–121.)

surgical procedures. Contraindications for urethral catheterization include patients with acute prostatitis, blood at the urethral meatus or suspicion of urethral injury, and patients with severe urethral strictures, and fistulas.

Equipment and Technique

Urethral catheterization is an invasive procedure and the patient should be informed of the reason

for catheterization. It is important to prepare and drape the urethra in a sterile fashion in order to decrease introduction of skin and genital flora into the urinary tract. In conscious males, it is helpful to insert 2% lidocaine jelly to anesthetize and lubricate the long urethra. The equipment needed for urethral catheterization includes a urethral catheter, povidone-iodine solution (or a similar antiseptic solution in a patient with a known iodine allergy), lubricating or lidocaine jelly, urinary drainage bag, 10 ml syringe, sterile gloves and drapes, and normal saline (Box 30-1).

Although intubating the urethra seems relatively simple, this procedure nevertheless can cause significant morbidity in an already ailing patient. The most common complications from urethral catheterizations include creation of a urethral perforation (false passage) and

---

Table 30-1 Indications for Urethral Catheterization

Diagnostic	Therapeutic
Collection of urine for culture	Acute or chronic urinary retention
Measurement of postvoid residual urine	Urinary output measurement
Urodynamic studies	Management of hematuria and clot evacuation
Measurement of intra-abdominal compartment	Intravesical chemotherapy
Retrograde instillation of contrast agents for cystograms or cystourethrography	Bladder decompression after surgical procedures

---

Box 30-1 Technique for Urethral Catheterization

- Start the procedure with positioning the patient. Men can be catheterized in the supine position with the penis stretched perpendicular to the body; in females it is very helpful to place the patient in the frog-leg position (Figures 30-2 and 30-3). Alternatively, elderly women or women with recent orthopedic surgery who are unable to abduct the thighs can be flexed at the hips to provide direct access to the urethra (often an assistant should help maintain this position in women who are incapable of assisting).
- Swab the urethra with povidone-iodine.
- In men it is critical to retract the foreskin and clean the glans penis thoroughly. In addition it is easier to inject 10 ml of 2% lidocaine jelly into the urethra in order to facilitate catheter passage through the long urethra.
- After the urethra is prepped and draped grasp the catheter with the dominant hand after lubricating it with lubricating jelly.
- Using steady and gentle pressure advance the catheter into the urethra.
- In females the urethra is short (3–5 cm) and after the catheter is advanced 8–10 cm through the urethral meatus urine will be brought forth. At this point inflate the balloon with 5–10 cm³ of normal saline and connect the urethral catheter to a urinary drainage bag.
- In males, it is critical to advance the catheter up to the balloon hub and only inflate the balloon when urine is returned. If urine is not returned irrigate the catheter to confirm placement in the bladder before inflating the balloon.
- In males it is also critical to replace the foreskin at the end of catheterization in order to prevent a paraphimosis from developing.

bladder decompression in patients with acute retention include hypotension and postobstructive diuresis. Early hypotension is typically a result of a vasovagal response to the acute decompression of a distended bladder.

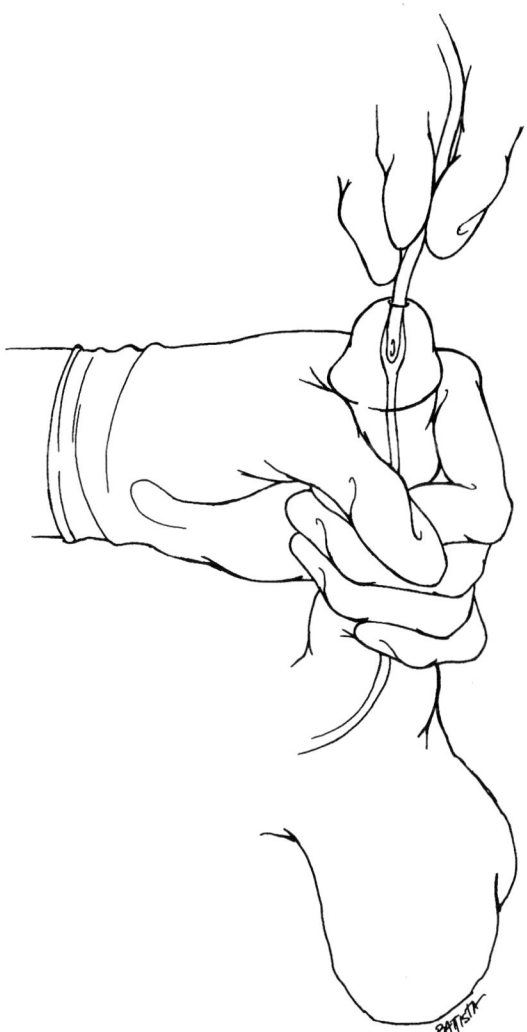

Figure 30-2 Proper positioning of the hand while trying to place a urethral catheter into the penis. It is very helpful to keep the penis stretched and perpendicular to the patient's body. Using steady and gentle pressure the catheter is advanced into the urethra. (Used with permission from Han M: Urological procedures. In Chen H, Sonnenday CJ, editors: *Manual of Common Surgical Procedures*, ed 2, Philadelphia: Lippincott Williams and Wilkins, 2000, pp 205–236.)

hematuria with traumatic catheterizations. If a false passage is suspected the balloon of the Foley catheter should never be inflated and the catheterization should be aborted. Urology should be consulted as this may be best evaluated by bedside cystoscopy. Hematuria caused by traumatic Foley catheter placement is caused by the disruption and damage to the small mucosal vessels of the urethra and prostate. The treatment of traumatic Foley catheter placement usually consists of IV fluid hydration, catheter irrigation, and monitoring. In addition, bleeding from prostatic origin usually will need continuous bladder irrigation with a three-way Foley catheter (see Figure 30-1). Other physiologic complications that can occur after

---

CLINICAL CAVEAT

Urethral Catheterizations

- Catheter size is usually referred to using the French scale (1 Fr = 0.33 mm in diameter). Therefore an 18 F catheter is approximately 6 mm in diameter.
- Usually an 18 F Foley is recommended for male patients and a 16 F Foley is recommended for female patients.
- A large 22 or 24 F three-way Foley should be placed for patients who have gross hematuria and are at risk from obstructing clots resulting in the need for manual clot evacuation or continuous bladder irrigation.
- Coudé or curved tip catheters are specifically designed to help bypass areas of the male urethra that are difficult to negotiate such as the prostatic urethra in a patient with prostatic enlargement.
- Difficulty in catheterizing the male patient can result from various causes including BPH or prostatic adenocarcinoma, urethral strictures (including urethra meatal stenosis, and bladder neck contractures). If the initial attempt for Foley placement has failed in a patient who has a history of or is suspected of having one of the above mentioned pathologies, further attempts at catheterization should be avoided and urology consulted for urethral evaluation and placement.

Cystourethroscopy

Cystourethroscopy is the technique that permits direct visualization of the lower urinary tract through a cystoscope. In the ICU setting this is easily accomplished with a flexible cystoscope and can be performed at the patient's bedside (Figure 30-4). Often anatomic or functional lower urinary tract pathologies such as benign prostatic hyperplasia (BPH), anterior or posterior urethral obstruction, urethral strictures, and spasms of the external urinary sphincter do not allow successful passage of the catheter into the bladder. If a Coudé catheterization is not successful it is sometimes possible to negotiate the obstruction with a flexible cystoscope. The advantages of a flexible cystoscope over the conventional rigid cystoscope include greater comfort for the patient, ability to perform the procedure while the patient is supine or bedridden, ease of passing the instrument over an elevated bladder neck or through an enlarged prostate with minimal bleeding, and the capacity to inspect many angles of the urethra and bladder with deflection of the tip of the instrument. The flexible

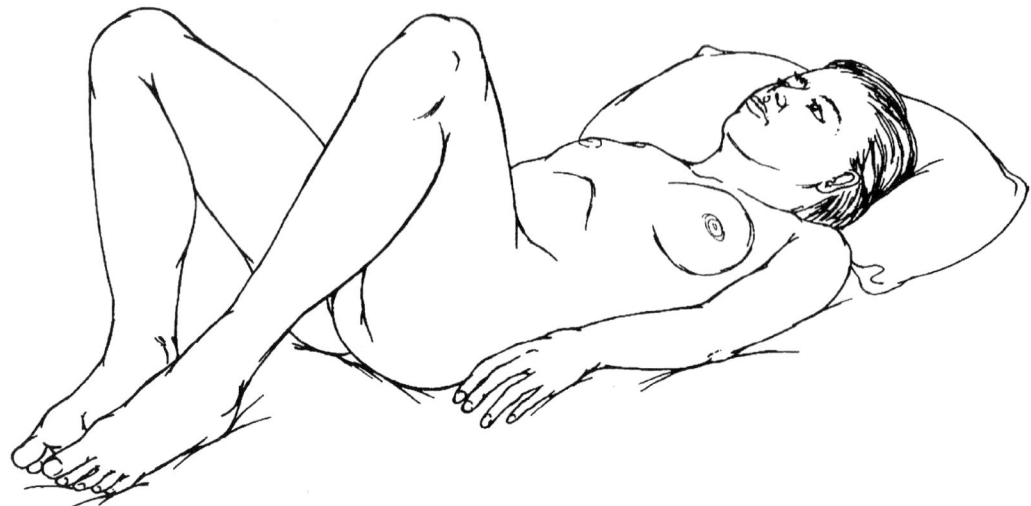

Figure 30-3   Proper positioning of a female patient in the frog-leg position for urethral catheterization. (Used with permission from Han M: Urological procedures. In Chen H, Sonnenday CJ, editors: *Manual of Common Surgical Procedures*, ed 2, Philadelphia: Lippincott Williams and Wilkins, 2000, pp 205–236.)

cystoscope can be passed under direct vision into the bladder or to the level of the obstruction where a guide wire can be placed through the compromised urethral lumen into the bladder through the working port of the cystoscope. After visualizing the wire in the bladder the flexible cystoscope is withdrawn making sure not to remove the guide wire simultaneously from the bladder. A specialized catheter hole puncher is then used to create a hole at the tip of a straight urethral catheter (Figure 30-5). The hole punch creates a smooth hole at the tip of the urethral Foley catheter which is much easier to pass through a narrowed urethra than the more jagged opening

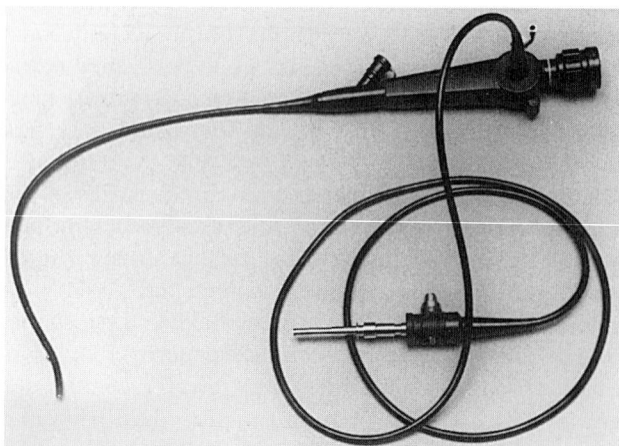

Figure 30-4   Flexible cystoscope with an attached light source and a deflectable tip. (From Carter HB: Basic instrumentation and cystoscopy. In Walsh PC, Retik AB, Vaughan D, Wein AJ, editors: *Campbell's Urology*, ed 8, Philadelphia: WB Saunders, 2002, pp 111–121.)

created by a scissors or scalpel blade. Alternatively, a Council-tipped catheter, a Foley catheter manufactured with a smooth edged hole at the tip, can be used if available. The lubricated catheter is then passed over the guide wire into the bladder. When urine drains the balloon is inflated and the guide wire is withdrawn. Patient preparation and equipment is identical to that of urethral catheterization in addition to the equipment needed for cystoscopy, which usually includes a flexible cystoscope, light source with fiber-optical light, 0.035 or 0.038 F flexible tip guide wire (so that the wire does not perforate through the bladder wall), 1 liter of normal saline or sterile water irrigant, and transurethral resection ("TUR") tubing. If the obstruction is caused by a tight urethral stricture or bladder neck contracture, urethral dilation may be needed prior to insertion of the Foley catheter of sufficient luminal size to drain a bladder particularly if bleeding and clots are anticipated. Dilation is performed with Heyman serial dilators that are more rigid than a rubber or latex catheter but still flexible enough to negotiate urethral curves and bends. Serial dilations in the bladder (so there is a return of urine) are done starting at 8 F and increasing by 2 F sizes until a dilator 2 F sizes larger than the catheter to be placed is passed. This ensures smooth catheter passage.

If the patient is receiving anticoagulation (e.g., full-dose heparin) urethral dilation can induce significant bleeding and should be avoided and alternative access should be sought. It is important to ensure that the patient does not have an active urinary tract infection as urethral instrumentation can worsen the infection and make the patient bacteremic and/or uroseptic. If cysto-urethroscopy is needed, the patient should receive

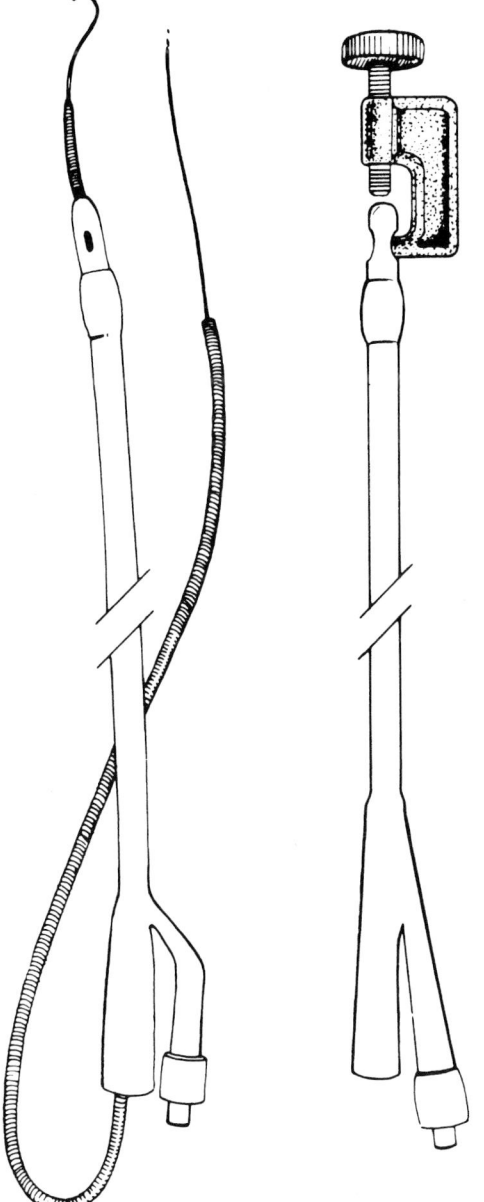

Figure 30-5   Left, Council catheter with end-hole passed over a guide wire. Right, Creation of an end-hole in a Foley-type catheter with a catheter hole puncher. (From Carter HB: Basic instrumentation and cystoscopy. In Walsh PC, Retik AB, Vaughan D, Wein AJ, editors: *Campbell's Urology*, ed 8, Philadelphia: WB Saunders, 2002, pp 111–121.)

antibiotics (preferably before as well as after instrumentation) making sure to adequately cover Gram-negative microbes.

Suprapubic Cystotomy Catheter

When it is not possible to bypass bladder outlet obstruction secondary to an enlarged prostate, bladder neck contracture, nonpassable urethral strictures, or proximal

Table 30-2 Indications and Contraindications for Percutaneous Suprapubic Cystotomy Catheter	
Indications	**Contraindications**
Urethral strictures	Prior midline infraumbilical incision*
False passage	Nondistended bladder*
Repeated catheterizations with inability to pass urethral catheters	Coagulopathy
	Pregnancy
	Carcinoma of the bladder
Acute prostatitis	Pelvic irradiation*
Traumatic urethral disruption	
Periurethral abscess	

* If an ultrasound machine is available then a suprapubic cystotomy can be placed under ultrasound guidance in these situations with extreme caution.

urethral disruption by using the above mentioned procedures, placement of a percutaneous suprapubic cystotomy catheter is recommended and preferable to repeated attempts at urethral catheterizations in order to avoid urethral trauma. Furthermore, repeated attempts at urethral catheterizations can cause the creation of false passages which can make subsequent catheterizations impossible and lead to urethral stricture disease or even fistula. Table 30-2 lists the indications and contraindications for performing this procedure. Currently there are two common commercial available types of percutaneous catheters: the Bonanno percutaneous suprapubic catheter set (Becton-Dickinson and Co., Franklin Lakes, NJ) and the Stamey percutaneous suprapubic catheter set in 10 F, 12 F, or 14 F (Cook Urological, Spencer, IA).

The basic approach of this technique involves percutaneous puncture of the bladder through the anterior abdominal wall with an obturator and catheter together. Upon entering the bladder, the obturator is withdrawn leaving the draining catheter in the bladder.

Equipment and Technique

As with all bedside or surgical procedures consent should be attained for placement of a suprapubic catheter. The equipment needed includes a percutaneous suprapubic catheter, as mentioned above (Figure 30-6), sterile prep solution, drapes and gloves, an 18–24 gauge 3-inch spinal needle, injectable 1% lidocaine, needle driver with 0 or 2-0 permanent (e.g., silk) suture, scalpel, and a urinary drainage bag (Box 30-2).

Before one places a suprapubic catheter it is critical that coagulation profiles are normalized and the patient's platelet count is adequate. If there has been prior abdominal or pelvic surgery, past trauma to the lower abdomen, pelvic irradiation, and an empty bladder it is helpful to use ultrasound for bladder localization. Complications of suprapubic catheter placement include bowel injury,

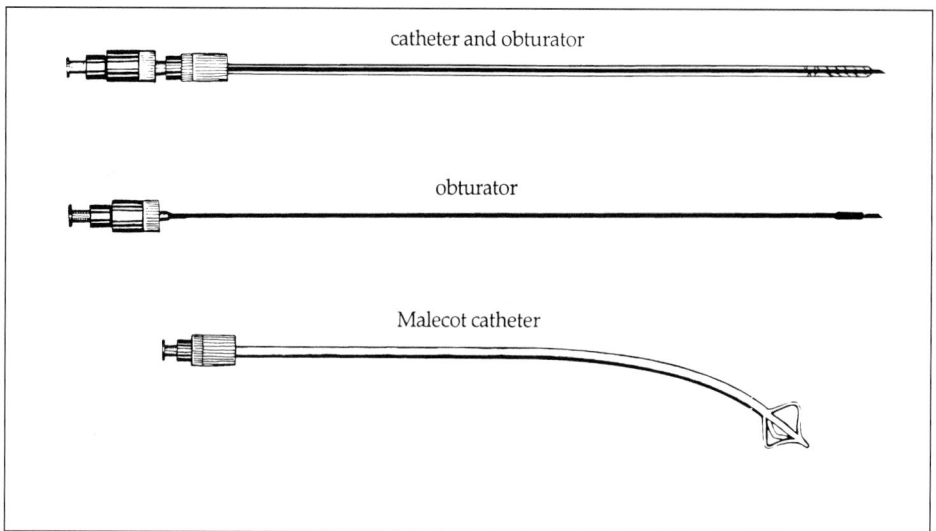

Figure 30-6   Stamey percutaneous cystotomy set with obturator and catheter. (From Carter HB: Basic instrumentation and cystoscopy. In Walsh PC, Retik AB, Vaughan D, Wein AJ, editors: *Campbell's Urology*, ed 8, Philadelphia: WB Saunders, 2002, pp 111–121.)

Box 30-2   Technique for Percutaneous Suprapubic Cystostomy Catheter

- Start the procedure with positioning and prepping the patient. The patient is placed in the supine position and the suprapubic area is percussed in order to confirm an adequately distended bladder. If the bladder is not distended the patient's bladder can be filled by injecting normal saline through the urethra until the bladder is filled. Using a catheter tip syringe gently close the distal urethra around the tip to prevent escape of the solution through the urethral meatus. Alternatively, if available an ultrasound can be used to localize the bladder. This is especially useful in patients who have had previous abdominal surgery or pelvic irradiation.
- The suprapubic area is shaved, prepped with povidone-iodine solution, and draped in a sterile fashion.
- The percutaneous tract and the surrounding area (2–3 cm above the superior margin of the pubic symphysis in the midline with a 2 cm radius) should be anesthetized with 1% lidocaine (**Figure 30-7**). Infiltration of local anesthetic should reach to the anterior rectus abdominus fascia.
- The catheter of choice (Bonanno or Stamey) is assembled
  - For the Bonanno catheter: the disposable catheter sleeve is advanced over the radiopaque catheter thereby straightening the J of the distal catheter. After the catheter is straightened the 18-gauge needle is inserted into the catheter. Once the bevel of the needle is seen extending from the end of the catheter, the disposable catheter sleeve is removed.
  - For the Stamey catheter: the needle obturator is guided into the catheter tip to stretch and straighten the self-retaining mechanism of the Malecot catheter. The catheter is then locked in place by turning the Luer lock thereby closing the Malecot wings.
- An 18–24-guage 5-inch spinal needle with a 10 ml syringe is then inserted perpendicular to the anesthetized skin and advanced while withdrawing on the syringe (see Figures 30-7 and 30-8). Correct placement is usually 4 cm above the pubic symphysis in the midline. The needle is usually directed using a 45–60° angle (**Figure 30-8**). Correct placement of the needle is confirmed by withdrawing urine into the syringe.
- Some people find it useful to leave the spinal needle in place as a guide.
- The catheter is then placed in the same tract or adjacent to the spinal needle if left in and is inserted into the bladder. The suprapubic catheter is then advanced until the bladder is punctured and urine will be seen emerging from the catheter. Once urine is brought forth, the catheter can be advanced another 1–2 cm.
- The next step involves the disengagement of the suprapubic catheter from the obturator and final advancement of the catheter into the bladder.
- For the Bonanno catheter: the needle is stabilized while the catheter is advanced over it. The catheter should be advanced until the suture disk lies flush with the skin.
- For the Stamey catheter: the catheter is stabilized and the white hub of the needle obturator is rotated counterclockwise opening the Malecot wings. The catheter is then fully advanced as with the Bonanno tube. The catheter is then slowly withdrawn until the Malecot wings meet resistance of the bladder wall.
- Aspirate as needed to confirm correct intraluminal placement (Figure 30-8). The catheter is then secured to the skin with permanent suture (2-0 silk or nylon suture can be used). The tube is then attached to the urinary drainage bag utilizing a gentle curve so that it is not kinked. Abdominal fixation in multiple sites may be necessary to avoid kinking.

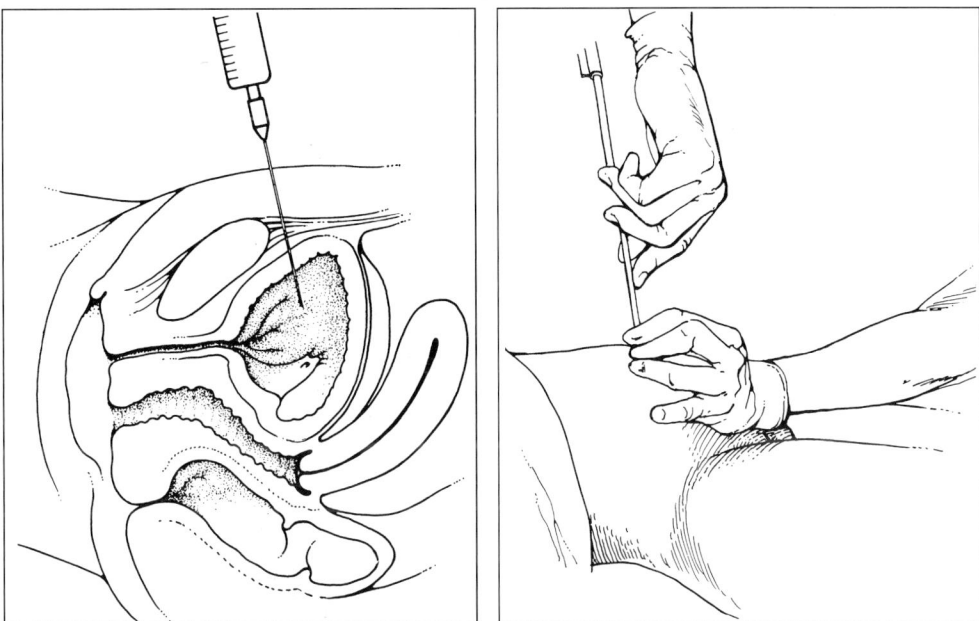

Figure 30-7   Localization of the bladder with a spinal needle placed percutaneously above the pubic bone (left). Placement of a percutaneous cystotomy catheter with obturator (right). (From Carter HB: Basic instrumentation and cystoscopy. In Walsh PC, Retik AB, Vaughan D, Wein AJ, editors: *Campbell's Urology*, ed 8, Philadelphia: WB Saunders, 2002, pp 111-121.)

transient hematuria, and leakage around the catheter site. Bowel injury is the most feared complication. If bowel is entered, one may exchange the needle and continue with the procedure. In order to minimize bowel injury, the bladder should be adequately distended with the patient placed in the Trendelenburg position thereby displacing any loops of bowel that encroach on the dome of the bladder. Ultrasound guidance is also helpful in preventing injury to the bowel. Transient hematuria is also common with suprapubic

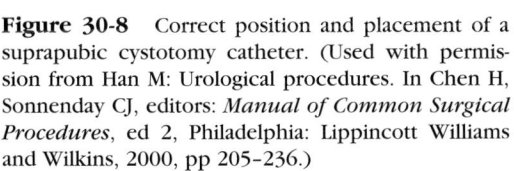

Figure 30-8   Correct position and placement of a suprapubic cystotomy catheter. (Used with permission from Han M: Urological procedures. In Chen H, Sonnenday CJ, editors: *Manual of Common Surgical Procedures*, ed 2, Philadelphia: Lippincott Williams and Wilkins, 2000, pp 205-236.)

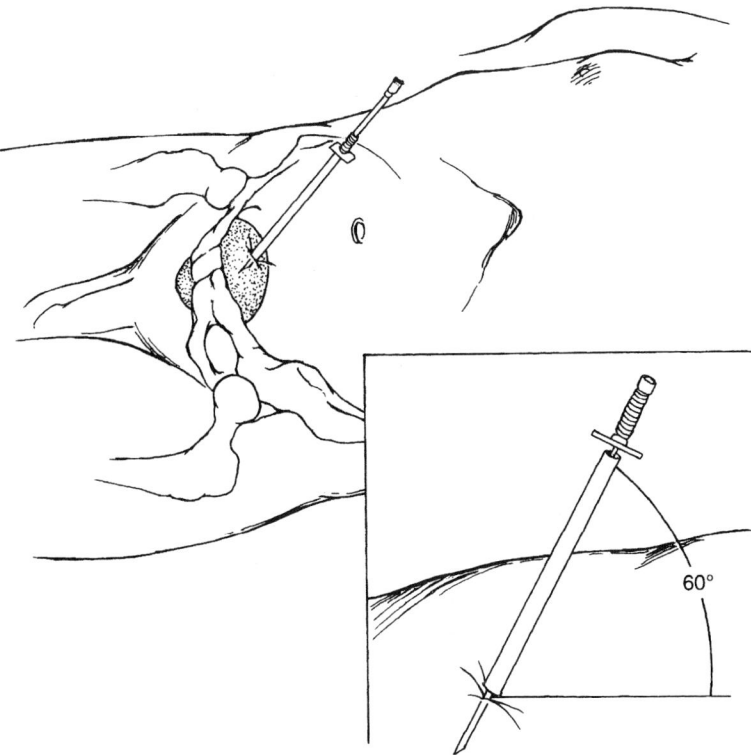

catheter placement. If the bladder is filled with clots there is a possibility for the smaller catheters to become obstructed. This can usually be relieved with gentle irrigation of the catheter with normal saline. Leakage around the catheter may indicate catheter damage or plugging, obstruction, bladder spasms, or that the tube has become partially dislodged where some holes are in the bladder and others are intramucosally located, or even outside the wall of the bladder. Administration of antimuscarinic agents such as oxybutynin or tolterodine can assist with reducing bladder spasms.

Percutaneous Nephrostomy Catheter

A percutaneous nephrostomy tube is an alternative method of gaining access to and diverting urine away from (or simply draining) the urinary system. Originally, percutaneous tube placement was considered to be a substitute for surgical nephrostomy in critically ill patients or as a temporizing measure prior to definitive surgery. With advancement of percutaneous experience and instruments and improved radiographic imaging, the clinical benefits of percutaneous access to the renal collecting system have been expanded (Table 30-3). Frequently in the ICU setting patients have postrenal failure and develop hydronephrosis secondary to supravesical ureteral obstruction. Moreover, patients in the ICU who have multiple medical comorbidities can develop supravesical obstruction with primary or superimposed renal infection, leading to urosepsis, which requires

Table 30-3	Indications and Applications of Percutaneous Nephrostomy Tube

Obstruction
  Pyonephrosis
  Acute and obstructive pyelonephritis
  Renal or ureteral calculi
  Fungus ball or sloughed papillae
  Renal abscess, urinoma, lymphocele
  Obstructing neoplasms
Diversion
  Urinomas
  Fistula and fibrosis
  Infection and abscesses
Functional assessment
  Oliguria and azotemia
  Renal salvage
Collecting system access
  Stricture dilation
  Culture, biopsy, and cytology
  Stent placement
  Calculus therapy
  Drug instillation
  Nephroscopy
  Intrarenal surgery

emergent percutaneous drainage. Under semi-urgent and elective tube placement the following contraindications for percutaneous nephrostomy tube placement exist: uncorrected coagulopathy, hyperkalemia (>7 mEq/l), urothelial neoplasms, and anatomical variations that may preclude the procedure. However, there are many times when urgent tube placement is performed in light of these relative contraindications as in the situation in which drainage may be necessary to reverse intravascular coagulopathy arising from urosepsis.

In most centers, percutaneous nephrostomy tube placement is performed in an interventional radiology suite. Patients must be hemodynamically stable enough to lie prone for roughly one hour. In ICU patients this often requires nursing and respiratory staff to accompany them for the procedure. Under conscious sedation, fluoroscopic or computed tomography (CT) guidance is used with the administration of intravenous contrast to visualize the opacified collecting system. Alternatively, ultrasound guidance can also be used in patients with contrast allergy, pregnant women, or patients with high-grade obstruction necessitating urgent decompression. Usually an 8 to 10 F catheter is placed for urgent decompression with larger tubes reserved for drainage of thick, purulent, or bloody material. The technique is performed by placing a needle or catheter-sheathed needle into the pelvicaliceal system via a translumbar approach (Figure 30-9). The needle should not go directly into the renal pelvis, but instead go first through the renal cortex, because the decompressed renal pelvis is often too flimsy in its own right to permit the somewhat firm tube in place. After radiographic (fluoroscopic) confirmation of needle placement is obtained, a J-shaped guide wire is then passed through the needle into the renal pelvis and the needle or sheath is pulled out, leaving the guide wire in place. The tract is then serially dilated with a 6 to 10 F Teflon fascial dilator and a pigtailed 8 F catheter is passed through the dilator into the renal pelvis. Because this provides direct access to the upper collecting system, urine for culture and/or cytology can be obtained simultaneously. The tube is then locked in place causing the tube to curl or pigtail in the renal pelvis, and is then sutured to the skin (Figure 30-10). Urinary drainage is ensured by the multiple side holes in the pigtail portion of the nephrostomy tube which resides within the renal pelvis.

Complications of nephrostomy tube placement include bleeding, worsening or development of urosepsis, pneumothorax or hemothorax, and bowel, vascular (e.g., inferior vena cava or major renal vessels), or visceral injury. If access to the necessary calyx is over the twelfth rib there is an increased chance of lung and splenic injury, pneumothorax, and hemothorax. As with all other surgical procedures any coagulopathy must be corrected and an adequate platelet count is needed prior to percutaneous tube placement.

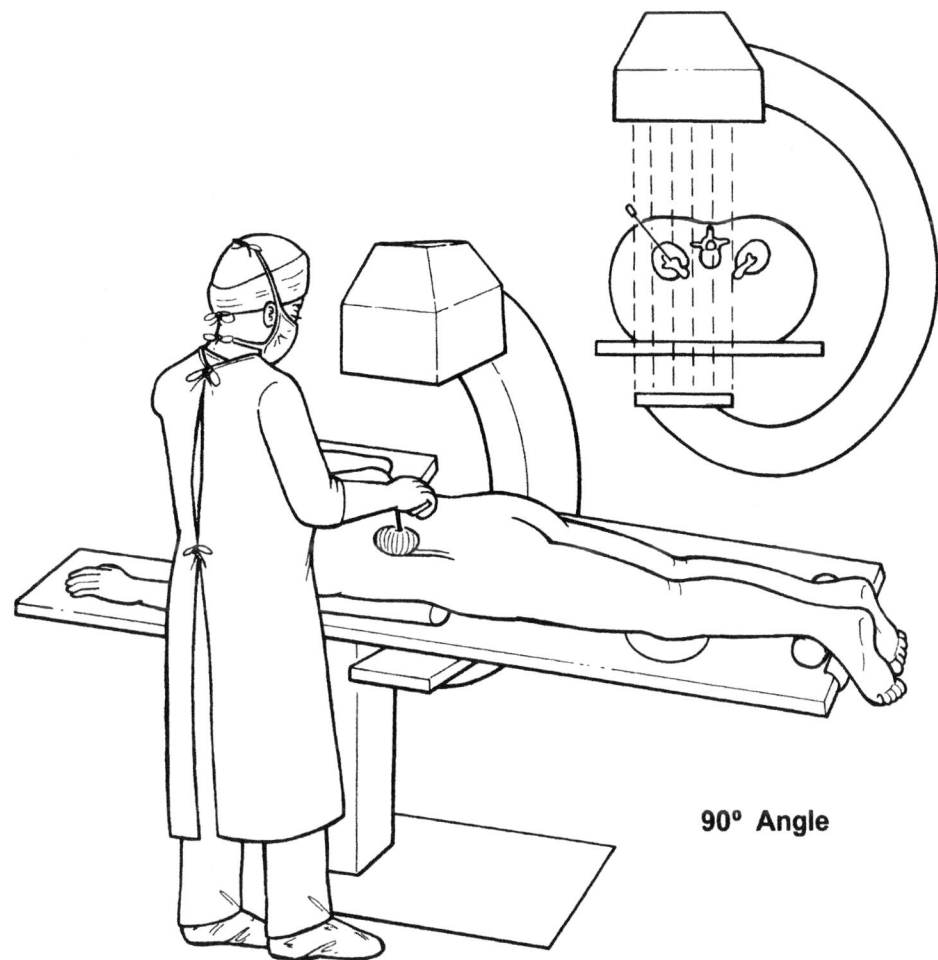

90° Angle

Figure 30-9   Typical patient position during percutaneous nephrotomy placement in an interventional radiology suite. (From McDougall EM, Liatsikos E, Dinlenc CZ, Smith AD: Percutaneous approaches to the upper urinary tract. In Walsh PC, Retik AB, Vaughan D, Wein AJ, editors: *Campbell's Urology*, ed 8, Philadelphia: WB Saunders, 2002, pp 3320–3360.)

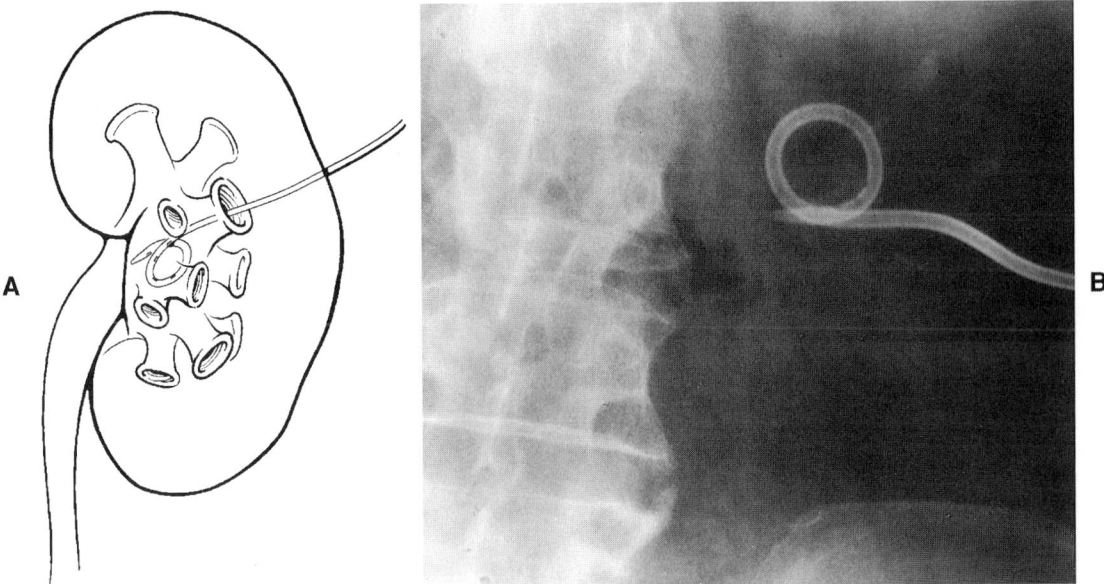

Figure 30-10   Self-retaining nephrostomy tube in place. A, Diagram of a standard self-retaining nephrostomy tube in place with the tip coiled in the renal pelvis. This catheter has a string that forces it to maintain its pigtail configuration. B, Radiograph demonstrating the typical radiographic appearance of a standard self-retaining percutaneous nephrostomy catheter. (From Zagoria RJ, Tung GA: Interventional genitourinary radiology. In Zagoria RJ, Tung GA, editors: *Genitourinary Radiology – The Requisites*, ed 1, St. Louis: Mosby-Year Book, 1997, pp 371–399.)

MANAGEMENT OF UPPER URINARY TRACT OBSTRUCTION

Bacteremia and sepsis from urologic origin in patients in the ICU may occur in a variety of settings. Therefore, appropriate imaging is essential when excluding urinary obstruction and intrarenal or perinephric abscesses as the cause. Subsequently if a source is found, prompt elimination is critical for full recovery of the septic episode.

Lower urinary tract obstruction, as may occur in patients with complicated urinary tract infections and/or bladder outlet obstruction, can usually be relieved with successful placement of a Foley urethral catheter (either by direct urethral catheterization or by flexible cysto-urethroscopy; see above) or by percutaneous suprapubic cystotomy catheter. In the setting of upper urinary tract obstruction and sepsis it is critical to decompress urgently the upper urinary tract and relieve the obstruction. Upper urinary tract obstruction is usually diagnosed by an elevation in serum creatinine and with subsequent imaging (usually ultrasound or CT scan) revealing hydronephrosis with a possible etiology such as an obstructing calculus or extrinsic compression of the ureter. Table 30-4 lists common causes of upper tract obstruction in patients in the ICU.

Obstructive pyelonephritis is a true urologic emergency that warrants immediate decompression of the collecting system to prevent life-threatening sepsis. If the obstructed collecting system is not decompressed, the process can progress to pyonephrosis which carries a high risk of renal scarring and mortality. Other indications for upper tract drainage include prevention or treatment of urinary extravasation, management of urinary tract fistulae and perforation, extrinsic compression from nonurinary malignancies (e.g., ovarian, cervical, colonic, lymphomatous, pancreatic, and gastric cancers), and relief of intractable pain. In addition, there are certain urologic pathologies that can cause rapidly progressive bacteremia and life-threatening sepsis if they are not expeditiously managed. Emphysematous pyelonephritis, which is commonly caused by aerobic and facultative anaerobic coliform microorganisms, causes life-threatening sepsis in poorly controlled diabetics. Acute papillary necrosis, also routinely seen in the diabetic among other populations, can cause significant upper tract obstruction as the papillae slough off and occlude the renal pelvis and ureter. It is critical to remember that the absence of pyuria or bacteriuria in bladder urine does not entirely exclude upper tract obstruction as complete obstruction may render the urine in the bladder free from bacteria or white blood cells.

In the setting of upper urinary tract obstruction, effective and emergent urinary drainage can be accomplished by either percutaneous nephrostomy or retrograde ureteral stent placement. The selection of nephrostomy tube placement versus ureteral stent placement depends on various factors including rapidity of access and availability to a cystoscopy or interventional radiology suite, expertise available, availability of anesthesia, or the presence of a coagulopathic state which may preclude the procedure from occurring. Both are widely used and accepted methods for decompression of the upper urinary tract. Although urinary drainage and decompression is of paramount importance, the question that remains is – Are all types of drainage equal? The optimal choice (assuming both procedures are readily available) for upper tract drainage is controversial. Proponents of percutaneous drainage claim that placement of large-caliber tubes during percutaneous nephrostomy allows for better drainage of the thick and viscous purulent fluid. These larger-caliber tubes (12 to 14 F tubes as compared to 6 to 8 F internal ureteral stents) are less likely to become occluded by the viscous material and subsequently will allow for a rapid resolution of the infection. Another advantage of percutaneous nephrostomy tube placement includes the ability to assess accurately and monitor the drainage from the affected kidney. By close monitoring of the affected kidney, the adequacy of drainage and recovery can be assessed. Alternatively, because most ureteral stents are internalized, an accurate assessment of drainage from the pathologic kidney is not possible. Furthermore, the development of pyonephrosis usually occurs secondary to ureteral obstruction. Therefore, ureteral stenting is often difficult or impossible. Attempted passage of a ureteral stent through an obstructed ureter increases the risk of worsening sepsis and/or ureteral perforation. Finally, placement of a percutaneous tube allows for the possibility for a delayed nephrostogram with identification of the site of obstruction thereby facilitating planning of definitive treatment. Advocates for ureteral stenting argue the greater comfort and decreased morbidity of an internal tube, thereby reducing the need for urgent definitive management. In addition, placement of the ureteral stent usually is faster and requires less radiation

Table 30-4	Causes of Upper Urinary Tract Obstruction

Obstructive pyelonephritis and pyonephrosis
Impacted proximal ureteral stone or staghorn calculi
Ureteral stricture or fistula
Lower urinary tract obstruction
Emphysematous pyelonephritis
Acute papillary necrosis
Intrinsic obstruction by ureteral or renal pelvis carcinoma
Extrinsic compression of the ureter
  Neoplastic processes (usually nongenitourinary malignancy)
  Retroperitoneal hematoma

than nephrostomy tube placement. Moreover, they cite the decreased risk of major complications such as hemorrhage, pneumothorax, and visceral injury that exists with percutaneous nephrostomy tube placement. Table 30-5 reviews the advantages and disadvantages of ureteral stent versus percutaneous nephrostomy for drainage of an obstructed upper urinary tract.

As seen from Table 30-5, the choice for drainage is controversial since each procedure has significant advantages and disadvantages. Despite strong arguments on both sides of the controversy, only two prospective, randomized studies have directly compared the efficacy of both drainage procedures for decompression of an obstructed, infected urinary system. The first trial was performed by Pearle and colleagues, who randomized 42 patients presenting with acute urinary tract obstruction with signs and symptoms of infection due to ureteral calculi to either percutaneous nephrostomy placement or cystoscopic ureteral stent placement. There was one treatment failure in the percutaneous nephrostomy arm, which was salvaged by ureteral stent placement. Neither treatment modality demonstrated superiority in promoting a more rapid recovery from acute obstruction after drainage. The two treatment arms were comparable with regard to time to clinical improvement including normalization of temperature, time to normal white blood cell count, and length of hospital stay. Procedure and fluoroscopic time were significantly shorter in the stent group, while cost analysis demonstrated an advantage to the percutaneous nephrostomy group, which was half as costly as stent placement. As expected, this was largely due to the higher costs of anesthesia, the operating room, and its staff. Patient satisfaction was also evaluated using a visual analog pain scale. Flank pain was noted to be greater in the nephrostomy tube arm with the need for a significantly increased amount of parenteral narcotics. This result was probably confounded by the general anesthesia and pain medication received in the operating room in the stent group. Finally, there was no significant difference between the duration of pain medication needed after the procedure between the two groups. The authors concluded that the choice of drainage can be individualized according to the patients and institutional characteristics.

The second study was performed by Mokhmalji and associates who randomized 40 patients with stone-induced hydronephrosis to either percutaneous nephrostomy tube or ureteral stent placement. Unlike the Pearle study, only 65% of the patients had signs and symptoms of infection. The rest of the patients had a procedure done for other reasons including persistent renal colic, elevated creatinine, and the presence of large obstructing calculi. In this study all patients in the nephrostomy group had successful nephrostomy tube placement, while only 80% of the stent patients randomized to stent placement were able to be successfully stented. Percutaneous tube placement was associated with a significant decrease in indwelling tube drainage time, with over

Table 30-5	Advantages and Disadvantages of Ureteral Stent versus Percutaneous Nephrostomy Tube Placement for Upper Urinary Tract Decompression	
Procedure	**Advantages**	**Disadvantages**
Percutaneous nephrostomy	Large-caliber tubes (with no size limitation) for external drainage External access allows for accurate measurement of drain output Access to the catheter allows for irrigation and possible management of clotted off tubes Can be performed with local anesthesia or IV sedation Avoids manipulation of the ureter and possibility for worsening sepsis No irritative bladder symptoms Possibility for access to the nephrostomy tract for subsequent definitive treatment	Morbidity of an external drain Need for mandatory care of an external tube Risk of hemorrhage Risk of pneumothorax Greater risk for injury to the surrounding organs Radiologist-driven Impossibility to perform this procedure in a coagulopathic patient
Ureteral stent	No external collection device Low risk of injury Can be performed in coagulopathic state Less urgency to perform a definitive procedure	Irritative voiding symptoms Incontinence or reflux Suprapubic and/or flank pain High failure rate for extrinsic compression Unable to monitor urinary drainage from affected kidney No way to manually unobstruct the stent Can require the possibility to manipulate an obstructed ureter causing bacteremia and sepsis Ureteral erosion or fistulization High chance for stent encrustation

half of the stented patients and only 20% of the nephrostomy patients requiring an indwelling tube for 4 weeks. In addition, the duration of antibiotic use was longer in the stented group, although the difference did not reach statistical significance. Unlike the Pearle study, a trend for a reduction in the quality of life was seen in the patients with stents compared to those who underwent percutaneous nephrotomy tube placement. This was most pronounced for male patients and patients younger than 40 years of age. Other trends seen were a shorter x-ray exposure time and decreased analgesic use in the percutaneous nephrostomy tube arm. Based on the findings that the nephrostomy tube arm had a shorter indwelling tube time and antibiotic usage as well as a marginally higher quality of life score, the authors concluded that percutaneous nephrostomy tube placement was favored over cystoscopic stent placement for drainage of an obstructed upper tract.

In our opinion, the optimal choice for drainage of an obstructed, infected upper urinary tract remains a matter of controversy, as the current prospective trials fail to show a clear-cut advantage of either procedure. Currently, the choice for which procedure we use depends on multiple factors including patient preference, availability of a skilled endoscopist or interventional radiologist, patient clinical parameters (which may preclude anesthesia), and availability of an operating room. Larger prospective, randomized trials with adequate patient numbers and ability to perform subgroup analyses are awaited.

NONOPERATIVE MANAGEMENT OF GENITOURINARY TRAUMA

Although recent developments of trauma systems and centers have contributed to the declining rates of mortality from major traumatic injuries, the best care provided to a patient with polytrauma comes from the organized team of specialists including members of the trauma ICU. As trauma to the genitourinary tract occurs in 10% of all serious traumatic injuries the urologist is a critical member of this team. In the majority of cases traumatic injury to the genitourinary tract when encountered in an ICU setting will be managed nonoperatively. The following sections discuss the nonoperative management of renal, bladder, and urethral injury. Injuries to the ureter, testicles, and penis are not included as in the majority of cases they are operatively managed.

Renal

Out of all injuries to the genitourinary tract, renal injuries are the most common. It has been estimated that renal trauma occurs in 1–3% of all trauma patients and

up to 5% in patients with abdominal trauma. Renal injury management has evolved over time as a result of the increased use of CT scans in the trauma setting. This has allowed for better radiologic staging of renal trauma thereby permitting the vast majority of these injuries to be managed nonoperatively. Nonetheless, certain injuries will require surgical management. Overall, the main objective in dealing with patients with renal trauma is to prevent significant hemorrhage while retaining as much kidney function as possible in order to avoid end-stage renal failure.

The approach to any patient with renal trauma involves assessing whether the cause of the injury is due to penetrating or blunt trauma. This is extremely important, as the management of the injury will be quite different. Ninety percent of real injuries occur from blunt trauma including falling from heights, motor vehicle accidents, and violent assaults. Most renal injuries occurring from blunt trauma are minor and rarely, if ever, require surgical intervention. Alternatively, penetrating trauma, which compromises 10% of patients with renal trauma, requires surgical exploration unless there is definitive clinical and radiographic evidence establishing the extent of injury. In one study of a level III trauma center, only 2% of renal injuries resulting from blunt trauma required surgical intervention. Therefore, nonoperative management of renal trauma has been espoused by multiple level III trauma centers that have significant experience managing kidney injuries.

Physical Examination

Initial work-up of renal trauma follows the same assessment and resuscitation algorithms as established by the American College of Surgeons Trauma Life Support program (ATLS). After assessing for adequate airway, breathing, circulation, disability, and exposure, as outlined by the well-known mnemonic "ABCs of trauma," a more detailed physical examination to assess for renal trauma can be performed. External evaluation of the abdomen, back, and chest should be performed as abdominal and flank tenderness, contusions and abdominal and flank ecchymosis, lower rib fractures, and penetrating wounds of the upper abdomen, flank, and lower thorax have all been associated with renal trauma. A palpable flank mass should cause the evaluating examiner to suspect retroperitoneal and renal injury.

Urinalysis should be quickly performed in patients suspected of having renal injury. Hematuria (macro- and microscopic) is the most common sign of penetrating and blunt renal trauma. It has been estimated that dipstick urinalysis can detect the presence or absence of hematuria in over 97% of cases. A key point to remember is that the presence and amount of hematuria does not correlate with the degree of renal trauma. Moreover, the absence of hematuria does not preclude renal injury as its absence has been reported in 25–36% of patients with thrombosis of the renal artery and in 33% of patients with ureteropelvic junction injury. If urine is microscopically analyzed the presence of greater than 5 red blood cells per high-powered field indicates the possibility for renal trauma. The presence of hematuria in patients presenting to a trauma center usually signifies a significant renal injury with estimated rates of grade IV and V injuries around 25%.

Imaging and Radiographic Staging

Patients that have hematuria and are stable enough to undergo imaging can safely be staged with a radiographic procedure. The different imaging modalities that have been used to assess the extent of renal injury include contrast-enhanced CT scan, intravenous pyelography, angiography, retrograde pyelography, ultrasonography, radionuclide scintigraphy, and magnetic resonance imaging (MRI). With the advance of CT scanners, CT scan is the procedure of choice to detect renal injury in the trauma setting. CT scans are noninvasive, readily available in most trauma centers, and can rapidly and accurately detect the severity and depth of renal injuries, the presence of urinary extravasation and perirenal hemorrhage, and determine the status of the renal vascular pedicle. Furthermore, they provide information about the contralateral kidney and the extent of devitalized renal parenchyma, and the state of neighboring viscera which are important factors needed when a management plan is being formulated. Thus, CT scans have replaced intravenous pyelography as the primary modality for the assessment of renal injuries. Indications for radiographic imaging in patients with abdominal trauma include:

- All patients with penetrating injuries to the flank, abdomen, and lower back
- Blunt trauma associated with gross hematuria
- Microscopic hematuria with and without shock or a positive diagnostic peritoneal lavage

The advances of current CT scanners have contributed to the highly accurate organ injury grading scale of renal injuries developed by the American Association for Surgery of Trauma (AAST). The scale classifies renal injuries into five grades which correlate with patient outcome and permit selective management to be undertaken (Figure 30-11). Moreover, the scale has been prospectively validated and found to correlate directly with the need for surgical intervention. Table 30-6 reviews the renal injury scale. Overall, grade I injuries are subcapsular

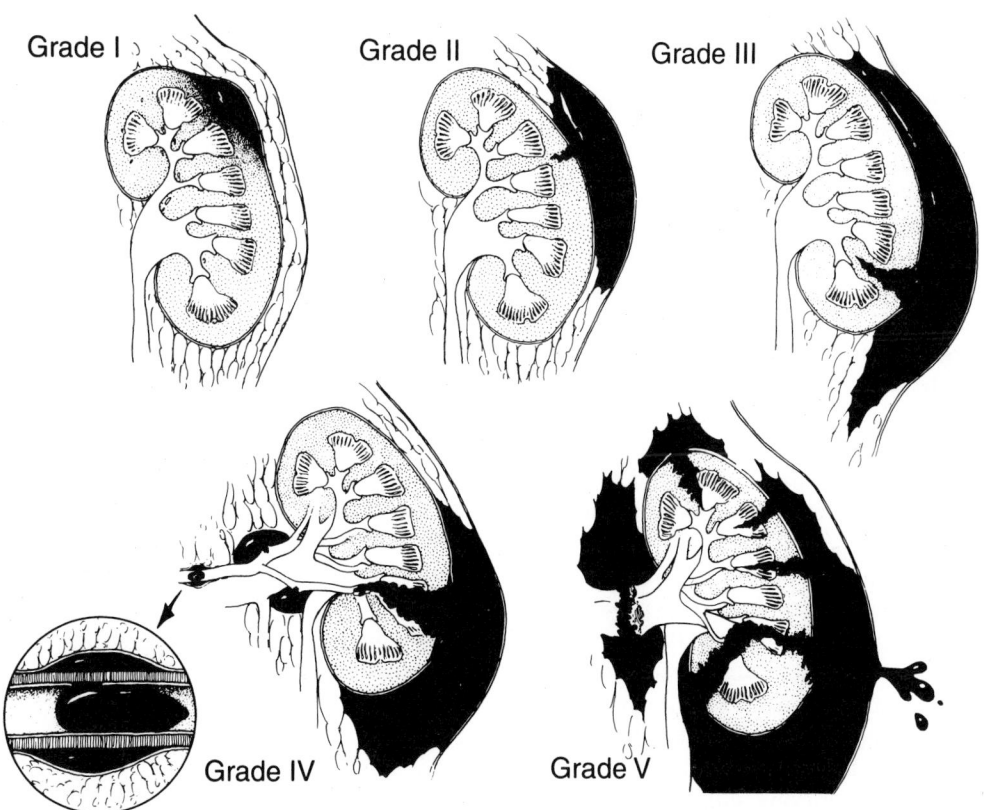

Figure 30-11   Classification of renal injuries by grade based on the organ injury scale of the American Association for the Surgery of Trauma. (From McAninch JW, Santucci RA: Genitourinary trauma. In Walsh PC, Retik AB, Vaughan D, Wein AJ, editors: *Campbell's Urology*, ed 8, Philadelphia: WB Saunders, 2002, pp 3707–3744.)

Grade	Injury Description
I	**Contusion:** Microscopic or gross hematuria with normal findings of imaging studies
	Hematoma: Subcapsular, nonexpanding hematoma without parenchymal laceration
II	**Hematoma:** Nonexpanding perirenal hematoma confined to renal retroperitoneum
	Laceration: Cortical (superficial) laceration <1 cm parenchymal depth of renal cortex without extension into the collecting system
III	**Laceration:** Deep, >1 cm parenchymal depth of renal cortex without extension into the collecting system or urinary extravasation
IV	**Laceration:** Laceration extending through the renal cortex, medulla, and collecting system with or without a devascularized segment
	Vascular: Main or segmental renal artery or vein injury and/or thrombosis with contained hemorrhage
V	**Laceration:** Completed shattered kidney
	Vascular: Avulsion of the renal hilum and pedicle

Table 30-6 Renal Injury Scale of the American Association for Surgery of Trauma

hematomas and renal contusions, while grade II injuries are small parenchymal lacerations into the renal cortex. Grade III injuries are parenchymal lacerations that extend through the corticomedullary junction, and grade IV injuries are those that involve the collecting system and/or vascular injuries with contained hemorrhage. Grade V injuries are completed shattered kidneys and pedicle avulsions of the great vessels.

Nonoperative Management

Fortunately, the vast majority of renal injuries are contusions or minor lacerations which are now adequately staged with the increased use of CT scanners in the trauma setting. Significant injuries (grades II–V) have been estimated to occur in only 5.4% of renal trauma cases. Most trauma surgeons and urologists would agree that grades I and II renal trauma are managed nonoperatively and only require conservative management. Extensive perirenal and large subcapsular hematomas rarely require surgery. These hematomas become organized and eventually reabsorb in a 2–3 month period. Periodic CT scan with frequent creatinine evaluations on an outpatient basis can ensure the hematoma is resolving with no damage occurring to the affected kidney. With appropriate and radiologically confirmed staging of grades III–V renal trauma there is controversy as to what is the most appropriate method of management. The only absolute indication for surgical exploration is massive life-threatening hemorrhage from a macerated and severely injured kidney (grade V renal trauma). Consequently, there are multiple reports from many trauma centers that show appropriately staged blunt and penetrating renal injuries can undergo selective nonoperative management, including major lacerations and some collecting system injuries.

The nonoperative course of a ruptured (grade III or IV) kidney requires strict hemodynamic monitoring and diligent follow-up with routine hematocrit or hemoglobin checks (e.g., hemoglobin checks every 6 hours for 48 hours while vital signs are stable, which can then be tapered to every 12 hours and then once a day) and a repeat CT scan 3–7 days after the injury to evaluate for size of the hematoma, urinary extravasation, and perfusion of the kidney laceration or fragment. It is also critical to obtain delayed images in order to ensure that the contrast can be seen flowing through the renal pelvis and down the ureter. Between 3 and 7 days after the original insult, marginally perfused kidney lacerations and fragments that can recover will appear as recovering while devitalized tissue will become more apparent. Furthermore, minor urinary extravasation will disappear by this time, while larger leaks will become more readily identified. These can be controlled either by percutaneous nephrostomy tube placement or internal ureteral stent placement. It is also important to realize that expectant management does not invariably lead to nonsurgical management and active monitoring can indicate when conservative management has failed. Therefore the urologist should be actively involved with the ICU team in the patient's progress and the possibility for surgical intervention. Indications for deferred open surgical treatment are recurring or persisting related bleeding particularly with hemodynamic instability despite adequate fluid resuscitation, and secondarily infected hematomas that have to be evacuated and surgically drained. A summary algorithm for initial nonoperative management of renal trauma is shown in Figure 30-12.

Bladder

Bladder injuries in trauma patients usually occur from a blow to the abdomen when the bladder is distended (mostly from motor vehicle accidents, crushing injuries, falls, or violent blows to the lower abdomen) or in

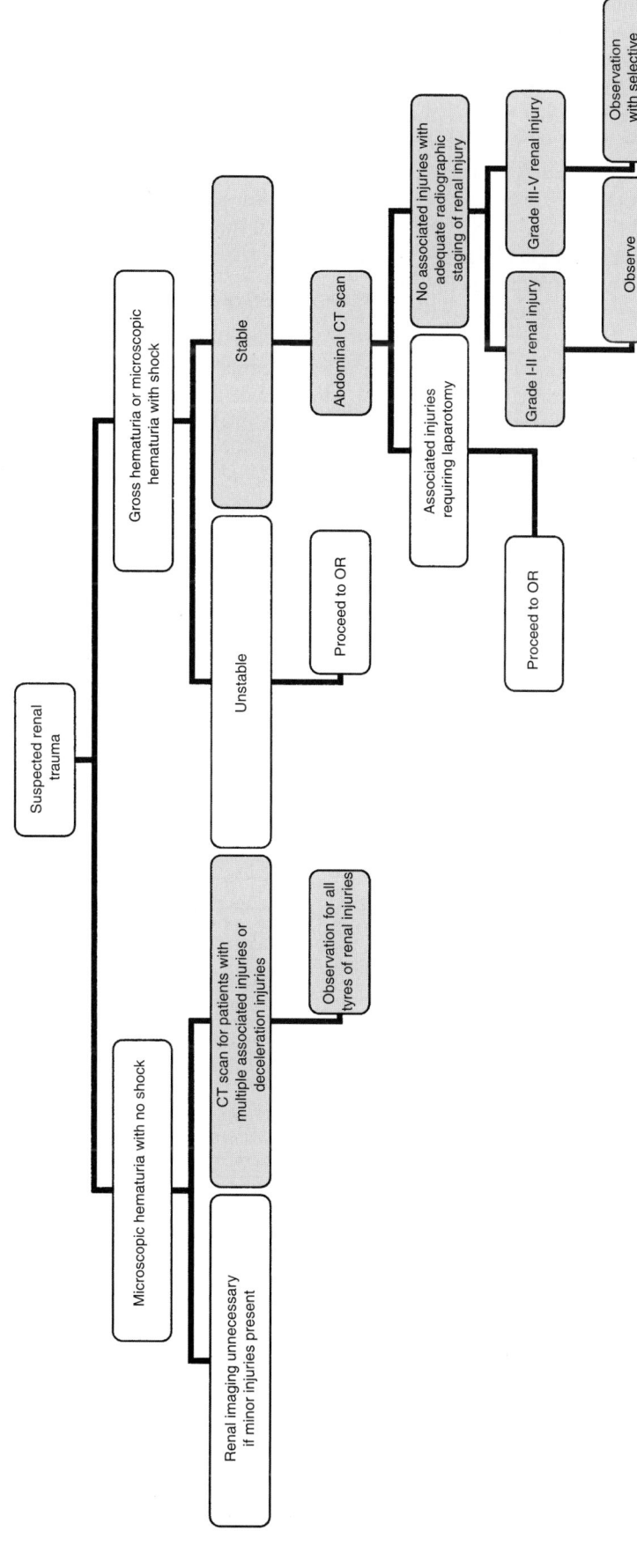

Figure 30-12 Decision-making algorithm for adult patients with renal injuries.

combination with pelvic fractures. In these cases the normal protective barrier of the pelvic ring is lost and the shearing forces of the injury may tear the bladder from its attachments. It has been estimated that in greater than 80% of patients with bladder injuries there is an associated pelvic fracture. Although rare, penetrating and blast injuries can injure the bladder during gunshot wounds to the lower abdomen.

Physical Examination and Radiologic Imaging

Gross hematuria (95%) is the hallmark finding in bladder injury. In addition the patient may also complain of suprapubic tenderness. If there is a concomitant urethral injury (see below) there may be blood at the urethral meatus or a history of an inability to urinate. Definitive diagnosis of a bladder laceration can be obtained by conventional cystography or CT cystography. Conventional cystography uses conventional x-rays or fluoroscopy, while CT cystography can be performed during the abdominal and pelvic CT scan performed for evaluation of other organ injuries. We routinely perform CT cystography in our center as it is quick and does not need an additional trip to the radiology suite after CT scans are obtained for nonurologic reasons. It is important to remember that the bladder needs to be distended adequately in order to show bladder leakage; an inadequately distended bladder can cause a false negative result. The procedure is usually done by using retrograde filling of the bladder with a minimum of 350 cm³ of diluted contrast (5%) and axial images are obtained through the pelvis. If urethral injury is suspected a retrograde urethrogram should first be performed to rule out urethral damage. It is crucial that even with CT scans, images also be obtained after the bladder is completely drained to make sure that no extravesical pooling of contrast is identified. With conventional cystography, oblique and lateral images during filling and after drainage are also mandatory. The adequacy of cystography for the diagnosis of traumatic bladder injury has varied in different studies from 85 to 100%. To achieve a high degree of accuracy careful attention to proper technique must be performed. Radiologically, bladder injuries can be classified as being extra- or intraperitoneal depending if the rupture is in the peritoneum or not. Intraperitoneal ruptures account for one-third of major bladder injuries, while two-thirds are extraperitoneal or combined.

Nonoperative Management

Extraperitoneal bladder ruptures are the most frequent type of bladder injury and can usually be conservatively managed by urinary catheter drainage. These injuries are usually handled by placing a Foley catheter (see Box 30-1 and Figures 30-1–30-3) for 10–21 days allowing the bladder to heal. Afterwards a cystogram is performed in order to ensure that any leakage has ceased

and the bladder is well healed. If the bleeding does not clear during this three-week time period or if multiple clots are formed not allowing for adequate urinary drainage, conservative management should be aborted and surgical correction undertaken. In general, all intraperitoneal and penetrating wounds to the bladder need to undergo prompt surgical correction. A summary algorithm for nonoperative management of bladder and urethral trauma is shown in Figure 30-13.

Urethra

Traumatic injuries to the urethra resulting from external trauma are the most devastating and debilitating injuries of the lower urinary tract. The potential complications of urethral trauma are associated with considerable long-term morbidity including incontinence, impotence, strictures, and fistula formation. The reported incidence of urethral injury with pelvic fracture in the world literature ranges from 1.6 to 25% (mean 10%)

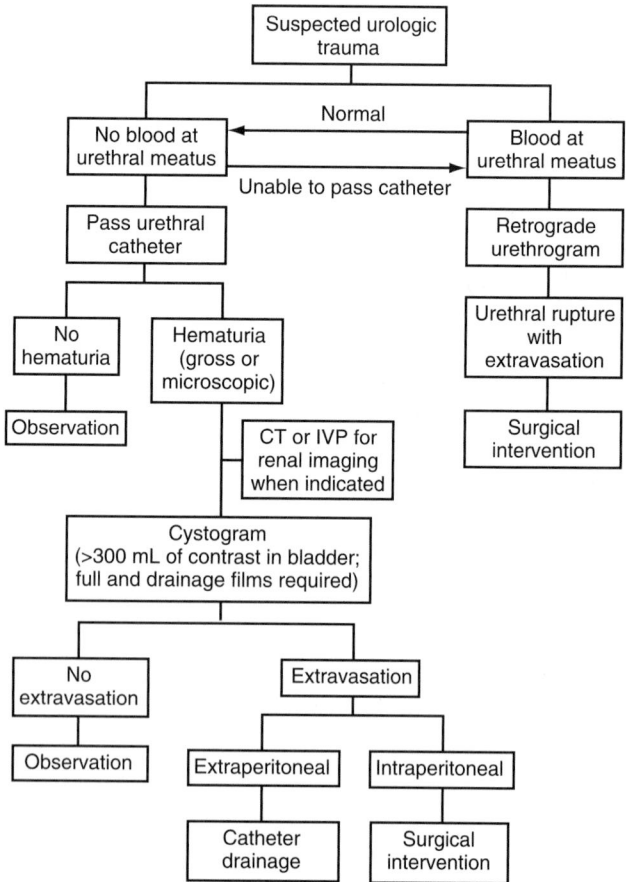

Figure 30-13 Decision-making algorithm for patients with pelvic fracture and suspected bladder or urethral injury, or both. (From McAninch JW, Santucci RA: Genitourinary trauma. In Walsh PC, Retik AB, Vaughan D, Wein AJ, editors: *Campbell's Urology*, ed 8, Philadelphia: WB Saunders, 2002, pp 3707–3744.)

with 66% of them being complete posterior urethral ruptures. The primary aim in the management of posterior urethral disruption is the re-establishment of a continuous urinary tract while minimizing the incidence of long-term complications. Double vertical fractures, fractures and dislocations involving the pubic symphysis, and Malgaigne's fractures (fracture through the ipsilateral ischiopubic rami or pubic symphysis and usually associated with massive posterior disruption through the sacrum or ilium) are among the fractures associated with highest incidence of urethral trauma.

Physical Examination and Radiologic Imaging

Clinically, urethral disruption is suspected by the triad of blood at the urethral meatus, inability to urinate with a palpable full bladder, and a high-riding prostate on digital rectal examination. When blood at the meatus is discovered or these clinical symptoms suggest urethral disruption it is mandatory to perform a retrograde urethrogram to rule out urethral disruption. If the contrast does not leak and makes its way into the bladder in a retrograde manner without evidence of extravasation, a urethral catheter can be placed. If urethral disruption is suspected, a urethral catheter is not inserted to avoid converting a partial rupture into a complete one and a suprapubic cystotomy catheter is placed as mentioned above (Box 30-2 and Figures 30-6–30-8).

Nonoperative Management

The treatment of traumatic urethral disruptions is controversial and still remains unresolved, mainly due to the complications that may arise during the initial treatment. Some urologists advocate primary urethral alignment while others favor initial suprapubic cystotomy and delayed urethroplasty. The various series reported in the literature along with recent advances in endoscopic and radiologic procedures has fueled the controversy even further. Currently, the most widely accepted approach in the management of posterior urethral disruption, and the approach we use in our center, is delayed repair in order to re-establish urethral continuity under controlled circumstances. A suprapubic cystotomy tube is quickly placed in the trauma bay and the injury conservatively managed. After three months the patient is re-evaluated and scheduled for delayed urethroplasty. A summary algorithm for nonoperative management of bladder and urethral trauma is shown in Figure 30-13.

CLINICAL CAVEAT

Nonoperative Management of Genitourinary Trauma

- Fortunately, the vast majority of renal injuries are contusions or minor lacerations which are now adequately staged with the increased use of CT scanners in the trauma setting.
- Most renal injuries are conservatively managed with serial hemoglobin or hematocrit checks and delayed reimaging.
- Extraperitoneal bladder ruptures are the most frequent type of bladder injury and can be conservatively managed by urinary catheter drainage for 10–21 days. Afterwards a cystogram is performed in order to ensure that any leakage has ceased and the bladder is well healed.
- Traumatic injuries to the urethra resulting from external trauma are the most devastating and debilitating injuries of the lower urinary tract.
- Clinically, urethral disruption is suspected by the triad of blood at the urethral meatus, inability to urinate with a palpable full bladder, and a high-riding prostate.
- Currently, the most widely accepted approach in the management of posterior urethral disruption is initial immediate placement of suprapubic catheter and delayed repair in order to re-establish urethral continuity under controlled circumstances.

SELECTED READING

Altman AL, Haas C, Dinchman KH, Spirnak JP: Selective nonoperative management of blunt grade 5 renal injury. J Urol 164(1):27–31, 2000.

Chandhoke PS, McAninch JW: Detection and significance of microscopic hematuria in patients with blunt renal trauma. J Urol 140(1):16–18, 1988.

Corriere JN Jr: Extraperitoneal bladder rupture. In McAninch JW, editor: *Trauma and Reconstructive Urology*, ed 1, Philadelphia: WB Saunders, 1996, pp. 269–274.

Corriere JN Jr, Sandler CM: Bladder rupture from external trauma: diagnosis and management. World J Urol 17(2):84–89, 1999.

Follis HW, Koch MO, McDougal WS: Immediate management of prostatomembranous urethral disruptions. J Urol 147:1259, 1992.

Frontera R: Intraperitoneal bladder rupture. In McAninch JW, editor: *Trauma and Reconstructive Urology*, ed 1, Philadelphia: WB Saunders, 1996, pp. 275–286.

Harris AC, Zwirewich CV, Lyburn ID, Torreggiani WC, Marchinkow LO: CT findings in blunt renal trauma. Radiographics 21:S201–214, 2001.

Husmann DA: Diagnostic techniques in suspected bladder injury. In McAninch JW, editor: *Trauma and Reconstructive Urology*, ed 1, Philadelphia: WB Saunders, 1996, pp. 261–267.

Kawashima A, Sandler CM, Corl FM et al: Imaging of renal trauma: a comprehensive review. Radiographics 21(3):557–574, 2001.

Koraitim MM: Pelvic fracture urethral injuries: the unresolved controversy. J Urol 161:1433, 1999.

Matthews LA, Smith EM, Spirnak JP: Nonoperative treatment of major blunt renal lacerations with urinary extravasation. J Urol 157(6):2056-2058, 1997.

McAninch JW, Santucci RA: Genitourinary trauma. In Walsh PC, Retik AB, Vaughan D, Wein AJ, editors: *Campbell's Urology*, ed 8, Philadelphia: WB Saunders, 2002, pp 3707-3744.

Mokhmalji H, Braun PM, Martinez Portillo FJ et al: Percutaneous nephrostomy versus ureteral stents for diversion of hydronephrosis caused by stones: a prospective, randomized clinical trial. J Urol 165(4):1088-1092, 2001.

Moore EE, Shackford SR, Pachter HL et al: Organ injury scaling: spleen, liver, and kidney. J Trauma 29(12):1664-1666, 1989.

Morehouse DD, Mackinnin KJ: Management of prostatomembranous urethral disruption: 13-year experience. J Urol 123:173, 1980.

Mundy AR: Pelvic fracture injuries of the posterior urethra. World J Urol 17:90, 1999.

Palmer JK, Benson GS, Corriere JN Jr: Diagnosis and initial management of urological injuries associated with 200 consecutive pelvic fractures. J Urol 130:712, 1983.

Pearle MS, Pierce HL, Miller GL et al: Optimal method of urgent decompression of the collecting system for obstruction and infection due to ureteral calculi. J Urol 160(4):1260-1264, 1998.

Podestá ML, Medel R, Castera R, Ruarte A: Immediate management of posterior urethral disruptions due to pelvic fracture: therapeutic alternatives. J Urol 157:1444, 1997.

Rosenstein D, McAninch JW: Update on the management of renal trauma. Contemp Urol 15(7):42-53, 2003.

Sandler CM, Goldman SM, Kawashima A: Lower urinary tract trauma. World J Urol 16:69, 1998.

Webster G, Mathes G, Selli C: Prostatomembranous urethral injuries: a review of the literature and a rational approach to their management. J Urol 130:899, 1983.

Wessells H, McAninch JW, Meyer A, Bruce J: Criteria for nonoperative treatment of significant penetrating renal lacerations. J Urol 157(1):24-27, 1997.

Wessells H, Suh D, Porter JR et al: Renal injury and operative management in the United States: results of a population-based study. J Trauma 54(3):423-430, 2003.

TRAUMA AND ETHICS

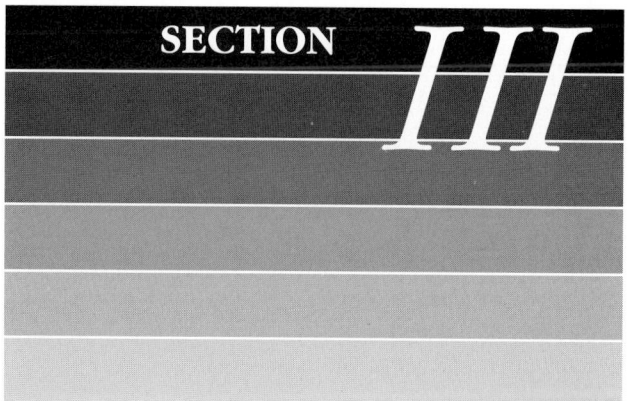

CHAPTER 31

Trauma: The Golden Hour, Principles of Assessment, and Resuscitation

MARC J. SHAPIRO, M.D., F.A.C.S., F.C.C.M.

The field of trauma, or injury, is continuously evolving as knowledge is gained into therapeutic management. Currently trauma is the leading cause of death in the USA of individuals under 44 years of age and the fourth leading cause of death overall. Of the approximately 60 million injuries annually occurring in the USA, half, or 30 million, require some form of medical care. About 12% of these injured patients, or 3.6 million, require hospitalization, with many of these patients residing in the intensive care unit (ICU). Approximately 9 million of these injuries lead to various types of disabilities, with 450,000 being serious and permanent, such as paraplegia. In the USA 150,000 victims die as a result of their injury; thus there is a 3:1 ratio of permanent disability to death. Fifty one percent of all injury deaths are a result of motor vehicle crashes in the USA. The annual cost related to trauma is over $400 billion annually and is in part accounted for by medical expenses, lost wages, insurance-related costs, property damage, fire loss, employer costs, and indirect loss from work-related injuries.

There is a trimodal distribution of death due to trauma. Early or immediate death (45%) occurs at the scene of the incident and is related to a devastating and catastrophic injury such as cerebral herniation, aortic transection, or cardiac rupture. Other than preventive measures, there is little medically that can be done. Although rapid transport from the scene has allowed some of these patients to arrive in extremis in the

emergency room, lethality is uniform. The second group (35%) are those that arrive in the emergency department (ED) and require aggressive evaluation and therapy. These patients will be discussed as part of the term "golden hour" below. The third mode of death (20%) occurs days or weeks after admission in patients who usually reside in the ICU. These patients progress to severe sepsis, hypotension, and even multiple organ failure before succumbing to death. In the following sections on trauma assessment and resuscitation, methods of care are discussed so as to prevent the progression to this most serious of clinical conditions.

THE GOLDEN HOUR

CLINICAL CAVEAT

The Golden Hour
- Try to be thorough but expeditious
- Do not spend too much time in the radiology department
- Hemodynamically labile patients need expeditiously to have determined the etiology of hypotension and have it treated. This may involve moving the patient to the operating room, ICU, or interventional radiology

When the term "golden hour" was first utilized and popularized by R. Adams Cowley, one of the founders of MIEMS, the Maryland Institute of Emergency Medical Services, in Baltimore in 1963, the approach to the trauma patient was relatively straightforward, with a limited number of diagnostic tests available as part of the initial evaluation. Most trauma centers try to adhere to this concept; however, frequently those seriously ill

337

require other types of procedures, generally radiographic, to be performed and this takes the patient out of the ED and ICU environment. Once a patient arrives, a rapid, though thorough, examination needs to be completed and disposition of the patient should be decided. There is certain information that can be obtained while the patient is in the ED to help with decision-making.

The advanced trauma life support (ATLS) course developed by the American College of Surgeons' Committee on Trauma provides an extensive discussion of the algorithm used to approach a multiply and seriously injured patient. By following the steps outlined below, little will be missed. Any life-threatening injuries need to be identified early and addressed, even if out of sequence of the algorithm. The team in the emergency room must be assigned before arrival of any injured patient to certain responsibilities. If staffing levels allow, nursing should be responsible for charting, obtaining equipment, obtaining vital signs, and beginning two large-bore cannulas, initially in the antecubital fossa if possible.

The fact that many prehospital support systems now are "scooping and running" to the ED prior to IV access being established has allowed critical savings of time at the scene, and in urban areas is being seen more frequently with transported critically injured patients. Once the vein is cannulated, it is imperative that a trauma panel be obtained, including a complete blood count, electrolytes, blood urea nitrogen, creatinine, blood sugar, type, and cross for 4–6 units of packed cells, prothrombin time (international normalized ratio), partial thromboplastin time, amylase for blunt trauma, and drug and alcohol screen when appropriate. However, the role of clinical laboratory values in assisting in the management of patients early on in their resuscitation may be misleading. Even though the hematocrit may be normal early on after the injury, it may be elevated due to dehydration from the environment or as a result of polyuria from an intoxicated patient. The hematocrit may also be low due to the effects of dilution from the resuscitation. However, a low hematocrit in the acute setting implies that there is blood loss and blood should be given. The white blood cell count is also elevated after injury due to the demargination of leukocytes from the effects of cortisol, glucagon, and epinephrine. The inability to normalize elevated lactate, correct a significant base deficit, or correct a metabolic acidosis is a poor prognostic sign. An arterial blood gas can be beneficial, although this requires another puncture. Once the laboratory values are obtained, fluids, as discussed below, can be given.

The role of gastric tonometry to guide resuscitation remains unfounded due to its limitations to distinguish between intramucosal carbon dioxide and that residing within the gastric lumen. There also remains debate as to whether the mucosal bicarbonate level is equal to the easily measured arterial level. Tissue oximetry, which allows for the direct measurement of tissue PO_2, remains strictly a research tool.

Box 31-1 Rapid Sequence Intubation
• Lidocaine – 1 mg/kg
• Norcuronium – 0.01 mg/kg
• Versed – 0.05 mg/kg or etomidate 0.3 mg/kg
• Succinylcholine – 1–2 mg/kg

Primary Survey

Beginning with the primary survey upon arrival, a rapid glance over of the entire patient is performed as well as trying to obtain as complete a history from the prehospital support personnel as rapidly as possible. Identification of the following life-threatening conditions requires urgent intervention:
- Tension pneumothorax
- Pericardial tamponade
- Respiratory insufficiency
- Hemorrhage
- Shock
- Massive hemothorax

The algorithm "ABCDE" has been used for the primary survey. Coincident with the drawing of laboratory studies, the airway of the patient needs to be assessed. If there is evidence of respiratory insufficiency or hypoxemia, an airway needs to be established. Acutely a nasopharyngeal or oral airway may not be enough to allow the patient to maintain a patent airway or to clear secretions and endotracheal intubation is necessary. Although the prehospital support population is beginning to get away from rapid sequence intubation (RSI), it is still popular in the emergency room. Box 31-1 presents one formula used with preoxygenation on 100% oxygen.

CLINICAL CAVEAT

Primary Survey and the ABCs
- Airway with cervical spine control
- Breathing
- Circulation with hemorrhage control and cardiac care
- Disability with rapid neurologic evaluation
- Exposure of the patient without inducing hypothermia
- Resuscitate, draw serum chemistries, place a gastric and bladder drainage tube if no contraindication

CURRENT CONTROVERSY

Rapid Sequence Intubation
- There are many thoughts on whether RSI is necessary. Various centers uses various methods of RSI
- Some centers do not use a nondepolarizing neuromuscular blocking agent
- Succinlycholine can cause an increase in ICP, intragastric pressure, and intraocular pressure and is avoided generally in burn patients due to potassium mobilization

Under emergent conditions an orotracheal tube should be placed. This route should also be used for any trauma victim with a head injury or maxillofacial injuries. If these conditions and findings are not present and the intubation is semi-elective, the nasal route can be considered. In situations where the anatomic landmarks are indistinct, or oral intubation is not possible to be accomplished for whatever reason, a surgical airway should be created. A large needle/catheter cricothyroidotomy can be performed, ventilating the patient with small tidal volumes and a rapid rate. A cricothyroidotomy can also be performed with a small tracheostomy or endotracheal tube. A CO_2 device can be used to confirm correct position of the airway access in addition to pulse oximetry, auscultation, end tidal CO_2 if available, and bronchoscopy, if the tube size will allow.

Once the airway has been established, breathing, or ventilation, must be instituted. Although the neurologic examination is lost with narcotic sedation or chemical paralysis, these agents may need to be administered in order to ventilate adequately the patient. Manual ventilation should ensure that there is minimal resistance and that oxygenation can be accomplished. If this is not feasible then a checklist of possible problems includes malposition of the tube, a pneumothorax, hemothorax, or an occluded tube.

Circulation involves two aspects to be addressed. If the patient is hemorrhaging, the bleeding needs to be controlled. Pelvic fractures with lateral displacement can be tamponaded by using a bed sheet folded and placed around the anterior and posterior superior and inferior iliac crest. A beanbag molding the pelvis, manually reduced, may also work. Otherwise external fixation, internal fixation, or even angiography to try to identify and embolize the bleeding may be helpful. If there is major bleeding coming from a transected extremity vessel due to a penetrating injury or from a large scalp injury, pressure should be applied to control the bleeding while operative intervention is being arranged. One study which looked at hypovolemic resuscitation for penetrating torso trauma demonstrated that until the bleeding is controlled, if the patient gets over resuscitated and even hypertensive, bleeding may be further exacerbated, leading more rapidly to hypothermia and coagulopathy.

The other "C" in the algorithm is cardiac. If the intravascular volume is low, the cardiac output will be compromised. If myocardial contractility is compromised, such as in a patient who had an MI and this led to a the motor vehicle crash, then a cardiac work-up is in order, possibly including coronary angiography. However, anticoagulation may be contraindicated if there is also an intracranial bleed or an injury that has a major bleeding tendency with anticoagulation, such as a pelvic fracture or hepatic laceration.

Disability is a rapid neurologic examination which consists of talking to the patient to see how they respond, checking the pupil reactivity and size, evaluating for evidence of otorrhea or rhinorrhea, and tabulating a Glasgow Coma Scale (GCS) which ranges from a worst possible score of 3 to a best possible score of 15 in evaluating the three categories of Box 31-2.

The Brain Trauma Foundation in collaboration with the Joint Section on Neurotrauma in Critical Care of the American Association of Neurological Surgeons and the Congress of Neurological Surgeons performed an evidence-based review of the literature and of the 13 clinical recommendations found three that they considered to achieve the level of standards. (See Clinical Caveats:

Box 31-2   Glasgow Coma Scale

EYE OPENING

Spontaneous: 4
To speech: 3
To pain: 2
None: 1

BEST MOTOR RESPONSE

Obeys commands: 6
Localizes pain: 5
Normal flexion (withdrawal): 4
Abnormal flexion (decorticate): 3
Extension (decerebrate): 2
None (flaccid): 1

VERBAL RESPONSE

Oriented: 5
Confused conversation: 4
Inappropriate words: 3
Incomprehensible sounds: 2
None: 1

Neurologic Evidence-Based Recommendations box.) Other recommendations included:

- Intracranial pressure (ICP) monitoring in severe head injury with a GCS of 3–8
- Initiation of therapy at an ICP of 20–25
- Avoidance of hypotension
- Avoidance of hypoxia
- Maintenance of cerebral perfusion pressure > 70 mmHg
- Providing 140% of resting-metabolism caloric support in nonparalyzed, brain-injured patients (100% in chemically paralyzed patients), using feedings that contain ≥15% of calories as protein, by the seventh day after injury
- Consideration of high-dose barbiturate therapy in hemodynamically acceptable, salvageable head-injury patients with refractory intracranial hypertension
- Use of mannitol in intermittent boluses for control of intracranial hypertension

---

CLINICAL CAVEAT

Neurologic Evidence-Based Recommendations
- Recommendation against the use of prophylactic antiseizure medications to prevent LATE posttraumatic seizures
- Avoid chronic, prolonged hyperventilation in the absence of increased ICP
- Avoid glucocorticoids in the treatment of severe head injury

---

The National Acute Spinal Cord Injury Study found that in traumatic patients a 30 mg/kg bolus of methyl prednisolone followed by 5.4 mg/kg for 24 hours, and for another 24 hours in those having treatment initiated at 3–8 hours after injury, had an improved functional outcome although there was an increased incidence of pneumonia and severe sepsis with the 48-hour administration.

The "E" in the algorithm is for exposure, in that the patient must be examined front to back and top to bottom and in order to do that the anatomy must be available. Hypothermia is a real concern, however, and patients should remain covered to prevent a loss in temperature.

Coincident with resuscitation should be gastric decompression and bladder decompression. Only after the patient has had a rectal examination, and in the male there is no evidence of a scrotal hematoma, a high-riding prostate, or blood at the urethral meatus, should a Foley catheter be inserted. If there are any of these findings, a urethrogram should be performed and, if normal, a Foley can be placed, followed by a cystogram. Although urethral injuries in females are rare due to the short length, a pelvic examination should be performed and if abnormal

blood is present at the meatus or there is concern due to a severe pelvic fracture a urethrogram should be performed. If normal, a Foley catheter can be placed and a cystogram should be performed.

Secondary Survey

By convention, the secondary survey, which is a more in-depth evaluation of the entire patient from top to bottom and front to back, may then be accomplished, while the patient is in the emergency room. If any life-threatening injuries are identified, they should be treated. Limb-threatening injuries should also have an action plan by this point.

CLINICAL CAVEAT

Secondary Survey
    Examine the patient head to toe and front to back, repeating the primary survey as you go along.

Tertiary Survey

This process identifies and catalogues all injuries within 24 hours. Some injuries are identified as a result of repeated examinations, clinical suspicions confirmed by radiography, or other diagnostic modalities. As patients begin to normalize after resuscitation, they may have new complaints or distracting injuries become less distracting. Additional lacerations and possibly underlying bony injuries may be discovered. The oral cavity may reveal loose teeth, which could possibly be aspirated if dislodged. A mandible fracture may be palpated. Seat belt marks may become more obvious, raising suspicion of hollow viscous injury, blunt cervical carotid, or brachial plexus injury. As many of these patients arrive in the ICU still with a cervical collar in place, laryngeal fracture as well as clearing of the cervical spine should be accomplished. Figure 31-1 shows one method to try to clear the cervical spine early. Occasionally fractures of the digits, ankles, or even fibula are found at this point.

The hemodynamically labile patient may not be able to be transported safely out of the ICU. Thus high-quality radiographs, computed tomography (CT) scanning, and multiplanar angiography may have to be delayed or alternative studies, such as portable radiographs, fluoroscopic on-table angiograms, ultrasound, or even diagnostic peritoneal lavage, will have to be performed as bedside procedures.

Depending on the need for neuromuscular blocking agents, anxiolytics and analgesics will also alter the ability to perform a complete neurologic examination. The level of sedation or somnolence can also be assessed through such methods as the Ramsay Scale, allowing for the

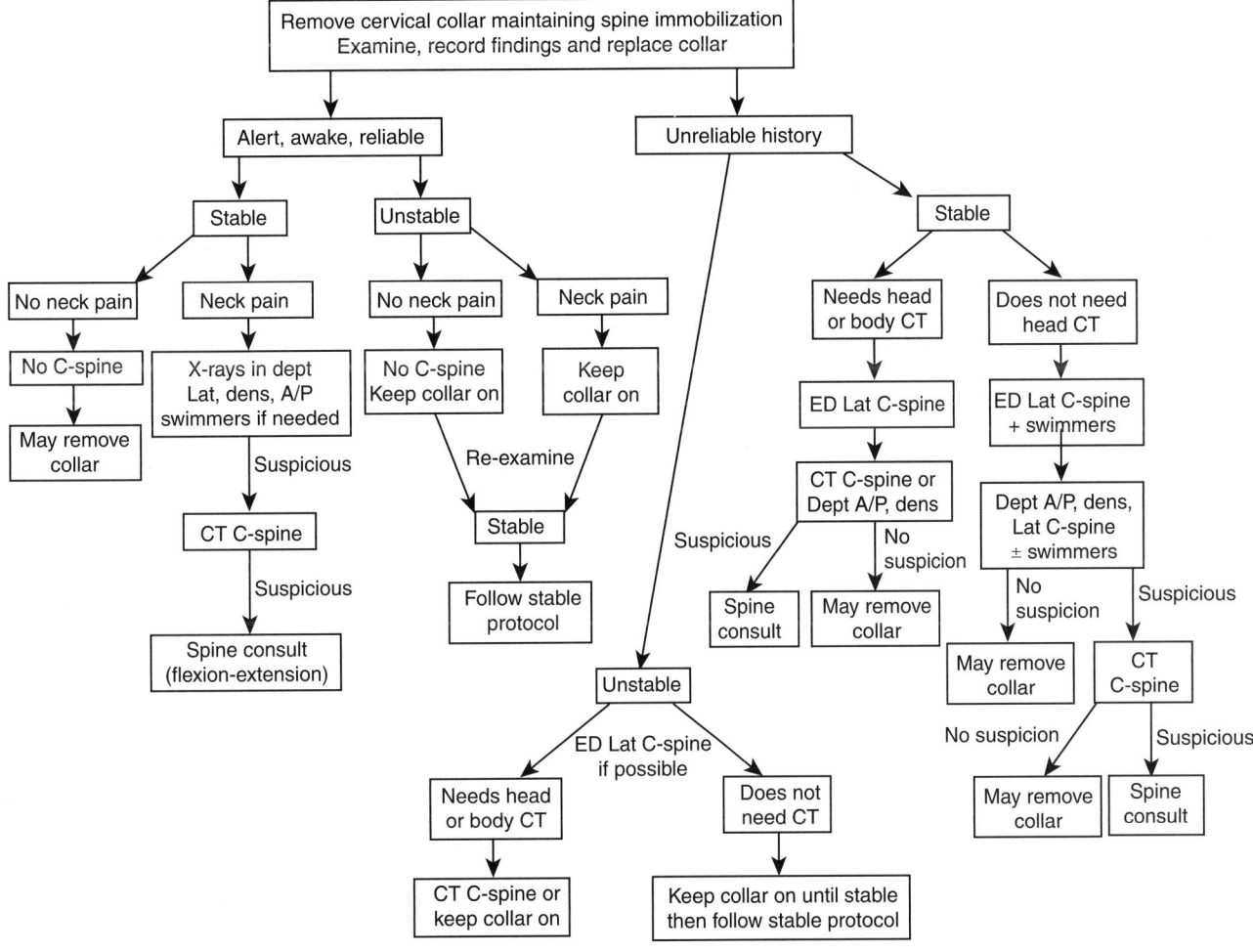

Figure 31-1   Protocol for clearing blunt trauma C-spines.

titration of these medications. There are also some short-acting, although more expensive, agents such as diprovan, which has a short half-life; however, as a fat emulsion it can precipitate pancreatitis and has been associated with elevated ICP in patients with intracranial bleeding. In addition stress gastritis prophylaxis should be instituted early as well as lower extremity compression devices for deep venous thrombosis (DVT) prophylaxis. Chemical antithrombotic prophylaxis should also be started if the patient is nonbleeding or has no other injuries or clinical conditions that would preclude its use.

CLINICAL CAVEAT

Tertiary Survey
- This more leisurely review of systems may lead to delayed recognition of injuries
- Do not jeopardize resuscitation by sending the patient prematurely out of the ICU where monitoring is less than ideal

Ancillary Studies

In addition to the serum laboratory tests obtained as the intravenous catheters are being placed and in addition to the cardiac monitor and pulse oximetry, an abdominal ultrasound, the focused assessment with sonography for trauma (FAST), can be performed. This rapidly looks at four areas: the pericardium, the pubic region, Morison's pouch which is the right hepatorenal space, and the left splenorenal space, looking for blood in the abdomen or around the heart. For the most part the FAST examination has replaced diagnostic peritoneal lavage (DPL) in the ED to evaluate for unexplained hypotension due to blood loss or pericardial tamponade. In addition a portable chest radiograph is also performed to look for a pnemothorax, hemothorax, mediastinal widening, or other pathology. The pelvic radiograph looks again for occult bleeding since a patient may lose up to half of their intravascular volume from a closed pelvic fracture. The third portable plain film obtained early on in the ED is the lateral cervical spine, looking for misalignment. Spinal cord injury can rapidly lead to profound vasodilatation and shock, necessitating aggressive volume resuscitation.

CLINICAL CAVEAT

Ancillary Studies
- The FAST (focused assessment with sonography for trauma) examination is a rapid screening for pericardial fluid and intra-abdominal fluid and is replacing diagnostic peritoneal lavage
- CT scan remains the gold standard for intra-abdominal evaluation in the trauma setting, short of surgery
- The radiology department is not a substitute for the ICU and as such attention to and provision of care is difficult to match in radiology. Beware of hemodynamic lability in a patient in which there is limited access, such as with angiography

---

Although these studies in general can be obtained quickly, further studies may delay a critically injured patient from going to the ICU. Thus the so-called golden hour can become four hours or longer and may not be in the patient's best interest to adhere to in some situations. The dynamic helical CT scan is rapid and capable of evaluating the entire body in relatively short order. In addition as a screen, the dynamic chest CT with contrast injection screens for aortic injury and has supplanted conventional angiography to large measure. However, interventional angiography with embolization, coiling, and stent graft placement has opened windows for nonoperative approaches to vascular lesions.

RESUSCITATION

In general adult victims of serious trauma who are in shock require aggressive resuscitation. By administering fluids rapidly it appears the incidence of end-stage organ dysfunction and ischemia can be ameliorated, if not halted. Access to the circulation is crucial and although routinely two large-bore antecubital vein lines are sought, rapid access and administration via nine French introducer sheaths placed in the femoral, subclavian, or internal jugular veins provides this access. Using a pressure infuser for two large-bore central cannulas, up to 5 liters of crystalloid can be given warmed to core temperature in 2 minutes or 5 liters of blood warmed to core temperature in 2½ minutes. Initially 2 liters of crystalloid is given rapidly and if the hemodynamics do not return to the patient's baseline, a further 2 liters are given as blood is being requested.

CLINICAL CAVEAT

Resuscitation
- Use two large-bore cannulas
- Warm the fluids and give the fluids rapidly
- In general 4 liters of crystalloid are given, followed by blood
- Begin blood immediately if actively bleeding
- Surgical bleeding belongs in general in the operating room

The crystalloids of choice are either lactated Ringer's (LR) solution or normal saline. The author's personal preference is LR due to the fact that there may be a theoretical, although not scientifically proven, advantage. When compared to normal saline the pH of LR is one log higher (pH = 6), sodium and chloride concentration is closer to that of serum, and the lactate gets converted by a functioning liver to bicarbonate. Both solutions cost the hospital under a dollar per liter. In a hypotensive trauma victim these fluids should be administered wide open and if after 4 liters the patient still is tachycardic, blood should be given. Typed and cross-matched blood is preferred, but this takes at least 30 minutes to process and that lag time may not be acceptable. Type-specific blood takes about 15 minutes to obtain, leaving O-negative blood that most commonly given urgently. Its administration should be given under pressure and warmed, given as rapidly as possible, and as much as needed. In the meantime bleeding sites should be sought and attempts to control them initiated. Although the arterial blood gas may give the hemoglobin value, this may not be reliable, and transfusion should be based in the initial period on the clinical condition.

Other blood components may also have to be administered, such as fresh frozen plasma if the number of units of packed cells exceeds 10 or there is on-going nonsurgical bleeding, platelets for profound thrombocytopenia, in the vicinity of 50,000, and cryoprecipitate for patients with factor deficiencies. This aggressive

---

CURRENT CONTROVERSY

Resuscitation
- The literature in general recommends crystalloids initially, although there is interest in hypertonic saline. Currently this is not the fluid of choice
- There is very little difference between LR and normal saline, although LR has some theoretical advantages
- Factor VIIa has been successful only anecdotally and is not a substitute for operatively correcting surgical bleeding
- Blood substitutes, although attractive, are still under investigation

resuscitation should continue in the ICU and should include crystalloids and blood early on. The use of albumin and hydroxyethylstarch as colloid volume is usually initiated in the ICU. These more expensive agents than crystalloids have not been shown to have an advantage early on in the trauma patient.

Other agents that have been used with limited success with nonsurgical coagulopathic bleeding is factor VIIa, which is given in the dose of up to 90 units/kg. It works temporarily for a couple of hours, which might be enough to warm and further resuscitate the patient and allow assessment of whatever might be bleeding. As a procoagulant factor VIIa may also cause vascular thrombosis, but in combat situations has been found to stop, albeit temporarily, bleeding.

A human and a bovine blood substitute are currently undergoing investigation in the trauma setting. One thought is to give these compounds in the prehospital setting so as to begin resuscitation with a compound providing oxygen-carrying capacity early and to cut down on the number of allogeneic blood transfusions.

Monitoring

Once the patient has been placed in the ICU, monitoring is crucial. There are advantages to getting trauma victims quickly from the ED to the ICU for continued, aggressive resuscitation. Patients with labile blood pressures may have to bypass departmental radiology studies such as CT scans or plain films. The latter can be done in the ICU, but foremost is to try to return the patients' vital signs to their normal physiologic level. Warm fluids rapidly given are continued. Pulse oximetry and EKG monitoring are routine as is frequent vital sign recordings. End tidal CO_2 monitoring may also be useful if available. An arterial line should be placed after ascertaining the best location. The radial artery is a common choice if the Allen's test reveals a patent palmer arch. The femoral

artery can also be used. Arterial access allows for continuous blood pressure monitoring and access for blood gasses and serum chemistries. However, it has been shown that the presence of an arterial cannula leads to increased phlebotomy, so serum chemistries should be drawn judiciously with as little blood as possible.

Central venous pressure (CVP) may provide a crude measure of central pressure. The pulmonary artery catheter is helpful when used early, although its popularity, even in trauma patients, has diminished. The volumetric pulmonary artery catheter calculates right ventricular end diastolic volume as a reflection of preload. It correlates fairly well with cardiac index and our practice is a goal of 120–150 ml/m². In addition these catheters can provide information used to calculate oxygen delivery and consumption index with goals of 150 and 600 ml/minute/m², respectively. These catheters are placed in the operating room or the ICU.

CURRENT CONTROVERSY

Pulmonary Artery Catheter
  Although there are studies showing that right ventricular end-diastolic pressure index correlates well with cardiac index, others still use pulmonary artery wedge pressure, oxygen delivery, or oxygen consumption to guide goal-directed therapy.

If there is no concern of esophageal injury, transesophageal cardiac monitoring can be utilized, providing information on filling pressures and cardiac performance. Transthoracic or transesophageal echocardiography can assess preload by evaluating end-diastole cardiac chamber size. However, in most institutions it requires specialists to perform the test, and is operator dependent, is variable in reproducibility, must be repeated for further evaluations, and is expensive. Esophageal Doppler sonography, in which an ultrasound probe is placed within the esophagus and positioned at the level of the descending thoracic aorta, measures blood flow velocity to calculate flow. This allows cardiac index determinations on a continuous basis and can help in goal-directed therapy.

Thoracic bioelectric impedance using surface electrodes is still being investigated in the ICU setting.

CLINICAL CAVEAT

Monitoring
- EKG and pulse oximetry monitoring should be done in the ED
- An arterial line can be useful for blood pressure monitoring; however, beware of over-phlebotomization
- A CVP is a poor method to monitor preload in the trauma setting
- Less invasive methods of cardiac monitoring such as esophageal Doppler can be used successfully as the use of the pulmonary artery catheter is decreasing
- The utility of bioimpedance is still being evaluated

The Elderly Trauma Victim

The elderly represent the fastest growing segment of the population. As one ages there is a decrease in fixed expiratory volumes over 1 second (FEV_1), functional vital capacity (FVC), FEV_1/FVC, and peak expiratory flow rate (PEFR). These changes all lead to a predictable decrease

---

Box 31-3 Risk Factors for Mortality Following Significant Blunt Trauma in the Elderly

- Pedestrian hit by a motor vehicle
- Initial systolic blood pressure < 130 mmHg
- Acidosis (pH < 7.35)
- Multiple long bone fractures
- Head injury

---

in arterial oxygen tension with age which may be expressed as $PaO_2 = 103.7 - 0.24$ (Age) ± 7.9 mmHg. As one ages there is also a decrease in cardiac reserve with a limited ability to compensate for shock or respiratory failure. Pulse rate decreases with age as does cardiac index. Although these patients are aggressively resuscitated, the amount needed may have to be decreased to avoid congestive heart failure and pulmonary edema. Once the volume status has been judged to be adequate, vasopressors may need to be instituted. A low threshold for noninvasive and invasive monitoring, including a pulmonary artery catheter, should be kept in mind and in addition to myocardial performance and other vital signs, lactate levels may be useful. If the lactate is clearing, then coupled with clinical history and examination, the patient should be improving. Due to other comorbidities in the elderly even what may be considered minor injuries can have devastating consequences. This alone frequently necessitates an ICU admission (Box 31-3).

Although ethical issues are important for all patients, all health care providers must be aware whether the trauma victim has an advanced directive. Many elderly have voiced concerns on the level of heroics and thus have limited the scope of care provided. If this information is available, it should be followed, if possible. In all other circumstances aggressive care continues unless there is an indication to limit this aggressive care, such as a patient with a neurologically devastating injury or inability to be resuscitated.

CLINICAL CAVEAT

Elderly Trauma Victim
Although the elderly have diminished pulmonary function and increased comorbidities, evaluation and resuscitation should be aggressive.

SELECTED READING

American College of Surgeons. *Advanced Trauma Life Support for Doctors*, Chicago, IL, 1997.

Cornwell EE: Trauma and critical care. J Am Coll Surg 186:115-121, 1998.

Dabrowski GP, Steinberg SM, Ferrara JJ, Flint LM: A critical assessment of endpoints of shock resuscitation. Surg Clin North Am 80:825-844, 2000.

Ledgerwood AM, Lucas CE: A review of studies on the effects of hemorrhagic shock and resuscitation on the coagulation profile. J Trauma 54:S68-S74, 2003.

Milzman DP, Rothenhaus TC: Resuscitation of the geriatric patient. Emerg Med Clin North Am 14:233-244, 1996.

Shapiro MJ: Traumatic shock: nonsurgical management. In Parillo JE, Dellinger RP, editors: *Critical Care Medicine: Principles of Diagnosis and Management*, ed 2, Philadelphia: Mosby, 2001, pp 501-512.

Webb AR, Shapiro MJ, Singer M, Suter P, editors: *The Oxford Textbook of Critical Care*, London: Oxford University Press, 1999.

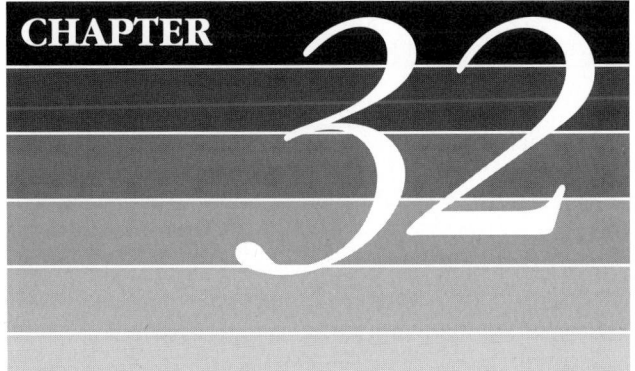

CHAPTER 32

Treating Thermal Injury and Smoke Inhalation

CHRISTOPHER W. LENTZ, M.D., F.A.C.S.

DINA M. ELARAJ, M.D.

Thermal injury is a major cause of morbidity and mortality in the USA. The USA has the fourth-highest fire death rate of all industrialized countries with 75–85% of all fire deaths related to residential fires. Approximately 2 million fires occur annually resulting in 1.4 million injuries. Burn injuries result in about 54,000 hospital admissions and 5000 deaths each year. Fires related to smoking are the leading cause of fire-related deaths, and flame injury is the predominant type of injury seen in patients admitted to burn centers. Most fire-related deaths, however, are due to inhalation of smoke and toxic gases with only about 25% due to the actual burn. Initial resuscitation of the burn patient, therefore, requires a high index of suspicion for inhalation injury and airway compromise.

Although the more severe burns are likely referred to a regional burn center, half of the admissions for thermal injuries are to hospitals without burn care facilities. It is therefore essential that physicians caring for these patients have some expertise in the initial management of thermal injury. Also, it is necessary to understand when referral to a regional burn center is appropriate.

ASSESSMENT OF DEPTH OF INJURY

Thermal injury causes coagulation necrosis of cutaneous tissue to variable depths. The degree to which tissue injury occurs depends on the temperature to which the tissue is exposed, the duration of contact, and the thickness of the exposed skin. The depth of the burn correlates with its clinical behavior and burns are often classified as first, second, third, and fourth degree. First- and second-degree burns are also classified as partial-thickness while third- and fourth-degree burns are classified as full-thickness injuries. Partial-thickness burns affect the epidermis and dermis and heal by migration of epithelial cells from preserved dermal appendages such as sebaceous glands, sweat glands, and hair follicles. Full-thickness burns affect the epidermis, entire dermis, and, in cases of fourth-degree burns, deeper tissues, destroying the dermal appendages and thus requiring skin grafting for closure. Deep partial-thickness burns may also require skin grafting for closure to avoid the development of a hypertrophic scar. Table 32-1 lists distinguishing characteristics of partial- and full-thickness burns.

The depth of the burn is usually established at the time of the injury. There are certain physiologic changes in the burn wound, however, that can result in the burn becoming deeper after the offending agent has been removed. Since the skin is frequently the first organ compromised in shock, failure to resuscitate a burn victim can result in ischemia of the burned skin, therefore causing a deeper burn wound. Furthermore, thromboxane A_2, a potent vasoconstrictor, is released by platelets in the burned skin. This, too, causes vasoconstriction of dermal vessels, impairing the oxygenation of burned tissue and expanding the zone of thermal injury. The temporary vasoconstriction caused by thomboxane A_2 also results

Table 32-1	Characteristics of Burn Wounds			
	Depth of Injury	**Appearance**	**Sensation**	**Healing**
PARTIAL THICKNESS				
First degree	Epidermis	Hyperemic	Painful/hypersensitive	Scarless within 7 days
Second degree				
Superficial	Superficial dermis	Moist, blistering, blanching hyperemia with rapid capillary refill	Painful/hypersensitive	Minimal scarring within 2 weeks
Deep	Deep dermis	Pale pink or dark red, nonblanching hyperemia or with delayed capillary refill	Decreased pinprick sensation, intact pressure sensation	Hypertrophic scarring in many weeks
FULL THICKNESS				
Third degree	Entire dermis	Dry, pearly-white or leathery	Insensate	By contracture
Fourth degree	Deep tissues	Necrotic, with thrombosed vessels	Insensate	Requires debridement or amputation

in a reperfusion injury within the burn. This results in the formation of oxygen free radicals which can further potentiate the tissue injury.

PATHOPHYSIOLOGY OF BURN SHOCK AND SMOKE INHALATION

In addition to the local tissue injury, burns also have systemic effects. Burns with a percent total body surface area (%TBSA) greater than 20% can result in hypovolemic shock or burn shock. There are two main losses of intravascular volume in thermal injury victims. First, the direct thermal injury to the tissue causes changes in dermal collagen resulting in a hydrostratic vacuum in the burned skin. This effectively draws fluid into the interstitial space at a significant rate. Obviously, the larger surface area burned results in a greater loss of fluid into the wound.

The second etiology of burn shock is the increase in microvascular permeability to albumin. In burns with a %TBSA > 20% this increase in permeability occurs throughout the body in burned and nonburned tissue. An increase in microvascular permeability is observed due to the direct effects of heat as well as the release of factors such as histamine, thromboxane A_2, leukotrienes, bradykinin, serotonin, and cytokines such as interleukin (IL)-1, IL-6, and IL-8. These result in a net loss of fluid and protein from the intravascular to the extravascular space, thus causing the edema that occurs in the areas of thermal injury (as well as the edema that develops in unburned tissue as the resuscitation of large burns proceeds).

It is the combination of both hydrostatic forces and increases in microvascular permeability that produces the hypovolemic shock observed in thermal injury victims.

Patients with larger burns will have more significant shock due to the large loss of intravascular volume into the interstitium. This is the reason resuscitation formulas have been developed to estimate the fluid needs of a burn victim based on their weight and the %TBSA burned.

Smoke inhalation injury is present in approximately 20% of burn admissions and increases the mortality associated with burns of any size. Inhalation injury is due to the inhalation of the chemical products of combustion. There are three main components contributing to the pathophysiology of smoke inhalation. The first of these is carbon monoxide (CO) toxicity. Carbon monoxide causes a functional anemia, as hemoglobin will preferentially bind CO rather than oxygen (by a factor of 250-fold). The carboxyhemoglobin (COHb) that is formed will shift the oxyhemoglobin dissociation curve to the left, thus decreasing oxygen delivery to the tissues. Patients can therefore be severely hypoxemic, manifested by a low oxygen saturation (SaO_2), while maintaining a normal arterial oxygen tension (PaO_2).

Cyanide toxicity may also be present. Inhalation of hydrocyanide, produced when synthetic materials such as plastics are burned, leads to rapid systemic absorption and binding of the mitochondrial cytochrome a-a3 system, thus impairing ATP production and forcing cellular anaerobic metabolism. Cyanide toxicity should be suspected in a patient with a persistent metabolic acidosis despite adequate resuscitation and adequate urine output.

Finally, acrolein and aldehyde gases dissolved within the smoke are directly toxic to the airway epithelium. When these compounds come into contact with the airway, the pseudostratified ciliated epithelial cells literally fall off the trachea and bronchi, leaving a raw basement membrane. This raw surface then secretes a proteinaceous material which solidifies and forms obstructing airway casts if not removed. Unlike the immediate effects of carbon monoxide and hydrogen cyanide, the airway damage from acrolein and aldehyde persists until the airway epithelium heals (which can take several weeks). Also, acrolein and aldehyde set off an inflammatory cascade in the airway circulation which affects the lung parenchyma. This results in the development of acute respiratory dysfunction syndrome (ARDS).

INITIAL MANAGEMENT PRIORITIES

Stop the Burning Process

The approach to the evaluation and treatment of a burn patient is similar to that of a trauma patient and, in fact, the patient should be assessed for concomitant trauma. The initial goal should be to stop the burning process. The patient's clothing should be removed and the burn wounds should be irrigated with cool water. The use of ice or ice water can cause vasoconstriction and can potentially cause ischemia to the burned skin, thus making the burn deeper. Acid burns cause a coagulation necrosis and should be irrigated for at least 30 minutes. Alkali burns cause liquefaction necrosis and are therefore more destructive. These types of burns should be irrigated for 60 minutes. Powdered chemicals should be brushed off and not irrigated. If a powdered chemical goes into solution, the surface area of skin damaged will be significantly increased. Eye burns require continuous irrigation with normal saline for up to 1 or 2 hours.

Burn patients are at great risk for developing hypothermia. The damaged skin has limited ability to regulate blood flow and therefore the convective loss of heat from a thermal injury victim is great. Since the majority of the above-mentioned techniques require wetting the patient, every effort should be made to insulate the patient and to increase the ambient temperature of the environment to minimize the risk of hypothermia.

Airway/Breathing

The airway should be initially assessed to ensure patency. The presence of stridor is an immediate indication for endotracheal intubation. Burns to the face are not at immediate risk for airway compromise; however, subsequent edema formation in addition to resuscitation fluids can make securing an airway more difficult later. It is therefore recommended that patients with facial burns be prophylactically intubated with a 7.5 mm internal diameter (i.d.) endotracheal tube or larger. This caliber of endotracheal tube will permit flexible bronchoscopy for diagnosis and therapeutic lavage if needed.

Patients burned in an enclosed space or found unconscious in a burning structure should be suspected of having smoke inhalation. Smoke inhalation is highly unlikely in patients injured outdoors since the smoke dissipates quickly. Findings that may be associated with inhalation include a history of hoarseness, wheezing, facial burns, singeing of facial hair, carbon deposits in the oropharynx, or carbonaceous sputum. Patients with significant smoke inhalation will have a COHb level of >10%. Chest radiography is useless in diagnosing inhalation injury. It is typically obtained to exclude underlying pulmonary pathology or evidence of thoracic trauma and therefore should be obtained. A definitive diagnosis of inhalation injury is made by bronchoscopy; if positive, carbonaceous deposits, hyperemia, edema, superficial sloughing, and/or ulceration of the mucosa will be seen below the level of the vocal cords.

If there is a suspected CO exposure, 100% oxygen should be administered. Patients with COHb levels <15% are frequently asymptomatic and smokers can have COHb levels of 5–7%. The classic cherry-red skin color is rare and can be difficult to evaluate if the skin is burned. A baseline COHb level and arterial blood gas should be obtained if CO exposure is suspected. Table 32-2 gives symptoms associated with varying levels of COHb.

If, despite adequate resuscitation, the patient has a progressive metabolic acidosis, cyanide toxicity should be expected. Blood cyanide levels of >0.1 mg/l should be immediately treated. The antidote for cyanide poisoning requires two interventions. First, sodium thiosulfate (125–250 mg/kg) is administered to transfer sulfur to the cyanide ion. Next, hydroxycobalamin (4 g) is given to chelate the cyanide to permit excretion.

Large surface area burns also require intubation and ventilatory support. Patients with large burns become hypercatabolic and produce large amounts of carbon dioxide. If the patient is unable to increase and maintain an adequate minute ventilation, hypercapnia ensues. Patients with underlying pulmonary pathology associated with an increase in physiologic dead space are more prone to this complication.

Circumferential third-degree torso burns can restrict respiratory excursion due to the constricting effects of the burned skin. This restriction is not usually present

Table 32-2 Carbon Monoxide Effects

COHb (%)	Signs and Symptoms
0–10	None
10–30	Headache
30–50	Dizziness, weakness, presyncope
50–70	Syncope, coma, cardiovascular depression
70–80	Further cardiovascular depression
80–100	Death

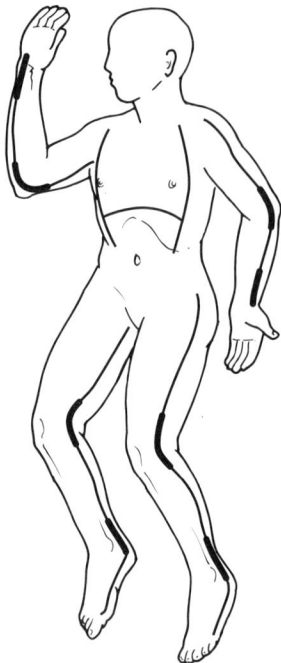

Figure 32-1   Correct placement of esharotomy incisions.

initially, but becomes more problematic during fluid resuscitation. Progressive tissue edema below the burned skin decreases total thoracic compliance and eventually impairs ventilation. This is manifest by a *gradual* increase in peak airway pressures and worsening respiratory acidosis. The treatment is a chest wall *escharotomy*; a cut into the burned chest skin along the right and left anterior axillary lines and joined horizontally across the costal margin. This will improve respiratory excursion and therefore improve compliance. Figure 32-1 illustrates the placement of escharotomy incisions along the anterior axillary lines connected by a subcostal incision. An escharotomy should only be performed by a knowledgeable surgeon.

CLINICAL CAVEAT

Acute increases in peak airway pressures in patients with circumferential torso burns should *first* be evaluated for airway obstruction, right main stem intubation, or pneumothorax prior to considering chest wall escharotomy.

Anticipation and treatment of pulmonary complications is necessary in order to decrease the morbidity and mortality associated with large burns (with or without smoke inhalation injury). Patients with smoke inhalation injury are at risk for pneumonia, ARDS, bronchiectasis, tracheo-malacia, and subglottic stenosis. Humidified oxygen, encouraging the patient to cough, and chest physiotherapy

assist in the clearing of airway secretions. Bronchodilators may be helpful to relieve bronchospasm. Mechanical ventilation may be required. Ventilator management strategies in patients with smoke inhalation injury include a pressure mode of ventilation with longer inspiratory times at lower peak pressures and positive end-expiratory pressure (PEEP) to improve compliance, recruit alveoli, and maintain an adequate functional residual capacity. Permissive hypercapnia may also be necessary to limit airway pressures.

Circulation

Since burned tissue swells, all constricting clothing and jewelry should be removed to prevent circulatory compromise. Finger rings should be removed as soon as possible since swelling of the digits may make removal later more difficult. Earrings should also be removed since increasing edema of burned ears could lead to pressure necrosis.

Burns with %TBSA greater than 20% will require resuscitation. It is necessary, in these patients, to secure adequate intravenous (IV) access. Large-bore (at least 16-gauge) IV catheters should be placed, preferentially through unburned skin, although this is not always possible. Catheters can be placed through burned skin, but since adhesive tape will not adhere to the burn, they should be secured with sutures. Central venous catheters provide more definitive venous access. Due to the high incidence of catheter colonization and infection, antibiotic-impregnated central venous catheters should be used if available. An indwelling urethral catheter should be placed to monitor urine output during resuscitation.

Resuscitation formulas have become the standard for initiating and conducting the treatment for burn shock. The most commonly used formula is the Parkland (or Baxter) formula. Correct application of this formula requires an estimation of the second- and third-degree %TBSA involvement and the patient's weight. The extent of the burn can be approximated using the "Rule of Nines" (Figure 32-2), a guide to estimating %TBSA burned based upon dividing the adult body into 11 regions each corresponding to 9%TBSA. The head and each upper extremity represent 9% of the TBSA; the anterior torso, posterior torso, and each lower extremity represent 18% of the TBSA. Children under 30 kg require a slightly different approximation of %TBSA due a disproportionately larger head; a child's head represents 18% of the TBSA and each lower extremity represents 14% of the TBSA. A rough estimate for irregular burns is that the patient's palm (not including the fingers) represents about 1% of the TBSA. A computerized estimation of the %TBSA burned may be generated at the website www.sagediagram.com.

Fluid resuscitation with lactated Ringer's (LR) solution should be guided by the Parkland formula which directs

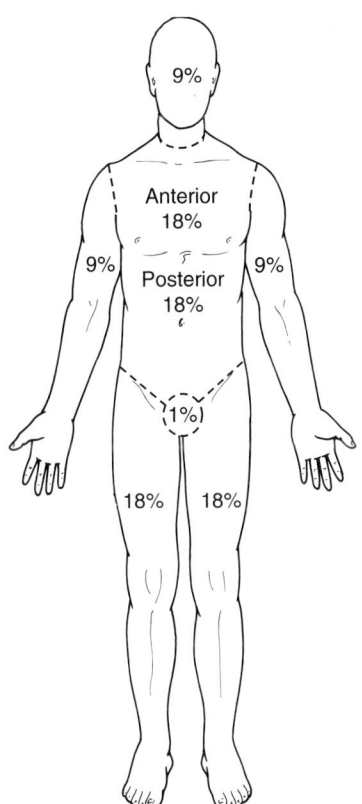

Figure 32-2   The "Rule of Nines," a guide to estimating the percent of the total body surface area (%TBSA) burned based upon dividing the adult body into 11 regions each corresponding to 9%TBSA.

that a fluid volume of 4 ml/kg/%TBSA burned be administered over the first 24 hours following the time of injury; half of this volume should be administered over the first 8 hours and the other half administered over the next 16 hours. Although this is the classic teaching of the application of the Parkland formula, it is impractical. Reducing the IV fluid rate to half after an arbitrary 8 hours does not estimate the physiologic need for fluid after being burned. Most burn centers use the Parkland formula to calculate the initial IV fluid rate. Then, physiologic parameters are used to titrate the IV fluid down over the next 24 hours. Practically speaking, this calculation provides a starting rate for IV fluid administration; this rate is then titrated up or down to maintain a urine output of at least 0.5 ml/kg/hour. The fluid is titrated down to a maintenance rate at 24 hours from the time of injury.

The presence of a smoke inhalation injury will increase IV fluid resuscitation requirements by anywhere from 40% to 75%. Other factors that may contribute to increased IV fluid requirements include large burns (>50% TBSA), alcohol intoxication, hepatic insufficiency, electrical injuries, and a history of chronic diuretic use. At 24 hours postinjury, adequate resuscitation will allow the patient

to be treated with IV fluids at a maintenance rate (30 ml/kg/day) plus 1 ml/kg/%TBSA burned to account for evaporative losses through the open burned wound. In large surface area burns this estimate of insensible loss can be quite significant.

> **CLINICAL CAVEAT**
>
> The rate of IV fluid administration should be calculated from the time of injury. For example, if a patient sustains a burn 3 hours prior to instituting IV fluids, half of the calculated 24-hour fluid requirement should be administered within the first 5 hours.

If the above resuscitation strategy is unsuccessful by 12 hours postinjury and the patient remains hypotensive (mean arterial pressure < 80 mmHg), tachycardic (heart rate > 120 beats per minute), or oliguric (urine output < 0.5 ml/kg/hour) despite increasing the rate of IV fluid administration, colloid should be administered. A variety of colloid solutions can be used; commonly used solutions include 5% albumin (0.3–0.5 ml/kg/%TBSA burned over 18 hours), 6% dextran-70 (0.5–1.0 ml/kg/%TBSA burned, not exceeding 33 ml/kg over any 24 hour period), and 6% hetastarch (0.5–1.0 ml/kg/%TBSA burned).

Electrical burns often require more extensive IV fluid resuscitation than calculated by the Parkland formula because the extent of subcutaneous and deep tissue involvement is usually underestimated by the apparent cutaneous injury. In addition, rhabdomyolysis may occur as a result of muscle necrosis, leading to myoglobinuria. Patients with myoglobinuria should be treated with LR at a rate of at least 1000 ml/hour to prevent acute tubular necrosis and ensure a urine output of at least 100 ml/hour. A sample of the patient's urine should be obtained initially and kept with the patient for comparison to subsequent samples to assess clearing of the pigment. Patients who sustain electrical injuries should be monitored with telemetry for at least 24 hours due to an increased risk for cardiac arrhythmias. Patients with electrical burns must also be assessed for neurologic injuries and concomitant musculoskeletal, especially spine, trauma, as these injuries are commonly associated with electrical injuries.

After appropriate wound care, extremity burns should be elevated and splinted in a position of function. Peripheral circulation should be monitored using a Doppler ultrasonic flow meter as circumferential full-thickness extremity burns may compromise distal perfusion and require escharotomy. Patients who sustain electrical injuries are at risk for the development of a compartment syndrome and may require fasciotomy to decompress tissue compartments. Doppler flow should be monitored on an hourly basis at the most distal aspects of the extremities, i.e., the palmar arch and digital vessels of the hands and the pedal vessels of the feet. One should not await the presence of neurologic signs such as paresthesias, pain, or paralysis to make the diagnosis of impaired distal perfusion. Figure 32-1 illustrates placement of escharotomy incisions along the lateral and medial aspects of the extremities and over the dorsal aspect of the hand. A lateral incision is made first; if no improvement in Doppler flow is detected within 5–10 minutes, the medial incision is then made. It is important that the escharotomy incision is made along the entire length of the full-thickness burn and that it crosses the joints.

BURN WOUND CARE

Basic principles of burn wound care involve keeping the wounds clean, moist, and protected. It is essential that the patient be kept in a warm environment above 30°C. Burns should be cleansed with a warm chlorhexidine solution. First-degree burns may be treated with any moisturizing cream. Superficial or deep partial-thickness burns to the face or neck should be treated with petrolatum. This should be reapplied several times per day to maintain moisture. Burns to the ears should be treated with mafenide acetate (Sulfamylon) cream if cartilage is exposed. Large blisters, especially those located over the palms or the soles should be evacuated but left intact and dressed with a moisturizing ointment and gauze dressing.

Superficial partial-thickness burns elsewhere on the body may be treated with petrolatum or temporary skin substitutes such as xenografts, cadaveric allografts, Apligraf (collagen/fibroblast matrix with overlying keratinocytes), Biobrane (collagen/nylon mesh with an outer silicone film), or Trancyte (human newborn fibroblasts cultured on the nylon mesh of Biobrane). These temporary skin substitutes promote reepithelialization and reduce wound pain, evaporative losses, and edema, and are left in place to adhere to the wound bed until healing occurs.

Deep partial-thickness and full-thickness burn wounds should be treated with a topical antimicrobial agent to decrease the risk of developing an invasive burn wound infection. Table 32-3 lists distinguishing characteristics of four commonly used topical antimicrobial agents. One effective treatment strategy is to treat deep partial-thickness or full-thickness wounds with silver sulfadiazine (Silvadene) or Acticoat (an ionic silver-coated polyethylene fabric). Wounds treated with silver sulfadiazine should be cleansed once or twice daily and the cream reapplied. Wounds treated with Acticoat need to be moistened with water (not saline, as this will cause the dressing to dry out) several times a day and the dressing changed every 3–4 days.

Infected full-thickness burns should be treated with mafenide acetate, as this is the only agent that can penetrate the eschar, and the dressings changed twice daily. Note that mafenide acetate is a strong carbonic anhydrase inhibitor and can cause a hyperchloremic metabolic acidosis.

OTHER CONSIDERATIONS

Systemic Wound Management

Ibuprofen should be administered on a scheduled basis (1200 mg loading dose followed by 800 mg every 8 hours) for the first 72 hours after a burn injury occurs to decrease thromboxane A2 production and the resultant dermal vasoconstriction.

Tetatus toxoid should be administered if the patient's last immunization was more than 5 years previously.

There is no role for the administration of prophylactic systemic antibiotics.

Pain Control

Partial-thickness burns are associated with a significant amount of pain due to the exposure of pain fibers

---

Table 32-3   Characteristics of Topical Antimicrobial Agents Used in the Treatment of Deep Partial- and Full-Thickness Burns

Agent	Spectrum of Activity	Eschar Penetration	Disadvantages/Side Effects
Silver sulfadiazine, 1% cream (Silvadene)	Gram positive, Gram negative, yeast	Poor	Transient leukopenia in 5–15%; some Gram-negative organisms, e.g., clostridia, are resistant
Ionic silver fabric dressing (Acticoat)	Gram positive, Gram negative, yeast	Poor	None
Mafenide acetate, 11.1% cream (Sulfamylon)	Gram positive, Gram negative	Good	Painful; carbonic anhydrase inhibitor causing acidosis
Silver nitrate, 0.5% solution	Gram positive, Gram negative, yeast	Poor	Can cause hyponatremia, hypokalemia, hypochloremia, hypocalcemia, and met-hemoglobinemia; stains environment, equipment, and personnel

in the dermis; adequate analgesia is essential and can usually be achieved by the intermittent administration of small amounts of IV narcotics. Patients requiring mechanical ventilation are commonly treated with a continuous infusion of IV narcotics. Patients with full-thickness burns usually have decreased narcotic requirements as these burns have destroyed the pain fibers in the dermis.

Nutritional Support

Patients with extensive thermal injury will experience a hypermetabolic state with increased oxygen consumption and catabolism resulting in the wasting of lean body mass. Patients with burns of >20%TBSA will have a resting energy expenditure (REE) 1.5 to 2 times normal and will require supplemental nutritional support. One formula for calculating the REE (in $kcal/m^2/hour$) in a burn patient, developed at the US Army Institute of Surgical Research, is:

$$REE = BEE \times [0.89 + (0.014 \times \%TBSA \text{ burned})]$$

where BEE is the basal energy expenditure and can be calculated from the Harris–Benedict equation:

for males, $BEE = 66 + (13.7 \times wt) + (5 \times ht) - (6.8 \times age)$

for females, $BEE = 65 + (9.6 \times wt) + (1.8 \times ht) - (4.7 \times age)$

where wt is weight in kilograms and ht is height in centimeters. Protein requirements may be in the range 2.5–3 g/kg/day.

Enteral feeds represent the optimal route of caloric support; however, patients with a >20%TBSA burn may have an ileus in the early postburn period and will not tolerate enteral feeds. These patients often require nasogastric tube decompression until the ileus resolves; gastrointestinal motility usually returns by the third to fifth day postinjury. Serum glucose levels should be monitored every four hours once feeds begin as burn patients will experience some degree of peripheral insulin resistance. Continuous insulin infusions may be necessary to control hyperglycemia. These patients are also at risk for the development of stress gastritis and should be prophylactically treated with antacids, H_2 receptor antagonists, or proton pump inhibitors.

CONCLUSIONS

The USA has one of the highest rates of fire-related deaths. The successful management of a burn patient requires an understanding of the pathophysiology associated with thermal injury and a high index of suspicion for smoke inhalation injury. Continued assessment of the airway, adequate IV fluid resuscitation, pain control, nutritional support, and appropriate wound care are essential components of the care of patients with thermal, chemical, or electrical burns. The anticipation and treatment of complications associated with different burn injuries play an equally important role in the management of these complex patients.

SELECTED READING

Demling RH: Burn care in the immediate resuscitation period. In Wilmore D, editor: *American College of Surgeons Surgery: Principles & Practice*, New York: WebMD Corporation, 2002, pp 49–61.

Demling RH: Burn care in the early postresuscitation period. In Wilmore D, editor: *American College of Surgeons Surgery: Principles & Practice*, New York: WebMD Corporation, 2002, pp 479–489.

Demling RH: Burn care after the first postburn week. In Wilmore D, editor: *American College of Surgeons Surgery: Principles & Practice*, New York: WebMD Corporation, 2002, pp 491–503.

Demling RH: Miscellaneous thermal injuries. In Wilmore D, editor: *American College of Surgeons Surgery: Principles & Practice*, New York: WebMD Corporation, 2002, pp 505–515.

Herndon DN, editor: *Total Burn Care*, ed 2, Philadelphia: WB Saunders, 2001.

Lentz CW, Peterson HD: Smoke inhalation is a multi-level insult to the pulmonary system. Curr Opin Crit Care 3:221–226, 1997.

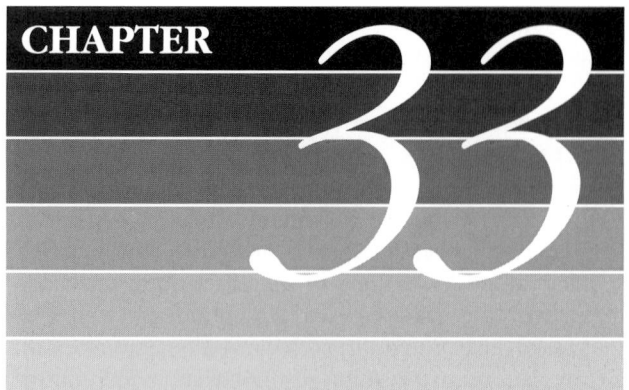

CHAPTER 33

Environmental Threat and Disaster Response: Natural Disasters and Biological, Chemical, and Nuclear Threat

JAMES E. SZALADOS, M.D., J.D., M.B.A.

The probability that civilian physicians will treat civilian casualties within the USA due to biological, chemical, and nuclear exposure continues to increase daily. The likelihood of such an attack outweighs that of conventional weapons in the civilian arena primarily because of accelerated terrorist activities. The impact of these agents is fourfold. The first is mortality and incapacitation of directly exposed individuals, the second is the psychology of mass panic and hysteria, thirdly civil disruption is superseded by post-traumatic stress disorders, and finally there are the lingering effects of agents on chronic health and genetic mutation in survivors. The key to effective response is based in education, index of suspicion (situational awareness), and response planning (standard operating procedures).

Physicians and other health care providers in civilian practice settings do not presently have sufficient training to participate in the frontline management of environmental threat scenarios. Physicians practicing in life-support specialties such as anesthesiology, emergency medicine, and critical care have a key role in the immediate and long-term public health response.

The general principles for the management of environmental threat are similar to the management principles for natural disasters, industrial accidents, or epidemics. Since these principles can be learned, education is fundamental to public policy initiatives regarding preparation of the health care system.

TYPES OF ENVIRONMENTAL THREAT

- Artificial versus natural. For example, a biological agent released either during or as a terrorist act versus natural epidemic of either an established or emerging biological organism.
- Point source versus line source. For example, release of an agent at a particular location versus multiple releases simultaneously or in sequence.
- Immediate versus sustained release.
- Human target versus infrastructure target. Humans as targets of environmental threat versus food sources or technology.
- Direct effect versus indirect effects. The immediate or discernible effect of environmental threat on humans versus insidious contamination, genetic effects, or vector-mediated diseases.

Toxins are biological substances produced by animals, plants, or microbes. Toxins are more difficult to manufacture on a large scale than are synthetic chemical weapons. Mass casualty biological weapons (MCBWs) are toxins capable of being used in attacks against the civilian or military infrastructure. The method of dispersion (e.g., aerosol, gas, ingestion) differentiates agents based on method of delivery. Inhalation, ingestion, and dermal activity differentiates agents based on the method of introduction.

LD_{50} refers to the dose required to cause death in 50% of patients, or the dose that results in a 50% chance of survival or death in a person receiving it. LD_{50} is a measure of toxity and also defines the practical applicability of agents as potential MCBWs.

The effects of agents must be considered. Lethality is only one index of effect; short-term and long-term incapacitation and public panic and anxiety are also important.

GENERAL PRINCIPLES OF CONTAINMENT

PEARLS

Principles of Response
Situational awareness:
- Index of suspicion
- Education and familiarity with potential problems
- Communication
Response deployment:
- Coordination and leadership
- Chain of command
Source control:
- Perimeter establishment
- Quarantine and isolation
- Disinfection and decontamination
- Antidotes and antibiotics
- Supportive critical care

The first priority of disaster medicine is the prevention of secondary casualties. Caregivers who are inexperienced in disaster or military medicine are especially vulnerable. The disaster plan is an operations blueprint that defines the policies and procedures to be implemented in the event of an emergency. The plan must include every conceivable aspect of mass casualty care including a contact hierarchy and contact information, personnel assignments, internal and external communication protocols, decontamination procedures and equipment, quarantine and lockdown, evacuation plans, and supply management. The effectiveness of any disaster plan will depend on the weakest link.

The chain of command is the hierarchy for various professionals involved in the response. Responsibilities are based on training and experience. Although health care providers are experienced in providing medical care in general, they lack the specialized training required to manage disasters. Inexperienced providers risk becoming casualties.

Law enforcement, the fire department, emergency medical systems, environmental agencies, public health organizations, and the military are included in the command structure.

The first principle of management is containment with a perimeter. Multiple circumferential perimeters are defined by threat levels. Quarantine may be necessary to prevent continued spread of offensive agents. Quarantine refers to a compulsory physical separation of affected persons and the definition further extends to a restriction of movement and to segregation as an affected group. Isolation is less restrictive and refers to separation and confinement of affected individuals known or suspected to be affected with an infectious agent. Disaster management assistance teams (DMATs) are disaster relief personnel usually deployed within 24–48 hours.

A variety of command posts may need to be established for various services and teams or locations. Command posts report to a command center which has operational control over disaster management personnel. Individual command centers report to a tactical command center which coordinates the allocation of personnel and resources. A strategic command center, usually geographically removed from the immediate disaster area, usually coordinates government agency activities. Communications are critical and likely to be extremely vulnerable. Communications may be targeted. Landline telephone communications may be physically compromised or overwhelmed by excessive use. Efficient communication requires prioritization and organization. Access overload control for cellular radio telephones (ACCOLC) assigns priority to cellular phones used by emergency personnel during periods of circuit overload. Cellular, radio (UHF and VHF), and internet communications provide redundancy. A system of couriers can be locally effective in the setting of a total communications breakdown. External communication is also necessary with local, state, and federal agencies; with the media; and with families.

Methods for cataloging the injured must be in place.

Principles of disaster response form the basis for a disaster plan. Disaster plans exist at the institutional, community, state, regional, and federal levels. Knowledge of the plan and repetitive rehearsal are important to the plan's success. Preparation activities increase organizational capacity in the event of a disaster. Preparation includes resources (material and personnel) inventories, prearranged agreements with suppliers and personnel, staff orientation and training, and drills. Response activities control the situation when it occurs. The first level is organizational and requires internal leadership and coordination with local and regional agencies. The second is a coordinated and dedicated staff response.

GENERAL PRINCIPLES OF MEDICAL MANAGEMENT

Natural Disasters

A "disaster" is defined as a "situation or event which overwhelms local capacity, necessitating a request to national or international levels for external assistance" or a sudden event which "causes great damage, destruction, and human suffering." Natural disasters can include hurricanes, tornadoes, volcanoes, earthquakes, flood, fire, or drought. Natural disasters can have both initial and secondary impact. Initial impact is the result of trauma or environmental exposure. Secondary injuries may occur as a result of impact on technological infrastructure, damage to nuclear, toxic chemical, or biologic facilities with leakage of hazardous materials, the precipitation of dangerous conditions, loss of power, and spread of disease. Initial priorities will include evacuation, evaluation and resuscitation, and containment of casualties.

Public health issues include the availability of basic services (water supply, food supply, electricity, sanitation and waste disposal, housing and shelter, and disposition of human and animal remains). Medical care ranges from trauma resuscitation to vaccination and treatment of secondary illnesses. Psychological support may be necessary to minimize post-traumatic stress disorder (PTSD) or crisis incidence stress disorder (CISD) and long-term psychological impact of the disaster. The purpose of psychiatric intervention is twofold: to provide immediate relief and early return to normal activities, and to prevent the development of chronic syndromes.

Vector control may be necessary to prevent spread of disease by mosquitoes, flies, and rodents.

Conventional Weapons

Explosives remain the most likely mass casualty cause in the USA and elsewhere. Explosives directly cause blast, burn, and penetrating trauma. Additionally, explosive devices will indirectly cause other injuries and fatalities depending on the arena in which the explosives are deployed: buildings, subways, airplanes, industrial complexes, for example. Since the US health care system is currently functioning near or at capacity, special plans must be in place for the care of large numbers of acute casualties.

Biologic Agents

PEARLS

Clues Signaling a Biologic/Chemical/Toxicologic Event
- Large numbers of patients with a similar syndrome
- Large numbers of patients with an unusual disease or syndrome
- A higher morbidity or mortality than expected with common disease
- A single case of a very uncommon disease
- An unusual clinical presentation of a known disease
- An unusual geographic or seasonal distribution

- A sudden or increased incidence of a stable endemic disease
- A similar genetic type of organism isolated from different times or locations
- A simultaneous cluster of outbreaks in noncontiguous geographic areasx

Overview

Throughout history epidemics have killed countless millions, eliminated cultures, defeated empires and their armies, and thereby irrevocably altered the course of civilization. That the power of infectious agents could be strategically and tactically directed for political and military purposes is a logical extrapolation. Bacteria, viruses, fungi, and their biological toxins, as well as newer chemical toxins could be deployed to kill or disable combatants or cripple the civilian or agricultural infrastructure of enemies.

The key advantages of such agents are that they are relatively inexpensive to produce, allow for the preservation of structural integrity following attack, and allow for selective immunization, barrier protective, or antidotal defensive measures. In addition, such agents can be easily deployed, are difficult to detect, and it can be difficult to trace temporal, spatial, and causal origins when used for terrorist purposes. The key disadvantage remains epidemiological unpredictability.

A key function of health care providers will be the rapid diagnosis of index cases and communication with public health authorities. A key dilemma for public health authorities will be the differentiation of the presenting symptoms of the pathogens listed below from other diseases with similar symptoms, especially in the flu season, and to differentiate isolated endemic cases from index cases of potential epidemics. Biologic agents can be categorized as either infectious agents per se or biological toxins.

Infectious Agents

Infectious biologic agents used in biologic warfare or bioterrorism can include bacterial, viral, and atypical organisms. Almost any agent that incapacitates troops can be employed in the battlefield. The most effective terrorism agents are those which incite panic. Bacterial agents which have been successfully weaponized include anthrax (*Bacillus anthracis*), plague (*Yersinia pestis*), and tularemia (*Francisella tularensis*) (Boxes 33-1 and 33-2).

Anthrax is a spore-forming gram-positive bacillus that is endemic worldwide. Occupationally, cutaneous anthrax is contracted by individuals working with contaminated animal fibers such as goat hair. Gastrointestinal anthrax is enzootic in Third World countries with domestic ungulate herds. The use of anthrax as a germ-warfare agent requires that anthrax spores be concentrated, electrostatically stabilized, and disseminated at a target. An outbreak of

Box 33-1   Categorization of Agents

- The Center for Disease Control (CDC) categorizes agents as A–C based on ease of dissemination, impact, and defensibility.
- A-type agents receive the highest priority because of ease of dissemination, person-to-person transmission, and high morbidity and mortality. These agents include anthrax, botulism, plague, smallpox, tularemia, and viral hemorrhagic fevers.

respiratory anthrax should be presumed to be a result of a threat until proven otherwise. The symptomatology of respiratory anthrax follows a biphasic clinical pattern; initially, there is nonspecific syndrome consisting of malaise, fatigue, myalgia, fever, nonproductive cough, and occasionally a sense of precordial fullness. Frequently, this prodrome is followed by signs of improvement after 2–4 days. The second phase of respiratory anthrax is characterized by the acute onset of hypoxia, dyspnea, and severe respiratory failure. Radiographic studies may reveal mediastinal widening and pleural effusion. Septicemia, septic shock, with or without meningitis, then usually develops within 24 hours. The pathophysiology of anthrax-related sepsis is due to toxins produced by the germinating spores. Vaccines, not completely effective, target the exotoxin components. Inhalational anthrax is very difficult to diagnose in its early, treatable stages. Paradoxically, antibiotic therapy must be initiated rapidly, and often empirically, with penicillin or fluoroquinolones such as ciprofloxacin. Spores are extremely tenacious and vigorous decontamination at the site of spore release is necessary.

Plague (bubonic plague, the "black death") eradicated a significant segment of the world's population during a series of pandemics in the Middle Ages. *Y. pestis* is a gram-negative bipolar-staining bacillus which belongs to the Enterobacteriaceae family. Plague is presently endemic worldwide and is also notably endemic in the southwestern United States. Plague is an enzoonotic infection which is transmitted from natural animal reservoirs to

Box 33-2   Anthrax

- Anthrax can present in three different forms: inhalational, cutaneous, and gastrointestinal. Inhalation anthrax is the most lethal form spread by inhalation of anthrax spores.
- Inhalation anthrax has incubation period of 1–7 days and affects the mediastinal lymphatic system causing death by hemorrhagic mediastinitis. There is no respiratory transmission between persons.
- Treatment of inhalation anthrax is with intravenous ciprofloxacin or doxycycline based on sensitivities.

humans by either contaminated tissues or insect vectors. Bubonic plague is characterized by bacterial proliferation in regional lymph nodes. Massive regional lymphadenopathy ("buboe") typically occurs 2–8 days following the bite of an infected flea. The groin is the most common site of buboes. The lymphadenopathy is typically followed by sepsis with high-density bacteremia, diffuse purpuric skin lesions, hemorrhage, and necrosis. Weaponized plague is most likely to be pneumonic plague which is spread by the intentional release of aerosolized bacteria, or by person-to-person droplet-mediated transmission. The incubation period for pneumonic plague is 1–6 days, and is manifested by progressive diffuse lymphadenopathy, hemoptysis, patchy bronchopneumonia or confluent consolidation, purulent sputum, septic shock, and respiratory failure. The mortality rate from pneumonic plague is extremely high. A formalin-killed vaccine is no longer commercially available. Early aggressive treatment with intravenous streptomycin, penicillin, or gentamicin may be effective; postexposure prophylaxis with doxycycline or ciprofloxacin is also recommended. The psychological effect of a widespread urban outbreak of plague is likely to be devastating.

Tularemia is a gram-negative coccobacillus, enzootic primarily in animals, and endemic worldwide, primarily within the northern hemisphere. Tularemia continues to be responsible for significant human morbidity and mortality, and is regionally referred to as either "rabbit fever," "water-rat trapper's disease," or "deerfly fever." The human host in tularemia is generally accidental, occurring through insect vectors. Tularemia can be typhoidal, pneumonic, or ulcero-glandular. The incubation period ranges from 1–21 days but usually starts abruptly with acute onset of fever, chills, headache, malaise, anorexia, and fatigue. Additional prominent symptoms include cough, chest discomfort, emesis, diarrhea, and dysphagia. Pneumonic tularemia occurs in only 7–20% of all tularemia cases, and therefore, a regional outbreak of pulmonary tularemia should suggest a threat. Approximately 25–30% of patients with pulmonary tularemia will not manifest the radiographic infiltrates or other clinical findings for pneumonia. Pulmonary tularemia is characterized by a dry cough, minimal sputum production, pleuritic chest pain, substernal tightness, and only occasional respiratory failure requiring mechanical ventilation. Tularemia is more likely to be incapacitating than lethal. However, severe disease may be complicated by disseminated intravascular regulation, rhabdomyolysis, hepatitis, meningitis, and renal failure. The diagnosis is basically one based in a high index of suspicion. The drug of first choice for all forms of tularemia except meningitis is streptomycin, but gentamicin is an acceptable substitute. A vaccine for tularemia is currently under review by the FDA. Person-to-person transmission of tularemia is unlikely.

Smallpox, caused by the *Variola major* virus, is probably the most feared viral bioterrorism agent.

Because smallpox is considered to have been eradicated worldwide since 1977, even a single case of smallpox would likely indicate a terrorist attack. Smallpox has an incubation period ranging from 7 to 17 days, with an average of 12 days; the illness typically follows a brief prodromal period of 2-4 days during which the virus can be isolated from the blood. The prodromal symptoms are flu-like and include fever, myalgias, nausea, and vomiting. The disease typically begins with a centrifugal rash which progresses in a uniform pattern from maculopapules to vesicles to pustules and scabs over a 1-2 week period. It is important to note that the centrifugal distribution and the homogeneity of the rash are key differential diagnostic points: in chickenpox, lesions are distributed evenly over the body beginning on the trunk and in chickenpox, individual lesions form and scab over at different times. In its most prominent form, death may occur before the rash becomes manifest, and in its most discreet form, the disease may follow its full course to recovery. The mortality in the past has ranged from 25-50%; however, those statistics reflect mortality within a partially immunized population. Vaccination has been shown to be effective up to four days after exposure. Treatment is supportive. Notably, monkeypox is another *Orthopoxvirus* disease caused by a variola virus. It is endemic in African monkeys and can rarely be spread to humans.

Viral hemorrhagic fevers include Marburg and Ebola, which belong to the *Filovirus* class. The incubation period for filovirus fevers ranges from 2 to 19 days and symptoms begin with the abrupt onset of fever, myalgia, and headache. Progression of symptoms to gastroenteritis, pneumonitis, pancreatitis, pharyngitis, and encephalitis is common. With further progression, petechiae, diffuse hemorrhage, and a truncal maculopapular rash may become evident. Typically, in the second week, the patient will either defervesce and improve rapidly, or will die in shock from multiorgan failure. The mortality of Marburg at the present time is approximately 25%. Ebola has higher mortality depending on the subtype of virus: Sudan subtype has mortality of 50%, and Zaire subtype has a much higher mortality of 90%. There are no vaccines or similar preventive measures; antiviral chemotherapy such as Ribavirin may be effective as treatment. Management is supportive and extensive quarantine precautions are indicated. These viruses can be weaponized for aerosolized dissemination.

The viral encephalitides include a variety of agents such as the *Togavirus* subclass of alphaviruses (Eastern equine, Western equine, Venezuelan equine); the flaviviruses (West Nile, Dengue, St. Louis); the Bunyaviruses (Rift Valley); the *Arenaviruses* (Lassa, Junin, and Machupo). Patients with viral encephalitis tend to have signs and symptoms of meningeal inflammation but, in addition to headache, fever, and nuchal rigidity, the patients with encephalitis also have alterations in consciousness. Infections may be acute, subacute or chronic. Treatment is

generally symptomatic unless the cause is otherwise identified to not be viral, in which case specific therapy is usually available and should be instituted as soon as possible.

Q fever, caused by *Coxiella burnetii*, is an enzootic illness in ungulates with worldwide distribution. Humans are infected by inhalation of contaminated aerosols or by insect vectors. *C. burnetii* is a pleomorphic coccobacillus with a gram-negative cell wall which possibly enters host cells. Person-to-person transmission is possible, especially in the pneumonic form of the disease. The incubation period for Q fever is 14-40 days and once again, the prodrome and clinical illness are nonspecific. Clinical manifestations range from pneumonia, to endocarditis, hepatitis, osteomyelitis, encephalitis, and meningitis. The radiographic appearance of Q fever pneumonia is variable; however nonsegmental and segmental pleural-based opacities are common findings. A pleural effusion is found in approximately 35% of cases. The pneumonia is rarely fatal. The treatment of choice is doxycycline or tetracycline, which can also be used for postexposure prophylaxis. An investigational vaccine is currently under development.

Community surveillance and centralized reporting form the basis for a bioterrorism response. Potential indications for intentional release of a bioweapon include unusual temporal or geographic presentations, unusual severity, and rapid epidemiologic spread.

Rapid diagnosis can be achieved using either immunologic testing or electron micrography for many agents. Containment and prevention of secondary spread are vital. Access to the National Pharmaceutical Stockpile for treatment will be managed by the Center for Disease Control in the armed forces. Rapid immunization or dispensation of prophylactic medication will help contain centers of outbreak.

Toxins and Chemical Agents

A disaster that involves the release of toxic chemicals and widespread toxic exposure of a population can occur in two different scenarios: first, the intentional release of a chemical warfare agent directed against the population; and second, the accidental or intentional spillage of stored or transported toxic chemicals in a populated area. A third potential scenario is chemical terrorism directed at the food supply chain, a scenario of which is discussed below.

Broadly speaking, a chemical attack could occur through the use of either toxins or synthetic chemical agents. The toxins represent a category of agents related to biological agents and also chemical agents. The toxins are products of biological processes or organisms which must be concentrated and weaponized prior to deployment. In general, toxins are proteins with high affinity to cellular binding sites. The toxins represent chemicals that include some of the most potent and deadly compounds known. Similar to chemical agents, toxins can be inhaled, ingested, or dermally absorbed.

Toxins

Botulinum toxin is the most potent toxin known (Box 33-3). It is a naturally occurring product of *Clostridium botulinum* and is comprised of seven different molecular toxins. The LD_{50} is 0.001 μg/kg. The mechanism of action of botulinum toxin is through binding to the neuronal cell membrane at the nerve terminus, followed by endocytosis, then the light chain of botulinum toxin cleaves specific sites on SNARE proteins preventing assembly of the symmetric fusion complex and blocking the release of acetylcholine. The intensive care unit (ICU) at Unity Health System in Rochester, New York, recently cared for a patient exposed to botulinum toxin who was in the ICU for almost a year. Botulinum toxin produces a flaccid paralysis. A pentavalent antidote available from the US Department of Defense must be administered early.

Clostridium tetanii produces tetanus toxin. The LD_{50} is 0.002 μg/kg. Tetanus produces a rigid, tetanic paralysis.

Ricin is a protein byproduct of castor bean processing in the production of castor oil. Ricin is a toxic byproduct of castor oil fermentation and affects cellular protein synthesis. Inhalation exposure produces symptoms within 4-8 hours manifested by pulmonary edema and respiratory tract necrosis. Treatment is supportive. Processing yields 3-5% ricin by weight and there is thus a large amount of ricin available. The LD_{50} is 3.0 μg/kg. Inhalation causes acute respiratory distress with pulmonary lesions; ingestion causes gastrointestinal hemorrhage with necrosis of the liver, spleen and kidneys; intramuscular injection

causes localized pain, and muscle and regional lymph node necrosis.

Staphylococcal enterotoxin B is a seven-component pyrogenic protein toxin isolated from *S. aureus*. The toxin classes and subclasses stimulate T-cells and cause fever and myalgia, nonproductive cough and interstitial edema, headache, and gastrointestinal complaints. The LD_{50} is 0.02 μg/kg.

Chemical Agents

Chemical agents are classified as vesicants, nerve agents, toxic inhalants, cyanogens, or riot control agents.

Vesicants

Vesicants include the mustards (HD, HT, HN), Lewisite (L), and phosgene (CX) and are defined to be agents that produce blisters or vesicles. These agents have been available since World War I. The mustards enter the body through the mucous membranes or the skin and react with proteins and nucleic acids. DNA replication is inhibited. There are no immediate signs or symptoms on contact, inhalation, or ingestion, unless direct exposure to concentrate occurs. Odor is variable. Symptoms occur 2-24 hours after exposure and include destruction of the spleen and bone marrow. The eyes are extremely sensitive to mustard gas. Mucosal sloughing of the lower respiratory tract followed by pneumonia and pulmonary edema result from heavy exposure. The mustards are also teratogenic.

Lewisite inhibits multiple enzymes by reacting with either glutathione or sulfhydryl groups. Lewisite contains arsenic and reacts with enzymes to cause pulmonary edema, diarrhea, fever, and lethargy. Lewisite causes immediate pain and irritation on contact, with erythema and blistering. Although Lewisite also inhibits DNA replication, it generally spares the bone marrow. It causes more severe tissue destruction. Death is usually from respiratory failure, bronchospasm, or pneumonia. The clinical effects are similar to mustard gas exposure and include profound shock from plasma leakage. Lewisite has an odor similar to that of geraniums. The specific antidote is Dimercapterol (2,3-dimercaptopropanol), otherwise known as British Anti-Lewisite (BAL), and aggressive intravenous fluid management. Iodophors and topical antibiotics may limit skin damage. Lewisite, like the mustards, is teratogenic.

Phosgene is commonly grouped with the blister agents and is a urticant causing extreme irritation of tissues. Phosgene has not been previously used in warfare. Like the vesicants it also inhibits DNA replication. Epithelial sloughing occurs from the skin and the respiratory, gastrointestinal, and genitourinary tracts. It is a potent pulmonary irritant. There is immediate pain on contact and ocular exposure results in conjunctivitis and keratitis. The main lesion is pulmonary edema with necrotizing bronchiolitis and thrombosis of pulmonary vessels. There is no laboratory test or antidote. Rapid topical

---

Box 33-3 Botulism

- Botulism results from the ingestion of botulinum toxin types A–G which are produced by *C. botulinum* and two other clostridial species. Botulinum toxin is the most potent neurotoxin known and affects the presynaptic releases of the acetylcholine, blocking neuromuscular transmission. The onset of botulinum toxin is generally slow and incapacitation is progressive ending in respiratory fatigue and generalized paralysis in 24-72 hours. Specific antitoxin therapy is available.

- The onset of botulism ranges from 24 hours to several days depending on the dose ingested. Person-to-person transmission is not generally an issue. Botulism can be treated using an equine polyvalent antitoxin if administered early. In the setting of established botulism, long-term mechanical ventilatory support and routine critical care management are necessary.

decontamination is essential. An effective decontaminant is 0.5% sodium hypochlorate if immediately available; otherwise copious water irrigation should be used. Iodophors may limit toxicity. Treatment is decontamination and supportive care.

Nerve Agents

Nerve agents include Tabun (GA), Sarin (GB), Soman (GD), and VX. The effects of nerve agents occur in seconds to minutes depending on the concentration of vapor. Biotoxicity is a function of acetylcholinesterase inhibition in the plasma, on red blood cells, and at the synapses. Accumulation of acetylcholine causes symptoms within minutes. Symptoms are therefore both nicotinic and muscarinic, being due to both nicotinic and muscarinic overactivity and include bronchorrhea, rhinorrhea, and bronchoconstriction; miosis; bradyarrhythmias; nausea, vomiting, and diarrhea; muscle fasciculations; and loss of consciousness and apnea. GB and VX are odorless, and GA and GD smell fruity. Sarin has an LD_{50} that is 26 times less than cyanide gas. Antidotes include atropine (6 mg IV/IM), diazepam, and pralidoxime hydrochloride (2-PAM). MARK and nerve agent antidote kits (NAAKs) contain these antidotes.

Toxic Inhalants

Toxic inhalants include phosgene (CX, CG), diphosgene (DP), chloropicrin (PS), and chlorine (Cl). The toxic inhalants/pulmonary agents specifically attack the lung tissue and cause pulmonary edema; their specificity differentiates these agents from the vesicants, which incidentally involve the respiratory tract. CG and DP are colorless and have the odor of green corn or freshly mown hay. These agents have a latent period of several hours. Pulmonary edema occurs due to an acetylation reaction which precipitates acute leakage at the alveolar–capillary membrane. Treatment is supportive and often requires airway maintenance, fluids/vasopressors, theophylline, and methylprednisolone.

Cyanogens

Cyanogens are variants of cyanide and include hydrogen cyanide (AC) and cyanogen chloride (CK). These compounds combine with the iron molecule of cytochrome a3 and precipitate anaerobic glycolysis and lactic acidosis due to cellular hypoxia. Cyanogens may have the odor of bitter almonds. The onset of effect is within 15–30 seconds and includes vomiting, convulsions, and respiratory failure. Antidotes consist of thiosulfate and sodium nitrite which form thiocyanate and methemoglobin, binding cyanide.

Riot Control Agents

Riot control agents are used by police departments and include lacrimants and irritants. Riot control agents include chloroacetophenone (CN), ortho-chlorobenzylidene-malononitrile (CS), dibenz(b,f)-1,4-oxazepine (CR), and Adamsite (DM). The riot control agents are lacrimants, skin irritants, and vomiting agents. Effects occur immediately on exposure and usually last 15–30 minutes. Treatment is supportive; however, asthmatics may require bronchodilator therapy and persistent ocular irritation may require ophthalmology consultation. Agent 15 is a nonlethal psychotomimetic agent which causes incapacitation from delirium. It can be ingested, inhaled, or absorbed. Symptoms are anticholinergic (delirium, temperature, dry mouth, and papillary dilatation). Physostigmine is an antidote.

Other Chemicals

A large variety of hazardous materials are stored near populated areas and are transported on public roads every day. These include hydrocarbons, corrosive agents, oxidizing agents, compressed gases, insecticides, and heavy metals. Examples include ammonia, pentaborane, potassium cyanide, sodium superoxide, and vanadium tetrachloride.

General Principles of Chemical/Toxic Response

The critical points regarding the medical response are (a) that medical personnel typically do not have the training or experience to become involved at "ground zero" and that the best of intentions may have disastrous effects, (b) that in any chemical or biological disaster there will be some patients who present without decontamination or treatment, (c) that the medical response must be prepared to triage, continue supportive care, specifically identify the threat, and institute antidotal therapy, and (d) the leadership of the hospital-based care team (Box 33-4).

Protective containment actions are (a) the initial isolation zone: surrounds the incident and includes upwind and downwind areas; and (b) the protective actions zone: areas downwind from the incident. These areas are considered perimeters. The key purposes of a perimeter are minimization of secondary injury and spread of the toxin. Protective actions also include the use of protective gear including the battledress overgarment (BDO) and the mission-oriented protective posture (MOPP) suits. In some circumstances protective action can also include prophylactic administration of antidotes

---

Box 33-4 Management

- Continued medical education is fundamental to an effective and concerted disaster response and national security.
- Mass simultaneous casualties in a concentrated area with the same or similar presenting symptoms raise immediate suspicion for chemical or toxin exposure.
- General management principles include decontamination, ventilation, antidote administration, and supportive therapies.

to chemical agents prior to entry into an "event" zone. Protective containment also requires an understanding of prevailing and forecast meteorologic conditions. Evacuation requires the movement of people from a threatened area to a safer place. This may include decontaminated survivors. Meteorologic conditions are important to dispersal and containment. Wind influences dispersal whereas rain can remove toxin particles from the air. Shelter in place should be considered when the risk of evacuating exposed patients could pose greater public harm than keeping them in place and treating them when they are. This can include isolation and/or quarantine.

PEARLS

- Contaminated clothing must be removed since it is a source of continued exposure
- Antidotes may need to be administered immediately on exposure
- Survivors of the initial exposure can then be managed to minimize injury
- Decontamination by dilution with large quantities of water is the first line of therapy
- The spread of agents will be largely determined by environmental conditions
- Evacuation is in the downwind direction
- Approach to the affected area is from upwind

The fundamental principle of decontamination after chemical or toxic exposure is dilution. Dilution can be accomplished by copious irrigation with water but can also include using soap and dilute solutions of sodium hydrochlorite (bleach). Decontamination procedures are essential and relatively easy consisting of the removal of residual agents from clothing and skin. Dry decontamination employs absorbant powder, whereas wet decontamination works by dilution. Mild soap or bleach solutions can increase the effectiveness of wet decontamination. It is important to remember that those performing decontamination must protect themselves from exposure to toxic agents. Decontamination logistics must also include the decontamination facility, water supply, personnel and protective gear, and potentially drainage control (Box 33-5).

Nuclear Threat

Although nuclear attack in the form of warfare remains an ever-present possibility, the indiscriminate global ramifications have made retaliation a sound mutually accepted deterrent strategy. Nuclear casualties are most likely to arise from a reactor mishap, inadvertent spillage of contained nuclear waste, or a terrorist attack (Box 33-6).

Box 33-5 Intensive Care Unit Care

Following decontamination provisions for intensive cardiovascular support for mass casualties will be necessary. The doses of atropine required to treat nerve agent exposure are massive. Immediate treatment with specific antidotes can be lifesaving. In the case of nerve agents and cyanogens, antidotes are available. The understanding of symptoms and their management is also important. Since ventilators are not likely to be available for all casualties, AMBU ventilation via endotracheal tubes may be necessary. Mouth-to-mouth resuscitation can be dangerous and expose rescuers to residual nerve agents, especially VX. Anesthesiologists possess specialized knowledge regarding airway management, chemical ventilation, fluid management, hemodynamic support, and assessment of central nervous system and neuromuscular function. Additional supportive care may include topical application of Betadine to limit the effects of vesicants, burn and wound care, and antibiotics where indicated.

Nuclear radiation refers to ionizing radiation and includes alpha, beta, and gamma radiation, and neutrons. Ionizing radiation directly interacts with cellular water to produce highly reactive free radicals and with nucleic acids to affect cell replication and tissue regeneration.

The unit for exposure is the roentgen, symbol R, equal to 2.58×10^{-4} coulombs/kg of air. The unit for absorption is the rad, which is equal to 100 ergs per gram of energy deposited. The unit for tissue effects is the dose equivalent, which is equal to absorbed dose $\times$ quality factor.

Clinical acute radiation syndrome follows the acute absorption of 2000–4000 rad, has immediate onset, and is usually rapidly lethal. An absorption of 70–2000 rad equates with a fair chance of survival and is manifested by severe nausea, vomiting, bloody diarrhea, severe capillary leak, and hypovolemia. Lower doses cause bleeding, immunosuppression, vomiting, and severe fatigue. Potassium iodide (KI) can protect the thyroid if it is administered within 3–4 hours of radiation exposure. Paradoxically, KI administered after radioactive iodine has become concentrated in the thyroid will actually block the elimination of radioactive iodine and worsen its effects. Decontamination is with soap and water and requires protective gear.

Box 33-6 Dirty Bomb

The "dirty" bomb is a high-yield conventional explosive contaminated with radioactive material such as uranium, cobalt-60, cesium-137, plutonium, or thorium.

Food and Water Supply

Food and water supplies are vulnerable to contamination by chemical, biologic, and nuclear agents. Dilution naturally protects the water supply to some extent. Diversity of ingredients and diverse food sources make large-scale food contamination difficult. Specific contamination of a point food source such as a salad bar has occurred (i.e., the Dalles, Oregon). Such contaminations are similar to other "outbreaks" of food poisoning and are differentiated by the intent behind the occurrence. Contamination of fertilizers or the introduction of pathogens such as hoof-and-mouth disease or s pongiform encephalopathy ("wasting disease") are possible, but logistically difficult, easily detectable, and can be intercepted early. A high index of suspicion, communication, and situational awareness is always necessary.

SELECTED READING

Arnon SS, Schechter R, Inglesby TV et al: Botulinum toxin as a biological weapon. JAMA 285:1059–1070, 2001.

Barbera J, Macintyre A, Gostin L et al: Large-scale quarantine following biological terrorism in the United States: scientific examination, logistic and legal limits, and possible consequences. JAMA 286(21):2711–2717, 2001.

Borio L, Inglesby T, Peters CJ et al: Hemorrhagic fever viruses as biological weapons: medical and public health management. JAMA 287(18):2391–2405, 2002.

Henderson DA, Inglesby TV, Bartlett JG et al: Smallpox as a biological weapon: medical and public health management. JAMA 281(22):2127–2137, 1999.

Inglesby TV, Dennis DT, Henderson DA et al: Plague as a biological weapon. JAMA 283:2281–2290, 2000.

Inglesby TV, O'Toole T, Henderson DA et al: Anthrax as a biological weapon, 2002: updated recommendations for management. JAMA 287(17):2236–2252, 2002.

Mayer TA, Bersoff-Matcha S, Murphy C et al: Clinical presentation of inhalational anthrax following bioterrorism exposure: report of 2 surviving patients. JAMA 286(20):2549–2553, 2001.

Novick LF, Marr JS: *Public Health Issues in Disaster Preparedness*, Gaithersburg, MD: Aspen Publications, 2001.

Sidell FR, Takafuji ET, Franz DR: *Textbook of Military Medicine. Part I. Medical Aspects of Chemical and Biological Warfare*, Washington, DC: TMM Publications, Office of the Surgeon General, Walter Reed Army Medical Center, 1997.

Szalados JE: Chemical terrorism response and the anesthesiologist: conventional agents, emerging threats, and management principles. TraumaCare 14(1):15–23, 2004.

Walker RI, Cerveny TJ: *Textbook of Military Medicine. Part I. Medical Consequences of Nuclear Warfare*, Washington, DC: TMM Publications, Office of the Surgeon General, Walter Reed Army Medical Center, 1989.

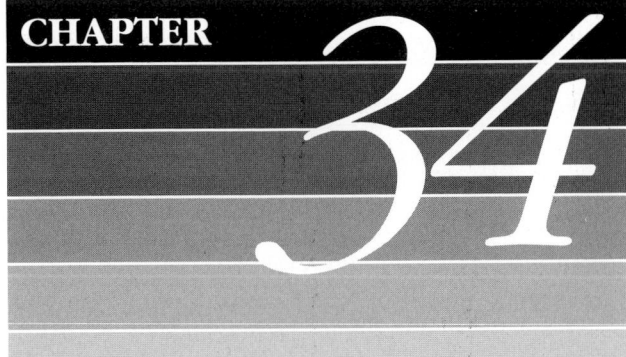

Poisoning

JOSEPH DOOLEY, M.D.

Patients suffering from either intentional or accidental poisoning frequently require an admission to the intensive care unit (ICU). Poisoning may also be associated with traumas, such as carbon monoxide with burns, and illegal drugs with motor vehicle accidents. Resuscitation and stabilization should be the first priority when treating the poisoning victim. It is then important to limit absorption of the toxin, identify the toxin, and initiate specific therapy. This chapter focuses on these points and examines the identification and treatment of specific agents. A discussion of the treatment of patients exposed to chemical weapons completes the chapter.

RESUSCITATION AND STABILIZATION

Identifying the toxic agent should never delay the resuscitation of the patient. Using basic life support guidelines, the patient's airway, breathing, and circulation should be assessed and problems treated. Many agents can cause respiratory insufficiency and therefore supplemental oxygen should be administered. In some cases tracheal intubation and mechanical ventilation are required. If a patient is at risk for aspiration, due to a depressed level of consciousness, the airway should be protected. In most cases this would be accomplished with a rapid sequence induction and oral intubation. Next, attention is turned to the cardiovascular system. Many agents can cause hypotension (usually by increases in venous capacitance). Therefore, hypotensive patients should have IV access established and be treated with isotonic crystalloid solutions to correct intravascular volume deficiencies. Certain agents are associated with life-threatening tachycardia and hypertension, which would require pharmacologic intervention. When the patient is hemodynamically stable with adequate oxygenation and ventilation, attention should be turned toward identifying the toxic agent and the extent of the exposure. In addition, a patient presenting with an unexplained depression of level of consciousness should receive intravenous thiamine (100 mg), intravenous dextrose (ampule of D_{50}), and intravenous naloxone (0.4–2 mg).

DIAGNOSIS

After the initial resuscitation, attention should be turned toward determining the responsible toxin(s). When possible, the administered substance (ingestion, injection, inhalation) and extent of exposure (quantity, timing, and chronicity) should be determined. Sources for this information include the patient, family members, and friends. Next, a physical examination should be performed, which could supply useful information, since many toxins produce predictable physiologic changes (see Tables 34-1 and 34-2). In addition, there are constellations of symptoms that characterize certain poisoning syndromes. These are known as "toxidromes" (Table 34-3).

Laboratory examinations may be of benefit in the evaluation and treatment of patients suffering from poisoning. These examinations include an arterial blood gas, qualitative toxicology screens, quantitative analyses, and, perhaps, an EKG. An arterial blood gas is useful for

Table 34-1	Clues to Diagnosis in Poisoning: Vital Signs	

Vital sign	Increased	Decreased
Blood pressure	Amphetamines Cocaine Anticholinergics Sympathomimetics	Antihypertensives Cyclic antidepressants Narcotics Organophosphates Sedatives/hypnotics
Heart rate	Amphetamines Cocaine Anticholinergics Ethanol Sympathomimetics Theophylline	Barbiturates Beta-blockers Cholinergics Digoxin Sedatives/hypnotics
Respiratory rate	Amphetamines Anticholinergics Carbon monoxide Hydrocarbons Organophosphates Salicylates	Alcohol Barbiturates Narcotics Sedatives/hypnotics Gamma-hydroxy- butyrate (GHB)
Temperature	Amphetamines Cocaine Anticholinergics Beta-blockers Cyclic antidepressants Salicylates Sympathomimetics	Sedatives/hypnotics Barbiturates Carbon monoxide Ethanol Hypoglycemics Narcotics Sedatives/hypnotics Gamma-hydroxy- butyrate (GHB)

Reproduced with permission of the Society of Critical Care Medicine from Zimmerman JL: Poisoning/overdose. In Dries DJ, editor: *5th Critical Care Refresher Course*, ed 5, Des Plaines, IL: Society of Critical Care Medicine, 2001, pp 123-136.

several reasons. Determining hypoxia, hypercarbia, and anion gaps may be useful in determining the offending agent. In addition, the information gained may prompt emergent treatment such as securing the airway and providing mechanical ventilation. Qualitative toxicology screens are performed on urine samples and report only the presence or absence of a substance. They are limited

Table 34-2	Clues to Diagnosis in Poisoning: Neurologic Findings

Pinpoint Pupils (Miotic)	Dilated Pupils (Mydriatic)
Cholinergics	Alcohol
Narcotics	Anticholinergics
Organophosphates	Antihistamines
Phenothiazine	Phenytoin
Phencyclidine (PCP)	Sympathomimetics

Reproduced with permission of the Society of Critical Care Medicine from Zimmerman JL: Poisoning/overdose. In Dries DJ, editor: *5th Critical Care Refresher Course*, ed 5, Des Plaines, IL: Society of Critical Care Medicine, 2001, pp 123-136.

Table 34-3	Toxidromes

Drug Class	Symptoms
Cholinergics	Salivation, lacrimation, urination, defecation, GI upset, emesis (SLUDGE); also, bradycardia, fasciculations, confusion, meiosis
Anticholinergics	Dry skin, hyperthermia, mydriasis, delirium, thirst
Sympathomimetics	Hypertension, tachycardia, seizures, CNS excitation, mydriasis
Narcotics	Miosis, respiratory depression, depressed level of consciousness
Sedatives/hypnotics	Depressed level of consciousness, respiratory depression, hyporeflexia

Reproduced with permission of the Society of Critical Care Medicine from Zimmerman JL: Poisoning/overdose. In Dries DJ, editor: *5th Critical Care Refresher Course*, ed 5, Des Plaines, IL: Society of Critical Care Medicine, 2001, pp 123-136.

to the particular tests performed at individual institutions. The "tox screen" is often of limited utility, since it rarely changes therapy and many toxins are not detectable. Quantitative serum levels are useful in the treatment of acetaminophen and salicylate overdoses. Other potentially useful quantitative levels include carboxyhemoglobin, ethanol, methanol, ethylene glycol, theophylline, phenytoin, lithium, barbiturates, digoxin, cyclic antidepressants, lead, mercury, and arsenic.

TREATMENT

After the initial stabilization of the patient, efforts are turned toward decreasing the exposure to the agent through gastrointestinal (GI) decontamination and/or enhanced elimination. During this time it is important to continue efforts to support the airway and ventilation and to maintain hemodynamic stability.

GI decontamination can be accomplished through several modalities. This includes gastric emptying procedures, adsorption of drugs, and increasing transit through the GI tract. Gastric emptying procedures include ipecac-induced emesis and gastric lavage. Ipecac-induced emesis has very limited utility. It is not used when managing adult poisoning victims. It is contraindicated in patients with depressed level of consciousness or when corrosive substances or hydrocarbons are ingested. Complications of induced emesis include aspiration pneumonitis, esophageal rupture, and Mallory–Weiss tear (upper GI hemorrhage). Gastric lavage with a large-bore (36–40 F) orogastric tube has been used. It is contraindicated in caustic and hydrocarbon ingestions, in patients at risk of GI perforation, in combative patients, and in patients with severe coagulopathies. The current recommendation is that gastric lavage only be used for life-threatening quantities of poison when the therapy can be instituted within 60 minutes of the ingestion. There is no good evidence showing the benefit of gastric lavage (although the highest risk patients are often excluded from the studies). The decision to perform gastric lavage must be made on a case-by-case basis. Its use is limited.

Single-dose activated charcoal is the most common technique used for GI decontamination. The activated charcoal adsorbs the toxin in the GI tract thus limiting systemic absorption. The usual dose is 1 g/kg. Activated charcoal is not effective in adsorbing iron, lithium, cyanide, strong acids and bases, alcohols, and some hydrocarbons. Activated charcoal is contraindicated in patients with depressed levels of consciousness who do not have airway protection, or if a GI perforation is known or suspected. Studies suggest that the maximum benefit of activated charcoal is obtained when it is administered within one hour of the ingestion.

Cathartics and whole bowel irrigation have been used in poisonings. It is felt that limiting the contact time with the GI tract may be of some benefit in limiting absorption. There is no clinical evidence showing the benefit of either technique.

The other major treatment category for managing toxic exposures is enhanced elimination. Enhanced elimination can be achieved with multiple-dose activated charcoal (MDAC), urinary alkalinization, and renal replacement therapies.

MDAC is used to adsorb agents that are initially absorbed but then reenter the GI tract. Toxins (or their metabolites) reenter the GI tract either through the enterohepatic circulation (present in bile) or through active secretion or passive diffusion distal to the stomach. There is no strong evidence demonstrating the efficacy of MDAC. However, it has been recommended that MDAC be used in the cases of life-threatening ingestion of carbamazepine, dapsone, phenobarbital, quinine, or theophylline. MDAC is administered either as bolus doses (0.5–1.0 g/kg every 4 hours) or a continuous infusion (0.25–0.5 g/kg/hour, not less than 12.5 g/hour).

Urinary alkalinization has been of proven benefit in poisoning involving weak acids such as salicylates, phenobarbital, and primidone. The weak acids are ionized in the alkaline urine where they are trapped in the renal tubules, and then cleared. Urinary alkalinization is achieved by administering a sodium bicarbonate drip. The drip can be made in multiple ways including adding three ampules of sodium bicarbonate to 1 liter of sterile water or varying amounts of sodium bicarbonate (e.g., 75 mEq) in D_5W. The drip rate is then adjusted to achieve a urinary pH of 7.5–8.5. Electrolytes should be monitored and corrected as needed.

Renal replacement techniques used to enhance elimination include intermittent hemodialysis, intermittent hemoperfusion, continuous hemofiltration (CVVH), and continuous hemodialysis (CVVHD). Hemodialysis should be used early in the treatment of toxicities involving methanol, ethylene glycol, salicylates, lithium, boric acid, and thallium. Hemoperfusion involves passing whole blood through an adsorbent containing (charcoal) cartridge. Charcoal hemoperfusion is the preferred method for eliminating carbamazepine, phenobarbital, phenytoin, and theophylline. Continuous renal replacement techniques are of primary benefit for patients who are not hemodynamically stable enough to tolerate intermittent techniques.

SPECIFIC TOXICITIES

Clearly there is a large variety of substances that can cause toxicities. An exhaustive discussion of many different agents is beyond the scope of this chapter. This chapter examines substances that are more likely to be associated with critically ill patients in the ICU. Although not yet seen in the West, a terrorist attack using nerve agents is a distinct possibility. These agents will be briefly discussed.

Acetaminophen

Acetaminophen (N-acetyl-p-aminophenol (APAP)) toxicity is commonly seen. The reason for this is multifactorial. Clearly, it is easily available to individuals wishing to harm themselves. In addition, it is present in a large number of medications, which may not be known to many patients. For example, patients taking percocet for pain may supplement themselves with acetaminophen and easily achieve toxic doses. Many lay people are unaware of the potential toxicity of APAP. APAP can lead to hepatotoxicity and potential mortality that is preventable. APAP toxicity is the second leading cause of acute liver failure in the USA and is the leading cause in the UK. APAP is metabolized in the liver to the toxic metabolite N-acetyl-p-benzoquinoneimine, which results in liver cell injury and death. Maximal hepatic cell injury occurs at 72–96 hours postingestion. Initial symptoms include right upper quadrant pain and abnormal liver function tests. The severity of symptoms is somewhat variable and depends on the quantity of ingestion. Toxicity may occur when 7.5–10 g are ingested over 8 hours. Fatalities are rare for doses less than 15 g. Symptoms may progress to encephalopathy, coagulopathy, jaundice, and renal failure. When patients develop encephalopathy (fulminant hepatic failure), they have a mortality approaching 80%. At this point, liver transplant may be their only option (60–80% survival). The treatment for APAP toxicity beyond the supportive measures described earlier is to administer *N*-acetylcysteine (NAC (mucomyst)). For acute, single ingestions an APAP level is obtained at 4 hours after ingestion (or immediately on admission if the time of the ingestion is unknown). The Rumack–Matthew nomogram is used to determine whether or not to institute NAC therapy. The initial dose of mucomyst is 140 mg/kg administered orally (PO or NG) followed by 70 mg/kg doses every 4 hours for 17 doses. The treatment duration and dosing should be coordinated with the local poison control service.

Salicylates

Salicylate toxicity should be suspected if a metabolic acidosis with an anion gap is present on blood gas analysis. Initial symptoms include tinnitus and nausea/vomiting. Tachypnea, respiratory alkalosis, and hyperthermia are seen. Symptoms may progress to include depressed level of consciousness, coma, seizures, coagulopathy, transient hepatotoxicity, and hypoglycemia. Treatment includes alkalization of the urine and administering activated charcoal. In severe cases hemodialysis may be required.

Carbon Monoxide

Carbon monoxide (CO) poisoning is common and could be the result of accidental exposure (car/structure fires, poorly ventilated heaters, poorly ventilated generators, etc.) or intentional exposure. CO binds to hemoglobin with an affinity 200–250 times greater than oxygen. This results in poor oxygen delivery to the tissues which leads to cell hypoxia and possibly cell death. Clinical manifestations are nonspecific and may be confused with other illnesses unless the exposure is known or suspected. Common symptoms include headache, nausea, and vomiting. Other signs and symptoms include confusion, arrhythmias, angina, syncope, seizures, tachycardia, and tachypnea. Clearly, death can be the result of severe exposures. Of those that recover from acute CO exposure, 10–30% have delayed neuropsychiatric sequelae. Many may have a permanent neurologic injury. Quantitative CO levels should be obtained on either arterial or venous blood gases. Management includes administering 100% oxygen until CO levels return to normal and treating clinical abnormalities (cardiac ischemia, arrhythmias, acid–base disorders, etc.). In severe cases hyperbaric oxygen therapy may be instituted. This can decrease the half-life of carboxyhemoglobin from 40 to 80 minutes (with isobaric 100% oxygen) to 15 to 30 minutes. Hyperbaric oxygen therapy is not widely available, which limits its use. Furthermore, outcome studies have not shown a benefit of hyperbaric oxygen therapy on

the long-term sequelae and mortality associated with CO poisoning.

Cocaine and Amphetamines/ Metamphetamines

These drugs are widely used and abused in the USA and may be seen in patients presenting to the ICU. Clearly use of these agents may lead to severe trauma, which would then complicate the treatment of the patient's injuries. Adverse sequelae of the use of these drugs have complicated the course of routine surgical procedures. The most severe sequelae include cardiovascular complications (severe hypertension, arrhythmias, myocardial ischemia, and aortic dissection) and neurovascular complications (seizures, cerebral infarction, and intracranial hemorrhage). The management of these complications is largely supportive (managing hypertension, cardiac ischemia, arrhythmias, seizures, etc.).

Beta-blockers and Calcium Channel Blockers

Occasionally, overdoses of beta-blockers and calcium channel blockers are seen. The most common manifestations include bradycardia, hypotension, and atrioventricular conduction abnormalities. Central nervous system (CNS) abnormalities, such as lethargy, confusion, and coma, are sometimes seen. The cardiovascular abnormalities are difficult to manage with traditional inotropes and vasopressors. Initial management includes isotonic intravenous fluid, atropine, and glucagon. Glucagon stimulates cyclic adenosine monophosphate (cAMP) thus bypassing the adrenergic receptors. In some cases high-dose vasopressors/inotropes may be required.

Other Agents

Other agents that may be seen in toxic levels in the ICU include benzodiazepines, opioids, digoxin, etc. Benzodiazepines and opioids are commonly used in the hospital for sedation and analgesia. Patients may receive excessive dosages of these agents. Treatment primarily involves respiratory support until serum levels decrease. Occasionally, a benzodiazepine antagonist (flumazenil) or narcotic antagonist (naloxone) may be used to treat overdoses. Caution should be used with both. Flumazenil use has been associated with seizures. Complete block of narcotic receptors in the setting of severe injury or surgery will result in severe pain with possible hypertension, tachycardia, and pulmonary edema. If naloxone is used, small doses should be administered until the respiratory status improves while maintaining adequate pain control. Toxic digoxin levels are occasionally seen in the ICU especially in patients on chronic doses who develop renal insufficiency. Manifestations include a large variety of cardiac arrhythmias, anorexia, nausea/vomiting, and hyperkalemia. The standard of care for life-threatening digoxin toxicity is to administer digoxin-specific antibody fragments (digibind). There are many other agents that can cause toxicity in the ICU. When unexpected symptoms are encountered, an investigation of agents used/exposed to should be undertaken and treatment initiated. This often involves consultation with the local poison control service.

CHEMICAL WARFARE AGENTS

In the current world situation a major chemical attack in a large populated area is a distinct possibility. There were 27,000 casualties due to the use of chemical weapons (including mustard gas and tabun nerve agent) by the Iraqis during the Iran–Iraq war. Even more concerning, there were several fatalities and hundreds of casualties when the Aum Shinrikyo cult released sarin nerve gas in a Tokyo subway. These agents could be used in a terrorist attack in the future. It is therefore reasonable for physicians managing ICUs to have knowledge of the identification and treatment of these agents.

There are several classes of chemical weapons that may be employed. These include the nerve agents (sarin, tabun, soman, VX), blistering agents (mustard gas, Lewisite), choking agents (chlorine, phosgene, chloropicrin), blood agents (hydrogen cyanide and cyanogen chloride), and toxins (saxitoxin, ricin, and botulinum toxin). It is beyond the scope of this chapter to discuss all of the agents. This chapter briefly discusses the more likely agents, namely the nerve agents and blistering agents.

Nerve agents are irreversible anticholinesterases of high potency and are chemically related to organophosphate insecticides. They inactivate acetylcholinesterase (AChE), which causes accumulation of acetylcholine at muscarinic, nicotinic, and CNS synapses. The muscarinic effects include miosis, glandular hypersecretion (salivary, bronchial, and lacrimal), sweating, bradycardia, atrioventricular block, QT prolongation, bronchoconstriction, diarrhea, and incontinence of urine/stool. The effects on the nicotinic receptors progress from fasciculations to skeletal muscle weakness to paralysis. AChE inactivation in the CNS results in irritability, giddiness, ataxia, fatigue, amnesia, hypothermia, lethargy, seizures, coma, and respiratory depression. Death can occur through a variety of mechanisms. Treatment must be instituted rapidly if there is going to be any chance of survival.

Like other poisonings, attention to basic resuscitation (intubation, controlled ventilation, etc.) must be made. Atropine and oximes are effective antidotes but need to be administered early (i.e., in the field). If the patient survives to the ICU, continued treatment will probably be necessary. Atropine antagonizes the muscarinic and CNS effects. It is preferable to glycopyrrolate, which does not cross the blood–brain barrier. The initial dose of atropine is 2 mg IV and should be repeated every 5-10 minutes until pupillary dilation occurs and heart rate rises above 80 beats/minute. An atropine infusion (0.02–0.08 mg/kg/hour, up to 1000 mg/day) may be required for persistent bradycardia. The oximes (pralidoxime) reverse nicotinic receptor dysfunction and thus reduce or reverse skeletal muscle weakness. They reactivate AChE by cleavage of phosphorylated active sites, detoxify unbonded nerve agent molecules by direct action, and have an endogenous anticholinergic effect. Irreversible bonds between the nerve agents and AChE form after 2 minutes of exposure to soman, after 5 hours for sarin, after 13 hours for tabun, and after 48 hours for VX gas. This gives time to administer the pralidoxime for most of the agents. Other potential treatments include diazepam (control seizures and limit long-term neurologic sequelae), clonidine to control CNS cholinergic symptoms, and magnesium to reduce presynaptic ACh release.

Mustard gas is the most likely used vesicant. It causes NAD^+ depletion, which disrupts glycolysis and causes the release of destructive proteases. There is a latency period between exposure and the development of symptoms. Therefore, close observation is required for all suspected exposures. The clinical symptoms include cutaneous manifestations, ocular symptoms, respiratory complications, and bone marrow suppression. The cutaneous manifestations are universal and range from first-degree chemical burns to severe edema, vesication, and necrosis. Management includes decontamination, burn care, fluid resuscitation following burn protocols, pain control, and perhaps antibiotic therapy. Ocular symptoms (85% of victims) include pain, blurred vision, lacrimation, corneal edema, and vesication. Management includes copious irrigation and standard corneal abrasion treatment. Respiratory compromise occurs in over 70% of the victims ranging from tracheobronchitis to pulmonary hemorrhage and pulmonary edema. Management is primarily supportive with endotracheal intubation and mechanical ventilation. The lung injury may be permanent. Bone marrow suppression occurs with severe exposure and may result in immunosuppression and increased bleeding risk. Bone marrow suppression is a poor prognostic sign.

It is hoped that the ICU physician will not have to deal with mass casualties from a terrorist chemical attack. This is not an exhaustive discussion, but covers the more likely agents. For both nerve agents and mustard gas it is important to be aware of potential provider exposure to these agents. Decontamination should be accomplished prior to ICU admission.

CONCLUSION

Poisoning and toxicity problems are common problems in the ICU. As in all cases, attention to the basics of resuscitation (airway, breathing, and circulation) should be the clinician's first priority. After stabilization, attention should be turned toward agent identification, limiting absorption, and administering antidotes. Early and aggressive treatment in the ICU can limit morbidity and mortality.

SELECTED READING

Abraham RB, Rudick V, Weinbroum AA: Practical guidelines for acute care of victims of bioterrorism: conventional injuries and concomitant nerve agent intoxication. Anesthesiology 97:989–1004, 2002.

White SM: Chemical and biologic weapons. Implications for anesthaesia and critical care. Br J Anaesthesia 89:306–324, 2002.

Zimmerman JL, Rudis M: Poisoning. In *Critical Care Medicine*, ed 2, Mosby, 2001, Chap 73.

Ethics in Critical Care

DAVID KAUFMAN, M.D., F.C.C.M.

JEFFREY SPIKE, Ph.D.

An appreciation for medical ethics arms the intensivist with the ability to dissect the frequent dilemmas that arise in the intensive care unit (ICU). The ICU is replete with controversy and situations that require a formal understanding of the basic principles used to guide us through the quagmire that often arises when life and death hang in the balance.

From a practical standpoint, medical ethics is the art of resolving conflicts that arise around treatment and treatment decisions. The conflict may involve the patient, family, caregivers, or society. An approach to these conflicts is as necessary as, say, an approach to hypotension or oliguria. Without an approach we would be ignoring

---

Box 35-1 Principles of Medical Ethics

- Autonomy
- Beneficence
- Nonmaleficence
- Justice

---

the mechanisms that led to the conflict or problem in the first place. A little preparation will allow one to be more comfortable when confronting these situations, making responses more likely to be useful (and less likely to make things worse).

There are four basic principles of medical ethics that give us the tools to begin to resolve some of these conflicts: autonomy, beneficence, nonmaleficence, and justice. The weight we give each of these four different principles is often determined by our individual and societal morals (Box 35-1).

PRINCIPLES OF MEDICAL ETHICS

Autonomy

Autonomy is the principle that most often supersedes the other principles in the USA. Whether or not this fact is justified depends on one's moral beliefs and how consistent they are with the majority. It is based on the belief that, if at all possible, we should let each individual determine his or her own destiny.

Capacity is presumed in an adult and one does not need a psychiatrist to make this determination. In addition, a patient may have capacity for one decision and not for another, so understanding the complexity of a decision is extraordinarily important. Thus patients may still be able to communicate a choice of health care agent, even when they cannot make a medical decision.

In the ICU, however, we often work through a surrogate to determine the patient's wishes when capacity is not present. Ideally the surrogate is chosen by the patient and becomes their health care agent. In that case a living will is a document that directs the health care agent. The documents together, the appointment of a health care agent and the living will, comprise the health care proxy. It is important to realize that it is in the province of the health care agent to interpret the living will. Although it is important for physicians to guide patients and their surrogates through this difficult process, it is also important to accept the authority of the health care agent over the living will should the physician believe they are in conflict.

If no health care agent is selected, most intensivists will rely on a next-of-kin to help direct care. It is important to know that, although this is a widely accepted practice, it is justified by the ethical assumption that the next-of-kin can represent the patient's wishes. If there is someone who knows the patient well, but is not a "blood relative," and the family are all distant (or worse, estranged), then this same assumption would justify letting the close friend make decisions.

The health care agent is supposed to pattern their decisions after the choice the patient would have made if they had capacity. Unfortunately, this is often not the reality. Many people are unable or unwilling to stop treatment for someone else even when they know the person would have stopped it himself or herself. Sometimes they are unwilling to accept the burden of the decision and sometimes they are unwilling to accept the reality that continued treatment is approaching medical futility. Someone tried to put a humorous spin on this once by saying that, unfortunately, patients often choose for their agent the one person who cannot live without them.

In situations where one has reason to believe a health care agent or other surrogate is not following the patient's wishes, the best recourse is time: one should put aside as much time to talk to the surrogate as the surrogate needs, and ask them to think about which of the available options the patient would choose, if the patient could sit up and talk for one moment of clarity. They should be given some time to think about it, and time set to meet again to make a decision. If possible, they should be given some signs to look for which would make their decision easier, such as the improvement or worsening of blood pressure or oxygenation. (There have been rare cases of agents being removed from power even though they were chosen by the patient, but only when it was painfully obvious that their decisions were totally contrary to the patient's wishes. In general this should be viewed as an unneccesarily adversarial move, not to mention one likely to fail in court.)

The doctors the family will remember kindly in such a personal crisis are the ones who show they understand why the family is having a difficult time, and help them to deal with it. Communication skills, trustworthiness (including honesty and patience, and just being on time), and compassion are the personal qualities that are needed to become an exemplary intensivist. In modern medicine it is very often only after arriving in the ICU that the family gets this chance to establish a relationship with a physician.

Beneficence and Nonmaleficence

Beneficence is the concept that we will treat the patient to try to *benefit* them. This principle is the most subject to interpretation of all the principles because benefit may be defined differently for the same patient by different physicians. Nonmaleficence is the concept in medicine that physicians should attempt to not cause any harm. This approach often means that nothing should be done unless the potential benefits outweigh the risks of a treatment. Together these principles represent the traditional ethics of the Hippocratic Oath (which gave no weight to patient autonomy).

Often beneficence and nonmaleficence are in direct conflict. Suppose a patient, without capacity or a surrogate, has marginal renal function and requires a study with intravenous contrast. If the physician believes the benefits outweigh the risks the physician will make the beneficence argument and proceed with the study. If, on the other hand, the physician believes the risks outweigh the benefits, the physician will make the nonmaleficence argument and not perform the study. There may be much clinical judgment involved in this decision.

The lesson to keep in mind here is that it is not always best to "do everything." Indeed, that term is one that should never be used with patients or surrogates, because it is so vague. It is better to think that one can aggressively try to "cure" a patient, or just as aggressively try to "care" for a patient, and those may require different interventions (so one cannot do both, i.e., "everything"). It should be remembered that the words "intensive care" have hints of both possible goals of treatment. Many patients die in the ICU, and ethical practice would require clinicians to be skilled in the care of those patients as well as those who live. (For similar reasons, one should never say, "There's nothing more we can do," or suggest that one will "withdraw care." There are things that can be done that show one still cares about the patient right through pronouncing death and care delivered to the body until the person is taken to the morgue.)

Justice

The concept of justice incorporates the greater good of society into the ethical equation. This principle is difficult to accept if applied to the individual patient at the bedside rather than to a group of patients. Is it fair for one intensivist to deny admission to the ICU for a patient in a persistent vegetative state and yet another intensivist accepts the patient in to another ICU? Ideally, society as a whole should make justice decisions and we should not leave this principle solely in the hands of a single physician.

Intensivists are often faced with an expensive new therapy and need to decide who should receive this therapy. For example, activated protein C was recently approved for the treatment of septic shock and costs between $6000 and $10,000 for a course of therapy. Should the price play a role in our decision to use this novel new drug? Do we give activated protein C to someone who is 100 years old and suffering from severe septic shock and, we believe, is unlikely to survive more than a couple of hours? Do we give it to someone who is young and who is suffering from very mild septic shock and is very likely to survive with standard therapy? Tackling justice at the bedside is a prickly path that, if taken, must be done consciously and cautiously. It can be very tempting to use one's authority to impose one's own value judgment, and it is important to remember that not everyone has the same values.

Arguments

These four principles serve a very practical function. They allow the clinician to view an ethical dilemma from different perspectives. They are not meant to provide a simple solution to problems, so much as helping in understanding the source of the problem. The four principles are independent, meaning there is no reason to expect them to lead to a single answer to a dilemma. Once a problem is analyzed using this scheme the conflicting positions in a dilemma are better appreciated. Even if the dispute continues after the analysis, at least the problem can be understood from more than one perspective. This appreciation for other perspectives may lead to softening of firmly held positions and make an eventual compromise easier, even if it does not lead to an immediate resolution.

An argument in philosophy means a conclusion with premises that provide support, like evidence for a scientific theory. A dilemma is when there are arguments for two incompatible conclusions. The goal of analyzing ethical dilemmas is not to prove only one view is right, but to show persons holding each position that the other position is also reasonable. Which course to follow may be decided by which argument has better support, or by which person has more at stake or more authority to make the decision or will suffer the consequences of the decision.

Case Studies

There are many unique ethical situations that arise in the ICU that deserve mention. Three situations, however, bring out special features of this environment and are particularly illustrative. We will use them to investigate the different view obtained from the vantage point of the four basic principles of medical ethics discussed above.

The Jehovah's Witness

A 58-year-old woman who is a Jehovah's Witness presents to the ICU after a skiing accident that led to a splenic laceration. Given the fact that she would not accept a transfusion at a presenting hemoglobin of 6.0 g/dl a splenectomy was performed with her consent rather than observation. Postoperatively she had unexpected bleeding and her hemoglobin dropped to 2.3 g/dl. At this point she developed a lactate level of 3.5 mmol/l and a delirium. Her husband, who is not a Jehovah's Witness, demands that a blood transfusion be given. She has not filled out a health care proxy.

This case, like many in the ICU, does not have an obvious answer. The principle of autonomy would dictate that we follow her initial wishes but we cannot be sure that she would not choose a transfusion if she was so morbidly anemic. We could even speculate that by not appointing a proxy, she knew her husband would be asked to decide, and she preferred it that way.

The principle of beneficence could also be interpreted in different ways. Should we say that it is in her best interests to have a blood transfusion or is it in her best interests not to have a blood transfusion because it goes against her religious beliefs? It is most important when facing this situation to realize that many Jehovah's Witnesses never change their mind, and accept death over transfusion, but that some do change their mind (and even make subtle provisions to enable that to happen). The tone of the family meeting should be a quiet enquiry into which of these scenarios is the more likely, without calling into doubt the scientific validity of the metaphysical beliefs of the faithful.

The Transplant

A 23-year-old woman presents to the emergency department and is transferred to the ICU following an overdose of acetaminophen. This is her third suicide attempt. Despite appropriate therapy, she develops fulminant hepatic failure. A liver is identified and she is scheduled for a transplant. She has hepatic encephalopathy and does not presently have capacity. The anesthesia resident on rotation asks why a patient that has tried to commit suicide is scheduled for a transplant when donated livers are such a limited resource.

The issue of justice is woven into every transplant decision. Since organs are a limited resource, for each person who receives a vital organ somebody else must be denied the organ who will die as a result. Ranking systems are attempts to remove justice from bedside decision-making and, appropriately, place them in the hands of society. Since this patient does not have capacity we would turn to her health care agent or, more likely if she did not a have a health care proxy, her next-of-kin to make a decision. Since it was a suicide attempt the agent would be invoking the principle of beneficence over autonomy since she may very likely refuse a transplant if she had capacity.

A waiting list for livers may include many patients who have potential contraindications: an active alcoholic with cirrhosis, a person with a genetic disease that would eventually destroy the transplanted liver, a prisoner, or a patient with viral hepatitis that may recur. The best reason to have a centralized rating system such as the United Network for Organ Sharing (UNOS) is to prevent these decisions being made according to random variations in social biases.

Brain Death

A 20-year-old woman presents following a gunshot wound to the head and is pronounced dead by brain criteria following appropriate examinations and confirmatory tests. Her family is informed and they do not accept these criteria. They believe as long as there is a heartbeat she is alive and that they will consult a lawyer if an attempt is made to disconnect her from the ventilator.

Death by brain criteria (as opposed to cardiorespiratory criteria) is an accepted method of declaring death in the USA. As a society we have been unable to define life to everyone's satisfaction so it should be no surprise that we have been unable to define death without some controversy. Indeed, it is amazing that the criteria for brain death have not been steeped in more controversy. In this situation the interpretation of the principles of autonomy, beneficence, nonmaleficence, and justice depends entirely on whether or not one accepts this definition of death. If it is believed she is dead there can be no issue of autonomy, beneficence, or nonmaleficence unless one believes it is harming her not to fulfill any known wishes regarding her death she is believed to have held while alive. Justice and the use of resources for someone who is dead is the only active principle that can be invoked. While it would be justified to stop all interventions as soon as the diagnosis of death is made, in the case of brain death it is common to allow the family to visit with the patient before discontinuing treatment. This may give them some comfort, but it should not be done in a way that makes them think that the patient is still alive, or it may lead to resistance to withdrawal of treatment.

It is very important to be careful with the terms that the staff uses in the ICU. Even some very experienced doctors and nurses will occasionally say "brain dead" when they mean "irreversibly and profoundly brain damaged, with no hope of a significant recovery" or "persistent vegetative state" (PVS). If families confuse these various concepts, the differences should be explained to them. PVS patients have eye movements, sleep–wake cycles, and can be kept alive for months, years, and sometimes even decades with little more than good nursing care and occasional antibiotics for infections. The decision of whether to continue or discontinue life-sustaining treatment for PVS patients is left to the patient's surrogate.

General Comments

There are other ways to approach medical ethics besides using these four basic principles. Some experts have advocated learning ethics from case studies alone. This is known as *casuistry*. As might be imagined, it is often criticized as relying too heavily on the ethical equivalent of anecdotal evidence. Other experts have advocated what is called virtue theory, emulating persons we recognize as role models in order to hone our insight and judgment in ethically complex cases. This too has its critics, who are concerned that it will weigh traditional values too heavily, and not allow room for moral progress. As in other fields in medicine, these different methods are models that allow us to move closer to the truth, but we are still looking at shadows. Each model may help to understand medical ethics, and none should be ignored. However, from a practical perspective the four principles do help determine why well-meaning people disagree, and that may be why they have been the most commonly used model for the past 30 years.

CAPACITY

When determining capacity the physician must take into account the patient as well as the proposed decision. Patients may have capacity for one decision and not another. The most important element of capacity is whether the patient understands the consequences of the choice they make, whether that choice is to accept or refuse a treatment option that has been offered (or even recommended).

Additionally, a patient may not be able to make a decision but would understand a decision that has been made. In this situation the patient should be informed of the decision. The patient's response may help one solidify or rethink the determination in the first place.

Telling a patient that he or she has been made DNR may feel impossible to do, but with experience it can be done. It should always be remembered that capacity is presumed in an adult. Hence, while the right of physicians unilaterally to "lift" a DNR order agreed to by a patient is ethically questionable, the right of a patient to refuse DNR status is not. Here, as above, communication and honesty are all important. DNR does not mean stopping anything currently being provided – it means not escalating the level of interventions should there be a sudden turn for the worse. And the justification for DNR is that cardiopulmonary resuscitation would not work in this situation, or would be likely to leave the patient in a worse condition. Every intensivist should be familiar with the literature around success rates of DNR for various classes of patients.

CHOICE OF A HEALTH CARE AGENT

Most people choose a health care agent who is closest to them. It seems appropriate to choose a wife or adult child for such a potentially momentous task. The theory, however, is that this person will make *the patient's own* decision should they be without capacity. Many agents know that the patient would not want their present and future life but are afraid to make a decision to withdraw or limit treatment or are afraid to continue their own life without this person, and so choose to keep the person alive. Perhaps it would make more sense to suggest to patients that they choose someone who knows them well *but can live without them*.

The ideal surrogate exists in textbooks but rarely in real life. It is not realistic to expect a surrogate to come to the table free of any of their own agendas. The education of the patient's family is an important role for the intensivist. Surrogates must be frequently but gently reminded that they are making *their loved one's decision* rather that making *a decision* for their loved one.

FUTILITY

Futility is a word frequently evoked in the ICU but rarely defined. We tend to use the word as if it were a mathematical absolute rather than a statistical probability. Many experienced intensivists have had the experience of telling the family of a patient that continued treatment was "futile," only to have the patient improve and survive to a quality life. Besides, it is often unclear what we mean by futility. Are we implying that the patient is so moribund that death is imminent? Are we implying that the patient will not survive the ICU admission? Or are we implying that if the patient does survive his or her quality of life will be very limited?

It is probably best to avoid the term futility and focus on providing the family with more descriptive and individualized terms. An in-depth discussion with time to answer questions will be more beneficial than using terms that are confusing and possibly misleading.

Sometimes "futility" needs to be determined during a code. Some physicians believe that attempts at resuscitation need to be attempted for a specified period of time. The truth is that some judgment is involved and there is no magic period of time or duration of a particular rhythm that is defining.

Recently there has been discussion about whether the family should be allowed to be present during a resuscitation attempt. The traditional rule that the family is asked to leave has a paternalistic air, and can create suspicion in the mind of the family if the attempt fails. There is increasing acceptance of allowing the family to remain in the room if they request to do so, assuming there is enough room and they are not likely to interfere with the process. Many families do not want to watch their loved one in this situation, but for some others this will provide them with the conviction that death was inevitable.

INFORMED CONSENT

Ideally all patients and their surrogates should be informed about the potential risks and benefits for all procedures performed and all medications given. Increasingly, this includes blood transfusions. Here, once again, judgment must be used given the sheer number of procedures and medications ordered in the ICU. It is also important to remember that one's responsibility is to offer only reasonable alternatives, and that families should not be asked to micromanage or allowed to make unreasonable choices, such as accepting high-risk interventions while refusing low-risk ones with equal or better efficacy.

PHARMACEUTICAL CONNECTION

The pharmaceutical industry frequently buys gifts for physicians, claiming they are interested in dialogue and education. It must always be remembered that drug companies are for-profit businesses and they must, ultimately, answer to their shareholders and not care givers. They know the gifts they buy influence prescription patterns, whether the recipients believe it or not. Research by independent agencies shows that drug companies now spend more money on detailers and advertising than on research and development, totaling about $9000 per physician per year. Many physicians falsely believe their colleagues are susceptible to this kind of influence, but not them. The only way to be certain one is not being influenced is to realize there is *no "free lunch."*

SELECTED READING

Beauchamp T, Childress J: *Principles of Biomedical Ethics*, New York: Oxford University Press, 2002.

Lo B: *Resolving Ethical Dilemmas: A Guide for Clinicians*, Philadelphia, PA: Lipincott Williams and Wilkins, 2000.

McCullough L, Jones J, Brody B: *Surgical Ethics*, New York: Oxford University Press, 1998.

CHAPTER 36

Safety, Quality, Scoring Systems, and Legal Issues in Critical Care

JAMES E. SZALADOS, M.D., J.D., M.B.A.

Physicians subscribe to the Hippocratic Oath and strive to provide the highest quality of medical care to their patients; a professional atmosphere of caring, respect, and trust within the physician–patient relationship; and are therefore patient advocates of the highest order. Health care accounts for approximately 14% of the US gross domestic product (GDP) and yet paradoxically almost 50% of Americans have limited access to health care because they either do not have health insurance or have coverage limitations. Critical care medicine (CCM) alone accounts for approximately 0.5% of the GDP, 13% of hospital costs, 4.2% of national health expenditures; furthermore, most of these costs are accrued within the last year of patients' lives.

Since physicians have traditionally placed paramount importance on their fiduciary responsibilities to patients, they have been slow to accept health care costs as measures of quality. However, medical care, especially CCM, represents a significant cost to society and there is thus a reasonable request for social accountability. Increasingly, individual providers and health care systems are being held accountable for the quality they provide in return for health care dollars spent. The trend is one of increasing scrutiny. In all areas of medicine, incremental measures of value added will be used to justify incremental costs.

The outcome of health care can be assessed retrospectively using any one of a myriad of measures ranging from crude mortality to more complex quality-of-life indices. Measures of outcome must be risk-adjusted (e.g., comorbidities, severity of illness) and account for variables such as functional status at discharge, quality of life, and cost of care. Although vitally important to the medical education and continuing medical education process, medical quality assurance in the form of morbidity and mortality rounds has largely failed in itself to provide either minimum quality standards or a means for system-wide performance improvement.

Individual provider or departmental performance becomes meaningful only when it is aggregated in databases that provide for longitudinal trending, risk adjustment, statistical analysis, and external comparisons. External comparisons are especially important to differentiate reliably "best practices" which potentially form the basis for outcomes-based standards of care which can be published, disseminated, and thereafter continually improved upon. Guidelines and practice parameters, and protocols and pathways are examples of standards of care. These tools are developed and disseminated by medical societies and colleges, regulatory organizations, lawmakers, and developers of health policy.

The topics of safety, quality, severity of illness and case mix, and risk management and medical liability are closely related and inter-related. An understanding of safety, process improvement, and legal requirements not only improves clinical patient care but also optimizes teamwork and communication in the health care setting and minimizes risk exposure. Physicians must be "citizens" of the institutions and systems in which they practice. Involvement or leadership requires an understanding of the support systems, processes, and the vocabulary of teamwork.

SAFETY

Heightened societal awareness regarding the incidence and impact of errors in medicine resulted in the widespread focus on a "culture of safety." Error management focuses on the principles of prevention, recognition, and mitigation-of-effect. Prevention is best accomplished via multiple tiers of decision-support and verification. General systems theory suggests that the use of algorithms, checklists, and team-based practice creates a more optimal environment for error prevention. Decision-support systems also include the availability of information at the point of prescribing, such as PDAs, intranet and internet access, and reference texts. Multiple levels of verification include nurses, pharmacy, and colleagues. According to the Agency for Health Care Research and Quality, adverse drug events (ADEs) cause approximately 777,000 injuries and deaths annually and cost $1.5 million to $5.6 million annually per hospital depending on hospital size. In addition, ADEs increase hospital length of stay by 8–12 days per patient affected and increase hospitalization cost by up to $24,000 per event. Medication dosage errors account for 28% of all hospital-related errors. The Institute of Medicine has highlighted the problem and proposed changes. Hospitals that do not proactively implement plans to reduce medical error will risk losing market share and increase their medical–legal liability. Examples of practical implementations of safety measures include resident work hours and supervision requirements, computerized position order entry and point-of-care decision support systems, and communication facilitation models such as crew resource management. Medical errors are also common in CCM, perhaps as a result of the intensity of care. The team model of critical care practice is a key component of the "culture of safety" and encourages collaboration and input.

PEARLS

Examples of Patient Safety Improvement Opportunities
- Adverse drug reactions (ADRs)
- Venous thromboembolism (VTE)
- Stress-related gastrointestinal bleeding
- Unplanned extubations
- Ventilator weaning protocols
- Sedation and pain management protocols
- Falls, restraints, and related injuries
- Failure to honor patient DNR preferences
- Communication issues
  - Wrong surgery/site
  - Informed consent
  - Abnormal laboratory or radiology results
- Nosocomial infections
  - Ventilator-associated pneumonia (VAP)
  - Central venous catheter-related infections
  - Surgical site infections
- Contrast-induced nephropathy
- Malnutrition and related complications
- Unanticipated mortality

Computerized physician order entry (CPOE) is a computerized order entry system whereby physicians and other licensed providers enter medication and plan-of-care orders directly into a computer terminal. CPOE has an impact on patient safety by eliminating transcription errors, and automatically crosschecking for patient drug allergies and sensitivities, end-organ dysfunction and dosing, and drug interactions. Electronic medical records can potentially increase patient safety by delivering accurate and legible medical information to many health care providers simultaneously at any point of care. Decision support systems (DSSs) include digitalized reference materials, formularies, internet access to search engines, and guidelines and protocols available at the point of care through digital area networks. DSSs can also automatically initiate physical/occupational therapy evaluations, social work consultations, and discharge planning, for example.

Crew resource management (CRM), originally called cockpit resource management, is a model of active team participation at all levels of decision-making. In essence, based on the safety practices of airlines, "any crew member can question or stop takeoff." CRM is based on the concepts of situational awareness, interpersonal communications, and standard operating procedures, and debriefing to optimize operational integrity and safety. Fully trained and credentialed providers and appropriate staffing ratios are important to outcomes.

Leadership defines the culture. The impact of leadership style, attitude, commitment, and willingness to adhere to the team model of critical care is fundamental to nurturing a culture of safety and quality. Continuous learning is essential. Medicine and especially critical care is a field where significant changes and advances occur frequently. Distillation of information and a dedication to education in both academia and private practice alike is a key component of safety and quality.

Data also reveal that patient safety varies in the same institution between days, nights, and weekends. There is a significantly higher incidence of errors, slower response to critical incidents, and poorer outcomes during "off-shifts." Fatigue impairs data assimilation and decision-making ability. Although standard operating procedures and other support systems can mitigate the effects of fatigue, the imposition of mandatory rest times is becoming uniform practice.

QUALITY

A precise definition of "quality" is elusive but may be best defined as an error rate, although both frequency and magnitude of errors must be considered. Maximization of quality may be considered to represent minimization of the variation from an accepted standard. Health care reform of any nature must be based in a delivery system based in data and information. The challenge is to determine what is sufficiently important to be measured and how best to measure it. Measurement is the basis for any systematic safety or quality program; thus, there is an overlap between the concepts of safety and

PEARLS

Continuous Quality Improvement Process

Data
↓
Practice pattern measurement
↓
Benchmarking
↓
Dissemination of information
↓
Protocol and pathway development
↓
Interventions
↓
Ongoing practice pattern monitoring

Box 36-2 Root Cause Analysis

- Root cause analysis (RCA) is a method of incident analysis and quality improvement which focuses on identifying the causes of adverse events. The RCA employs the scientific method, verbal and visual dialogue, and systems attempting to identify cause and effect relationships.
- The RCA has become the prevalent model of incident analysis for both quality and risk management activities.
- The importance of RCA is that it focuses not on a single event or person as a root cause of an adverse event, but upon the systems and processes that were absent or failed to detect an unsafe situation, provide appropriate backup, or mitigate the extent of injuries.

quality management. The public is increasingly aware of safety and quality issues and will be a driving force for changes in this arena (Box 36-1).

Peer review is a legislatively mandated review of adverse clinical events and outcomes. Morbidity and mortality (M&M) conferences represent a type of peer review. Peer review is subject to legislation such as confidentiality, privilege, and antitrust.

Intensive care unit (ICU) staffing may also have an impact on quality, as reflected in patient outcome. ICU staffing by a dedicated full-time intensivist has been shown to improve significantly clinical care and patient outcomes, measured as the efficiency of resource utilization, mortality, morbidity, or patients' and staff satisfaction. Nursing staff-to-patient ratios are important to both quality and safety initiatives. The State of California enacted mandatory nursing staffing ratios in an effort to improve patient safety and quality of care.

Credentialing of providers ensures that minimum educational, training, and certification requirements have been met. Advanced cardiac life support (ACLS) and fundamental critical care support (FCCS) are examples of advanced credentialing. Continuing medical education (CME) is also an important basis for continued

PEARLS

Underlying Root Causes of Adverse Events
- Human
  - Fatigue
  - Training
  - Communication
- Technical
  - Equipment failure
- Systemic
  - Workplace ergonomics
  - Decision support systems and backup
  - Production pressure
  - Lack of policies and procedures
  - Organizational culture

credentialing. Credentialing is also regulated by state legislation and hospital bylaws (Box 36-2).

Publication of a guideline, protocol, or pathway presupposes a certain level of consensus within the scientific community regarding its validity. Guidelines are statements from specialty societies that define practice parameters based on extensive literature review by experts. Guidelines are published and become important "standards" but are not absolutely binding.

The American College of Cardiology/American Heart Association guidelines on perioperative cardiovascular evaluation for noncardiac surgery is one example of a comprehensive clinical guideline that has been widely accepted and adopted. Protocols are statements-of-care plans that are based on best practices. Protocols and pathways reduce variation and increase the cost-effectiveness of clinical care.

Systematic expert analysis of published medical literature is necessary because the medical literature is replete with published studies of questionable scientific validity. Sophisticated critical appraisal is necessary to

Box 36-1 Quality Management

- Quality management refers to any one of a number of terminologies for a system of quality maximization. These terms include quality improvement (QI), quality assurance (QA), continuous quality improvement (CQI), total quality management (TQM), and performance improvement (PI), among others.
- Quality measurement and improvement has its basis in clinical epidemiology.
- The purpose of quality management in medicine is to clarify the implications of variations in medical practice and suggest improvements based on data.

determine the relevancy and applicability of the studies to clinical situations.

INTENSIVE CARE UNIT SCORING SYSTEMS

Scoring systems have been developed in response to a need for comparative analysis of patient outcomes within a single institution over time and to assess the impact of continuous quality improvement (CQI), and for inter-institutional analysis to identify best practices. Scoring systems are also used to estimate prognosis and outcome, to justify triage decisions, and to optimize resource allocation.

Many commonly accepted medical practices have been implemented which had not been subjected to rigorous scientific clinical investigation. The lack of convincing evidence supporting the efficacy of interventions or medical therapies has resulted in diverse individual practitioner beliefs or practices with large variations in clinical outcome. Increasingly, these beliefs are being questioned and challenged in large prospective randomized multicenter clinical trials resulting in accepted evidence-based standards. Theoretically, each and every intervention used in intensive care should be subjected to randomized controlled trials to determine its clinical effectiveness.

Data-driven evidence-based practices are supplanting traditional teachings. ICU scoring systems allow fairly accurate predictions regarding clinical outcomes in populations of patients but cannot accurately and reliably predict the probability of individual survival.

A scoring system describes the association between an independent variable such as case mix or severity of illness and a dependent variable such as survival or functional status. A scoring system is developed using retrospective outcome data from large populations of patients and is a mathematical model capable of being prospectively applied to new populations to predict outcome. Development of the scoring system is accomplished through multiple logistic regression analyses which describe the strength of the association between combinations of independent variables while simultaneously accounting for the effects of other independent variables in the system.

Scoring systems are most commonly used for research studies and for general inter-institutional comparisons. The use of scoring systems for inter-institutional outcome and performance comparisons is very controversial both because of the unknown underlying assumptions in the statistical modeling and because outcomes other than survival and mortality are important. Descriptors of outcomes include measures such as mortality, morbidity, functional status, quality of life, and cost.

A scoring system must function independently of treatment, be disease specific and yet function over a

Box 36-3 Examples of Organ-Specific Measures

- Glasgow Coma Scale (GCS) for central nervous system injuries
- Child–Pugh Score for cirrhosis
- Ranson's Criteria for pancreatitis
- Lung Injury Score (LIS) for respiratory failure

range of diseases, be clinically credible, be capable of measuring severity at multiple points along the care continuum, be relatively easy to implement, and provide statistically valid information. All predictive indices currently in use have a false classification rate of 10–15%. Therefore, 10–15% of patients predicted to survive will die, and vice versa.

Data can be quantitative, quantal, or qualitative. Quantitative data refers to measured quantities. Quantal data refers to attributes that may be classified.

A distribution curve is a frequency distribution of the incidence of specific values. A normal or Gaussian curve has values evenly distributed around the mode; a multimodal curve is a frequency distribution curve with more than one mode. Many populations are normally distributed but many critical care populations cannot be described using a normal distribution curve.

However, the fundamental issue regarding mortality and survival is the appropriate time interval (30 days, 6 months, 5 years, etc.) at which the endpoint represents a valid quality indicator.

Applications of scoring systems include comparative audit, evaluative research, development of standards, and clinical care. Limitations of scoring systems include data accuracy, population sampling, data interpretation, and clinical applicability.

Examples of critical care scoring systems include organ-specific measures (Box 36-3) and general severity-of-illness scoring measures.

The Glasgow Coma Scale (GCS) is an example of a simple scoring system used for the assessment of the extent of coma in patients based on eye opening (4), verbal response (5), and motor response (6). The scale is weighted in favor of motor response. The total GCS is the sum of each category and ranges from a minimum of 3 to a maximum of 15. GCS applications include prehospital triage and assessment of clinical change based on serial examinations. The GCS is an example of a descriptive scoring system which later evolved into a correlate of outcome. The GCS is incorporated into most contemporary general severity scoring systems including Acute Physiology and Chronic Health Evaluation (APACHE) II and III, Simplified Acute Physiology Score (SAPS) II, and Mortality Probability Model (MPM) II (Box 36-4).

> ### Box 36-4 Examples of Generalized Severity-of-Illness Scoring Systems
>
> - Trauma Increased Severity Score (TRISS)
> - Sequential Organ Failure Assessment (SOFA)
> - Acute Physiology and Chronic Health Evaluation (APACHE I–III)
> - Mortality Probability Model (MPM I and II)
> - Simplified Acute Physiology Score (SAPS I and II)
> - Therapeutic Intervention Scoring System (TISS)
> - Multiple Organ Dysfunction Score (MODS)

Trauma Increased Severity Score (TRISS) was developed in 1983 and combined elements from the Trauma Score and the Injury Severity Score (ISS). The Trauma Score was replaced by the Revised Trauma Score which is used in the current model along with the ISS, age, and type of injury. APACHE I was the first version of the APACHE system developed between 1979 and 1981 to measure the severity of illness in ICU patients and consisted of two parts: (a) an acute physiology score reflecting the extent of 34 potential variables and (b) chronic health evaluation questionnaire which classified patients according to prior health status. This model correlated directly with hospital mortality but did not include probability calculations.

APACHE II is the second version of APACHE introduced in 1985 with several important changes: (a) the number of physiologic variables is reduced to 12, (b) acute renal failure receives double weighting, (c) the cost of coma scale is given greater weight, (d) a score is assigned to reflect the prognostic impact of emergency surgery, and (e) the chronic health questionnaire is dropped and scores are assigned to reflect diminished physiologic reserves related to aging, immune deficiency, and chronic cardiac, pulmonary, renal, and liver disease. APACHE II scores range from 0 to 71. APACHE III allows for (a) individual evaluative scoring and (b) predictive modeling to estimate the probability of death for individual patients at different times during their ICU stay. The scoring system is based on 17 physiologic variables, a coma scale, age, and comorbid conditions. APACHE III scores range from 0 to 299.

APACHE is expensive to implement and use. APACHE scores do not correlate well with resource utilization. APACHE scores may penalize patients with good end-organ reserve and good ward care, since they may not accumulate sufficient points to warrant ICU admission.

The MPM was developed by Lemeshow in 1985 and subsequently revised as MPM II in 1993. MPM incorporates a large number of variables: 137 at admission and 75 at 24 hours. Therefore, the MPM has a unique versatility in being applicable at admission and also 24 hours later. The MPM modeling population also excludes patients admitted with burns, cardiac surgery and coronary care patients, and patients less than 18 years old.

SAPS II was created in 1992. The model excludes patients who are admitted for burns, coronary care, and cardiac surgery. SAPS II uses 17 variables: 12 physiologic variables, age, type of admission (scheduled surgical, unscheduled surgical, medical), and three variables related to underlying disease (hematologic malignancy, AIDS, and metastatic cancer).

The Therapeutic Intervention Scoring System (TISS) was developed in 1989 and was originally proposed as a method for the quantitation of resource utilization in critically ill patients. The premise was that more seriously ill patients would require more therapeutic interventions independent of specific diagnoses. Therefore, the severity of illness could be determined from the number and complexity of monitoring needs and interventions. TISS has remained a method of analysis of expenditures and outcome. An advantage of TISS is its inherent simplicity.

MEDICOLEGAL ISSUES

Medicolegal matters of concern to critical care practitioners extend from medical malpractice to increasingly complex regulatory legislative law. The threat of legal liability based on a malpractice claim of negligence is an important concern and may drive defensive medicine practices as well as increasing health care costs. The trend is one of increasing judicial awards, increasing societal awareness of litigation as a forum for recovery of awards, and increasing malpractice insurance premiums. Adverse outcomes can range from dissatisfaction of patients and/or family to iatrogenic mortality. However, regulatory legislation is an important source of legal risk to both individual practitioners and institutions. For example, guidelines for documentation of services and coding and billing are associated with the risk of fraud in both teaching institutions and in private practice. Additionally, legislation intended to ensure patients' privacy protection will have significant impact on electronic medical records and databases, and the transmission of electronic information between providers. Trends such as the development of telemedicine and electronic mail communications with patients will continue to challenge the medical–legal relationship. The following should not be strictly construed as legal advice, since laws regarding medical practice vary by individual state. In general, patients may have legal recourse against physicians, hospital staff, hospitals, and payers individually or in combinations.

PEARLS

Liability – Risk Minimization Strategies
- Communication
- Documentation
- Dissemination of accepted guidelines and protocols
- Adherence to policy

Negligence and Professional Malpractice

Medical malpractice is a type of negligence. Under civil liability the tort of negligence requires that the plaintiff demonstrate four elements: duty, breach of duty, causation, and damages. In addition, the causation relationship must satisfy the proximate cause requirement whereby a breach of duty proximately caused either an injury or a lost opportunity for clinical recovery. Negligence is generally treated as a civil cause of action; however, under some rare circumstances, negligence in medical treatment law may rise to a level of criminal action.

Negligence is defined based on deviations from accepted medical practices but not errors of judgment. Duty is the primary element of the negligence theory of liability. Duty is created by the physician–patient relationship and requires that a physician act in accordance with the specific norms or standards established by the medical profession. Medical malpractice specifically refers to a medical care which represents a deviation from that care which would normally be rendered in the same or similar situation. Medical malpractice is not defined by a less than optimal outcome, unless the care rendered was otherwise substandard. Therefore, expert testimony is required to demonstrate medical malpractice by defining an appropriate standard of care. The standard of medical care is that which a prudent physician with similar qualifications would have rendered in the same or similar situation. The standard of medical care is determined from expert testimony. Breach of duty must be proved by the plaintiff. The plaintiff must demonstrate that the defendant-physician did not act in accordance with the standard of care required as a duty stemming from the physician–patient relationship. Causation refers to the reasonably close causal connection between the act and the injury. Causation is closely related to "legal cause" and "proximate cause."

Damages is a term that refers to the actual loss, injury, or harm suffered by the patient as a result of the physician's breach of standard of care. The purpose of awarding damages in a tort action is "to make whole again" the injured party and return him or her to a position or condition similar to that which existed before the tort. The damages awarded may be either compensatory or punitive. Compensatory damages may be special or general.

General damages include noneconomic losses such as "pain and suffering." Punitive or exemplary damages awarded in addition to actual losses to make an example of the egregious actions. Special damages compensate the plaintiff for hospital and long-term care costs, for example.

Consent for Treatment

Consent is a key element of the physician and patient relationship and may be considered as a type of contract which requires that there be an element of consideration (informed) and acceptance of a plan of care. Therefore, consent obtained under fraudulent pretenses or under duress, for example, may not be valid. Informed consent presupposes that patients must agree to be examined and/or treated; without such an agreement, there is potentially an invasion of privacy and possibly a tort of battery. The physician must disclose to patient information that is sufficient to enable the patient to make an "informed" decision about a potential treatment or procedure. In order for such an agreement to constitute informed consent there must be a clear documentation of the risks, benefits, and alternatives to the proposed intervention. Implied consent is consent that may be tacit, or implied, which is based in the situational context of the patient presenting for care. Implied consent is most often used to justify treatment interventions in the context of emergency and critical care. Whenever possible consent should be informed and express. The documentation of the basis on which consent was obtained is fundamental. Express consent is best documented in written form. However, documentation of a verbal discussion may be adequate under some circumstances. In order for consent to be informed and valid the consenter must have both capacity and competence. Both terms refer to the cognitive ability of the patient to understand the ramifications of his/her decision.

Capacity is generally considered to be contextual and situational and not fixed. For example, a patient who has received psychoactive medication may temporarily lack the capacity to form an informed decision. Competence is generally a fixed characteristic of the patient such as a cognitive limitation or an age of minority without emancipation or other potential modifiers.

Patients may also refuse treatment. Competent patients have the right to refuse particular elements of medical therapy (surgery, blood or blood product transfusions, other specific interventions) or all and any medical care. Refusal of one therapeutic intervention does not in itself constitute refusal of other alternatives.

Patients who make an informed decision to refuse all interventions may request to be discharged AMA or "against medical advice." A discharge AMA does not necessarily relieve practitioners of their obligations.

Box 36-5 Do Not Resuscitate

- "Do not resuscitate" (DNR) is also referred to as "do not attempt resuscitation" (DNAR) and is a type of informed refusal of treatment. Given the complexity of the term "resuscitation," a blanket DNR may be subject to scrutiny.
- DNR is no longer generally considered to be an absolute specification; it is necessary that it be further categorized and subclassified in order to best represent an individual patient's precise directives.
- Limited critical care DNR may allow mechanical ventilation and hemodynamic monitoring and support but may limit the use of cardiopulmonary resuscitation, defibrillation, or dialysis, for example.
- Conservative care DNR may allow dialysis and hemodynamic support but preclude intubation and mechanical ventilation, for example.
- Comfort care may restrict interventions to those measures maximizing comfort. It is important to realize that DNR is a type of consent that requires careful documentation. Additionally, DNR never means "do not treat" and even comfort care DNR patients require maximization of comfort and dignity.

Abandonment constitutes a breach of the duty to provide continuity of care once the physician–patient relationship has been established. Abandonment can become an issue where a discharge AMA does not well document the exact circumstances and does not provide for follow-up if needed.

Advance Directives and Do Not Resuscitate

Advance directives are requests made by capable and competent persons which become important when patients can no longer communicate. Examples of issues involving advance directives include living wills and health care proxies, and do not resuscitate (DNR) status. In the absence of a written designation of a health care proxy state laws often delineate the order in which relatives and decision-making authority occurs (Box 36-5).

Autonomy refers to an individual's right to decision-making regarding his or her own personal self-determination. Beneficence refers to the fiduciary duty of physicians to act in the best interests of their patients. Fiduciary duty is a special responsibility with which physicians are entrusted to act as agents on their patients' behalf. The word "duty" has both ethical and legal ramifications. Thus, physicians must balance the duty of care against the respect for individual autonomy. This means that it may be ethically more acceptable to err in resuscitating a patient who may have not desired it, rather than to erroneously assume the patient is DNR and inappropriately withhold life-sustaining treatment. It also means that the communication between physician, patient, and families regarding life support decisions must be clear, complete, and absolutely unambiguous. It is unfair to focus on issues of pain, discomfort, and dignity without clearly revealing that the alternative to life support is "death." Nonmaleficence expresses the guiding principle which underlines the fiduciary duty of medical care: primum non nocere; meaning "above all else, do no harm." Notably, harm can be defined either by omission or commission of acts which inflict emotional, psychological, or physical injury. Paternalism refers to the desire of health-care providers to make decisions on behalf of their patients. Where instinctive paternalism drives physicians to withhold information or disclose information selectively, it is inappropriate, and probably illegal, since consent to treatment or a refusal of treatment are not based on "informed consent." Thus, a DNR order, is essentially an informed consent document. In order to be truly valid, consent must equally disclose risks, benefits, and alternatives; and it must be obtained after full disclosure to a patient who is competent, without any duress or coercion. Documentation of a mental status examination has significant legal, medical, and ethical value where DNR discussions take place with patients whose capacity to understand and consent may later be questioned.

DNR orders are generally classified into three or more general categories reflecting specific levels of treatment that the patient consents to: (1) limited critical care, suggesting full life support but limiting CPR; (2) conservative care, suggesting full medical care short of mechanical ventilation and CPR; and (3) comfort care, suggesting treatment to maximize comfort only. However, these categories vary in their interpretation between providers and between institutions. Therefore, additional documentation, aside from simply "checking a box on a form" is usually required. Additionally, the DNR form should always be accompanied by a written note in the body of the chart reflecting the basis of the decision, the alternatives discussed, and the patient's level of comprehension. Perhaps most importantly, it is necessary to realize that Do Not Resuscitate *never* means "do not treat." Additionally, withdrawal of life support *never* means "withdrawal of care".

The administration of medication with the intent of treating pain and anxiety within the comfort care context is not generally considered to be synonymous with either euthanasia or physician-assisted suicide. Medication doses are generally based on individual clinical effect and not absolute numerical values.

Withdrawal of life support usually requires either a determination of medical futility, brain death, or a change in DNR status to comfort care DNR. Brain death is a statutorily defined definition of death. The Uniform Brain Death Act (1978), the Uniform Determination of Death Act (1980), state legislation, and case law are all important considerations to the development of policy. Since state laws regarding brain death determination are not uniform, policy should be developed with the advice of counsel.

Triage and Rationing of Services

Triage refers to the prioritization of resource allocation to the individuals most acutely in need. Where scarce resources preclude an appropriate level of care to a critically ill patient, considerations for an appropriate transfer must be made. Triage in the ICU is commonplace and is often based on a subjective assessment of severity of illness and requirements for therapeutics and monitoring. Triage should probably be accompanied by an objective measure of severity of illness if possible.

The Health Insurance Portability and Accountability Act: HIPAA

Respect for the privacy and confidentiality of patients' medical information is a well-established principle of both medical ethics and health law. A respect for each patient's individual rights and dignity is essential to ensure trust and to promote the integrity and the completeness of health information disclosure within the scope of the physician–patient relationship. A "fiduciary duty" is one which a professional owes to a patient beneficiary, by virtue of knowledge, training, and experience. Fiduciary principles impose a heightened duty of loyalty, integrity, and devotion upon professionals. The physician's duty of confidentiality dates from the Hippocratic Oath, is codified within the Principles of Medical Ethics of the American Medical Association, and has been reiterated in legislative statutes such as the Federal Privacy Act of 1974, in the Guiding Principles of the Joint Commission for the Accreditation of Health Care Organizations (JCAHO), and, most recently within HIPAA. Multiple levels of law govern the privacy of health-care information and existing civil causes of action can include breach of privacy, breach of confidentiality, breach of contract, breach of loyalty, and other statutory violations.

The broad goals of HIPAA are to: (1) increase the efficiency of electronic health-care transactions; (2) ensure the continuity of an employee's health insurance coverage during the process of changing jobs; and (3) mandate widespread privacy protection measures for ensuring the security of individually identifiable health information. HIPAA is increasingly necessary as "electronic data interchange" (EDI) is used to transmit personal health information via electronic and digital media.

Additionally, digitally stored information is vulnerable to threats such as worms, viruses, and Trojan horses which can eradicate digital data or compromise their security. HIPAA is characterized by three intra-related parts: (1) the administrative simplification provisions; (2) the privacy rule, which sets security standards and policies; and (3) the security rule which governs relationships between health-care business associates. HIPAA increases the level of control that individual patients have over their personal health information (PHI) by requiring notice regarding the proposed uses of their personal information, allowing patients the right to inspect, amend, and copy medical records, receive an accounting of disclosures of their PHI, and also restrict the use of their information. HIPAA privacy regulations protect only that health information which is individually identifiable. De-identified data, on the other hand, can be used or shared, generally without restrictions, for research, organizational strategic planning, and teaching.

The penalties for violation of HIPAA provisions are strict. The Office of Civil Rights has the authority to receive and investigate complaints, and the United States Department of Justice imposes penalties at $100 per violation to a maximum of $25,000 per year for each violation. Intentional or malicious disclosures which fall under the category of criminal violations range from $50,000 to $100,000 and up to five years in prison for false pretenses; and $250,000 and 10 years in prison if the information is sold for commercial advantage, personal gain, or malicious harm.

Billing, Coding, the False Claims Act

The economic realities of practice management require not only the highest possible level of quality in patient care, but also an analysis of costs and reimbursement to achieve an optimum balance between revenue and expenses without compromising quality. Critical care is defined by the U.S. Health Care Financing Administration (HCFA) to be the direct delivery by physicians of medical care for a critically ill or critically injured patient. Critical illness or injury acutely impairs the function of one or more vital organ systems such that there is a high probability of a sudden and clinically significant deterioration by which survival of the patient is jeopardized. A high level of professional preparedness is necessary to intervene urgently. Critical care also involves frequent assessment, and high complexity decision-making to assess, manipulate, and support vital organ functions. ICU admission in itself is insufficient justification for claiming reimbursement for critical care services unless other explicit criteria of medical necessity, physician attendance, and therapeutic complexity are met as well as documented. Additionally, the standard for procedural supervision is such that the attending physician must be physically present and immediately available in the case of difficulty. Although otherwise credentialed residents may be sufficiently technically proficient to perform independently, the requirements for procedural billing are more stringent. Misrepresentation of patient care rendered in a teaching hospital setting as 'supervised' when in fact it was not closely supervised, represents fraudulent billing and is subject to civil and/or criminal penalties. Since hospitals are reimbursed independently by the Centers for Medicare and Medicaid Services (CMS) for resident teaching, hospitals and providers may not bill for services provided independently by residents alone. Also, time spent teaching residents cannot be claimed toward critical care time unless the physician and residents are together directly engaged in patient care. Billing for critical care services requires diagnostic codes which must match the verbiage documented within the medical record. Thus, documentation is the key to accurate and timely claims review and payment by insurers, defensibility in the event of a bad outcome, and a pivotal tenet to billing compliance standards. The submission of claims for any component of critical care, procedure, or other evaluation and management for which the attending physician was not directly present may constitute fraud and abuse under the False Claims Act. Submission of a bill for services at a level of service greater than that which was actually provided represents "up-coding;" whereas, submission of a claim a level of service lower than that actually provided represents "down-coding." Both up-coding and down-coding represent mis-coding and are both illegal. Although, the False Claims Act has traditionally been enforced by the government against hospitals and providers in the setting of inappropriate billing for services rendered to Medicare patients, there is an increasing trend towards monitoring for billing fraud, and enforcement action, by private insurers.

Other issues within the scope of health-care fraud and abuse include restrictions on self-referral under the Stark Law, and the relationships between physicians and hospitals under the "anti-kickback" statute.

SELECTED READING

Bogner MS: *Human Error in Medicine*, Hillsdale, NJ: Lawrence Erlbaum, 1994.

Classen DC, Pestotnik SL, Evans RS et al: Adverse drug events in hospitalized patients. JAMA 277:301–306, 1997.

Cook DJ: Evidence-based critical care medicine: a potential tool for change. New Horizons 6:20–25, 1998.

Iezzoni LI: The risks of risk adjustment. JAMA; 278:1600–1607, 1997.

Institute of Medicine: *Crossing the Quality Chasm: A New Health System for the 21st Century*, Washington, DC: National Academy Press, 2001.

Institute of Medicine: *To Err is Human: Building a Safer Health System*, Washington, DC: National Academy Press, 2000.

Layde PM, Maas LA, Teret SP et al: Patient safety efforts should focus on medical injuries. JAMA 287:1993–2001, 2002.

Marshall JC, Cook DJ, Christou NV et al: Multiple Organ Dysfunction Score: a reliable descriptor of a complex clinical outcome. Crit Care Med 23:1638–1652, 1995.

Szalados JE: Critical care medicine: essentials of the reimbursement process. NYSSA Sphere 53:22–28, 2001.

Szalados JE. Health information privacy and HIPAA: The Health Insurance Portability and Accountability Act. Curr Rev Clin Anesth 25(1):1–16, 2004.

Szalados JE. Age and functional status as determinants of intensive care unit outcome: sound basis for health policy or tip of the outcomes iceberg? Crit Care Med 32(1):291–293, 2004.

Szalados JE. Intensive care unit resource utilization by Medicare patients: margin and mission meet public policy and practice economics. Crit Care Med 32(11):2351–2352, 2004.

Szalados JE. Do Not Resuscitate and end-of-life care issues: clinical, ethical, and legal principles. Curr Rev Anesth 24(5): 47–53, 2003.

Internet Resources

Agency for Healthcare Research and Quality: www.ahrg.org

American Board of Quality Assurance and Utilization Review Physicians: www.abqaurp.org

American College of Legal Medicine: www.aclm.org

American Health Quality Association: www.ahqa.org

Leapfrog: www.leapfroggroup.org

National Committee for Quality Assurance: www.ncqa.org

Project Impact: www.sccm.org/pi

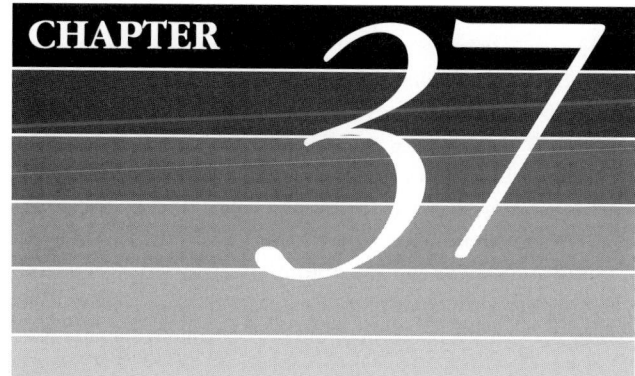

Scoring Systems

SANJEEV V. CHHANGANI, M.D., M.B.A.

Critical care consumes a disproportionate share of hospital resources. While intensive care unit (ICU) beds comprise between 5 and 10% of total hospital beds, critical care accounts for as much as 25–34% of total hospital costs. Quality and cost of care are emerging as growing concerns among health care buyers, policy makers, regulators, and the public at large. As a result there is increased scrutiny and pressure to improve ICU care processes and outcomes. Critical care, by virtue of its high cost, high complexity, and high mortality, lends itself to measurement of ICU performance and quality of care. Given the relatively high mortality in ICU patients, death is a sensitive and meaningful measure of outcome. Therefore, mortality still remains a "gold standard" as an outcome measure for critically ill patients. Scoring systems have been developed in response to an increasing emphasis on the evaluation and monitoring of critical care services.

ROLE OF SCORING SYSTEMS

The purpose of scoring systems in ICUs is to take into account the characteristics of patients that could affect their risk of a particular outcome and account for factors that are outside the control of those providing the care. Various patient-related factors associated with an increase in risk of death in ICUs include increasing age, greater severity of illness, emergency surgery, and presence of concurrent severe medical conditions. Accounting for such patient characteristics or "case mix" is essential for proper comparisons of outcome. Outcome is usually measured as death before discharge from hospital after critical care. The role of scoring systems is based on the quantification of case mix and the development of mathematical models to estimate probabilities of outcome for ICU patients. The association between the independent variables (case mix) and the dependent variable (death) is described in the form of a multiple logistic regression model. Applying the model, the probability of death before discharge from hospital after critical care can be estimated for each patient and summed for all patients to yield the expected hospital death rate for the group of patients. The expected hospital death rate can then be compared with the actual hospital death rate. Standardized mortality ratio (SMR) is the ratio of actual to expected deaths. SMR can be used as a measure of quality of different providers or ICUs. An SMR greater than 1.0 may reflect poor care and an SMR of less than 1.0 may reflect good care.

The major roles of ICU scoring systems include the following:

- *Perform comparative audits.* As mentioned above, the use of case-mix-adjusted outcomes as a measure of clinical effectiveness of ICUs assumes that an SMR of >1.0 may reflect poor care and an SMR of <1.0 may reflect good care. Local clinical audits must be performed to explain the reasons for any unexpected results. Severity models (Box 37-1) have been widely used as the basis for public report cards. Managed care organizations and group practices are keenly interested in outcomes reporting.
- *Perform evaluative research.* Scoring systems have been used to aid risk stratification in randomized

Box 37-1   Severity Models

Severity models present a "point estimate" of probability of hospital mortality.

controlled trials. Given the heterogeneity of ICU patients, it is proposed that stratification of using an accurate, objective estimate of the risk of hospital death might create a more homogeneous subset of patients to isolate better the effects of the intervention on the outcome. Therefore, in clinical trials severity scores may provide a number of functions including a way to evaluate entry or exclusion criteria, randomization balance, and risk-adjusted efficacy outcome measure.

- *Individual patient management.* Scoring systems have been used as a common, standard terminology to convey information rapidly about a patient and classify patients according to severity of illness. It is believed that an accurate, objective estimate of the risk of hospital death can provide an additional piece of information to help make clinical decisions about treatment plans for individual patients. It is important to mention that no model is accurate enough to predict that a given patient will certainly either survive or die, so the use of scoring system *alone* to direct therapy is not recommended.
- *Quality improvement*, like research, requires a severity-adjusted method to control for differences in the presenting characteristics of patients when one is assessing outcome. Resource utilization, cost variation, and reimbursement strategies can also be analyzed using a severity adjustment approach. In various quality improvement and/or cost strategies severity scoring systems can provide a benchmark for new initiatives.

CLINICAL CAVEAT

None of the ICU prediction models is accurate enough to predict that a given patient will certainly either survive or die, so the use of a scoring system *alone* to direct therapy is not recommended.

TYPES OF SCORING SYSTEMS

Scoring Systems based on Resource Utilization

Severity of illness can be ranked based on resource utilization, on the assumption that more severely ill patients

will need more ICU resources (nursing, monitoring, and therapeutic interventions). The Therapeutic Intervention Scoring System (TISS) quantifies the number of interventions to estimate severity of illness. The original TISS scored 57 therapeutic interventions with point values of 1 to 4, and patients at highest risk had scores of more than 40 points. Variations on TISS include the intermediate TISS, designed for step-down areas, and a simplified TISS-28, which reduces the number of variables. Because interventions can be driven by local practices, TISS scores generally are not used for prognosis or quality assessment.

Scoring Systems based on Physiologic Derangement

There are three major ICU scoring systems based on physiology. These models are all based on the assumption that more critically ill patients have values that deviate more from physiologic normal for a variety of common variables such as heart rate, blood pressure, and neurologic status, and that they also have altered physiologic reserve with advanced age and chronic illness.

Acute Physiology and Chronic Health Evaluation

In the early 1980s Knaus and colleagues first developed Acute Physiology and Chronic Health Evaluation (APACHE I) as a general ICU outcomes model. Initially, 34 physiologic variables thought to have an effect on outcome were selected. These were then reduced to 12 more commonly measured variables in APACHE II. The values that represent the greatest deviation from normal for the physiologic variables are collected during the first 24 hours after admission to the ICU. The final APACHE II score (Table 37-1) is the sum of the points assigned to each of the three components and range from 0 to 71, with an increasing score representing a greater severity of illness. In addition, coefficients are assigned to 42 specific disease designations that are considered to represent the majority of patients admitted to most ICUs. The patient's probability of dying is calculated with a logit equation that takes into account the APACHE II score and a disease coefficient with a weight added for emergent surgery. APACHE II represents a reduction in variables and an improvement in performance over the original APACHE based on multivariate regression analysis. Pediatric, burns, and coronary bypass patients are excluded from APACHE II. The relationship between APACHE II scores and hospital mortality differs for surgical and nonsurgical patients. APACHE II does not control for pre-ICU management. Admission source predicts hospital death irrespective of the APACHE II score.

APACHE III is the most recent version of the APACHE system. It addresses the limitations of APACHE II, specifically the impact of treatment location before ICU admission. This commercially available model includes

Table 37-1   APACHE II Score Form

Physiologic Variable	High Abnormal Range					Low Abnormal Range			
	+4	+3	+2	+1	0	+1	+2	+3	+4
1. Temperature, rectal (°C)	≥41	39-40.9		38.5-38.9	36.0-38.4	34-35.9	32-33.9	30-31.9	≤29.9
2. Mean arterial pressure = (2 × diastolic + systolic)/3	≥160	130-159	110-129		70-109		50-69		≤49
3. Heart rate (ventricular response)	≥180	140-179	110-139		70-109		55-69	40-54	≤39
4. Respiratory rate (nonventilated or ventilated)	≥50	35-49		25-34	12-24	10-11	6-9		<5
5. Oxygenation, A-aDO$_2$ or PaO$_2$ (mmHg)									
(a) FIO$_2$ > 0.5: record A-aDO$_2$	≥500	350-499	200-349		<200				
(b) FIO$_2$ < 0.5: record PaO$_2$					>70	61-70		55-60	<55
6. Arterial pH (if no ABGs record serum HCO$_3$ below*)	≥7.7	7.6-7.69		7.5-7.59	7.33-7.49		7.25-7.32	7.15-7.24	<7.15
7. Serum sodium	≥180	160-179	155-159	150-154	130-139		120-129	111-119	≤110
8. Serum potassium	≥7	6-6.9		5.6-5.9	3.5-5.4	3-3.4	2.5-2.9		<2.5
9. Serum creatinine (mg/dl); double point for acute renal failure	≥3.5	2-3.4	1.5-1.9		0.6-1.4		<0.6		
10. Hematocrit (%)	≥60		50-59.9	46-49.9	30-45.9		20-29.9		<20
11. White blood cell count	≥40		20-39.9	15-19.9	3-14.9		1-2.9		<1
12. Glasgow Coma Scale (score = 15 − actual GCS)	15 - GCS								
A. Total acute physiology score (APS)	**Sum of the 12 individual variable points =**								
*Serum HCO$_3$ (venous, mmol/l); not preferred, use if no ABGs	<52	41-51.9		32-40.9	22-31.9		18-21.9	15-17.9	<15

Glasgow Coma Scale (circle appropriate response)

Eyes open

4 - spontaneously
3 - to verbal stimulus
2 - to painful stimulus
1 - no response

Motor response

6 - to verbal command
5 - localizes to pain
4 - withdraws to pain
3 - decorticate
2 - decerebrate
1 - no response

Verbal - nonintubated

5 - oriented and converses
4 - disoriented and talks
3 - inappropriate words
2 - incomprehensible sounds
1 - no response

Verbal - intubated

5 - seems able to talk
3 - questionable ability to talk
1 - generally unresponsive

B: Age Points

Age	Points
<44	0
45-54	2
55-64	3
65-74	5
>75	6

Age points =

C: Chronic Health Points

If any of the 5 CHE categories is answered with "yes" give + 5 points for nonoperative or emergency postoperative patients

Liver	Cirrhosis with PHT or encephalopathy
Cardiovascular	Class IV angina or at rest with minimal self-care activities
Pulmonary	Chronic hypoxemia or hypercapnia or polycythemia of PHT > 40 mmHg
Kidney	Chronic peritoneal or hemodialysis
Immune	Immune compromised host

Chronic health points =

APACHE II Score

A + B + C (A = APS points, B = age points, C = chronic health points)

Total APACHE II Score =

17 physiologic variables that were determined to contribute independently to outcome. Five new variables (blood urea nitrogen, urine output, serum albumin, bilirubin, and glucose) were added, and serum potassium and bicarbonate were deleted from the score. The final APACHE III score is determined by the sum of the physiologic points together with age and chronic health points. The final APACHE III score can vary between 0 and 300, and a 5-point increase represents a significant increase risk of hospital death. The APACHE III scoring system has not been widely accepted or used.

Simplified Acute Physiology Score

The Simplified Acute Physiology Score (SAPS) I uses a subset of the original APACHE variables. SAPS is the European equivalent of APACHE. Like the APACHE system, SAPS uses the worst values collected during the first 24 hours after ICU admission, and excludes burn patients and cardiac surgery patients. The outcome measure for SAPS II is vital status for hospital discharge. This model includes 17 variables, including 12 physiologic variables, age, type of admission, and three underlying diagnoses (AIDS, metastatic cancer, and hematologic malignancies).

Mortality Probability Models

Mortality probability models (MPMs), like APACHE and SAPS, exclude pediatric, burn, and cardiac surgery patients and estimate hospital mortality risk based partly on physiologic derangement, but consider a smaller number of variables. MPM II uses data obtained at ICU admission (MPM_0) and at the end of the first 24 hours (MPM_{24}). The admission model contains 15 variables and the 24-hour model uses five of the 15 MPM_0 variables plus 8 additional ones. Age and chronic health status are included in both MPM_0 and MPM_{24}. MPM directly calculates a probability of survival from the available data. The final result for MPM II is expressed as a probability of death with a range from 0 to 1. The most important difference between MPMs and other systems is that the MPM_0, with the exception of information related to cardiopulmonary resuscitation, produces a probability estimate that is available at ICU admission and is independent of ICU treatment. MPM does not require specifying a diagnosis (Table 37-2).

Trauma Scoring Systems

The general scoring systems such as APACHE II, SAPS II, and MPM II perform poorly on trauma patients. The revised trauma score (RTS) consists of Glasgow coma scale (GCS), systolic blood pressure, and respiratory rate. The most abnormal value is recorded, and the RTS is the sum of the coded values multiplied by the weight for each of the variables. The injury severity score (ISS)

Table 37-2	Mortality Probability Model at Intensive Care Unit Presentation (MPM_0)

Physiology
  Coma/deep stupor
  Heart rate > 150/minute
  Systolic blood pressure < 90 mmHg
Chronic diagnoses
  Chronic renal disease
  Cirrhosis
  Metastatic neoplasm
Acute diagnoses
  Acute renal failure
  Cardiac dysrhythmias
  Cerebrovascular incident
  Gastrointestinal bleeding
  Intracranial mass effect
Other
  Cardiopulmonary resuscitation before ICU admission
  Mechanical ventilation
  Medical or unscheduled surgery
  Age

is an index of the severity and extent of anatomic injury. The trauma–injury severity score (TRISS) combines the RTS and the ISS, a classification of the type of injury (penetrating vs. blunt), and the patient's age. TRISS has become the most widely used and accepted scoring system for trauma outcome assessment. In patients with acute head trauma GCS still remains the most applicable severity scoring system.

Morbidity Scores

A number of studies have raised the concern about mortality rate as a sensitive outcome measure. There is growing interest in using morbidity as an outcome measure. In critically ill patients the development of one or more organ system dysfunctions represents the most important morbid event. Multiple organ dysfunction syndrome (MODS) represents a major cause of ICU and hospital mortality. The two most commonly used morbidity scores are the Multiple Organ Dysfunction (MOD) score (Table 37-3) and the Sequential Organ Failure Assessment (SOFA) score. Both are based on serial measurement of easily available parameters of organ dysfunction. The MOD score has the advantage of being relatively independent of any particular treatment practices. The maximal MOD score (the sum of the highest score achieved in each organ system during the patient's ICU stay) gives an estimate of cumulative organ dysfunction. The change in MOD score is thought to reflect the development of additional organ failure. There is fairly good correlation between the change in MOD score and ICU mortality. The method of scoring for SOFA is similar

Table 37-3   Multiple Organ Dysfunction (MOD) Score

Organ System	Score 0	1	2	3	4
Respiratory* (PO_2/FIO_2 ratio)	>300	226-300	151-225	76-150	≤75
Renal† (serum creatinine)	≤100	101-200	201-350	351-500	>500
Hepatic‡ (serum bilirubin)	≤20	21-60	61-120	121-240	>240
Cardiovascular§ (PAR)	≤10.0	10.1-15.0	15.1-20.0	20.1-30.0	>30.0
Hematologic¶ (platelet count)	>120	81-120	51-80	21-50	≤20
Neurologic** (Glasgow Coma Score)	15	13-14	10-12	7-9	≤6

* The PO_2/FIO_2 ratio is calculated without reference to the use or mode of mechanical ventilation, and without reference to the use or level of positive end-expiratory pressure.

† The serum creatinine concentration is measured in μmol/l without reference to the use of dialysis.

‡ The serum bilirubin concentration is measured in μmol/l.

§ The pressure-adjusted heart rate (PAR) is calculated as the product of the heart rate (HR) and the ratio of the right atrial (central venous) pressure (RAP) to the mean arterial pressure (MAP): PAR = HR × RAP/MAP.

¶ The platelet count is measured in platelets/ml × 10^{-3}.

** The Glasgow Coma Score is preferably calculated by the patient's nurse, and is scored conservatively (for the patient receiving sedation or muscle relaxants, normal function is assumed, unless there is evidence of intrinsically altered mentation).

to the MOD scores in most organs, except for cardiovascular dysfunction. The SOFA score utilizes a combination of hypotension and requirement for specific vasoactive drugs (Table 37-4).

SHORTCOMINGS IN SELECTING A SCORING SYSTEM

APACHE II remains the most widely used and recognized scoring system. The URL http://www.sfar.org/scores2/apache22.html can be used to download APACHE II. The criteria for selection of a scoring system should be based on the accuracy (validity and reliability) and

goodness-of-fit (calibration and discrimination) of the mathematical model used to estimate outcome. Discrimination, or the ability of a model to distinguish between a patient who will die and one who will live, is usually measured by the area under the measured receiver operator characteristic (ROC) curve. The total area under the curve is a good summary measure of predictive ability. Calibration compares the observed mortality with that predicted by the model within severity strata. Validity is the ability of the score to measure fully what it is intended to measure, and includes construct, content, and criterion validity. There is no "gold standard" to use as the basis for establishing the validity of scoring systems. Reproducibility is the ability of the score to be

Table 37-4   Sequential Organ Failure Assessment (SOFA) Score

Variable	SOFA Score 0	1	2	3	4
Respiratory (PaO_2/FIO_2, mmHg)	>400	≤400	≤300	≤200*	≤100*
Coagulation (platelets × $10^3/\mu l$)	>150	≤150	≤100	≤50	≤20
Liver (bilirubin, mg/dl)†	<1.2	1.2-1.9	2.0-5.9	6.0-11.9	>12.0
Cardiovascular (hypotension)‡	No hypotension	MAP <70 mmHg	Dop ≤ 5 or Dob (any dose)§	Dop > 5, Epi ≤ 0.1, or Norepi ≤ 0.1§	Dop > 15, Epi > 0.1, or Norepi > 0.1§
Central nervous system (Glasgow Coma Score)	15	13-14	10-12	6-9	<6
Renal (creatinine, mg/dl; or urine output, ml/dl)¶	<1.2	1.2-1.9	2.0-3.4	3.5-4.9 or <500	>5.0 or <200

* Values are with respiratory support.

† To convert bilirubin from mg/dl to μmol/l, multiply by 17.1.

‡ Dob, dobutamine; Dop, dopamine; Epi, epinephrine; MAP, mean arterial pressure; Norepi, norepinephrine.

§ Adrenergic agents administered for at least 1 hour (doses given are in μg/kg/minute).

¶ To convert creatinine from mg/dl to μmol/l, multiply by 88.4.

repeated with similar results in differing situations. A responsive score is one in which a change in the score correlates with a clinically important change in the gold standard. In general, APACHE II and III, SAPS II, and MPM II demonstrate good discrimination (ROC 0.83), but have poor calibration.

It is important to note that while scoring systems may apply to groups of patients they do not accurately predict death in an individual patient or the external data sets. This is due to the inability of a single model adequately to adjust risk for all case mixes across a long time period during which quality of care has changed.

SUMMARY

The ICU scoring systems provide us with the best available measures of "quality." The scoring systems can play a role in identifying the processes of care associated with best outcomes. Before an ICU scoring system is implemented, there must be an institution's cultural desire to change and an organizational commitment to measure processes and outcomes, and a commitment to standardized care. The scoring systems of the future are likely to be disease-specific, not generic, and be applicable to a more homogeneous population.

SELF-ASSESSMENT

QUESTION

The most appropriate use of a severity-of-illness model represents which *one* of the following?
A. As a screening tool for ICU admissions
B. To decide when "near" futile care should be stopped
C. Quality of care comparisons
D. To determine nurse staffing ratio

SELECTED READING

Buckley TA, Gomersall CD, Ramsay SJ: Validation of the multiple organ dysfunction (MOD) score in critically ill medical and surgical patients. Intensive Care Med 29:2216-2222, 2003.

Glance LG, Dick AW, Osler TM, Mukamel D: Using hierarchical modeling to measure ICU quality. Intensive Care Med 29:2223-2229, 2003.

Gunning K, Rowan K: ABC of intensive care: outcome data and scoring systems [clinical review]. BMJ 319(7204):241-244, 1999.

Marik PE, Varon JV: Severity scoring and outcome assessment. Computerized predictive models and scoring systems. Crit Care Clin 15(3):633-646, 1999.

Mourouga P, Goldfrad C, Rowan K: Does it fit? Is it good? Assessment of scoring systems. Curr Opin Crit Care 6:176-180, 2000.

POSTANESTHESIA
CARE UNIT

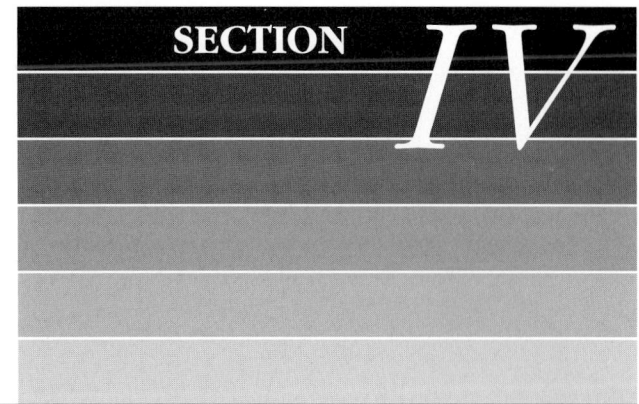

CHAPTER 38

Common Postanesthesia Care Unit Problems

ROGER R. NG, M.D.

STEWART J. LUSTIK, M.D.

The anesthesiologists' goal following surgery is to return their patients to normal physiologic states with minimal side effects. The transfer of patients from the operating room (OR) to the postanesthesia care unit (PACU) entails many challenges, including treatment of pain, nausea/vomiting, hypoxia, temperature disturbances, confusion, and hemodynamic instability. These PACU problems often lead to delays in discharge. The potential for complications following even the most benign anesthetics is 20–30%. This chapter reviews many common PACU complications and examines new strategies and therapeutic measures available for the recovery room practitioner. Hemodynamic complications in the postoperative patient are described in Chapter 40.

PAIN

Pain control in the perioperative period is always a high priority for anesthesiologists and patients. Postoperative pain is most common after orthopedic surgery (especially shoulder surgery) and surgery of more than 2 hours' duration. Inadequate pain relief can predispose a patient to a variety of postoperative complications, including increased sympathetic nervous system responses, nausea and vomiting, atelectasis, pneumonia, and deep vein thrombosis. Postoperative pain management begins with review of a patient's preoperative pain state and any treatments provided prior to surgery. Patients with longstanding pain associated with chronic medication use will have developed a tolerance especially notable in the perioperative period. The provider must consider not only the type and amount of preoperative pain medication, but also the level of pain control prior to surgery. Those patients without adequate pain control prior to surgery will be difficult to manage especially in the immediate postoperative period. Patients taking chronic opioid therapy should continue their regimen through the day of surgery and, if possible, throughout the postoperative period to assist with developed tolerance. Patients that received preemptive analgesia with analgesics or by regional or neuraxial blockade may have reduced postoperative pain; preemptive analgesia prevents the establishment of central sensitization caused by incisional and inflammatory injuries.

Before prescribing analgesics, the PACU practitioner must consider the type of the surgery and the intensity of pain expected. A patient's physical and psychologic state and cultural background may influence subjective perception of pain. Therefore, the provider must assess the patient in order to determine the severity of pain and course of treatment. Numeric pain scales and Visual Analog Pain scales (VAS; 0 being no pain and 10 being the worst pain ever noted) can assist in the treatment of pain by helping patients quantify their pain.

In addition to incisional pain, a patient may complain of nonsurgical pain, which must be elucidated before aggressive treatment is initiated. A headache, sore throat from airway instrumentation, and limb or back pain from prolonged positioning may distract the provider from adequate incisional pain relief.

Narcotics

Opioids are considered the mainstay for treatment for early postoperative pain. Opioids are potent analgesics that control moderate to severe postoperative pain. Binding to mu, kappa, and delta receptors spinally and supraspinally, opioids may cause respiratory depression, pruritis, nausea and vomiting, over-sedation, urinary retention, and prolongation of postoperative ileus.

Opioids such as fentanyl (12.5 to 50 μg), hydromorphone (0.125 to 0.5 mg), meperidine (10 to 25 mg), or morphine (1 to 4 mg) may be cautiously intravenously titrated at five-minute intervals until an adequate analgesic level is reached or respirations are 10 or less per minute. Although fentanyl has a quick onset (1 to 2 minutes) and rapid peak effect (3 to 5 minutes), its short duration of action compared with morphine results in higher pain scores and more need for oral analgesia when patients recover in phase II. In the face of residual postoperative sedation, PACU nurses should be acutely aware of respiratory depression and titrate opioid therapy carefully for patient comfort. Preoperative neuraxial morphine may last up to 24 hours (0.1 to 0.4 mg intrathecal, 3 to 5 mg epidural) and delivers good pain control in the recovery room. Pruritis and nausea are common side effects with opioid therapy and can be treated with nalbuphine and antiemetics, respectively. Intrathecal water-soluble opioids such as morphine may cause respiratory depression in the late postoperative period. Recently, more research has demonstrated good pain control with intra-articular opioids placed by surgeons at the completion of their procedures, with or without local anesthetics. Patient-controlled analgesia (PCA) most commonly involves a preprogrammed system of continuous and/or incremental dosage of opioids with a set lockout interval. PCA is often started in the PACU, where nurses can evaluate and initiate loading doses. PCA increases patient satisfaction and decreases opioid requirement compared to scheduled regimens. Morphine and meperidine should be avoided in patients with renal insufficiency due to the accumulation of active metabolites. PCA can be used with epidural infusions with combination techniques of local anesthetics and opioids or with local and opioid infusions independently. Naloxone 40 μg IV may be repeated as needed to reverse respiratory depression; care should be taken, as rapid reversal has been associated with catecholamine release and pulmonary edema.

Nonsteroidal Anti-inflammatory Drugs

The role of nonsteroidal anti-inflammatory drugs (NSAIDs) has changed as more anesthesiologists pursue regimens that can supplement or replace opioids, and thus decrease the incidence of opioid side effects. Effective as an analgesic, NSAID inhibition of cyclo-oxygenase (COX) expression has been associated with reduction of inflammatory mediators on peripheral nociceptors to promote preemptive analgesia. The use of NSAIDs has increased recently as studies have found equal efficacy between doses of NSAIDs and opioids without many of the deleterious central effects. Unfortunately, unlike opioids, there is a ceiling effect with NSAIDs. Contraindications to NSAID use include history of allergy, renal insufficiency, peptic ulcer disease, and platelet dysfunction. There has been great concern over the COX_2 inhibitor agents over the last year. The majority have been withdrawn from use. There may be increased risk for cardiovascular events. We therefore recommend that they not be used until further evaluation and risk benefit studies by the FDA.

Local Anesthetics

Local anesthetics block sodium channels and prevent the transmission of electrical nerve impulses and are widely recognized as effective agents in perioperative and postoperative pain management. Local anesthetics can be utilized at various sites for analgesia. In addition to nerve blocks performed by the anesthesiology team, intraoperative infiltration of incisions and joints by surgeons can reduce postoperative pain. Those at high risk for potential pulmonary complications can benefit from intercostal nerve blocks with local anesthetic seen commonly in thoracic and upper abdominal procedures. Extremity nerve blocks (e.g., interscalene, axillary, supraclavicular, and sciatic) provide excellent pain control that will last many hours beyond the patient's time in the PACU. Many patients without adequate pain control may be offered a nerve block in the PACU. Ultrasound guided blocks can be performed accurately and efficiently, with a lower incidence of complications. The toxicity of local anesthetics is reflected in the central nervous and cardiovascular systems. With careful management and vigilant dosing of local anesthetics, especially in the pediatric and geriatric populations, seizures and cardiac arrhythmias can be minimized. These potential toxicities are generally due to intravascular or inadvertent intrathecal injection. Neuraxial anesthesia involving the placement of local anesthesia into intrathecal, epidural, or caudal space can be performed throughout the perioperative period to help manage postoperative pain. Side effects include hypotension secondary to sympathectomy and difficulty ambulating due to motor blockade and loss of proprioception. Analgesia is enhanced when narcotics are added to local anesthetics in neuraxial blockade. Safety with caudal anesthesia with the pediatric population has been well documented in the one-shot bolus or continual infusion, with close observance to dosing.

NAUSEA AND VOMITING

Postoperative nausea and vomiting (PONV) remains the most common complication in the immediate postoperative period. Many patients acknowledge that PONV is the most distressing complication involved with the surgical experience, often more distressing than postoperative pain. The incidence of PONV has been found to be as high as 30–50% in the first 24 hours following surgery. As the number of ambulatory surgery centers and outpatient procedures continue to rise, the management of PONV becomes increasingly more important to both patients and the health care system. Delays in discharge, risk of pulmonary aspiration, increased cost of nursing and medical care, and the potential for unanticipated hospital admission following ambulatory surgery erode the cost savings of outpatient surgery. The debate continues regarding the timing and the efficacy of the many modalities for the prevention and treatment of PONV.

Nausea involves the subjective sensation of discomfort often associated with vomiting, but may occur independently caused by impulses from the gastrointestinal tract or from the cerebellum with motion sickness. The physiology of vomiting involves an intricate communications network centering on the emetic center located in the lateral reticular formation in the medulla. Afferent inputs involve chemical mediators from the chemoreceptor trigger zone, solitary tract nucleus, vestibular apparatus, cerebellum, and higher cortical areas, as well as input from the gastrointestinal system. Efferent impulses are transmitted through the vagus, phrenic, and spinal nerves and coordinate the diaphragm and abdominal musculature in the act of vomiting. The central chemical receptors involved include dopaminergic, muscarinic, serotoninergic, histaminic, and opioid.

The blockade of these receptors is the mainstay in the treatment of PONV.

Risk Factors

The risk factors involved in PONV can be subdivided into three areas: patient, surgery, and anesthesia. Patient-related factors include female gender, nonsmoking status, and previous history of PONV or motion sickness. School-age children have a higher incidence than adults, whereas younger infants have a lower incidence.

The type and duration of surgery are associated with the rate of PONV. Surgery with an increased incidence of PONV includes craniotomy; ear, nose, and throat procedures including tonsillectomies and adenoidectomies; ophthalmic, including strabismus surgery; major breast; laparoscopic, especially gynecologic; laparotomies; and orthopedic/shoulder operations. There is a 60% increase in the incidence of PONV for each 30-minute increase in surgical duration.

Anesthetic-related factors can be divided into preoperative, intraoperative, and postoperative management. Perioperative opioids have been associated with two to four times the incidence of PONV. However, inadequate analgesia in the perioperative period can cause increased PONV. Intraoperatively, the use of nitrous oxide has been shown to increase PONV, especially in the later postoperative period. The diffusion of nitrous oxide to the middle ear and bowel, stimulating the vestibular apparatus and bowel distention, activates the dopaminergic receptors in the cortical medullary system and endogenous cerebrospinal opioids from bowel distention. Modern volatile anesthetics increase the incidence of PONV, although less than previously used ether and cyclopropane. When propofol is used as an induction and maintenance agent, it reduces PONV in the early postoperative period with less benefit approximately 6 hours postoperatively. Propofol in low bolus doses (20 mg IV) in the PACU has been shown to assist in the treatment of PONV. Reversal of neuromuscular blocking drugs (NMBDs) with anticholinesterases, such as neostigmine and edrophonium, increases gastric motility and may increase PONV. PONV is more common at doses greater than 2.5 mg of neostigmine. Because anticholinergic medications are routinely given with anticholinesterases to reduce their muscarinic actions, there are reports that the use of tertiary agents like atropine, which cross the blood–brain barrier, may cause less PONV than those that do not (glycopyrrolate).

Recent research has found that oxygen at 80% during and possibly two hours following laparoscopic gynecologic surgery results in a twofold reduction in nausea and vomiting compared to 30% oxygen. It is thought that hyperoxia decreases dopamine release by the carotid bodies and decreases serotonin release by the intestines in periods of ischemia.

Although not conclusive, administration of intravenous fluids above maintenance rates (20 ml/kg) to ensure proper hydration reduces PONV. Dehydration, orthostatic hypotension, and dizziness can all promote postoperative emesis.

Postoperatively, there are numerous stimuli that may cause PONV. Following a general anesthetic, the vestibular apparatus may become sensitized by diffusion of nitrous oxide into the middle ear, causing emesis. Movement of those individuals by stretcher, wheelchair, or ambulation may cause PONV, especially in those individuals that received opioids. Environmental factors can reduce the incidence of PONV, especially those with a history of previous PONV or motion sickness. A quiet environment with minimal activity may prevent and reduce emesis.

Agents

There are a number of agents available in the prevention and treatment of PONV. There are opposing views regarding treatment of PONV prophylactically or with rescue medication. The cost effectiveness, side effect profile, and patient satisfaction must be considered, especially as newer and more expensive antiemetic agents are being developed and used regularly. Pretreating patients at low risk for nausea and vomiting is not cost effective; however, many providers agree that high-risk patients undergoing operations with a high likelihood of emesis should be treated aggressively with multiple agents. We will focus on each medication as a treatment for emesis and/or nausea, and the potential for effective combination therapy.

Dopamine Antagonists

Metoclopramide antagonizes central dopamine receptors and at high doses antagonizes 5-HT3 receptors. Although it is not recommended to treat or prevent PONV because of its minimal antiemetic effect, metoclopramide increases lower esophageal sphincter tone and motility through interactions of dopaminergic and cholinergic receptors. Droperidol interacts though heterocyclic, neuroleptic central dopaminergic receptors and is known to cause adverse effects similar to metoclopramide, including sedation, lethargy, agitation and extrapyramidal symptoms. These effects can be minimized by the use of lower dosing (0.625–1.25 mg) in adults; its low cost and high efficacy make it an attractive agent. Droperidol is contraindicated in patients with Parkinson's disease. Droperidol can be effectively dosed at 50–75 µg/kg in children. Droperidol has been much discussed with regards to the "black box" warning that was provided recently by the US Food and Drug

Administration, due to anecdotal reports that found the prolongation of QTc interval and fatal arrhythmias; one should consider alternatives in patients with a prolonged QT interval or at high risk of arrhythmias.

Promethazine and prochlorperazine are direct-acting dopamergic antagonists that work directly on the CTZ. Even at low doses, they appear to be very effective for PONV but are associated with sedation and extrapyramidal side effects.

Histamine H1 Antagonists

Commonly used in regimens for chemotheraputic-induced nausea and vomiting, the histamine H1 receptor antagonists are weakly antiemetic. Due to their low cost, H1 blockers have found resurgence in interest as antiemetic medication. Common side effects include sedation that may not be suitable for the postoperative period.

Muscarinic Antagonists

Receptors in the vestibular apparatus include muscarinic and histaminic receptors. Although many studies extrapolate the use of anticholinergics from the premedication period, atropine can cause irritable behavior, dry mouth, and blurred vision. Transdermal scopolamine, if placed well before the preoperative period, has been shown to lessen PONV, especially in patients receiving epidural opioids as well as children using a morphine PCA.

Serotonin Antagonists

Ondansetron is the prototypical serotonin antagonist and although it has structure similar to metoclopramide, it has no affinity at the dopamine receptor. Multiple studies have shown that ondansetron used to treat PONV is effective at a 1 mg dose and is effective in the prevention of PONV at a 4 mg dose. Many believe that ondansetron is more consistently an antiemetic than an antinausea agent. Side effects include headache, lightheadedness, dizziness, increased liver enzymes, and constipation. Ondansetron has been noted to be effective in children at a dose of 50 µg/kg. Although increasingly expensive, other agents in this class include granisetron 40 µg/kg and dolasetron 12.5–50 mg.

Corticosteroids

Although its exact mechanism of action is unknown, dexamethasone is an effective antiemetic at a dose 150 µg/kg for children and 8–10 mg for adults if given prior to incision. There is no proven benefit of dexamethasone in the PACU.

Postanesthesia Care Unit Regimens

After receiving a patient in the PACU with PONV, the care provider must examine the patient at the bedside and determine if there is a disease process causing PONV which needs immediate treatment such as cardiac ischemia, hypotension, hypoxia, abdominal obstruction, a nasogastric tube causing irritation, or residual blood or sputum in the airway. Next, it should be determined whether or not prophylaxis was given prior to completion of surgery. For patients who did not receive prophylaxis or only received dexamethasone, a 5HT3 receptor antagonist such as ondansetron 1.0 mg should be administered. If prophylaxis with 5HT or droperidol was attempted, it should not be repeated within the first 6 hours after surgery; propofol 20 mg or phenergan 12.5 mg are acceptable alternatives.

RESPIRATORY COMPLICATIONS

Postoperative hypoxemia is of great concern for anesthesiologists and the incidence of it ranges from 3 to 50%. Risk factors involved in predicting postoperative hypoxemia include increased ASA class, preoperative oxygen saturation, increased age, male gender, obesity, smoking history, coexisting lung disease, surgical site, and duration of surgery. Transferring patients emerging from general anesthesia to the PACU carries a significant risk of postoperative hypoxia if transferred without oxygen; approximately 30% of pediatric and adult inpatients will develop hypoxemia.

Diffusion hypoxia is most often seen in the first minutes following cessation of nitrous oxide. This most commonly occurs when a patient receiving nitrous oxide is switched directly to room air. Nitrous oxide is 30 times as diffusible as nitrogen and the inspired air is diluted with nitrous oxide and PAO_2 lowered. This can be prevented by routinely providing patients with supplemental oxygen following discontinuation of nitrous oxide. Although the differential diagnosis of hypoxia and/or hypercarbia in PACU patients is broad, a directed history and physical examination usually leads to the correct etiology and treatment (Table 38-1).

Hypoventilation

Following general anesthesia and early in the PACU, many studies have shown the need for ASA 1 and 2 patients to require supplemental oxygen therapy. It is estimated that approximately 50% of patients without supplemental oxygen will have an episode of postoperative hypoxemia within three hours after surgery.

Residual potent inhalational agents and narcotics given in the perioperative period may cause hypoventilation in the postoperative patient, especially in patients with underlying lung disease, such as chronic obstructive pulmonary disease (COPD). These drugs will depress ventilatory drive mainly at central locations and depress the body's normal response to hypoxemia and hypercarbia. Low levels of isoflurane and halothane

Table 38-1	Respiratory Complications in the Postanesthesia Care Unit
Hypoventilation	Residual medications
	Airway obstruction
	Residual neuromuscular blockade
	Pain with breathing
Increased shunt	Atelectasis
	Mucus plugging
	Preexisting anatomic shunts
Increased dead space	Pulmonary edema
	Aspiration
	Pulmonary embolism – thrombus, air, fat
	Pneumothorax
	Bronchospasm
	Decreased cardiac output
	Acute respiratory distress syndrome

(0.1 MAC) severely reduce hypoxic drive. Respiratory depression caused by opioids will present with a slow respiratory rate. Although sedation may be present, the patient is arousable and will follow commands. Normal oxygenation does not rule out significant hypoventilation, as high inspired oxygen concentrations may allow patients to remain adequately oxygenated with progressive hypercarbia.

Airway obstruction in the early postoperative period is commonly caused by decreased upper airway tone and possibly increased airway edema. Pharyngeal obstruction is commonly due to the tongue. Pharyngeal dilator muscle contraction activity is decreased due to residual medications in the semiconscious patient. Laryngeal obstruction may also occur secondary to laryngeal spasm or direct airway injury. Prolonged procedures, traumatic intubations, excessive bucking, and coughing during emergence may result in laryngeal edema. Hematomas are common causes for external compression of the trachea, following head and neck procedures, including surgery on the carotid artery and thyroid. Patients with history of obstructive sleep apnea are at increased risk of airway obstruction especially with sedation. Bilateral injury to the recurrent laryngeal nerve (e.g., during thyroidectomy) will result in unopposed vocal cord tension and stridor. Postoperative stridor may also be caused by acute hypocalcemia after unintentional removal of parathyroid glands, although this often presents after leaving the PACU. Laryngospasm may occur in a sedated patient due to secretions.

Recurarization, or residual neuromuscular blockade, is more common with long-acting neuromuscular blockade, such as pancuronium, although residual paralysis is common even two hours after administration of an intermediate-acting agent. Patients will have shallow breathing patterns and generally be tachypneic in the PACU. Many modalities have assisted with the monitoring of blockade including train-of-four ratio, sustained tetanus, and sustained head lift for 5 seconds. The ideal train-of-four ratio of >0.7 is not practical in the operating suite. Due to increased use of shorter-acting neuromuscular agents and more commonplace use of nerve stimulators, adequate reversal is more reliable and less postoperative residual blockade and upper airway obstruction is observed in the PACU.

Incisional thoracic and abdominal pain results in shallow rapid breathing and may result in a decrease in the forced vital capacity/vital capacity (FVC/VC) ratio postoperatively. Upper abdominal surgery will reduce diaphragm excursion musculature and decrease abdominal assistance to breathing, converting the work of breathing to the intercostals musculature. Pain can also prevent the coughing and deep breathing that is required to clear secretions and open closed airways.

V/Q Mismatch

Ventilation/perfusion mismatch may cause hypoxia or hypercarbia in the PACU. Shunt (low ventilation relative to perfusion) will cause a more significant hypoxemia, whereas deadspace (high ventilation relative to perfusion) may additionally cause hypercarbia. Intraoperatively, patient positioning will potentially worsen V/Q mismatch prior to surgical intervention. Nondependent areas of lung will be well ventilated but poorly perfused, while dependent areas will have better perfusion. These changes will linger into the early postoperative period and may cause hypoxemia.

Postoperative atelectasis can occur from bronchial obstruction due to secretions or blood in the airway, or poor inspiratory effort. This can occur in a segmental or diffuse pattern. Right to left intrapulmonary shunting will occur and the patient will develop a decreased functional residual capacity and smaller airway volumes, which increase airway collapse. Upper abdominal and thoracic procedures will commonly cause significant postoperative atelectasis. Following thoracic cases with endobronchial intubation, collapse of a patient's lung is a source of major atelectasis and if not corrected intraoperatively will be difficult to manage in the PACU without positive pressure ventilation to open up the collapsed airways.

Pulmonary edema may cause hypoxia in the PACU. Pulmonary edema is most common in patients with a decreased left ventricular ejection fraction, severe valvular disease, or myocardial ischemia, especially in the setting of acute rises in afterload or heart rate. Healthy patients with airway obstruction and hypoxia after extubation can develop negative pressure pulmonary edema from the sustained reduction in interstitial hydrostatic pressure. Pulmonary edema may also be due to increased capillary permeability after pulmonary injury, including aspiration, trauma, massive transfusion, sepsis, and acute respiratory distress syndrome.

Pulmonary embolus would be suspected in a patient with pleuritic chest pain, dyspnea, tachypnea, and decreases in PaO_2. Pulmonary hypertension, right-sided heart strain on ECG, elevated central venous pressures, and systemic hypotension may be apparent in those patients with a large pulmonary embolus. Patients at high risk include those who have been on prolonged bed rest prior to surgery. Petechiae may be present in patients with fat emboli, which may occur after long bone fractures.

Pneumothorax should be high on the differential diagnosis of hypoxemia in cases following central line placement, brachial plexus blockade, intercostal nerve blocks, trauma including rib fractures and chest tube placement, procedures which involve the head and neck, and diaphragm, especially in the retroperoneum. In addition to rarely causing a pneumothorax, upper extremity blocks may cause hypoxia from phrenic nerve paralysis.

Evaluation

Hypoxemia may present as hypertension, hypotension, tachycardia, bradycardia, agitation, or cardiac dysrhythmias. These signs and symptoms are nonspecific and may be subtle; thus, the pulse oximeter should be continued throughout the PACU period. Pulse oximeters are accurate in the range 70–100%, although they require pulsatile blood flow for differentiation of oxygenated and deoxygenated blood and are unreliable in periods of hypovolemia, hypothermia, and peripheral vasoconstriction. Pulse oximeters are poor monitors of other clinically important species of hemoglobin (Hb), including Met-Hb and carboxy-Hb, which may cause unreliable readings. If in doubt, the clinician should draw an arterial blood gas and measure the partial pressure of oxygen directly. The arterial blood gas will reveal the patient's oxygenation and ventilation status. In addition to careful lung auscultation, a chest x-ray will help define the etiology of a patient with suboptimal oxygenation despite supplemental oxygen and a reasonable respiratory rate and tidal volume.

Treatment

Many of the above diagnoses can be treated quickly with supplemental oxygenation. Concentrations of 30–60% generally will correct mild to moderate hypoxemia. Although this may help correct arterial hypoxemia temporarily, the practitioner must evaluate the patient and treat the underlying cause of hypoxemia.

Airway obstruction requires expeditious correction. Loud snoring and/or inspiratory stridor characterize partial obstruction. Total obstruction is characterized by lack of air exchange and loss of breath sounds. The patient will commonly attempt to use all respiratory musculature to assist in respirations. Nasal flaring, retractions of the substernal notch as well as intercostal muscles, and increased diaphragmatic/abdominal excursions, which may perform paradoxically to chest movement, may occur. These patients should receive supplemental oxygen while correcting the obstruction. The patient's head should be extended and jaw thrust forward to assist in pulling the tongue forward from the posterior pharynx. If needed, an oropharyngeal or nasopharyngeal airway should be placed to ensure a patent airway down to the vocal cords. The nasal airway may be better tolerated in the lightly sedated patient. Continuous positive airway pressure may be successful in some patients. If the obstruction is not relieved, one must then consider problems with the larynx. Laryngospasm is treated with the head tilt and jaw thrust maneuver, as well as manual pressure at the angle of the mandible and positive pressure ventilation with a tight fitting bag and facemask with 100% oxygen. Suction if secretions or blood is suspected. If the laryngospasm does not resolve, a small amount of IV succinylcholine (10–20 mg) should be administered to assist in the relaxation of the cords. If unsuccessful, endotracheal intubation may be necessary to reestablish adequate ventilation. While intubating, one should observe the vocal cords closely for edema or trauma. Laryngeal edema may be treated with humidified inspired gases and nebulized racemic epinephrine. Although not of immediate relief, dexamethasone 0.5 mg/kg IV can be given in cases of laryngeal edema.

Residual opioid effects can be treated by the administration of naloxone. Naloxone 40 µg every 2 minutes will allow the practitioner to titrate the opioid reversal to adequate ventilation without completely antagonizing the analgesic effects following surgery. Poor titration will not only cause pain but activate the sympathetic nervous system, including hypertension, nausea and vomiting, pulmonary edema, and myocardial ischemia. Naloxone has a much shorter half-life than most narcotic medications provided for analgesia; therefore, patients must be monitored closely following dosing for renarcotization.

The evaluation of a patient with suspected neuromuscular blockade should include a sustained head lift for 5 seconds, vigorous hand grasping, and adequate vital capacity. Double vision and difficulty swallowing may also occur. Neuromuscular blockade can be evaluated in a moderately sedated patient with a nerve stimulator by testing for acceptable response with no fade to a sustained tetanus. There are generally four reasons for residual neuromuscular blocking drugs. First, conditions that potentiate neuromuscular blockers include aminoglycoside antibiotics or magnesium therapy as well as hypokalemia or metabolic acidosis. Second, altered pharmacokinetics with hypothermia and liver or renal failure will cause delayed metabolism or excretion of certain neuromuscular agents. Third, pharmacologic reversal of the neuromuscular blockade may have been inadequate, causing prolonged paralysis in the PACU. Fourth, the patient may inadvertently receive a neuromuscular block bolus in the PACU when a previously obstructed IV line is cleared. Patients with residual neuromuscular blockade must be quickly treated with supplemental oxygenation, additional antagonist, if indicated, and ventilatory support as needed.

Wheezing, rales, diminished bronchial sounds, and rhonchi may be present in many forms of ventiliation/perfusion defects. Increased inspired oxygen concentration will overcome many of these defects, especially in patients with known preoperative obstructive or restrictive lung disease. Bronchospasm should be treated with nebulized inhaled beta agonists or through metered dose inhalers for intubated patients. Right to left shunting, including atelectasis, may not significantly improve with increased oxygen concentration. In intubated patients simple atelectasis without potentially catastrophic complications (i.e., lobar collapse, mainstem intubation, pulmonary edema, aspiration) may easily be corrected with simple maneuvers performed in the PACU. Humidified gases, lung opening procedures, and administration of continuous airway pressures and positive end-expiratory pressure may be necessary to reinflate closed lung units. Pulmonary edema of cardiac and noncardiac origin may be treated with diuretics, vasodilators, and dialysis, if necessary, in renal failure patients. Positive pressure ventilation may be indicated in cases of unresponsive severe hypoxemia or respiratory acidosis. Intubation and ventilation with positive pressure ventilation will improve oxygenation by expanding lung volumes. Continued ventilatory support may be necessary until definitive treatment is identified.

Following aspiration, gastric contents must be quickly removed from the airway in the orophayrnx with thorough suctioning. To protect the patient's airway, a rapid sequence intubation with cricoid pressure will prevent further aspiration. The newly placed endotracheal tube should be quickly suctioned to prevent passing of foreign material to the distal airways. 100% oxygen and positive pressure ventilation should be started as soon as possible following the above maneuvers to avoid transient hypoxia.

TEMPERATURE ABNORMALITIES

Patients that arrive in the PACU with a temperature less than 35°C are associated with a 30% increase in PACU duration. Factors involved in heat loss include radiation, convection, cutanous vasodilation, evaporative loss from the surgical field, and sweating. In addition, infusion of room temperature intravenous fluids or cold blood products will contribute to heat loss. Although cool room temperature greatly contributes to hypothermia, anesthetic-induced reduction in thermoregulatory control of a patient will add to postoperative hypothermia. Mild hypothermia is generally defined as 34–36°C.

Complications with hypothermia have been extensively studied. Notable are myocardial ischemia, coagulopathy, wound infection/healing, prolonged drug effects, increased recovery times, and thermal discomfort. Upon emergence of general anesthesia, shivering may cause a large increase in oxygen demand. This may not directly cause hypoxia, but with an increased shunt fraction, the patient will likely become hypoxemic. As the patient attempts to regain thermostatic equilibrium following a procedure, oxygen consumption will increase and cause cardiac output and CO_2 production to increase. Oxygen consumption may increase as much as 400–500% above baseline cardiac consumption, causing a significant decrease in mixed venous oxygen saturation. Postoperative cold-induced hypertension in the elderly is associated with a threefold increase in norepinephrine concentrations, which could lead to myocardial ischemia.

Elderly patients with prolonged surgery have an increased likelihood of being transferred to the PACU hypothermic. These patients are three times more likely to have hypothermic-related myocardial ischemia or ventricular arrhythmias. Platelet function, clotting factor enzyme function, and fibrinolytic activity are three general mechanisms that may cause hypothermia-induced coagulopathy. Platelet numbers are not affected by hypothermia directly; however, platelet function is seriously impaired. Coagulation tests are completed at 37°C even if the patient's temperature is much lower; therefore, prothrombin and partial thromboplastin times will not be prolonged by hypothermia. Fibrinolysis appears to remain normal in mild hypothermia; however, the inability adequately to form clot may be the cause of coagulopathy.

Wound infections have been a concern for both surgeons and anesthesiologists. Hypothermia can cause complications related to poor healing in two ways. First, hypothermia causes thermoregulatory vasoconstriction. Vasoconstriction markedly decreases oxygen tension to subcutaneous tissues, which directly correlates with wound infections. Second, mild hypothermia impairs normal immune function, especially T-cell-mediated antibody and neutrophil oxidative bactericidal activities. Reduced free oxygen radicals, which are oxygen dependent, is notable in areas of vasoconstriction and hypoxia.

The pharmacokinetics of many anesthetic-related drugs are retarded in hypothermia. Many enzymes that metabolize drugs are temperature sensitive and will be affected by hypothermia. These medications include muscle relaxants and volatile and intravenous agents. The duration of vecuronium is nearly doubled in patients with a reduction of 2°C of core temperature, and atracurium at 3°C below core temperature will have an increase in duration of about 60%. Tissue solubility of volatile agents increases with hypothermia. This will cause greater uptake by the body at lower temperatures, and, therefore, longer exhalation times to recover. Intravenous propofol and fentanyl will have concentrations approximately 10% and 5% greater, respectively, for every 1°C drop in temperature. These factors are related to the delay in discharge of patients from recovery units.

Thermal discomfort is notable for patients with mild hypothermia. Many patients in the recovery room will complain more about feeling cold than pain. Other concerns with hypothermia include hypokalemia and unreliable pulse oxygenation due to vasoconstriction.

Many PACUs will not discharge patients until their temperature reaches 36°C. Treatment involves an environment that provides a source of warming and prevents heat loss. Warming intravenous fluids will not actively warm patients, but rather sustain normothermia for a patient. Active cutaneous insulation and a forced air warming system will provide adequate warming. Most forced air systems include a powered heat blowing unit as well as a cover. These disposable covers warm patients through convection and radiant heat. Convection loss is common in the operative suite and is the most common source of heat loss, as cold air passing over skin will promote loss, as seen with wind chill. A warming blanket passing warm air over skin will increase heat gain. Radiant heat loss will be reduced, as the warm covering will replace the cool surfaces of the operating suite and PACU.

Hyperthermia

Iatrogenic hyperthermia is usually due to vigorous warming without monitoring by the anesthesiologist. The differential diagnosis of hyperthermia includes sepsis, inflammation, endocrine abnormalities, central nervous system abnormalities, drug effects, and ineffective heat loss.

Sepsis may cause hypotension and systemic vasodilation in a febrile patient. Inflammation mediated through cytokines will cause a systemic inflammatory reaction that will present with hyperthermia. Transfusion reactions related to immune reactions of incompatible blood products will cause a febrile reaction, hemolysis, and a leukoagglutinin reaction.

Endocrine abnormalities include catecholamine excess, such as pheochromocytoma, thyroid storm, Addisonian crisis, and cocaine or amphetamine use. There are several central nervous system sources of hyperthermia, including trauma, in which hypothalamic injury can result in an elevated thermoregulatory set point, intoxication, or postoperative delirium (resulting in agitation and uncontrolled muscular exertion) and status epilepticus.

Anticholinergics and medications with similar actions including antihistamines and antidepressants will diminish sweating, classically seen in heat stroke, as well as a delirium. Serotonin syndrome is caused when a combination of meperidine or dextromethorphan is given to a patient on a monoamine oxidative inhibitor (MAOI). Other combinations include a selective serotonin reuptake inhibitor or tricyclic antidepressant and MAOIs or lithium. Patients on ecstasy (3,4-methylenedioxymethamphetamine, MDMA) or other hallucinogenic amphetamines react similarly. The syndrome is characterized by altered mental status, myoclonus, shivering, hyperthermia, and muscle injury. Treatments involve supportive measures, including antipyretics, antihypertensive agents, sedatives, and steroids.

Malignant hyperthermia (MH) is a rare but deadly myopathic disorder triggered by volatile inhalational anesthetics or succinylcholine. Although MH usually occurs during administration of triggering agents, MH may begin to manifest in the PACU or several hours later. MH is an autosomal dominant of variable penetrance characterized by an increase of metabolism and sympathetic hyperactivity resulting in increased production of heat, carbon dioxide, and lactic acid resulting in a respiratory and metabolic acidosis. Hyperthermia is a late sign. The involved defect is found in sarcoplasmic reticulum, which has lost the ability to reuptake calcium causing an intracellular buildup of calcium and uncontrolled skeletal muscle contraction and metabolism. MH is a diagnosis of exclusion and may be confused with sepsis, thyroid storm, neuroleptic malignant syndrome (NMS), and pheochromocytoma, although a severe uncontrollable respiratory acidosis responsive to dantrolene is most consistent with MH. Possible complications from MH include cardiac arrest, cerebral or pulmonary edema, renal failure, and disseminated intravascular coagulopathy.

In most cases, the onset, diagnosis, and treatment of MH will begin in the operating room and continue in the PACU. Treatment includes:
- Stopping surgery and triggering agents.
- Hyperventilation with 100% oxygen to correct severe respiratory acidosis.
- Titration of dantrolene 2 mg/kg every 5 minutes up to total of 10 mg/kg.
- Bicarbonate approximately 2-4 mEq/kg if needed to assist with the buildup of lactate created by the increased metabolism.
- Treatment of hyperthermia by cooling measures, including iced fluids, core temperature cooling, cooling blankets.

- Treatment of hyperkalemia if needed, e.g., insulin (10 units regular IV and glucose 50 ml D50).
- Monitoring urine to ensure adequate output, with examination for myogloninuria.
- Consideration of arterial and central venous access.
- Monitoring for arrhythmias, electrolytes, arterial blood gases.

The treatment of MH will follow in the ICU with close observation for 48-72 hours. The PACU practitioner must be acutely aware of these patients and the many possible complications with treatment and resolution of the acute crisis.

NMS is associated with medications that antagonize the effects of dopamine, notably phenothiazides and butyrophenones. Signs and symptoms include altered mental status, myoclonus, sweating, rigidity, hyperthermia, rhabdomyolysis, and autonomic instability. Although NMS and MH appear to have similar signs and symptoms, the mechanism of action is different and does not appear to have a genetic basis, nor does NMS have an increased susceptibility to MH. There is no completely effective therapy for NMS. Bromocriptine and dantrolene have been variably successful in combination with cooling and supportive measures.

DELAYED AROUSAL

Emerging patients brought into the PACU often exhibit delayed responses and disorientation, confusion, agitation, and uncooperativeness. These patients must be immediately evaluated for hypoxia (pulse oximeter) and hypercarbia (adequate respiratory rate and tidal volume). Agitation may be due to pain in a patient not fully arousable. This may manifest as increased sympathetic tone that can cause hypertension and tachycardia, dangerous in patients with cardiac disease. The most common cause of delayed arousal is residual medication effects; however, one must also consider metabolic abnormalities and neurologic injury.

Residual Drug Effects

Residual drug effects are seen most frequently in the elderly and patients with hepatic or renal failure. Reviewing the anesthesia record for preoperative and intraoperative medications may assist in the diagnosis and treatment of delayed emergence. Inhalational agents, especially in long cases, may be the reason for delayed emergence. Although inhalational agents are eliminated mainly though the lungs, many of the inhalational agents can accumulate in body fat. Following emergence, decreased stimulation in addition to prolonged excretion out of the body fat of inhalational agents can depress mental status. Age, pregnancy, and hypothermia will reduce minimum alveolar concentration in those patients.

Narcotics and benzodiazepines may be reversed with nalaxone and flumazenil (0.2 mg IV every minute, up to 1 mg total), respectively, but barbiturates, anticholinergics, psychotropic drugs, and alcohol have no specific antagonists. Physostigmine (1.25 mg IV) has been used with variable success as a nonspecific treatment of delayed arousal.

Metabolic Abnormalities

Many metabolic and electrolyte abnormalities in the anesthetized patient will not become apparent until emergence from general anesthesia, presenting as decreased mental status or delayed emergence. Hypoglycemia, hyponatremia, and hypocalcemia are common disturbances that necessitate evaluation in the PACU.

A notable substrate for the brain to metabolize is glucose, and it is well known that hypoglycemia will cause confusion and potentially coma. Those patients at highest risk for abnormalities include patients with diabetes mellitus who take insulin or oral hypoglycemics, patients with hepatic dysfunction (low glycogen stores), and patients who have endocrine dysfunction including hypothyroidism, hypopituitarism, and insulinomas. Glucose test strips can quickly evaluate for hypoglycemia, which can be easily treated with intravenous 50% dextrose. Severe hyperglycemia may cause decreased arousal; however, nonketotic hyperosmolar hyperglycemic coma takes days to develop and would rarely present in the PACU, unless in patients who were debilitated prior to presenting for surgery.

Hyponatremia can be seen related to multiple events, including free water absorption following transurethral resection of the prostate (TURP), hysteroscopy, and syndrome of inappropriate antidiuretic hormone release (SIADH). Pulmonary carcinomas commonly secrete antidiuretic hormone (ADH). Positive pressure ventilation and stress following a surgical procedure also cause SIADH. Neurologic evaluation of patients with TURP procedures performed under spinal anesthesia can be easily observed; however, the free water absorption of glycine-based irrigating solution during general anesthesia is more difficult to evaluate. Depending on the degree of hyponatremia, confusion, seizures, dysrhythmias, and coma can occur. Acute, severe hyponatremia may be treated quickly with infusion of hypertonic saline, but minimally symptomatic hyponatremia may be corrected slowly with normal saline and furosemide. Chronic hyponatremia should not be rapidly corrected due to the risk of central pontine myelinolysis.

Hypocalcemia may occur following thyroidectomy or parathyroidectomy and in patients with pancreatic insufficiency and malnutrition. Rapid infusion of blood products decreases ionized calcium due to binding with citrate. Hypocalcemia is exaggerated by alkalosis, such as in a patient hyperventilating due to pain. Signs and symptoms include confusion, seizures, and coma. Dysrhythmias including QT prolongation and decreased cardiac contractility are commonly seen. Tetanus may also occur as well as laryngeal and diffuse muscle spasm. Treatment includes IV fluid hydration, correction of respiratory alkalosis, and replacement with intravenous calcium.

Neurologic Events

Postoperative confusion may occur from intraoperative neurologic events such as cerebral ischemia, seizures, and embolic or thrombotic events. Prolonged hypotension during anesthesia will have deleterious effects on perfusion and cerebral blood flow. Although the brain autoregulates to maintain constant perfusion at a mean arterial pressure range of 50-150 mmHg, patients who are above and below these values will have cerebral perfusion that is pressure dependent. This curve is shifted to the right in patients with hypertension and cerebral hypoperfusion may occur without significant hypotension. Patients with existing cerebrovascular disease have even less tolerance to hypotensive events, as stenotic areas decrease perfusion to already susceptible areas of the brain.

Embolic phenomena may occur during carotid endarterectomy, sitting craniotomy (paradoxical emboli if patent foramen ovale), or in patients with longstanding atrial fibrillation. Those with localized motor deficits on examination indicating a possible ischemic or hemorrhagic event must be evaluated appropriately with imaging and/or neurologic evaluation.

Any neurosurgical procedure will have the potential for seizure activity, as foci are potentially created with manipulation of the brain. Generally, those being treated for seizures will already have a depressed mental status due to the disease itself or seizure medications. Many anesthetic agents are indicated in the treatment of seizures including benzodiazepines and barbiturates; however, certain intravenous agents have the potential for lowering seizure thresholds, including methohexatol and ketamine. The postictal state can be treated conservatively including protection of the airway, maintenance of hemodynamic stability, and treatment with phenytoin. Although muscle relaxants will stop physical muscle activity, brain metabolic activity will continue and must be treated accordingly.

If the above diagnoses are ruled out, and postoperative delirium continues, sedation and/or psychotropic agents may be needed to manage the uncooperative patient. Benzodiazepines, barbiturates, and haloperidol are agents of choice. Both benzodiazepines and barbiturates have sedative effects and may potentially interfere with further examination of the patient; however, haloperidol is a butyrophenone neuroleptic agent and can be used in cases of extreme delirium, agitation, and disorientation. Haloperidol is a dopamine antagonist with minimal amounts of sedation and cardiac depressive effects and can be given 5.0 mg IM or 2.5 mg IV prn. Side effects include dysrhythmias, acute dystonic reactions, extrapyramidal symptoms reversed by diphenhydramine, tarditave dyskinesias, and NMS.

CASE STUDY

The case is a 78-year-old male, with longstanding diabetes mellitus, hypertension, s/p TURP under spinal anesthesia. The patient is somnolent upon arrival in the PACU and the report received by the anesthesiology resident is that the patient received a bupivicane spinal, 3 liters LR and a propofol infusion because the patient "did not want to hear anything." As the anesthetist prepares to leave for the next patient it is quickly stated that the propofol infusion was discontinued approximately 5 minutes prior to the completion of the procedure and the patient has been "sleepy" since. Notable on preoperative evaluation is that the patient does not remember if he had taken his insulin at night or in the morning, but finger stick blood glucose on the morning of surgery was 92. Your evaluation finds an elderly gentleman, somnolent, unarousable, BP 100/45 P 98, RR 10 SpO$_2$ 99% on 3L NC. How would you evaluate this patient?

This is an elderly patient with multiple medical problems presenting to the PACU with prolonged somnolence. His preoperative history appears unreliable and his baseline mental status may not be completely normal. Even so, following his procedure under spinal anesthesia and propofol, the patient should be more arousable. His vital signs, oxygenation, and ventilation appear stable. After evaluating the airway, if the patient continues to be unarousable, check for iatrogenic causes including residual propofol in the intravenous line, agents given to the patient for nausea, or anxiolysis prior to the short procedure. Blood glucose should be checked and electrolytes drawn and evaluated. Hypoglycemia should immediately be corrected with D50 and monitored closely. Hyponatremia can cause central nervous system (CNS) depression following a TURP, which can be corrected with normal saline. Another CNS abnormality which may be evaluated if indicated from the anesthesiologist's record of the procedure is a prolonged hypotensive period following the spinal and an ischemic event in a patient with hypertension and diabetes and most likely cerebrovascular disease. Neurologic evaluation and imaging studies would then be indicated in this case, especially if the patient exhibited localizing motor deficits.

SELECTED READING

Gan TJ, Meyer T, Apfel CC et al: Consensus guidelines for managing postoperative nausea and vomiting. Anesth Analg 97(1):62-67, 2003.

Goll V, Akca O, Greif R et al: Ondansetron is no more effective than supplemental intraoperative oxygen for prevention of postoperative nausea and vomiting. Anesth Analg 92:112-117, 2001.

Kissin I: Preemptive analgesia [Clinical Concepts and Commentary]. Anesthesiology 93:1138-1143, 2000.

McCrory CR, Lindahl SG: Cyclooxygenase inhibition for postoperative analgesia. Anesth Analg 95:169-176, 2002.

Rosenbaum HK, Miller JD: Malignant hyperthermia and myotonic disorders. Anesthesiol Clin North Am 20:3, 2002.

Sessler DI: Complications and treatment of mild hypothermia. Anesthesiology 95:531-543, 2001.

Tramer MR: A rational approach to the control of postoperative nausea and vomiting: evidence from systematic reviews. Parts I and II. Acta Anaesthesiol Scand 45:4-19, 2001.

Watcha MF: Postoperative nausea and emesis. Anesthesiol Clin North Am 20:3, 2002.

Pulmonary Surgery
Postoperative Care

SANJEEV V. CHHANGANI, M.D., M.B.A.

With the advent of new techniques and technology, there has been a tremendous growth in pulmonary surgery in the last two decades. The emergence of video-assisted thoracic surgery (VATS) and recent advances in anesthetic management, including routine use of intraoperative flexible brochoscopy, has allowed pulmonary surgery to be performed with less stress and lower risk of intraoperative hypoxemia, thereby resulting in faster convalescence and improved outcomes. The patient for pulmonary surgery presents with unique challenges as compared with the patient for cardiac and vascular surgery. Inherent with the nature of the disease pathology and pulmonary surgery, the major cause of postoperative morbidity and mortality in this group of patients is pulmonary complications. Just as in cardiac and vascular surgery, the issues for pulmonary risk are complex, but there are no universally agreed on algorithms. However, many factors can be identified in the preoperative assessment of these patients for risk stratification purpose and identification of the high-risk patient. Advances in surgical techniques, anesthetic preoperative assessment and intraoperative management, and mechanical ventilation have decreased postoperative (post-op) complications and improved the outcomes after pulmonary surgery.

This chapter presents a review of post-op care of pulmonary surgery patients. In addition to the routine post-op care of the pulmonary surgery patient, identification of the high-risk patient and management of post-op complications are discussed. Special scenarios such as lung transplantation and thoracic trauma are also addressed.

Recent advances in surgical techniques and perioperative management have expanded the scope of pulmonary surgery. As a result, surgical procedures, especially minimally invasive and palliative, are being offered to patients previously considered "inoperable." Respiratory complications such as atelactasis, pneumonia, and respiratory failure requiring mechanical ventilation represent risks specific to pulmonary surgery. In the high-risk pulmonary surgery patient, measures can be taken preoperatively to pre-optimize respiratory function as much as possible, prevent complications, and improve outcome.

Assessment of Respiratory System Impairment

Impairment in the patient's quality of life, physical activity, and exercise capacity closely correlates with the degree of impairment in the respiratory function. A detailed history is extremely important to determine which patients will require pulmonary testing. There is no single test of pulmonary function that can predict outcomes for all patients having pulmonary surgery. Assessment of respiratory system mechanics, gas exchange, and heart–lung interaction provides the "three-pronged" approach (Box 39-1) on which to base "operability" of a patient with "resectable" lung cancer.

Respiratory Mechanics

The most valid test to predict post-thoracotomy pulmonary complications is the predicted postoperative (ppo) forced expiratory volume in 1 second (FEV$_1$%) expressed as a percentage of predicted volumes for age, sex, and height. It is calculated as:

$$FEV_1(ppo) \% = preoperative\ FEV_1\% \left(1 - \% \text{ functional lung tissue removed}/100\right)$$

The majority of post-op respiratory complications occur in patients who are left with ppoFEV$_1$ of less than 40%. In the patient with borderline ppoFEV$_1$ (30–40%)

Box 39-1 The "Three-Pronged" Approach

The "three-pronged" approach to evaluate respiratory system impairment includes assessment of respiratory mechanics (FEV$_1$), efficiency of gas exchange (DLCO), and heart–lung interaction (VO$_2$ max).

postresection pulmonary function can be further defined using ventilation perfusion scintigraphy (V/Q scan). If the lung region to be resected is nonfunctioning or minimally functioning on V/Q scan, the ppoFEV$_1$ can be modified accordingly.

The right lung has 22 subsegments (6 in right upper, 4 right middle, and 12 in right lower lobe) and the left lung has 20 (10 in left upper and 10 in left lower lobe). For example, if a patient is having left lower lobe resected the ppoFEV$_1$ decrease will be 10/42 or 28%.

Gas Exchange

Diffusion capacity of carbon monoxide (DLCO) correlates well with the efficiency and total surface area of alveolar–capillary units. A ppoDLCO (using the same calculation as for the FEV$_1$) of less than 40% predicted correlates with a high probability of developing post-op respiratory as well as cardiac complications. The traditional criteria of gas exchange, with an arterial partial pressure of oxygen (PaO$_2$) less than 60 mmHg or an arterial partial pressure of carbon dioxide (PaCO$_2$) of greater than 45 mmHg remain as useful warning signals of increased post-op risk.

Heart–Lung Interaction

The maximal oxygen consumption (VO$_2$ max) with exercise is a very useful predictor of post-op respiratory complications. A VO$_2$ max of less than 15 ml/kg/minute is consistent with increased risk of post-op complications. VO$_2$ max less than 10 ml/kg/minute carries extremely high mortality following pulmonary surgery. The ability of the heart and lungs to interact physiologically in response to exercise can also be evaluated by two simple and reliable tests: 6-minute walk test (6MWT) and exercise pulse oximetry. A 6MWT of less than 2000 feet correlates to a VO$_2$ max of less than 15 ml/kg/minute as well as a fall in oxygen saturation (SpO$_2$) during exercise. Patients with a decrease of SpO$_2$ greater than 4% during exercise are at increased risk of post-op morbidity and mortality following pulmonary surgery.

Using echocardiography, evaluation of the right ventricular function at rest and with exercise can provide clues to the hemodynamic tolerance of pulmonary resection.

Coexisting Medical Conditions

Cardiac Disease

Second only to respiratory complications, cardiac complications are a common cause of post-op morbidity and mortality following pulmonary surgery. Coronary artery disease risk factors must be elicited in the patient having pulmonary surgery. Elective pulmonary surgery is generally considered as an "intermediate risk" with respect to perioperative cardiac ischemia. Atrial fibrillation is a well-recognized complication of pulmonary surgery. Continuing beta-blockers or calcium channel blockers (diltiazem) through the perioperative period may be protective against development of such dysrhythmia. Risk of post-op atrial fibrillation increases with the amount of lung tissue resected, age, intraoperative blood loss, and dissection of pericardium.

Renal Dysfunction

Renal dysfunction after pulmonary surgery is associated with increased post-op mortality. Factors associated with an increased risk of post-thoracotomy renal dysfunction include previous history of renal insufficiency, diuretic therapy, pneumonectomy, infection, and blood transfusion.

Age

In general, risk of respiratory complications and cardiac arrhythmias is greater in the older than in the younger population.

Chronic Obstructive Pulmonary Disease

Patients with chronic obstructive pulmonary disease (COPD) are more likely to retain $PaCO_2$, have right ventricular dysfunction, and develop nocturnal hypoxemia. The presence of these factors in a post-thoracotomy COPD patient is associated with increased risk of respiratory complications. Cessation of smoking, optimization of bronchospasm and heart failure, and education in chest physiotherapy in this group of patients will help minimize post-op complications.

Table 39-1 summarizes the risk factors in a high-risk pulmonary surgery patient.

ROUTINE POSTOPERATIVE CARE

The vast majority of patients who undergo pulmonary surgery are extubated in the operating room and have at least one chest tube. One of the most outstanding problems encountered in the post-op pulmonary surgery patient is impaired gas exchange. Most post-op pulmonary surgery patients can be cared for on a specialized ward with nurses and other ancillary personnel trained to address the unique needs of these patients. A few patients, especially if kept intubated, are brought to the intensive care unit (ICU). When the patient has been settled into the postanesthesia care unit (PACU) or ICU, a complete assessment is done to establish a baseline and a verbal report is given to the PACU or ICU nurse and staff outlining operative procedure, the patient's intraoperative course, patient's condition, and expected post-op course. Typical post-op orders include routine orders, ventilator

---

Table 39-1	Characteristics of a High-Risk Thoracic Surgery Patient

1. History
   - Advanced age
   - COPD (hypercarbia, hypoxemia, heart failure)
   - Impaired quality of life (poor functional capacity, limited exercise tolerance)
   - Renal impairment
   - Presence of dysrhythmia and multiple coronary artery disease risk factors
2. Pulmonary functions
   - ppoFEV$_1$ < 40%
   - ppoDLCO < 40%
   - VO_2 max < 15 ml/kg/minute
   - Decline in exercise SpO_2 > 4%
3. Amount of pulmonary tissue removed and laterality
   - Pneumonectomy
   - Right-sided surgery
4. Recent history of radiation or chemotherapy

COPD, chronic obstructive pulmonary disease; ppoFEV$_1$, predicted postoperative FEV$_1$; ppoDLCO, predicted postoperative diffusing capacity of carbon monoxide; VO_2 max, maximum oxygen consumption; SpO_2, peripheral oxygen saturation.

---

setting (if the patient is intubated), fluid orders, pain control orders, and a portable chest radiograph.

Monitoring

The level of monitoring is determined by the severity of impairment in cardiopulmonary function. Close clinical supervision of pulmonary surgery patients allows early institution of therapy and prevention of cardiopulmonary catastrophe. In general, most pulmonary surgery patients can be safely cared for on the hospital ward. A pulse oximeter is commonly utilized to monitor closely peripheral arterial saturation and response to oxygen therapy. Thoracic surgical patients are vulnerable to hypothermia. Hypothermia and shivering can increase oxygen consumption tremendously and result in metabolic acidosis, pulmonary arterial hypertension, and increased risk for bleeding. Therefore, hypothermia must be avoided in pulmonary surgery patients. Telemetry can be used for patients considered at high risk for cardiac arrhythmia. All patients with unstable blood pressure (BP), refractory hypoxemia, relative narcotic overdose, and mechanical ventilation must be transferred to the ICU. An intra-arterial and a central venous catheter are used for BP monitoring, drawing arterial blood gases, and measuring central venous filling pressure to guide fluid therapy. A pulmonary artery catheter is rarely required in a post-op pulmonary surgery patient.

Fluid Management

The goal of fluid management in post-op pulmonary surgery patients is to infuse the minimum amount of fluid that will maintain adequate end-organ perfusion and electrolyte balance. For hypotension not due to acute blood loss, vasoactive agents may be used. Liberal fluid replacement may be associated with hypoxemia due to increased pulmonary arterial hydrostatic pressure, especially when post-op increased pulmonary capillary permeability is present. In most patients with normal BP, a urinary output of 0.5 ml/kg is considered adequate.

Care of the Chest Tube

The chest tube and drainage system must be functioning properly, unclamped, and applied to water seal before transport. In many circumstances two chest tubes may be placed to drain both air and fluid from the pleural space. A chest radiograph is ordered to confirm proper chest tube position and identify kinks or residual pneumothorax. Modern chest tube drainage systems have three compartments as shown in Figure 39-1. The first compartment is a simple graduated collection chamber where the amount of blood and fluid can be measured. The second compartment is an underwater seal that serves as a simple, reliable one-way valve, which allows air to escape from pleural space, but not to enter the pleural space during the next inspiration. The third compartment controls, via an atmospheric vent, the amount of negative pressure that can be developed by the chest tube drainage system suction. Two factors determine the level of suction. First, the height of underwater depth of the central movable tube; and second,

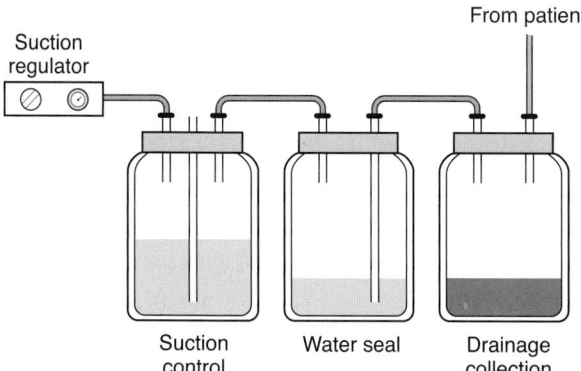

Figure 39-1 Chest tube drainage system showing three chambers for fluid collection, water seal, and suction control.

actual suction pump capable of generating low pressure (-15 to 20 cmH$_2$O and 10–15 l/minute flow) or high pressure (up to -60 cmH$_2$O with flows > 20 l/minute).

A blood loss up to 200 ml/hour via a chest tube is considered acceptable in the immediate post-op or post-trauma period. It should decrease with time. Persistent large-volume blood loss from the chest tube warrants re-exploration in the post-thoracotomy and trauma patient.

Chest Radiographs

Chest radiographs constitute an important part of the initial evaluation of the post-op pulmonary surgery or trauma patient. The following points are carefully evaluated.

Endotracheal Tube

The tip of the endotracheal tube (ETT) must be at least 3–4 cm above the carina. Too high or too low an ETT tip may risk accidental extubation and mainstem intubation, respectively. A double-lumen endobronchial tube, if left in place postoperatively, should be withdrawn until the tip is 3 cm above the carina. This will reduce the risk of coughing and tracheobronchial injury.

Pneumothorax

A small pneumothorax in the presence of a chest tube may be cleared by application of suction to the chest tube. However, continued pneumothorax may indicate a malfunctioning chest tube or the need for an additional tube due to bronchopleural fistula.

Mediastinal Shift

After lung resection, the mediastinum shifts toward the resected side and the diaphragm moves upward. Unusual shift may indicate atelactasis. After pneumonectomy, the mediastinum should be as near the center as possible. Too much air in the pneumonectomy space may compress the remaining lung and shift the mediastinum to the opposite side, making ventilation difficult (Figure 39-2). Aspirating air with a large-bore catheter, syringe, and stopcock can relieve too much tension in the pneumonectomy space. Combination of acute mediastinal shift and acute gastric dilatation can cause acute respiratory embarrassment.

CLINICAL CAVEAT

The combination of acute mediastinal shift and gastric dilatation in a postpneumonectomy patient represents impending respiratory failure and must be recognized and relieved immediately.

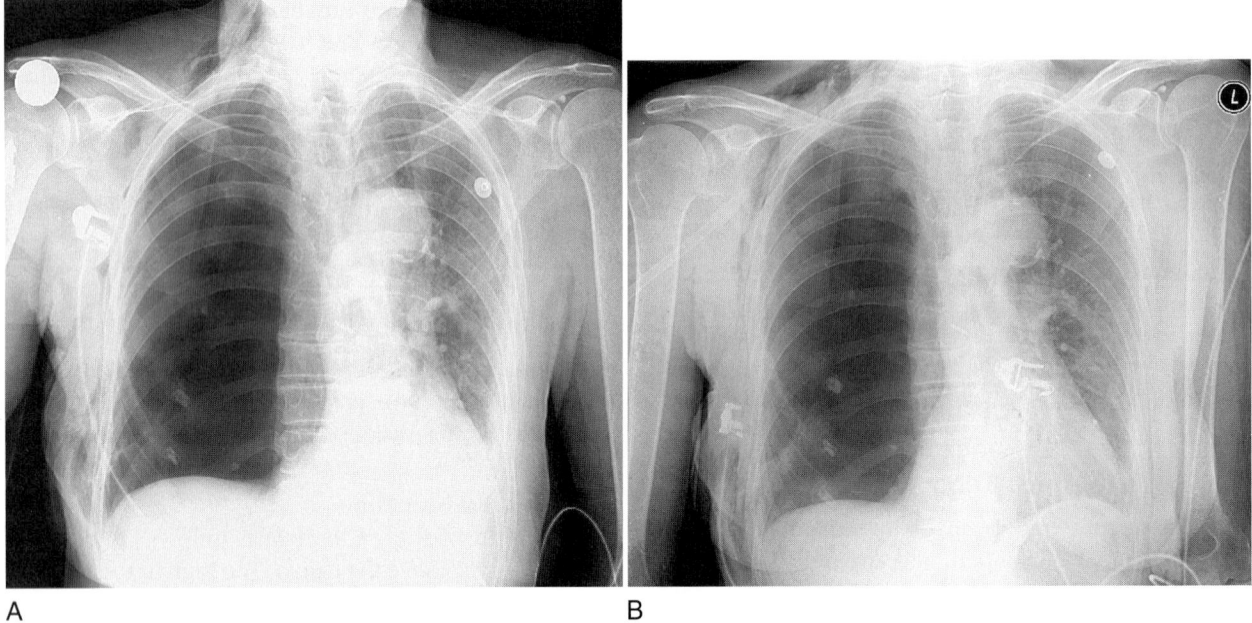

A   B

Figure 39-2 A chest radiograph taken immediately after right pneumonectomy. Panel A shows mediastinal shift to left. Panel B shows mediastinum returned to midline after aspiration of 1 liter of air from the right hemithorax (postpneumonectomy space).

Chest Physiotherapy

Thoracotomy surgically traumatizes the intercostal muscles and chest wall leading to ventilation/perfusion mismatching and hypoventilation from "inspiratory splinting."

The most common post-op pulmonary complication is atelactasis. Surgical factors, general anesthesia and paralysis, and the underlying medical condition of the patient all contribute to development of atelactasis. The functional residual capacity (FRC) declines by 35% after thoracotomy. Closing volume (CV), defined as the volume at which the flow from the dependent portions of the lung stops during exhalation during airway closure, increases in the post-op period due to a variety of factors, including fluid overload, advanced age, obesity, smoking, bronchospasm, and airway secretions. As the FRC declines and the CV increases, the lung is subject to airway collapse and atelactasis. In the low-risk patient, lung re-expansion can be achieved with nursing intervention such as coughing, deep breathing exercises, and ambulation. In higher-risk patients various devices such as incentive spirometry and intermittent positive pressure breathing are effective and cheap. Proper positioning of the patient helps to improve diaphragmatic excursion and postural drainage of secretions. Chest physiotherapy should ideally begin in the preoperative period with smoking cessation education, optimization of bronchospasm, teaching deep breathing, and coughing. Table 39-2 summarizes commonly used agents in post-op pulmonary care.

Mechanical Ventilation

The need for mechanical ventilation may arise due to acute or chronic $PaCO_2$ retention, excessive fluid or blood product administration, incomplete reversal of neuromuscular blockade, and excessive sedation. Ventilator settings, whether in volume- or pressure-limited mode, must limit peak pressure to less than 35 cmH_2O and plateau airway pressure to less than 25 cmH_2O. Settings resulting in high peak airway pressures or excessive positive end-expiratory pressure (PEEP) can produce barotrauma and result in disruption of bronchial anastomosis and bronchopleural fistula. COPD patients have a tendency to develop intrinsic PEEP, which can be minimized by using lower tidal volumes (6–8 ml/kg) and lower respiratory rates, high flow rates, and prolonged exhalation times. The patients must be appropriately sedated. Early extubation is always desired in a post-thoracotomy patient, especially after lung volume resection, pneumonectomy, or in the presence of a bronchopleural fistula.

Post-thoracotomy Analgesia

Pain control is integral to the care of patients having pulmonary surgery. When compared to open thoracotomy procedures, it is associated with significantly reduced post-op pain. Post-thoracotomy pain is transmitted via intercostal, phrenic, and vagus nerves. Effective post-thoracotomy analgesia may decrease perioperative

Table 11-4   Commonly Used Agents in Postoperative Pulmonary Care

Agent	Dosage	Route	Formulation	Comment
INHALED β-ADRENERGIC AGENTS				
Albuterol	2.5 mg (0.5 ml) in 3 ml NaCl q 4-6 h	Nebulized	0.5% solution	Predominant β_2, watch for hypokalemia with repeated doses
	4 puffs q 4-6 h	MDI	90 µg/MDI dose	
Terbutaline	1-2 puffs q 2-6 h	MDI	200 µg	Watch for hypokalemia, pulmonary edema, SVT
	0.25 mg	Subcutaneous injection	1 mg/ml	
Racemic epinephrine	0.5 mg in 3 ml NaCl q 1-4 h PRN	Nebulized	2.25% solution	Localized vasoconstriction reduces airway swelling
ANTICHOLINERGIC AGENTS				
Atropine sulfate	2.5-5 mg in 3 ml NaCl q 4-6 h	Nebulized	1 mg/ml	
Glycopyrrolate	0.2 mg in 3 ml NaCl q 6 h	Nebulized	0.2 mg/ml	
Ipratropium bromide	0.5 mg in 3 ml NaCl q 4-6 h	Nebulized	0.02% solution	
	2-4 puffs q 4-6 h	MDI	18 µg/MDI dose	
CORTICOSTEROIDS				
Hydrocortisone	2 mg/kg or	IV	50 mg/ml	
	2 mg/kg then	IV		
	0.5 mg/kg/h	Continuous infusion		
Methylprednisolone	60-125 mg q 6-8 h	IV/PO	40, 62.5 mg/ml	
Dexamethasone	4 mg q 6-8 h	IV/PO	4 mg/ml	Prophylactic for airway swelling
MUCOLYTIC AGENTS				
N-acetylcysteine	3 ml of 20% solution q 6-8 h	Nebulized	10, 20% solution	Use after nebulized β-agonist
Guaifenesin	100-400 mg q 6 h	PO	100 mg/5 ml	
NONSPECIFIC AGENTS				
Helium/oxygen mixture	70/30, 80/20 mixture	Face mask inhalation		Decreases turbulence of airflow via narrow airway

MDI, metered dose inhaler; SVT, supraventricular tachycardia; IV, intravenous; PO, oral; h, hours.

stress, reduce post-op pulmonary complications, and limit chronic post-thoracotomy pain syndrome. Post-thoracotomy analgesia begins with a thorough discussion of post-op events and course and analgesia choices. Typically, a multimodal analgesia regimen provides superior pain control compared to any single technique.

Intercostal Nerve Block

Before thoracotomy is closed, intercostal nerve blocks with 0.25% bupivacaine with epinephrine can reduce post-op pain and opioid requirement.

Systemic Opioids

Systemic opioids are generally given as part of a multimodal analgesia regimen, including nerve block and nonopioid analgesics. Patient-controlled analgesia provides better patient satisfaction. The benefit of analgesia must be carefully balanced against the risk of sedation, hypoventilation, and cough inhibition.

Nonsteroidal Anti-inflammatory Drugs

Nonsteroidal anti-inflammatory drugs (NSAIDs) block the synthesis of prostaglandins by inhibiting the enzyme cyclooxygenase. NSAIDs may be used for controlling ipsilateral shoulder pain after thoracotomy in patients with epidural analgesia. Gastrointestinal bleeding and decreased creatinine clearance are potentially serious side effects of NSAIDs. These drugs must be avoided in elderly patients and patients with preexisting renal disease, hypovolemia, and congestive heart failure.

Paravertebral Block

Paravertebral block can be established by a catheter placed surgically, at the time of thoracotomy, into the paravertebral space. Analgesia is usually supplemented with systemic opioids and NSAIDs. In spite of its simplicity, paravertebral block carries a failure rate of approximately 10%.

Interpleural Analgesia

After thoracotomy, dilution of local anesthetic with blood and loss of local of local anesthetic into the chest tube reduces the efficacy of interpleural block.

Epidural Analgesia

A thoracic epidural catheter provides effective and reliable post-thoracotomy analgesia and has been shown to be associated with decreased risk of post-thoracotomy respiratory complications and potentially improved outcome. The optimal site of insertion of the thoracic epidural catheter should be at the level of surgical incision. We use a mixture of 0.1% bupivacaine and 4 µg per ml fentanyl for epidural infusion at 6–10 ml per hour. A properly functioning thoracic epidural catheter is extremely valuable for post-thoracotomy analgesia in patients having lung volume reduction surgery or pneumonectomy. Epidural opioids may potentially cause urinary retention and delayed gastric emptying. One of the common concerns among surgeons of epidural analgesia is that it can potentially cause hypotension requiring excessive fluid administration.

Whether thoracic epidural analgesia reduces post-thoracotomy mortality is still a controversial topic. Current evidence, however, suggests that epidural analgesia can reduce post-op respiratory complications, decrease perioperative myocardial infarction, and reduce the incidence of thromboembolic events.

Management of Arrhythmia

Atrial tachyarrhythmias are common in a post-thoracotomy patient, with incidence ranging from 9 to 33%. The major arrhythmia in this population is atrial fibrillation (AF), followed by paroxysmal supraventricular tachycardia (PSVT), atrial flutter (A-Flutter), and multiform atrial tachycardia (MAT). The incidence of nonsustained ventricular tachycardia is approximately 15%.

The incidence of AF increases with amount of lung tissue removed (12–25% after lobectomy, 20–30% after pneumonectomy, and up to 40% after resection of malignant pleural mesothelioma) and advanced age (60 years or older). The onset of AF is greatest 2–3 days after thoracic surgery, with the majority reverting to sinus rhythm with appropriate therapy. Common clinical presentations of AF include dyspnea, palpitation, dizziness, and shortness of breath. With respect to the development of hypotension, younger patients tend to tolerate AF better than older patients. The proposed mechanisms of perioperative AF include preexisting atrial pathology (valvular

heart disease, congestive heart failure, advanced age), presence of triggering factors (atrial extrasystoles, increased sympathetic stimulation, acute atrial stretch), and surgical factors (atrial trauma, heightened sympathetic tone, inflammatory response).

A variety of drugs have been used to prevent post-op AF. Routine use of digoxin should be discouraged due to its lack of proven efficacy to prevent post-op AF. In a recent double-blind, placebo-controlled trial, Amar showed that diltiazem was effective in reducing AF by 50% in thoracic surgery patients. The rate of AF remains high despite extensive use of prophylactic beta-blockers. The routine use of amiodarone is not recommended due to its high cost and concern about pulmonary toxicity in thoracic surgery patients. The treatment of post-thoracotomy arrhythmias must begin with correction of reversible factors such as respiratory failure and hypoxemia, pain, and electrolyte imbalance. The initial goal is to establish hemodynamic stability, obtain a 12-lead ECG for diagnosis, and control the ventricular response. Patients with severe hypotension or signs of organ hypoperfusion must be emergently electrically cardioverted using synchronized DC cardioversion. Adenosine is used to treat PSVT and delineate the underlying arrhythmia. Recent evidence from cardiac surgery suggests that rate-controlling strategy may be superior to rhythm control. Beta-blockers (esmolol and metoprolol) or calcium channel blockers (verapamil and diltiazem) are commonly used rate-controlling drugs. Calcium channel blockers are avoided in patients with pre-excitation arrhythmia (Wolff-Parkinson-White syndrome). Caution should be exercised with beta-blockers in patients with known ventricular dysfunction and severe COPD. Pharmacologic conversion to sinus rhythm, if considered, must be used within 48 hours of AF due to the risk of developing left atrial thrombus with persistent AF and potential embolic complication with restoration of sinus rhythm. The examples of converting drugs include ibutilide, amiodarone, flecainide, and propafenone. Prophylactic magnesium administration before using any of these drugs will reduce the risk of torsades de pointes. The potential for thromboembolic complications increases if AF persists beyond 48 hours. Anticoagulation, using aspirin, heparin, or warfarin, is considered after weighing the risk of post-op bleeding.

MANAGEMENT OF SPECIAL CONDITIONS

Postpneumonectomy Pulmonary Edema

The syndrome of postpneumonectomy pulmonary edema (PPPE) refers to the development of an acute lung injury (ALI) or acute respiratory distress syndrome (ARDS) characterized by severe and often fatal pulmonary edema of unknown etiology. In spite of an increased awareness over the last two decades, a precise definition and pathogenesis of PPPE is lacking. The reported incidence of PPPE ranges from 2.5% to 14%. The incidence is greater after right pneumonectomy. It is universally fatal if unrecognized. It accounts for the majority of in-hospital mortality following lung resections. PPPE remains an equally challenging clinical problem for surgeons, anesthesiologists, and intensivists alike.

The diagnosis of PPPE is based on high index of suspicion and exclusion of factors known to cause ALI/ARDS. Among several conditions, the differential diagnoses include aspiration pneumonitis, pneumonia, cardiogenic pulmonary edema, pulmonary embolism, extrapulmonary sepsis, and drugs (amiodarone) and blood transfusions. The onset of symptoms usually occurs between post-op day 2 and 4, although radiologic findings may be seen earlier. Among many factors involved in the pathophysiology of PPPE, *volume overload* still remains an important topic of controversy between surgeons and anesthesiologists and has led to the dictum "Don't drown the down lung." The probable etiologies involved in the pathophysiology of PPPE include fluid overload, lung lymphatic injury, endothelial damage, increased pulmonary capillary pressure, hyperinflation of the lung, and right ventricular dysfunction. The role of oxygen toxicity and cytokines in PPPE is unclear.

CURRENT CONTROVERSY

In postpneumonectomy pulmonary edema *volume overload* still remains an important topic of controversy between surgeons and anesthesiologists and has led to the dictum "Don't drown the down lung."

The most important management strategy for PPPE is its prevention. The anesthesiologist and surgeon working together can take measures that will hopefully prevent the occurrence of PPPE in the post-op period. Among many considerations for the anesthesiologist include careful attention to perioperative fluid administration (not to exceed 20 ml/kg in the first 24 hours) and ventilation of the residual lung (limiting peak airway pressure to less than 35 cmH$_2$O and plateau pressure under 25 cmH$_2$O), use of vasopressors (instead of fluids) in the treatment of nonhemorrhagic hypotension, and minimizing the risk of hypotension due to epidural analgesia. Similarly, considerations for the surgeon include expeditious and hemostatic surgery and preventing residual lung compression or hyperinflation by establishing mediastinal centricity by aspirating excess air or fluid from the pneumonectomy space or using a balanced drainage system. Other supportive treatments include aggressive pain control measures using a multimodal

approach, supplemental oxygen to prevent hypoxemia during rest, sleep, and exercise, avoiding long periods with the residual lung in the dependent position, and lung protective ventilation with or without inhaled nitric oxide in patients requiring intubation. High-dose steroids may be considered in patients with a recent history of radiation or chemotherapy.

Bronchopleural Fistula

Air leak via a chest tube is initially common after lobectomy or segmental resection due to transection of small airways. With proper drainage via chest tube(s), moderate suction (20–30 cmH$_2$O), physiotherapy, and ambulation, the initial air leak normally subsides over 3–4 days. The development of a bronchopleural fistula (BPF) due to bronchial-stump disruption after pulmonary surgery is a serious complication. The etiologies of BPF include surgical reasons (poor suturing or stapling techniques or bronchial ischemia due to poor dissection) or post-op necrosis due to infection or tumor in the stump. Prompt re-operation and closure of the fistula are recommended for early bronchial-stump disruption. High-frequency jet ventilation (HFJV) or one-lung ventilation using a double-lumen tube may be required to facilitate healing and maintain adequate oxygenation and ventilation.

Lung Torsion or Infarction

Following lobectomy, torsion or infarction of the lung is possible if the blood vessels are twisted as the lung re-expands. Torsion usually occurs within the first 48 hours postoperatively. Venous engorgement may lead to tissue infarction. The middle lobe and lingua are more susceptible to torsion. Diagnostic findings include enlarging density on serial chest radiographs, hemoptysis, dyspnea, fever, and tachycardia. Bronchoscopy shows a distorted compressed bronchus. Immediate exploration and possible further excision of nonviable lung is required.

Cardiac Herniation

Cardiac herniation is a rare complication of pulmonary resection requiring wide surgical excision of the pericardium. Herniation occurs after chest closure in the early post-op period and may be related to differential pressures in two hemithoraces pushing (or pulling) the heart through the defect. Symptoms and signs may be sudden in onset and dramatic (cardiovascular collapse, hypotension, dysrhythmias, and myocardial infarction). Signs and symptoms are more profound with right-sided herniation due to the ease of superior vena caval obstruction. Immediate re-operation with correction of herniation and pericardial patching should be done.

Temporizing measures include discontinuing suction, placing the patient in the lateral decubitus position with the operative hemithorax uppermost, and minimizing PEEP and airway pressures in intubated patients.

Lung Transplantation

The major concerns relating to the post-op care of lung transplant recipients are hemodynamic and fluid management, respiratory management, management of renal function, ischemia reperfusion injury, allograft rejection, nutrition, and sepsis.

Respiratory Management and Mechanical Ventilation

After lung transplant, recipients have impaired cough reflexes due to the disruption of afferent nerve fibers and thus have difficulty mobilizing respiratory secretions. Aggressive pulmonary toilet is crucial. Frequent airway suctioning and inhaled bronchodilators are utilized in patients on or off the ventilator. After extubation, early ambulation, cough and deep breathing maneuvers, and bronchodilators help mobilize secretions and prevent atelactasis.

In uncomplicated cases most lung recipients can be extubated 24–36 hours after surgery. Adequate oxygenation is assured with supplemental oxygen and PEEP and $PaCO_2$ and pH adjusted based on minute ventilation. In general, during mechanical ventilation, lung protective ventilation using small tidal volumes (6 ml/kg adjusted body weight) and PEEP with close attention to prevent dynamic hyperinflation (auto-PEEP) is used. Recipients who were hypercapnic before remain so until medullary respiratory center readjusts over several weeks. At times, hyperinflation of a more compliant lung in a single-lung recipient with conventional ventilation necessitates differential lung ventilation utilizing a double-lumen endobronchial tube. Unrecognized hyperinflation can result in mediastinal shift and hemodynamic compromise. Weaning from the mechanical ventilator is initiated when the patient is warm, hemodynamically stable, and arterial blood gases show adequate oxygenation and ventilation using inspired oxygen 0.4 or less. A short trial of spontaneous breathing is performed using pressure support ventilation and pulmonary mechanics (negative inspiratory force and vital capacity) are measures prior to extubation. Weaning may be hampered by emergence of infection, phrenic nerve injury secondary to surgical procedure, ischemia reperfusion injury, and preexisting nutrition deficiency.

Hemodynamic and Fluid Management

The goals of hemodynamic and fluid management in a lung transplant recipient are to ensure adequate organ perfusion and prevent pulmonary edema. Vasoactive agents are added when appropriate, to maintain mean arterial pressure. Inotropic agents are needed to support cardiac output in recipients with preexisting right ventricular dysfunction. Vasodilators such as prostaglandin E_1 are used to control elevated pulmonary artery pressure, especially if it was being used preoperatively. Because of alterations in pulmonary capillary permeability, disordered fluid clearance related to disruption of pulmonary lymphatics, and therefore propensity to develop pulmonary edema, fluid administration is generally kept to a minimum. Blood and blood component replacement is undertaken as necessary. Echocardiography is useful in evaluating cardiac function and pericardial tamponade in an unstable patient.

Ischemia Reperfusion Injury and Allograft Rejection

The release of superoxide anions and oxygen free radicals and subsequent activation of neutrophils following reperfusion of the ischemic lung ultimately leads to increased capillary permeability, interstitial alveolar edema, altered vascular tone, and dysfunction of type-II pneumocytes. Clinically, lung injury induced by ischemia-reperfusion is characterized by nonspecific alveolar damage, pulmonary edema, and progressive hypoxemia within 72 hours of lung transplantation. Signs of resolution are usually apparent by day 4 and complete resolution is usually seen by day 14. If severe enough, it can lead to primary graft failure. Treatment is generally supportive and includes lung protective ventilation both during and immediately after surgery to protect the injured lung and prevent further worsening of acute lung injury and diuretics. Inhaled nitric oxide may be useful in the treatment of ischemia reperfusion injury by improving ventilation-perfusion mismatch without affecting systemic vascular resistance.

Acute rejection usually presents on days 4–5 following surgery and presents as worsening gas exchange, pulmonary infiltrates, and pulmonary hypertension. A transbronchial or open lung biopsy is required for definitive diagnosis. Current immunosuppressive regimens are based on the use of cyclosporine, azathioprine, and prednisone as the mainstay of therapy after lung transplantation. Immunosuppressive agents are continued and inhaled nitric oxide is used to decrease pulmonary vascular resistance without altering systemic resistance. Primary graft failure from ischemia-reperfusion may be so severe that it necessitates extracorporeal membrane oxygenation (ECMO) to support the patient until injury improves.

Management of Renal Function

Fluid restriction and diuretic and vasopressor use in conjunction with the use of nephrotoxic immunosuppressive and antimicrobial medications can lead to the development of acute renal failure in the post-op period. Dosing of all medications must be based on alteration in creatinine clearance. Low-dose nicardipine has been shown to be reno-protective in transplant recipients taking immunosuppressive agents. Some degree of renal insufficiency persists in these patients.

Nutrition

Stress ulcer prophylaxis is routinely used. Nutrition is a very important issue in lung transplant recipients. In general, enteral nutrition is desired. Metoclopramide can be used to treat gastroparesis, which is quite common in lung transplant recipients. Laxatives are used for regulation of bowel function.

Sepsis

Sepsis can be another problem in these patients. Prophylactic antimicrobials are important in preventing post-op infections. Common infections that are likely include bacterial pneumonia around day 2-3, acute rejection around day 4-6, and cytomegalovirus pneumonitis at week 4 following the surgery. Bacterial, viral, and fungal prophylaxis is based on culture data from the donor lung. After 1 month, trimethoprim-sulfamethoxazole is given as a prophylaxis against *Pneumocystis carinii* and acyclovir against herpes simplex virus.

Thoracic Trauma

Thoracic trauma accounts for 25% of all trauma deaths in the USA. With blunt or penetrating injury the basic principles of resuscitation are rapid restoration of airway, supplemental oxygen, needle decompression of a suspected tension pneumothorax, and coverage of an open pneumothorax wound.

Diagnosis

The initial evaluation is directed at diagnosing and treating life-threatening injuries related to the airway and cardiopulmonary system. A secondary survey should be rapidly done to search for other injuries. A combination of radiologic and clinical procedures is usually required to clearly define the nature and extent of thoracic injury. Despite its limitations, the initial chest radiograph represents the most important diagnostic tool in patients with thoracic trauma. Presence of pneumothorax, hemothorax, and rib fractures may be identified. A wide mediastinum on chest radiograph may indicate traumatic aortic injury. A computerized tomography scan of the chest is useful in diagnosing mediastinal hemorrhage, pulmonary contusion, and aortic rupture. Transesophageal performed intra-operatively may help in diagnosing traumatic aortic injury, traumatic rupture of the ventricular septum, cardiac tamponade, or wall motion abnormality seen with myocardial contusion in a hemodynamically unstable patient. A 12-lead ECG is required in monitoring all trauma patients. Unexplained arrhythmia may be an

initial clue to the presence of myocardial contusion. Aortography remains the "gold standard" for diagnosis of traumatic aortic injury in a hemodynamically stable patient. Bronchoscopy is the diagnostic test of choice in tracheobrochial trauma. The role of videothoracoscopy in the treatment and management of thoracic trauma patients has been expanding. The current indications for videothoracoscopy include evaluation of suspected diaphragmatic and mediastinal injuries, removal of foreign bodies, evaluation and treatment of persistent leaks and bleeding, and evacuation of a retained hematoma.

Management
Rib Fractures and Flail Chest

Simple rib fractures can be successfully treated with analgesics. Intercostal, interpleural, or epidural analgesia can be used in a high-risk patient. A flail chest occurs when the fracture of ribs at multiple locations produces discontinuity of a segment of thoracic wall and paradoxical motion with respiration. This results in increased work of breathing, decreased vital capacity, and hypoxemia due to V/Q mismatch. Invariably there is underlying pulmonary contusion in patients with flail chest. It is the underlying pulmonary contusion that plays the greater role in the patient's inability to oxygenate and ventilate. Key in the management of flail chest is pain relief. Conservative management including supplemental oxygen, epidural analgesia, and pulmonary physiotherapy may be used in patients with mild flail chest. Arterial blood gases may be drawn to monitor gas exchange. The patient with severe flail chest and pulmonary contusion requires mechanical ventilator support using lung protective ventilation strategy, along with adequate pain control, sedation, and careful attention to fluids. Pulmonary contusions are common after blunt thoracic trauma and may progress to full-blown ARDS.

Cardiac Contusion

Patients sustaining massive blunt chest trauma, with ECG abnormalities, and with a positive "steering wheel sign" on the anterior chest should be investigated for cardiac contusion. Patients with normal ECG can be managed on the regular ward. Stable patients with abnormal ECG should be admitted to a telemetry ward. All patients with unstable hemodynamic status must be admitted to the ICU. Antiarrhythmic and inotropic support is used for the treatment of arrhythmias and cardiogenic shock.

Tracheobronchial Injuries

Tracheobronchial injuries may be suspected in patients with thoracic trauma who develop massive subcutaneous and mediastinal emphysema or continuous air leak via chest tube. Laryngeal and tracheal injuries can be managed by endotracheal intubation with the cuff below the level of injury. HFJV can be used in to minimize airway pressure and inspiratory peak pressures to decrease the likelihood of suture line dehiscence after repair of distal tracheobronchial injury.

SUMMARY

The optimum post-op care of pulmonary surgery patients is challenging. Respiratory complications represent the major cause of post-op morbidity and mortality in this group of patients. Preoperative teaching in smoking cessation and pulmonary physiotherapy goes a long way in the prevention of post-op respiratory complications. Integral to routine post-op care of pulmonary surgery patients is good pain control. PPPE is universally fatal if unrecognized. The post-op period in patients with pulmonary trauma and transplant equally presents with unique challenges.

SELECTED READING

Alvarez JM: Postpneumonectomy pulmonary edema. In Slinger P, editor: *Progress in Anesthesia*, Philadelphia: Lippincott Williams & Wilkins, 2004, pp 187–220.

Amar D: Posthoracotomy arrhythmias. In Slinger P, editor: *Progress in Anesthesia*, Philadelphia: Lippincott Williams & Wilkins, 2004, pp 247–266.

Pennefather SH, Russell GN: Postthoracotomy analgesia: recent advances and future directions. In Slinger P, editor: *Progress in Anesthesia*, Philadelphia: Lippincott Williams & Wilkins, 2004, pp 163–186.

Slinger PD: Thoracic anesthesia. Anesth Analg 98(3 Suppl): A116–122, 2004.

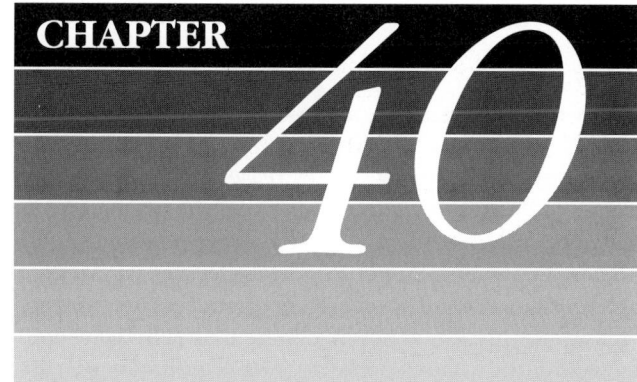

Hemodynamic Instability in the Recovery Room

D. JAY DUONG, M.D.

STEWART J. LUSTIK, M.D.

Hemodynamic instability is frequently encountered in the recovery room. Early recognition and treatment of hemodynamic instability in the recovering patient may prevent postoperative morbidity and mortality. For example, postoperative cardiac complications are the leading cause of postoperative death, and it may be in part due to the surgical stress hormone response that peaks in the recovery room. In patients with risk factors for coronary artery disease the estimated incidence of postoperative cardiac ischemia is 30–40% and is associated with increased mortality. Postoperative myocardial infarction results in a death rate of 30–70%. Other cardiac morbidities include heart failure and serious dysrhythmias. To prevent or minimize these potential complications it is essential to monitor vigilantly the patient with particular focus on the hemodynamics, followed by prompt treatment if indicated.

It is hoped that morbidity and mortality will improve with the advancement of surgical techniques and medical management, such as the perioperative use of beta-blockers to prevent coronary artery plaque rupture. This may be offset by surgical and medical advances that lead to patients with multiple severe medical problems, who were previously considered to be nonsurgical candidates, now receiving surgery, and, therefore, anesthesia. In addition, as longevity increases, the age of surgical patients may increase.

General and regional anesthesia can cause cardiovascular instability. The anesthesiologist is required to resuscitate continually the surgical patient, while concomitantly giving hemodynamically destabilizing anesthetic agents. Resuscitation extends into the postoperative care period when the residual effects of anesthetics are enhanced by the lack of surgical stimulation. Residual anesthesia can also mask the signs and symptoms of cardiovascular instability and attenuate or ablate the physiologic compensatory reflexes. The postoperative patient, therefore, needs to be closely and continually monitored in the recovery unit for the early prevention or detection and treatment of complications.

This chapter discusses the following cardiovascular complications encountered postoperatively: hypotension, hypertension, bradycardia, tachycardia, and tachyarrhythmias. Effective evaluation and treatment requires an organized and systematic approach. This begins with history gathering, consisting of reviewing the patient's preoperative evaluation (to determine the patient's baseline) and intraoperative course (to identify any complication or hemodynamic instability already encountered and the treatment). This is followed by an assessment of the patient's vital signs, a careful performance of a targeted physical examination, and a review of the patient's available laboratory data to formulate a differential diagnosis and determine an appropriate treatment. At times, the acuity of the instability requires immediate treatment to stabilize the patient while an etiology is sought.

HYPOTENSION

Hypotension is a frequently encountered complication in the postoperative setting. Hypotension is often defined as systolic blood pressure lower than 90 mmHg, or a decrease of 40% or greater from the patient's baseline blood pressure. If untreated, hypoperfusion of vital organs may lead to tissue ischemia or infarction. Some patients are at higher risk for developing hypotensive complications, such as patients with chronic hypertension, atherosclerotic disease of the coronary or carotid arteries, stenotic valvular disease, or increased intracranial pressure. Compensatory mechanisms act to preserve perfusion to vital organs; signs or symptoms of end-organ hypoperfusion, such as altered mental status, indicate the compensatory mechanisms are inadequate to overcome the degree of hypotension. Tissue hypoxia results in anaerobic metabolism and a lactic acid-induced metabolic acidosis and electrolyte derangements. If not treated, vital organ dysfunction can result, and a cycle of decompensation may ensue.

Determinants of Blood Pressure

To understand and control blood pressure one needs to understand the underlying physiology. Blood pressure (BP) is related to cardiac output (CO) and systemic vascular resistance (SVR) by the following equation:

$$BP = CO \times SVR \qquad (40\text{-}1)$$

This relationship is derived from rearranging the basic flow equation:

$$Q = \Delta P/R \text{ or } \Delta P = Q \times R \qquad (40\text{-}2)$$

where ΔP is the pressure difference between two points (mmHg), Q is the flow rate (volume/time), and R is the resistance to flow (mmHg × time/volume). This equation is a variant of Ohm's law. When applied to human circulation, ΔP represents blood pressure, Q describes cardiac output, and R is analogous to systemic vascular resistance. Equation 40-1 demonstrates that a decrease in blood pressure must be caused by either a decrease in cardiac output or a decrease in SVR.

The output of the left ventricle may be measured by themodilution using a pulmonary artery catheter, which approximates right ventricular output and when averaged over a period of time must be equal to left ventricular output. Cardiac output is directly related to heart rate (HR) and stroke volume (SV):

$$CO = HR \times SV \qquad (40\text{-}3)$$

Normal resting heart rate in the adult is 60–100 beats per minute. In patients with noncompliant ventricles (e.g., neonates or patients with left ventricular hypertrophy) HR is the primary determinant of cardiac output. Heart rate is regulated by the autonomic nervous system and influenced by hormones, such as thyroid hormone. A slow heart rate is desirable in patients with coronary artery disease, but significant bradycardia may result in a low cardiac output. A rapid heart rate increases myocardial oxygen demand and decreases diastolic time, and, thus, perfusion of the myocardium (the left ventricle receives most of its perfusion during diastole). Decreased diastolic time also may prevent adequate ventricular

filling, resulting in a reduced stroke volume and cardiac output.

Stroke volume is defined as the end-diastolic volume minus the end-systolic volume, or the volume of blood ejected with each ventricular contraction. Stroke volume is reduced if there is a decrease in preload or contractility. Preload is the myocardial tension at the end of diastole and may be estimated using multiple techniques. Ventilation-induced systolic pressure variation of greater than 15 mmHg accurately diagnoses low preload. Pressure in the left ventricle can be indirectly measured by the central venous pressure (CVP) or pulmonary capillary wedge pressure (PCWP). However, these pressure measurements may not accurately reflect left ventricular volume due to valvular heart disease or decreased left ventricular compliance. The right ventricular ejection fraction catheter uses a rapid thermistor and electrocardiogram electrodes to calculate end-diastolic volume without interference from ventricular hypertrophy or valvular disease. Preload is more accurately assessed using echocardiography, where the ventricular filling volume is directly visualized.

The amount of venous blood return to the ventricle and the venous vascular tone determine preload. The most common cause of inadequate preload is hypovolemia due to blood loss or inadequate fluid resuscitation. Impaired venous return can also be due to mechanical impedance such as positive pressure ventilation, diastolic dysfunction, inadequate ventricular filling time, stenotic valvular disease, abdominal compartment syndrome, pulmonary embolus, tension pneumothorax, or cardiac tamponade.

Contractility is the peak isometric tension that a cardiac muscle can generate for a fixed fiber length. The heart contracts more vigorously when the end-diastolic volume increases. This relationship is known as the Frank–Starling law of the heart. Contractility is affected by cardiac ischemia, the sympathetic tone, viable muscle mass of the ventricle, and inotropic drugs (e.g., dopamine, dobutamine, epinephrine, milrinone).

Blood pressure is also directly related to the SVR as shown in Equation 40-1. The factors that determine the resistance to fluid flow are described by Poiseuille's equation:

$$R = 8L\eta/\pi r^4 \qquad (40\text{-}4)$$

where L is the length of the tubing, η is the viscosity of the fluid, and r is the radius of the tubing. Poiseuille initially described this relationship for the flow of liquids through a glass tube. This relationship is applicable to the flow of blood in the circulatory system. The length of the vascular tubing can be considered to be a fixed variable. The viscosity of the blood, although it can be altered by hemoconcentration or hemodilution, is not regulated by the body on a minute-to-minute basis. Changing the radius through vasoconstriction or vasodilation is the primary means by which the body regulates vascular resistance, and, therefore, blood pressure. One can see from Equation 40-4 that if the radius is decreased by one-half, the resistance increases sixteen fold. This relationship holds for lamellar flow, where the maximum velocity of the fluid is at the center and zero at the walls. When there is a narrowing of the tubing such that lamellar flow becomes turbulent, the resistance to flow is even higher than that predicted by Poiseuille's equation. One can therefore appreciate that small changes in the vessel diameter can have significant impact on resistance.

Afterload is the ventricular wall tension during systole caused by the forces that oppose muscle fiber shortening. Afterload is proportional to arterial blood pressure and the chamber dimension, shape, and wall thickness. SVR can be readily altered and approximates afterload. The pulmonary artery catheter can be used to calculate SVR:

$$SVR = \frac{MAP - CVP}{CO} \times 80 \qquad (40\text{-}5)$$

where MAP is mean arterial pressure; the units for SVR are dyns/cm^5.

SVR is regulated by the autonomic nervous system and affected by inflammatory processes and temperature. A decreased sympathetic tone can be due to vasodilating properties of some medications or direct spinal cord inhibition of sympathetic nerves from intrathecal or epidural local anesthetics. Neurogenic shock, liver failure, spinal cord injury, carotid sinus dysfunction (S/P carotid endarterectomy), and adrenal insufficiency can also result in a low SVR. Systemic inflammation, such as sepsis or anaphylaxis, involves circulating factors that cause vasodilation. Bacteremia from urogenital procedures has caused fever and hypotension in the recovery room. Hyperthermia from excessive warming or malignant hyperthermia results in temperature-related vasodilation. Treatment is geared toward correcting the underlying cause and, if needed, instituting pharmacologic agents that augment vascular tone. Alpha-agonists are successful at increasing SVR and blood pressure, but the vasoconstriction may lead to decreased perfusion of vital organs.

Management of Hypotension

The management of hypotension begins with the elimination of erroneous blood pressure measurements, such as those caused by too large a cuff or calibration of a transducer above the level of the heart. An overdamped waveform can result in a falsely low systolic blood pressure; the MAP should be used in guiding therapy. It may be wise to check the blood pressure in the other upper extremity, particularly in patients with peripheral vascular disease that may have occlusions proximal to the cuff or arterial line. A careful review of the patient's history and intraoperative course will help determine if additional monitoring is needed prior to treatment.

The most common cause of postoperative hypotension is decreased preload from hypovolemia. Causes include inadequate replacement of intraoperative blood loss, postoperative bleeding, urinary losses, and third spacing of fluid. A simple test for hypovolemia is to use positional maneuvers that utilize gravity to augment venous return to the heart. Placing a patient in the Trendelenburg position can autotransfuse up to two units of blood volume. A rise in blood pressure suggests hypovolemia. Another useful test is to administer rapidly 250 ml of a crystalloid solution. If invasive monitoring is present, a rise in blood pressure with only a small increase in CVP or PCWP is suggestive of a hypovolemic state. This is followed by further fluid resuscitation as indicated. Vasopressors and positive inotropic agents are not indicated in this setting, except as a temporary means of treatment until intravascular volume can be adequately restored. Hypotension because of obstruction to venous return (e.g., cardiac tamponade) will often respond to fluid therapy, but the definitive treatment is eliminating the impedance.

If a fluid challenge results in rapidly rising filling pressures without much improvement in blood pressure, then the heart may be failing and further administration of fluids may be of little benefit. The pulmonary artery catheter (PAC) will indicate an elevated PCWP and SVR with a low cardiac output. Causes of cardiac dysfunction include hypocalcemia and myocardial infarction. Hypocalcemia should be suspected in any patient that received a large amount of blood products, especially in patients with liver dysfunction who will not efficiently metabolize citrate. If the ionized calcium level is low, intravenous calcium may correct the hypotension. Acute ST elevation indicates coronary artery occlusion and requires immediate and aggressive treatment (see Case Study box) including supporting blood pressure with inotropic agents in hypotensive patients. In contrast to ST elevation, new ST depression on the EKG may indicate cardiac ischemia secondary to the hypotension and the diastolic pressure should be raised (using phenylephrine) rather than employing the usual steps to maximize oxygen supply/demand (using beta-blockers and nitroglycerin). Other reversible causes of myocardial depression include acidosis and hypothermia.

A failure of hypotension to respond to a volume load may also be due to a significantly reduced SVR (Table 40-1). The PAC helps differentiate low SVR conditions from patients with decreased preload or decreased contractility.

Table 40-1	Causes of Low Systemic Vascular Resistance

Septicemia
Regional anesthesia
Medications
   Histamine releasers (e.g., morphine)
   Vasodilators
   Angiotensin receptor blockers
Impaired sympathetic nervous system regulation
Adrenal insufficiency
Anaphylaxis – blood products, medications (antibiotics)
Baroreceptor dysfunction s/p CEA

Common pharmacologic agents used to treat hypotension are listed in Table 40-2.

HYPERTENSION

Postoperative hypertension is common and must be considered in the context of the patient's preoperative and intraoperative blood pressure range. Treatment is indicated to prevent myocardial ischemia or infarction, left ventricular failure, or bleeding. However, treatment of hypertension must be balanced against the risk of overtreatment and the potential for end-organ hypoperfusion, as in patients with carotid artery disease or chronic uncontrolled hypertension, when blood pressures higher than normal may be required to maintain organ perfusion.

Prior to treatment, erroneous measurements must be ruled out; the size of the blood pressure cuff should be checked (a small cuff will give a falsely high reading) and if present the arterial line tracing should be observed for signs of an underdamped waveform. The most common causes of postoperative hypertension are heightened sympathetic activity, hypervolemia, and preexisting hypertension (Table 40-3).

Treatment is geared toward correcting the underlying cause prior to giving antihypertensive agents (Table 40-4). Hypoxia and hypercarbia can immediately be determined with the pulse oximeter and physical examination and treated as indicated. There are many modalities available to treat postoperative pain, including narcotics, intravenous ketorolac, and nerve blocks. Hypervolemia is typically due to aggressive fluid administration, excessive fluid absorption of irrigation fluids (e.g., transurethral resection of the prostate (TURP) syndrome), or renal failure. Clinical signs include jugular venous distention, pulmonary rales, and dilute urine. Treatment involves fluid restriction and use of diuretics; coexisting electrolyte abnormalities should be corrected.

Preexisting hypertension predisposes patients to postoperative hypertension. Patients that did not take their medications the day of surgery or loss of residual

Table 40-2	Common Pharmacologic Agents Used to Treat Hypotension		
Agent	**Therapeutic Category**	**Usual IV Dosage**	**Comment**
Phenylephrine	Alpha-adrenergic agonist	Children: 1–30 µg/kg/dose every 10–15 minutes; 0.1–0.5 µg/kg/minute infusion. Adults: 100–500 µg/dose every 10–15 minutes; 100–180 µg/minute initial infusion rate, followed by 40–60 µg/minute maintenance rate	May see reflex bradycardia
Ephedrine	Releases tissue stores of epinephrine	Children: 0.1–0.3 mg/kg/dose Adults: 5–25 mg/dose	Longer acting, but less potent than epinephrine
Epinephrine	Alpha- and beta-adrenergic agonist	Children: 0.05–0.1 µg/kg/minute infusion; titrate as needed Adults: 1–10 µg/minute infusion	
Norepinephrine	Alpha- and beta-adrenergic agonist	Children: 0.05–0.1 µg/kg/minute infusion; titrate as needed Adults: 1–10 µg/minute infusion	Requires cautious monitoring for extravasation
Dopamine	Dopaminergic and adrenergic agonist	1–20 µg/kg/minute, up to 50 µg/kg/minute; titrate as needed	Hemodynamic effects are dose-dependent
Vasopressin	Antidiuretic hormone analog	Children: 0.002–0.005 units/kg/minute; titrate as needed Adults: 0.2–0.4 units/minute; titrate as needed	Water intoxication requires discontinuation of the drug
Calcium chloride	Electrolyte supplement	Children: 10–20 mg/kg/dose Adults: 500–1000 mg/dose	Used in hypocalcemic states to improve myocardial contractions

Table 40-3   Causes of Hypertension
Preexisting hypertension
Heightened sympathetic activity due to
Pain
Anxiety
Restlessness
Surgical stress
Distended bladder
Hypothermia
Hypoxia
Hypercarbia
Endocrine abnormalities
Thyrotoxicosis
Pheochromocytoma
Cushing's disease
Hyperaldosteronism
Hypervolemia
Disorder of blood pressure regulation
Postcarotid endarterectomy baroreceptors dysfunction
Increased intracranial pressure
Exogenous causes
Cocaine
Medication or medication withdrawal

effects of medications already taken is not uncommon. The ideal agents for treating hypertension in the postanesthesia care unit (PACU) are agents that can be given with repeated intravenous boluses; continuous intravenous infusions will necessitate increased monitoring postoperatively. Beta-blockers have been proven to reduce perioperative morbidity and mortality and they should be used to treat postoperative hypertension unless there is a contraindication (uncontrolled congestive heart failure, advanced heart block, bradycardia, or history of significant bronchospasm). Other good options that will not need postoperative monitoring include nitropaste (1–2 inches topically), angiotensin converting enzyme (ACE) inhibitors (vasotec is available in intravenous form), labetolol (combined alpha and beta effects), and hydralazine. Short-acting antihypertensive infusions, such as nitroglycerine or nitroprusside, require arterial line monitoring and admission to an intensive care unit (ICU) or monitored care unit to continue their use.

The benefits and potential complications of each drug must be considered. Beta-blockers may precipitate bronchospasm in patients with reactive airway disease. Vasodilating agents may cause reflex tachycardia. ACE inhibitors decrease glomerular filtration and may depress renal function in the postoperative setting. Alpha-2 agonists may result in excessive sedation, particularly when used in the elderly or when combined with analgesics or anxiolytics. The choice of antihypertensive agent is considered in the context of the patient's underlying disease, comorbidities, and perioperative needs (e.g., same-day discharge, or ICU admission if continuous intravenous therapy is used).

Table 40-4 Common Pharmacologic Agents Used to Treat Hypertension			
Agent	**Therapeutic Category**	**Usual IV Dosage**	**Comment**
Esmolol	Beta-adrenergic blocker	Children: limited information Adults: 500 µg/kg over 1 minute loading dose; 50–200 µg/kg/minute maintenance	Short acting. All beta-blockers must be used cautiously in patients with bronchospastic disease or acute congestive heart failure
Metoprolol	Beta-adrenergic blocker	Adults: 5 mg/dose every 2 minutes, up to 3 doses	Beta-blockers can mask the signs and symptoms of hypoglycemia
Labetalol	Beta-adrenergic blocker	Adults: 0.25 mg/kg/dose; 2 mg/minute infusion, titrate as needed	Blocks alpha- and beta-adrenergic receptor sites
Diltiazem	Calcium channel blocker	Adults: 0.25 mg/kg over 2 minutes loading dose; 5–15 mg/hour maintenance	Use cautiously in hepatic/renal impairment
Hydralazine	Arteriole vasodilator	Children: 0.1–0.2 mg/kg/dose Adults: 10–20 mg/dose	Half-life is prolonged in renal disease
Enalaprilat	Angiotensin converting enzyme inhibitor	1.25 mg/dose	May impair renal function
Nitroprusside	Vasodilator	Children: 0.1–2 µg/kg/minute; maximum 5 µg/kg/minute Adults: 0.3–10 µg/kg/minute	High dose or prolonged administration can lead to cyanide toxicity
Nitroglycerin	Vasodilator, anti-anginal	Children: 0.25–0.5 µg/kg/minute; maximum 5 µg/kg/minute Adults: 5–200 µg/minute, ½–2 inch ointment	Commonly causes headaches
Furosemide	Loop diuretic	Children: 1 mg/kg/dose Adults: 20–40 mg/dose	Check serum potassium

BRADYCARDIA

Bradycardia, sinus or ventricular escape rhythms, may be the result of hypoxia, hypercarbia, hypothermia, myocardial ischemia, or medications. High spinal anesthetics or residual anticholinesterases from muscle relaxation reversal also result in an increased parasympathetic tone. Triggers of vagal tone include ocular pressure, carotid pressure, and Valsalva's maneuver. A patient after neurosurgery with bradycardia and hypertension may have increased intracranial pressure.

Bradycardia should only be treated if the patient is symptomatic or exhibits advanced heart block. Hypotension is initially treated with atropine 0.5 to 1.0 mg followed by dopamine (5 to 20 µg/kg/minute) or epinephrine (2 to 10 µg/minute) if needed. Cardiac pacing is indicated in high-grade AV nodal blocks, and may be effective if pharmacologic interventions do not adequately treat bradycardia and hypotension. Glucagon (0.15 mg/kg followed by 0.05–0.10 mg/kg/hour) has been demonstrated to counter effectively beta-blocker-induced bradycardia.

TACHYCARDIA/TACHYARRHYTHMIAS

In the postoperative period patients are predisposed to a variety of arrhythmias, especially in the presence of a heightened catecholamine state; the surgical stress response results in increased epinephrine levels that usually peak in the PACU. The commonly encountered dysrhythmias are sinus tachycardia, premature ventricular contractions, supraventricular tachycardia, and ventricular tachycardia. Tachycardia at a rate < 150 beats per minute is generally well tolerated except in patients with coronary artery disease or stenotic heart valves. Hemodynamic compromise associated with tachycardia is due to diminished stroke volume or decreased contractility from cardiac ischemia. Decreased stroke volume is a result of the shortened diastolic filling time. If a patient has coronary artery disease, decreased coronary artery perfusion coupled with increased oxygen consumption may result in myocardial ischemia and infarction if prolonged. Prompt diagnosis and correction of the underlying causes are essential in the recovery period.

Sinus tachycardia has many triggers and is also a compensatory mechanism for decreased oxygen delivery such as hypovolemia or severe anemia. Therapy should be aimed at treating the etiology of the sinus tachycardia (Table 40-5).

Tachyarrhythmias may present in the PACU, especially in patients with cardiomyopathies or history of arrhythmias. Cardioversion is indicated in patients exhibiting vital signs deterioration or symptoms associated with end-organ hypoperfusion. It is essential to identify correctly

Table 40-5   Causes of Sinus Tachycardia

Hypoxia
Hypercarbia
Pain
Anxiety
Hyperthermia
Infection
Hypotension
Acidosis
Medications – e.g., anticholinergics given with muscle
    relaxant reversal
Beta-blocker withdrawal
Alcohol withdrawal
Pulmonary embolus
Congestive heart failure
Thyrotoxicosis
Malignant hyperthermia

an arrhythmia and assess its hemodynamic consequence in order to determine the appropriate intervention and its urgency. If a diagnosis cannot be made by bedside telemetry, a 12-lead EKG, free of artifacts, may facilitate identification of the rhythm.

The causes of arrhythmias are variable. In the recovery period they commonly include preexisting heart disease, hypoxia, acid–base disturbances, myocardial ischemia, drugs, hypothermia, electrolyte abnormalities (potassium, calcium, and magnesium), and increased sympathetic tone. These physiologic disturbances increase myocardial excitability and irritability. General anesthesia lowers the threshold for dysrhythmias, and the recovering patient often has residual circulating anesthetics.

Inhalational anesthetics sensitize the myocardium to circulation catecholamines and premature ventricular contractions (PVCs) may be seen. Electrolyte abnormalities, acid–base disturbances, and hypoxia also cause PVCs. PVCs alone typically do not cause hemodynamic instability and management involves correcting any underlying cause listed above. PVCs generally resolve once residual anesthetics have worn off and do not require treatment with an antiarrhythmic.

Atrial flutter and fibrillation are the most common postoperative supraventricular tachyarrhythmias. Any physiologic alteration can precipitate atrial flutter or atrial fibrillation, even in the absence of underlying heart disease. This rhythm disturbance can result in a rapid ventricular response and hypotension. The loss of the atrial "kick" further decreases ventricular filling, particularly in patients with left ventricular hypertrophy (e.g., patients with aortic stenosis). In the stable patient treatment is first geared toward correcting reversible causes. Atrial fibrillation can be seen in the tachypneic patient with respiratory alkalosis and hypoxemia. Treating the hypoxemia and respiratory alkalosis will usually correct the dysrhythmia. If the rhythm is not corrected with treating reversible causes, attempts to convert atrial fibrillation or atrial flutter to normal sinus rhythm with amiodarone may be successful. To control the ventricular rate, pharmacologic intervention involves slowing the AV node with beta-blockers, calcium channel blockers, or digoxin. These medications should be avoided in patients with Wolf-Parkinson-White syndrome and digoxin should be used cautiously in patients with hypokalemia.

Ventricular tachycardia and fibrillation are commonly caused by acute myocardial infarction or ischemia. These rhythms are managed and treated as outlined in the advanced cardiac life support guidelines. Ventricular tachycardia that is unstable should be treated immediately with cardioversion, followed by drug therapy. Electrolyte and metabolic derangements should be promptly sought and corrected. Those without significant symptoms or hemodynamic instability may be treated with antiarrhythmic agents (amiodarone, lidocaine, or procainamide) and correction of underlying triggers. Patients with recurring ventricular tachyarrhythmias may develop cardiac death. Recurrence can be prevented by continuous infusion of an effective antiarrhythmic agent.

CONCLUSION

Hemodynamic instability is commonly encountered in the postanesthesia period. Vigilance in patient monitoring during this time is essential. Early identification of possible causes and institution of appropriate therapy may prevent the development of complications or death. A good understanding of the pathophysiology coupled with astute clinical skills are required to provide effective care for the recovering patient.

CASE STUDY

A 68-year-old woman with a history of hypertension and diverticulosis was admitted to the emergency room with abdominal pain and nausea with vomiting of one day duration. Work-up revealed an elevated white blood cell count of 14.6 and a perforated diverticulum in the sigmoid colon. Her remaining preoperative laboratory data showed hematocrit 36, potassium 3.8, and creatinine 1.2. EKG showed normal sinus rhythm at a rate of 92 beats per minute, and left ventricular hypertrophy by voltage criteria. She normally takes amlodipine for hypertension. She had an uneventful rapid-sequence induction, and her intraoperative

course was uncomplicated. Estimated blood loss was 300 ml, and she received 3000 ml of crystalloid. She was extubated at the end of the case, and was transferred to the PACU in stable condition.

After 35 minutes in the PACU she complained of chest pressure and dyspnea. Her vital signs were BP 145/86, HR 102, RR 24, O_2 sat 92% on room air. Telemetry revealed ST segment elevation. Physical examination revealed a woman in moderate discomfort. Lung examination was notable for new bibasilar crackles. Heart examination was notable only for tachycardia. A repeat 12-lead EKG showed sinus tachycardia with 2 mm ST segment elevation in leads II, III, and aVF consistent with an acute inferior myocardial infarction. Treatment was immediately initiated while cardiology was consulted. She was given 4 liters/minute of oxygen via nasal canula and her pulse oxymetry improved to 100%. She was also given nitroglycerin 0.3 mg × 3 sublingually with mild improvement in her chest pressure. This was followed by morphine 4 mg IV × 2 with good pain relief. Aspirin 325 mg PO and metoprolol 5 mg IV × 3 were administered. Stat labs for hematocrit, electrolytes, and cardiac enzymes were sent. Chest x-ray was clear. Heparin and thrombolytics were not administered due to concerns about bleeding. She was taken emergently to the cardiac catheterization lab where she successfully underwent angioplasty of her right coronary artery.

SELECTED READING

Azer S: Management of postoperative hypertension and hypotension in the recovery room. Mt Sinai J Med 48:365-368, 1981.

Bines AS, Landron SL: Cardiovascular emergencies in the post anesthesia care unit. Nurs Clin North Am 28:493-505, 1993.

Cullen DJ, Cullen BL: Postanesthetic complications. Surg Clin North Am 55:987-998, 1975.

Hines R, Barash PG, Watrous G, O'Connor T: Complications occurring in the postanesthesia care unit: a survey. Anesth Analg 74:503-509, 1992.

Malamed SF: The postanesthetic period. Dent Clin North Am 31:139-149, 1987.

Mecca RS: Complications during recovery. Int Anesthesiol Clin 29:37-54, 1991.

Rose DK, Cohen MM, DeBoer DP, Math M: Cardiovascular events in the postanesthesia care unit. Anesth 84:772-781, 1996.

Shander A, DeAngelis LJ: Cardiac instability in the recovery room. Int Anesthesiol Clin 21:59-75, 1983.

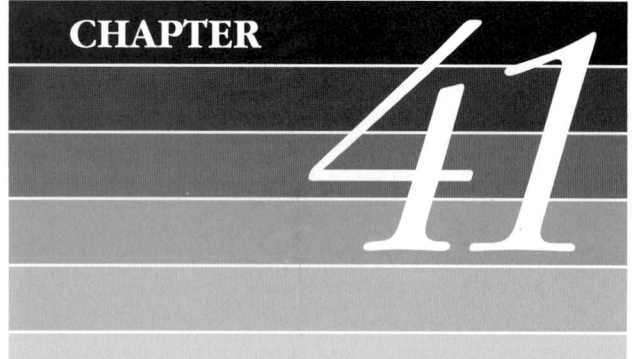

CHAPTER 41

Postoperative Transport to the Intensive Care Unit

JOSEPH DOOLEY, M.D.

The transport from the operating room to the intensive care unit (ICU) is a crucial time in the critically ill patient's care. In the operating room patients are managed one-to-one by an anesthesia care provider with full monitors. There is rapid access to emergency drugs, airway management equipment, IV infusion equipment, etc. In the ICU, the ICU team with 1:1 or 1:2 nursing coverage manages patients. During transport from the operating room to the ICU, these conditions may not exist. Optimal management of these patients during transport requires excellent communication between the operating room and ICU. In addition, conditions must be established that will provide for the safest possible transfer from the operating room to the ICU.

Before any discussion of transfer, clearly the need for a critical care bed must be established. This is not a trivial point. We all desire the optimal care for our patients. Unfortunately, ICU beds are often in short supply. Often the intensivist is faced with discharging a patient who would benefit from more time in the ICU in order to admit a new patient. The decision to admit a patient to the ICU should be made jointly between the surgical and anesthesiology teams. Clearly, a patient who requires more than a few hours of postoperative ventilatory support will need an ICU bed. These include those with large blood losses, evolving sepsis, long procedures with associated airway edema, etc. Patients who are extubated but have very marginal pulmonary function, are at high risk for respiratory failure and will need an ICU bed. There are patients who require intensive neurologic or vascular monitoring that can only be accomplished in an ICU. As soon as the need for an ICU bed is established, the critical care team should be contacted, so that preparations for the patient's arrival can be initiated.

COMMUNICATION

Communication between the surgical team and critical care team is one of the most important aspects of postoperative transport of the patient. Whether the patient is expected in the ICU after surgery or the need develops intraoperatively, contact with the ICU team should be made well in advance of patient transport. Issues discussed should include the surgical procedure, past medical history, blood loss, volume/product/vasopressor requirements, IV access, any significant intraoperative events, and special monitors (arterial line, Swan-Ganz catheter, etc.). In addition, anticipated postoperative ventilator requirements should be discussed. Ideally, the communication between the operating room and ICU should be physician to physician. However, it is important that the ICU physician communicate with the ICU nursing staff about the patient.

EQUIPMENT NEEDS FOR TRANSPORT

JACHO requirements for the ICU include having uniform monitor requirements for all ICUs for patient transport. At our institution, the monitors include EKG monitoring, pulse oximetry, and blood pressure monitoring. A defibrillator must be available. Since the patient transporting to the ICU from the operating room is an ICU patient, transport should be accomplished at a minimum with the above monitors. If patient requirements exceed the minimum required (such as pulmonary artery pressure monitoring, intracranial pressure monitoring, etc.), then they should be used. Beyond monitors, the physician transporting the patient should be prepared to manage any foreseeable problems the patient may develop en route to the ICU. This should include having a laryngoscope, endotracheal tube, stylette, AMBU bag, oxygen tank, IV fluid, and emergency drugs (including induction drugs, neuromuscular blockers, and vasopressors). Some patients present with or develop severe lung injury intraoperatively. These patients may have high oxygen and positive end-expiratory pressure (PEEP) requirements in order to oxygenate adequately. They may be very difficult to ventilate. Transport of these patients with an AMBU bag, with or without a PEEP valve, may be very unsafe. In these cases, transport should be accomplished using a ventilator.

THE TRANSFER

The transfer begins on the operating room table and ends in the ICU. Monitoring should not be interrupted during transfer of the patient from the operating room table to the ICU bed. Use of the transport monitor can start either before or after the patient is moved to the ICU bed. Care must be taken to protect the airway, IV access, and other implements (such as ventricular drains, epidural catheter, chest tubes, and Foley catheter) during the move from operating room table to ICU bed. At this point, the patient is ready to move. Before leaving the operating room, a final check for suitability for transfer should be made. The patient should be hemodynamically stable and adequately sedated for the period of transfer. Emergency equipment and drugs should be on the patient's bed. Lastly, the ICU should be contacted to ensure that it is ready to accept the patient. If the route to the ICU includes an elevator, this should be readied prior to leaving the room. Personnel for the transfer should include at least two individuals (one to monitor and treat the patient and one to move the bed). Upon arrival in the ICU, a detailed sign out should be given to the ICU staff.

DETOURS

Frequently, patients cannot be transferred directly to the ICU. The most common reason is the need for an admission to the postanesthesia care unit (PACU). This may include the need for postextubation respiratory monitoring, vascular monitoring, or neurologic monitoring. In this case, a detailed sign out should be given both to the PACU staff and telephonically to the ICU staff. It is important to establish the time when care will be transferred from the anesthesiology team to the ICU team. Confusion on the part of the PACU staff as to who is managing the patient could result in adverse outcomes.

Another common detour is to the radiology suite for a radiologic study or procedure. In this case the anesthesiologist should either continue to monitor and care for the patient or arrange for ICU personnel to care for the patient. Transfer of care to a member of the surgical team or the radiology staff during the study is strongly discouraged. These individuals are either not qualified to care for critically ill patients or unlikely to be familiar with anesthesiology equipment (monitors, infusion pumps, etc.) to make this a safe practice.

CONCLUSIONS

Communication is the most import factor in providing excellent continuity of care for patients leaving the operating room. At the University of Rochester, New York, we have established ICU transfer guidelines which are specific to our institution (see Box 41-1). These recommendations were agreed to by anesthesiologists and ICU directors (physicians and nurses). It is strongly recommended that institutions establish their own guidelines in order to facilitate the transfer of patients from the operating room to the ICU.

Box 41-1 SMH Department of Anesthesiology Guidelines for the Transfer of Intensive Care Unit Patients to and from the Operating Room

TRANSFER FROM THE ICU TO THE OPERATING ROOM

A. Patients will not be transferred until the anesthesia team responsible for the patient in the operating room gives direct approval to the operating room desk to send for the patient.

B. Patients will be accompanied from the ICU by a critical care nurse, who will remain with the patient until care is transferred to an anesthesia care provider (attending, resident, or CRNA). At times, the anesthesia team cannot immediately take over completely because of ongoing preparations for all aspects of anesthesia care.

C. The patient will be fully monitored (minimum EKG and pulse oximetry; add blood pressure for adults) and appropriately ventilated. Transfer equipment will include a defibrillator.

Continued

Box 41-1   SMH Department of Anesthesiology Guidelines for the Transfer of Intensive Care Unit Patients to and from the Operating Room—Cont'd

INTRAOPERATIVE

A. When it becomes clear that an ICU admission will be required, contact one of the following individuals to arrange for a bed.
    1. Adult, noncardiac: critical care fellow on call.
    2. Pediatric: PICU attending.
    3. Neonates: NICU attending.
B. Make sure that an ICU bed with monitor and defibrillator is available for the end of the procedure.

POSTOPERATIVE

A. Direct transfer to the ICU.
    1. Anesthesia care provider to contact ICU immediately prior to leaving the operating room.
    2. Anesthesia care provider will accompany the patient to the ICU.
    3. Full monitors and defibrillator for transfer.
    4. Direct sign out by anesthesia care provider to ICU team member detailing the operative course.
B. PACU admission prior to ICU admission.
    1. Certain situations dictate admission to PACU first (vascular checks, neurologic examinations, etc.).
    2. Anesthesia care provider will accompany the patient to the PACU and give sign out to the PACU nurse.
    3. Anesthesia care provider will contact the ICU physician to give sign out and transfer care as soon as feasible.
    4. For transfer to the ICU, a PACU nurse will accompany the patient with full monitors and defibrillator.
    5. Direct sign out to ICU team member detailing the perioperative course.
C. Indirect transfer to the ICU.
    1. Certain situations require procedures/studies outside of the operating room prior to transfer to the ICU (e.g., CT, MRI, angiography).
    2. Unless continued anesthesia is required, the anesthetist will not accompany the patient to an "off site" location.
    3. As soon as the need for the study/procedure is known, the ICU attending should be contacted to arrange for critical care nursing coverage during the procedure and thereafter. The ICU attending, in collaboration with the ICU and/or PACU nurses will arrange for coverage of the patient during the procedure.
    4. The place where care will be transferred will be arranged by mutual agreement between the anesthesia and critical care teams.
    5. If no ICU or PACU nurse is available, remain in the operating room.
D. ICU patients boarding in the PACU.
    1. When an ICU bed in not available, the patient will be boarded in the PACU.
    2. The critical care attending and ICU team will be responsible for the patient's care.
E. Nursing coverage in either the ICU or PACU is not available. The patient will remain in the operating room under the care of the anesthesiology team.

Department of Anesthesiology, University of Rochester, Rochester, New York.

Index

Please note as the subject of this book is critical care, all entries refer to this unless otherwise stated. Entries followed by "f" and "t" denote figures and tables respectively.